W. Kahle H. Leonhardt · W. Platzer

Color Atlas and Textbook of Human Anatomy

in 3 Volumes

Volume 1:

Locomotor System

by Werner Platzer

Translated by H. L. and A. D. Dayan
Edited by E. Palmer

202 colorplates with 763 drawings
by Lothar Schnellbächer and Gerhard Spitzer

1978
Year Book Medical Publishers
Chicago and London
Georg Thieme Publishers Stuttgart

Prof. Dr. med. *Werner Kahle*
Neurologisches Institut (Edinger Institut) der Universität Frankfurt/Main, FRG

Prof. Dr. med. *Helmut Leonhardt*
Direktor des Anatomischen Instituts der Universität Kiel, FRG

Univ.-Prof. Dr. med. univ. *Werner Platzer*
Vorstand des Anatomischen Instituts der Universität Innsbruck, Austria

Lothar Schnellbächer, Frankfurt/Main, FRG

Gerhard Spitzer, Frankfurt/Main, FRG

Hedi L. Dayan, M.B., and *Anthony D. Dayan*, M.D., Beckenham, Kent, UK

Dr. *Elisabeth Palmer*, Sistrans/Tirol, Austria

Distributed in continental North, South and Central America, Hawaii, Puerto Rico, the Philippines, United Kingdom and Eire, by Year Book Medical Publishers, Chicago and London.

Georg Thieme Verlag, Herdweg 63, P.O.B. 732, D-7000 Stuttgart 1
Typesetting: Tutte Druckerei GmbH, Salzweg-Passau, System: Linotype VIP,
Printed by R. Oldenbourg, München.

ISBN 3-13-533301-9 (Thieme)
ISBN 0-8151-4964-6 (Year Book)
LCCCN 76-51946
Book Code KK 1

Foreword

This pocket atlas is designed to provide a plain and clear compendium of the essential facts of human anatomy for the student of medicine. It also demonstrates the basic knowledge of the subject for students of related disciplines and for the interested layman. For all students preparation for their examinations and practice requires repetition of visual experiences. Text and illustrations in this book have been deliberately juxtaposed to provide visual demonstration of the topics of anatomy.
The pocket atlas is divided according to organ systems into three volumes: Volume 1 deals with the locomotor system, Volume 2 with the internal organs and Volume 3 with the nervous system and the organs of the special senses. The topographic relationships of the peripheral pathways of nerves and vessels are considered in Volume 1, insofar as they are closely related to the locomotor system; Volume 2 systematically describes the distribution of the vessels. The floor of the pelvis (pelvic cavity), which has a close functional relationship with the organs of the lesser pelvis, and the relevant topography are incorporated in Volume 2. The developmental anatomy (embryology) of the teeth is briefly mentioned in Volume 2 because it aids understanding of the eruption of the teeth. The common embryological origins of the male and female genital organs are also discussed because it helps to explain their structure in the adult, as well as their not infrequent variants and malformations. Certain problems connected with pregnancy and childbirth are mentioned in the chapter on the female reproductive organs. But these do not cover all the knowledge of embryology required by students. The notes on physiology and biochemistry are deliberately brief and only serve to provide better understanding of structural details. Reference should be made to textbooks of physiology and biochemistry. Finally, it must be emphasized that no pocket atlas can replace a major textbook or the opportunity to examine macroscopic dissections and microscopic preparations.
The reference list mentions textbooks and original papers as a guide to the more advanced literature, and it also cites clinical textbooks of relevance to the study of anatomy.
Those who require less detailed knowledge of the structure of the human body will find clear illustrations, too, of the anatomic bases of the more important methods of medical examination. To help the nonmedical reader, everyday English terms for the major organs and their parts have been supplied as far as feasible; these terms are also listed in the index.

Frankfurt/Main, Kiel, Innsbruck

The Editors

Preface to Volume 1

This volume provides a concise outline the topography of the related of the musculoskeletal system and peripheral pathways. It is meant to complement and not to replace larger textbooks of anatomy. Anatomy is best brought to life by visualizing it, so a particularly large number of illustrations has been included. They have been made from *specially* prepared specimens and, whenever possible, variants have been shown as they appeared in original dissection. For greater clarity the illustrations have been supplemented by schematic drawings, some of which have been taken from other monographs.

The publisher's artists deserve special thanks because it is only their skill that has allowed the author's intentions to be realized. G. S. Spitzer drew the most difficult preparations with sympathy and clarity, L. Schnellbächer was responsible for the skilled reproduction of the majority of the systematic illustrations, and D. Klittich undertook the legends and the production of some drawings.

The illustrators were dependent on skilled anatomical dissections for which the author wishes particularly to thank Dr. H. Maurer. The format of the publication has demanded some reduction in the scale of their endeavors, but for their experience, corrections and many hours of discussion I am most grateful to my indefatigable assistants, Dozent Dr. S. Poisel and Dr. R. Putz.

I wish to thank Prof. A. Ravelli, Head of the Department of Radiological Anatomy of our Institute, for the radiographs which have been used as the basis for many illustrations. Similarly, many others not mentioned here made great efforts to help this book to success, and I am grateful to all of them. *In the first place this book is intended* for medical students, but it will also provide information on human morphology for the interested layman. If there are a few mistakes or omissions I would appreciate suggestions and criticism from all my colleagues.

Particular mention must be made, too, of Dr. h.c. G. Hauff and his assistants, notably A. Menge, for their understanding and support. The publishers afforded all possible aid to further production of the book.

This volume is dedicated to my wife, whom I must thank for reading the proofs of the German edition, and to my daughters Beatrix and Ulrike.

Innsbruck

Werner Platzer

Contents

Vol. 2: Internal Organs by H. Leonhardt

Vol. 3: Central Nervous System and Sensory Organs by W. Kahle

General Anatomy

The body is divided into the trunk ('truncus' in the wider sense) and the upper and lower extremities. The trunk is divided into the head, the neck and the torso ('truncus' in the narrower sense). The torso consists of the thorax, abdomen and pelvis.

The upper extremity is joined to the trunk by the shoulder girdle and the lower extremity by the pelvic girdle. The shoulder girdle consists of the clavicles (**1**) and the scapulas (**2**) which lie on the trunk and move on it. The pelvic girdle, which consists of the two hip (coxal) bones (**3**) and the sacrum (**4**), forms an integral part of the trunk.

General Terms

Principal Axes

Vertical (longitudinal) axis, long axis (**5**) of the body, is vertical when the body is held in an upright posture.

Transverse (horizontal) axis (**6**) is perpendicular to the long axis and runs from left to right.

Sagittal axis (**7**) runs from the back to the front surface of the body in the direction of an arrow (sagittal) and is perpendicular to the other two axes.

Principal Planes

Median plane = the plane through the longitudinal axis and the sagittal axis and so is also called the median sagittal plane (**8**). It divides the body into two almost equal halves or antimeres (planes of symmetry).
Sagittal plane (**9**) = paramedian plane; any plane which is parallel to the median sagittal plane.

Coronal or frontal plane (**10**) = any plane which contains transverse axes and is parallel to the forehead and perpendicular to the sagittal planes.

Transverse planes (**11**) = these lie perpendicular to the sagittal planes and to the coronal planes. They are horizontal in the upright posture.

Directions in Space

cranial = toward the head (**12**)
superior = upward with the body erect (**12**)
caudal = toward the buttocks (**13**)
inferior = downward with the body erect (**13**)
medial = toward the middle, toward the median plane (**14**)
lateral = away from the middle, away from the median plane (**15**)
medius = in the midline (**16**)
median = within the median plane
central = toward the center of the body (**17**)
peripheral = toward the surface of the body
superficial (**18**)
anterior = toward the front (**19**)
ventral = toward the abdomen (**19**)
posterior = toward the back (**20**)
dorsal = toward the back (**20**)
proximal = toward the point of attachment of the limbs (**21**)
distal = farther away from the trunk (**22**)
ulnar = toward the ulna (**23**)
radial = toward the radius (**24**)
tibial = toward the tibia (**25**)
fibular = toward the fibula (**26**)
palmar = on or toward the palm of the
(volar) hand (**27**)
plantar = on or toward the sole of the foot (**28**)

Directions of Movement

flexion = bending
extension = stretching
abduction = away from the body
adduction = toward the body
rotation = pivoting or rotary motion
circum- = circular movement (a circum-
duction ferential movement)

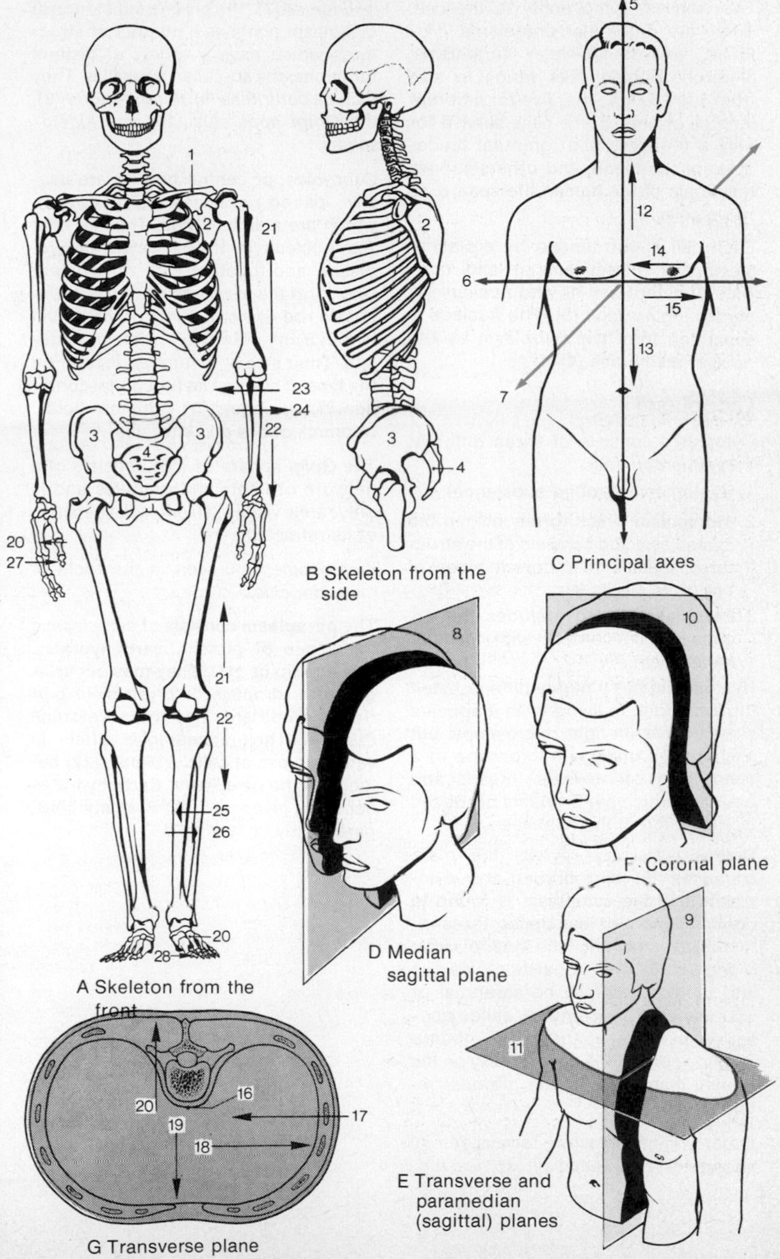

A Skeleton from the front

B Skeleton from the side

C Principal axes

D Median sagittal plane

F Coronal plane

E Transverse and paramedian (sagittal) planes

G Transverse plane

The smallest living entity is the cell. There are unicellular organisms, *protozoa*, and multicellular organisms, *metazoa*. Human cells range in size from 5 to 200 μm. They live for different lengths of time. Some cells survive for only a few days, e. g., granular leucocytes of the blood, and others survive the whole of the human life span, e. g., nerve cells.

Each cell is surrounded by a *plasma membrane* (plasmalemma) and consists of *cytoplasm* (**1**) and *nucleus* (**2**) containing *nucleoli* (**3**). The nucleus is separated from the cytoplasm by the nuclear membrane (**4**).

Cytoplasm

Cytoplasm consists of three different components:

1. **Hyaloplasm** (ground substance).
2. **Metaplasm** which forms later in the hyaloplasm and consists of the structures specific to different types of cell, e. g., fibrils, etc.
3. **Paraplasm** which includes the organelles concerned with cellular metabolism.

Hyaloplasm has a highly differentiated ultrastructure. In living cells it appears structureless on light microscopy, but examination under a microscope of a dead fixed cell reveals threads and granules which are artefacts produced by the action of the fixatives.

Electron microscopy reveals the *plasmalemma* (**5**) surrounding the cytoplasm, and the cytoplasm is found to contain a more or less dense, three-dimensional network, the *endoplasmic reticulum* (**6**). This consists of vesicles and tubules and may be agranular or granular (**6**). Fine granules, called *ribosomes* because of their high ribonucleotide content, lie superficially on the double membrane of the granular reticulum.

Other intracytoplasmic structures of variable size are called *cytosomes*, e. g., *lysosomes* (**7**). The ground substance of cytoplasm contains a number of structures which have a variety of distinct functions, the so-called **organelles**. They include *centrioles* (**8**), *mitochondria* (**9**), the *Golgi apparatus* (**10**) and *kinetosomes*.

Centrioles, or central bodies, are usually paired granules *(diplosomes)*, which are able to divide. They lie near the nucleus in the so-called *centroplasm*, and together with the nucleus they form the **microcenter**. *Mitochondria* (**9**) are rod-like structures of maximum length 5 μm, which may rotate or undulate. Their size and number depend on the type of cell and its functional condition. They consist of proteins, lipids, ribonucleotides and enzymes.

The *Golgi apparatus* (**10**) consists of a network of fibers and granules and is only rarely visible in living cells because of its refractility.

Kinetosomes are seen in the roots of cilia, *kinocilia*.

The **paraplasm** consists of cytoplasmic inclusions of protein, carbohydrates, fats and lipids (**11**). They may occur as granules, droplets or crystals. In part they are nutrients and in part storage material. Their appearance differs in various types of cells. *Melanin* (**12**) belongs to the paraplasm. Carbohydrates occur as *glycogen* (**13**) in many cells, particularly in liver cells.

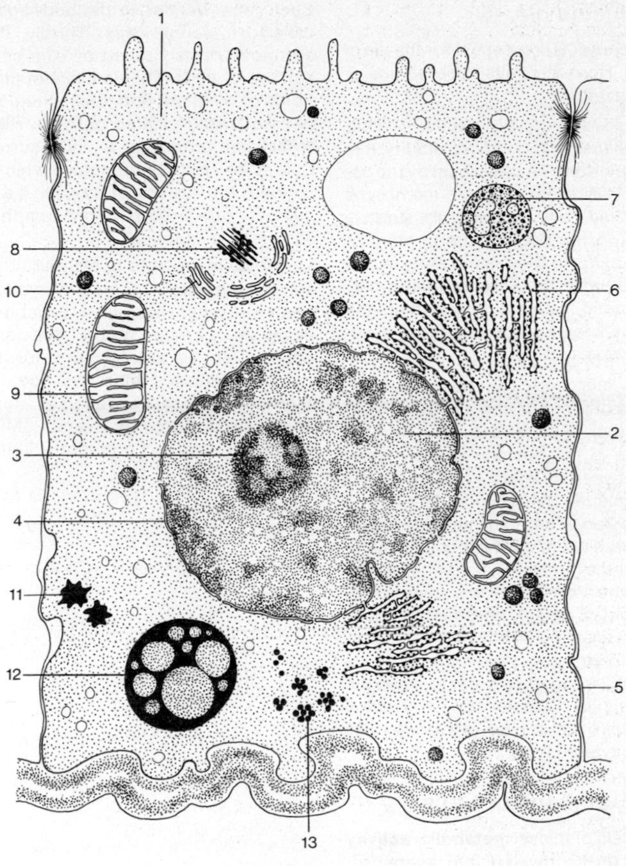

A Diagram of a cell as seen by electron microscopy (from Faller, A.: Der Körper des Menschen, 5th Ed., Thieme, Stuttgart 1972).

Cell Nucleus (A–C)

The **nucleus** (**1**) is essential for the life of the cell. Normally cells possess one or more nuclei.

The nucleus is usually visible in living cells because of its high refractility. It is separated from the cytoplasm by the delicate birefringent nuclear membrane (**2**). In fixed cells a **network-like structure** appears in the nucleus; its content of nucleic acids in the resting state is called *chromatin* (**3**). The chromatin carries genetic material from which the *chromosomes* are formed in the dividing nucleus.

The nuclear body (**4**), the *nucleolus,* consists of proteins and a large amount of ribonucleic acid (RNA). The number and size of the nucleoli varies a great deal between different cells. In the active nucleus, but only in females, a specific karyosome, the *sex chromatin* (**5**), lies adjacent to the nuclear membrane or the nucleolus. It may be used to decide the sex of a cell and hence of an individual. The sex chromatin is particularly easy to see in white blood corpuscles (granulocytes) where it is drumstick-shaped. In order to make the diagnosis of 'female sex' at least 6 drumsticks must be seen in 500 granulocytes.

Vital Functions of Cells

Every cell displays **metabolic activity** which can be divided into *anabolism* and *catabolism*. Anabolism is the ability of a cell to assimilate material it has taken up and to synthesize building materials for the cell. Catabolism comprises the processes required to sustain current cell function. The sum of oxidative processes in the cell is called *cell respiration*.

Cells are able to move. They show *plasma streaming* or movement within the cell of mitochondria, and *ameboid movement* initiated by *pseudopodia*, which are followed by the cell body. Such cells 'wander' in the body and are called *wandering cells*. Thirdly, there are movements caused by *cilia* on the surface of cells. They consist of motile fibrils (kinocilia), and the action of a layer of many ciliated cells (→ **ciliated epithelium**) produces a 'cilia current'. Cilia arise from kinetosomes which lie beneath the surface of the cell. If a cell has only one large strong cilium, this is known as a *flagellum.*

Lastly, cells are able to **reproduce** themselves by *mitosis, meiosis or amitosis*. Their reproductive ability is variable; for example, certain highly specialized cells, such as **neurons**, live for long periods and are unable to divide.

Further details may be found in 'Human Histology, Cytology and Microanatomy', by H. Leonhardt, Thieme, Stuttgart 1976.

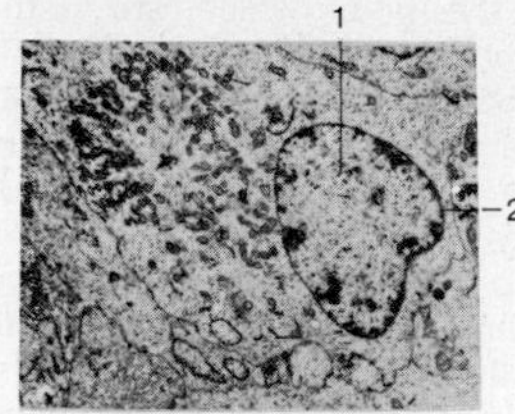

A Cell nucleus. Electron micrograph, X 6000.

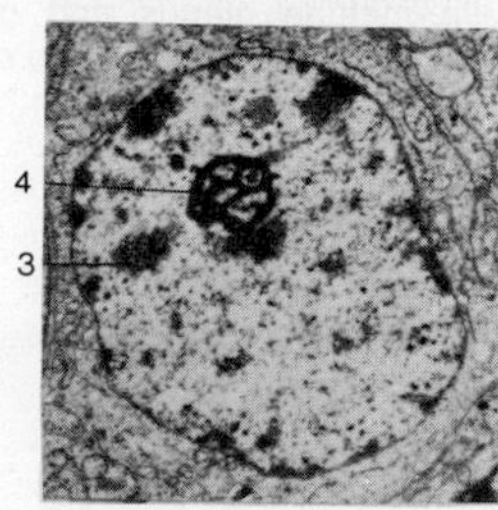

B Cell nucleus. Electron micrograph, X 12000.

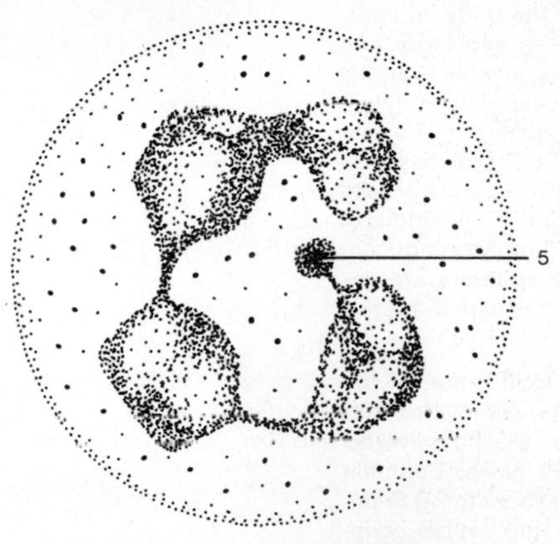

C White blood cell with sex chromatin attached to its segmented nucleus.
(Figs. A–C taken from Leonhardt, H.: Human Histology, Cytology and Microanatomy, Thieme, Stuttgart 1976)

A tissue is a collection of similar, differentiated cells and their derivatives. Several tissues may be associated to form an **organ**.

The manner in which different cells are associated determines the different types of tissues.

A common system of classifying tissues is based not on the manner of association of cells but on their histological structure and physiological functions. **Epithelial, supportive** and **muscular tissues** are described in this volume and nervous tissue is discussed in Vol. 3.

Epithelial Tissue (A–G)

Epithelial tissue serves several functions. Firstly, it provides a cover of **protective epithelium** for the inner and outer surfaces of the body and so prevents bacterial invasion, and it also prevents desiccation of the body. In addition, epithelia such as **secretory** and **absorptive epithelia** enable various substances to be exchanged, i.e., taken in from the outside (*absorption*) or excreted (*secretion*). Epithelial tissue is able to receive stimuli via the superficial epithelium (protective epithelium) in which specialized cells may be induced. Specialized **sensory epithelia** are described in detail together with the sense organs.

Depending on the organization of the cells, epithelia may be subdivided into *single-layered* (**A, B, C**), *multilayered* (**D**) and *stratified* (**F**) types. Epithelia may also be classified according to the shape of their cells into *simple squamous* (**A**), *cuboidal* (**B**) and *high columnar* (cylindrical) *epithelium* (**C**). Stratified epithelium is a true protective epithelium and may be *keratinized* or *non-keratinized.*

The outer surface of the skin is composed of keratinized, stratified, squamous epithelium, and those inner parts of the body which are particularly vulnerable, such as the mouth and throat, are covered by non-keratinized, stratified, squamous epithelium (**E**). The cells of high columnar epithelia may have processes, cilia, as in the respiratory tract, and are then known as *ciliated epithelium* (**F**). **Transitional epithelium** (**G**) is a special type in which the cells can withstand variable degrees of tension. Absorptive and secretory epithelia include glands and goblet cells (see Vol. 2), which produce secretions.

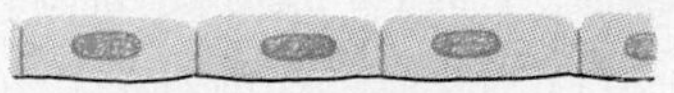

A Squamous (pavement) epithelium, single-layered

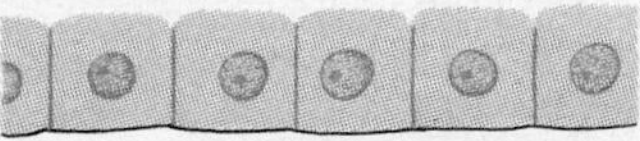

B Cuboidal epithelium, single layered

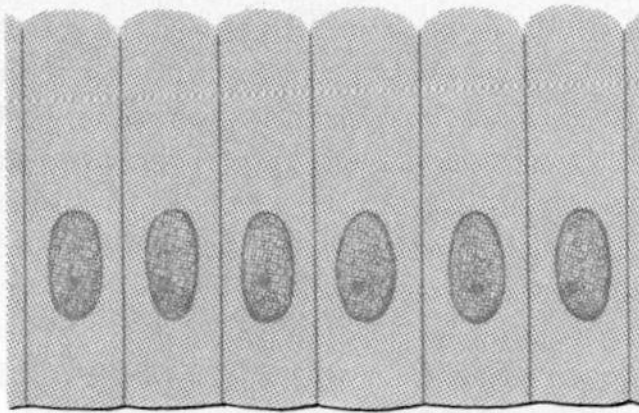

C Columnar (cylindrical) epithelium, single-layered

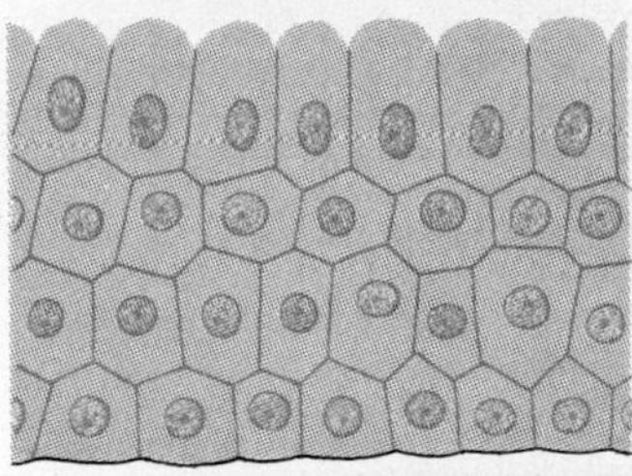

D Columnar (cylindrical) epithelium, multilayered

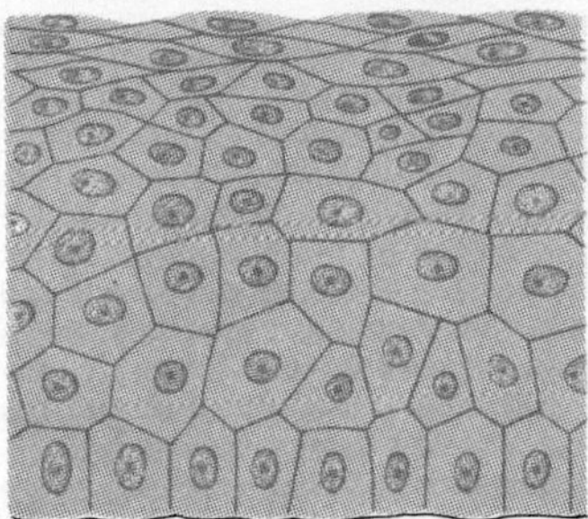

E Squamous epithelium (non-keratinized), stratified multilayered

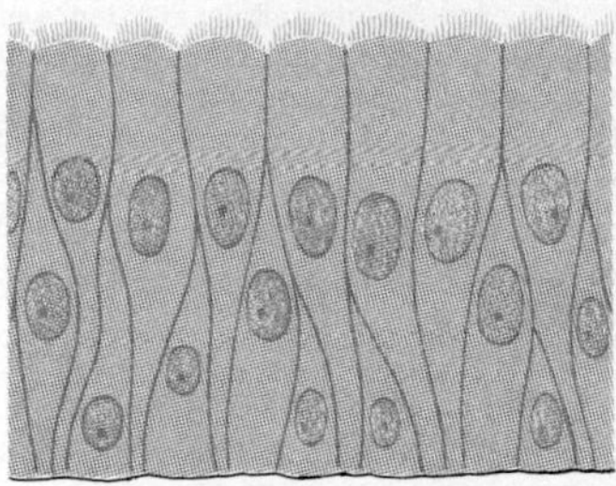

F Ciliated epithelium, multilayered

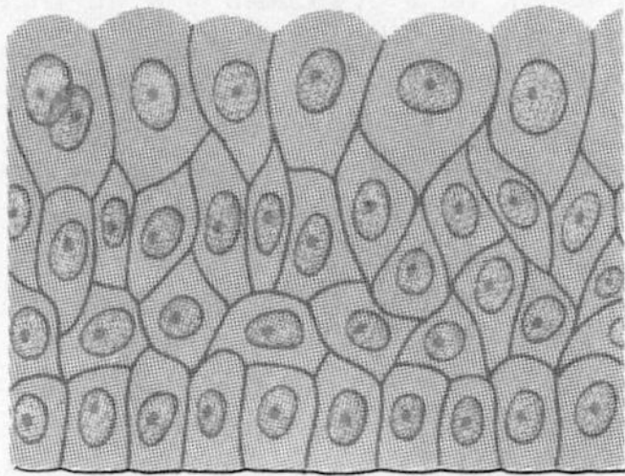

G Transitional epithelium

These tissues consist of complex combinations of cells, including **fixed** and **free cells,** and **intercellular substance.** The fixed cells are named according to the type of tissue, for example, connective tissue cells, cartilage cells, bone cells, etc. The intercellular substance in mature supporting tissue consists of *ground substance* and *differentiated fibers.*

Some of the principal types are:

Connective tissue: embryonic, reticular, interstitial and rigid connective tissue and fatty (adipose) tissue.

Cartilage tissue: hyaline, elastic and fibrocartilaginous tissue.

Bone.

Connective Tissue (A–B)

In addition to fixed and free cells, the intercellular substance contains reticular, collagen and elastic fibers and ground substance.

Fixed cells: **Fibrocytes** (many-branched cells. Their precursors, the fibroblasts, are able to produce intercellular substance and fibers), **mesenchymal cells, reticulum cells, pigment cells** and **fat cells.**

Free cells: **histiocytes** (polymorphic cells), **mast cells** (capable of amoeboid motion) and less commonly **lymphocytes, plasma cells, monocytes** and **granulocytes.**

The **intercellular substance** contains fibers – *reticular (lattice) fibers* – which resemble collagen in their structure (see below). They form fiber networks around capillaries, in basement membranes, around renal tubules and elsewhere. The second group of *collagen* fibers consist of fibrils held together by an amorphous cement substance. They are found in all kinds of supporting tissues. They are wavy, almost unstretchable and always occur grouped in bundles. This type is found particularly in tendons, the tympanic membrane, etc. Finally, there are the (yellowish) *elastic* fibers, which are also arranged in networks. They occur in arteries near the heart, certain ligaments (ligamenta flava, see p. 56) and elsewhere. The intercellular substance also includes the **ground substance,** which is partly produced by the tissue cells. It is involved in the exchange of materials between tissue cells and the blood.

Embryonic connective tissue: the most important type is mesenchyme.

Reticular connective tissue (A) contains *reticulum cells* which are able to phagocytize and store material. They have a remarkably active metabolism. This type of connective tissue can be divided into *lymphoreticular* (in lymph nodes, etc.) and *myeloreticular* (bone marrow) connective tissue.

Interstitial connective tissue is a loose tissue with no particular structure. Its main purpose is to fill gaps between individual structures (muscles, etc.) and it also forms a displacement layer. In addition to these functions, interstitial connective tissue takes part in general metabolism and regeneration. As well as cells it contains collagen, elastic and lattice fibers and ground substance.

Rigid connective tissue (B) contains a high proportion of collagen fibers and fewer cells and less ground substance than interstitial connective tissue. It is found in the palmar and plantar aponeuroses, in tendons, etc.

Fatty tissue contains large cells with a flattened nucleus lying at the cell margin. *Monovacuolar white fatty* (adipose) *tissue* should be distinguished from *plurivacuolar brown fat.* The latter is more common in infants than in adults, e. g., in the fatty capsule around the kidney. In addition to fat cells, it contains interstitial connective tissue and shows some lobular structure. There is **storage fatty tissue,** which is dependent on the nutritional state, and **structural fatty tissue,** which is independent of nutrition. The latter occurs in joints, bone marrow, the fat pads in the cheeks, etc. The storage type is most common in the subcutaneous fat layer. It is broken down according to requirements and the cells take on the form of reticular cells. After very marked weight loss (cachexia), their cytoplasm fills up with fluidserous fat cells.

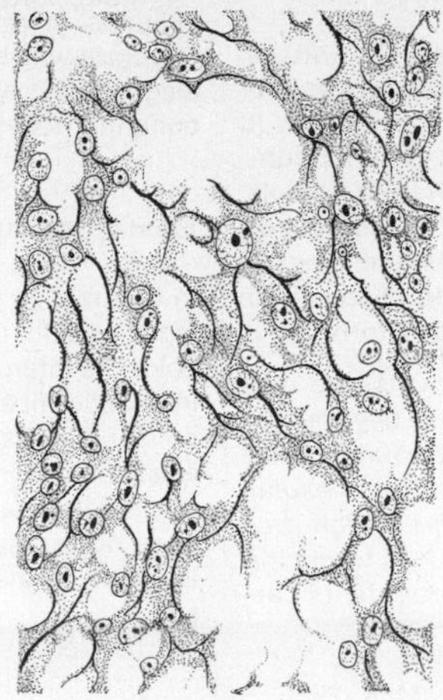

A Reticular connective tissue. Approximately X 300.

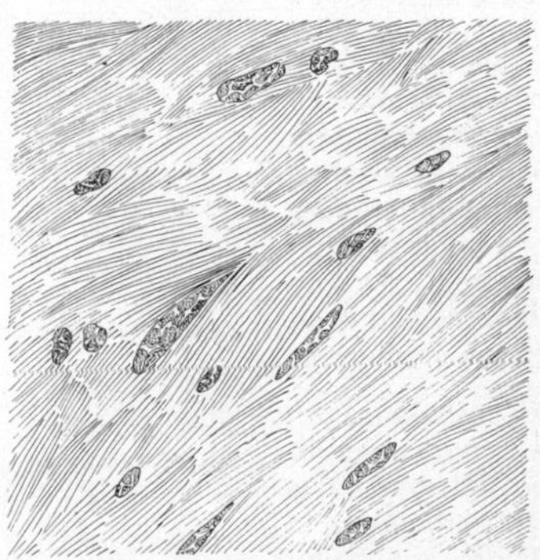

B Dense connective tissue in the corium. Approximately X 300. (Figs. A and B taken from Leonhardt, H.: Human Histology, Cytology and Microanatomy, Thieme, Stuttgart 1976)

Cartilage (A–C)

Cartilage is compressible as well as flexible, yet **resistant to pressure and to bending**, and soft enough to be cut. It consists of cells and intercellular substance, which is almost free of vessels and nerves. The nature of the intercellular substance determines the type of cartilage, which can be subdivided into **hyaline, elastic** and **fibrous** forms.

Cartilage cells, *chondrocytes*, are rich in water, glycogen and fat. They are vesicular in appearance, are rounded and have a round nucleus. The *intercellular substance*, which contains a high proportion of water (up to 70%), forms the basis of the supportive property of cartilage.

Hyaline Cartilage (A)

Hyaline cartilage is slightly **blue** and opaque in appearance. The intercellular substance contains many collagen fibrils and isolated elastic networks. The cells, which lie in spaces in the cartilage, are surrounded by a capsule and are separated from the intercellular substance by the so-called *cell halo*. These cells may be aligned in rows or columns (see p. 16) and together with the cell halo form a *chondrone*, each of which consists of the daughter cells produced by division of a single cell. Externally cartilage is covered by a thin layer – the *perichondrium*, which is almost in continuity with the cartilage.

The avascularity or poor vascularization of cartilage results in conditions suitable for the occurrence of degenerative processes. In addition, particularly in hyaline cartilage, calcium deposition occurs very early in life.

Hyaline cartilage is found in joint cartilage, rib cartilage, respiratory tract cartilage, in epiphysial disks and in the precursors of those parts of the skeleton that undergo chondral ossification.

Epiphysial disk cartilage contains columns or rows of cartilage cells, a structure which enables growth of cartilage (p. 16) and subsequently of the bone that follows it.

Elastic Cartilage (B)

In contrast to the bluish hyaline cartilage, elastic cartilage is **yellowish** in color. Its intercellular substance is rich in elastic fibers and contains fewer collagen fibrils. The large proportion of elastic fibers makes this type of cartilage particularly pliable and elastic. It does not contain calcified deposits. It is found in the auricle, the epiglottis, etc.

Fibrous Cartilage (C)

Fibrous cartilage, also known as connective tissue cartilage, contains fewer cells than the other types, but has many *bundles of collagen fibers*. It is found particularly in parts of the intervertebral disks (p. 54) and of the symphysis pubis (p. 22).

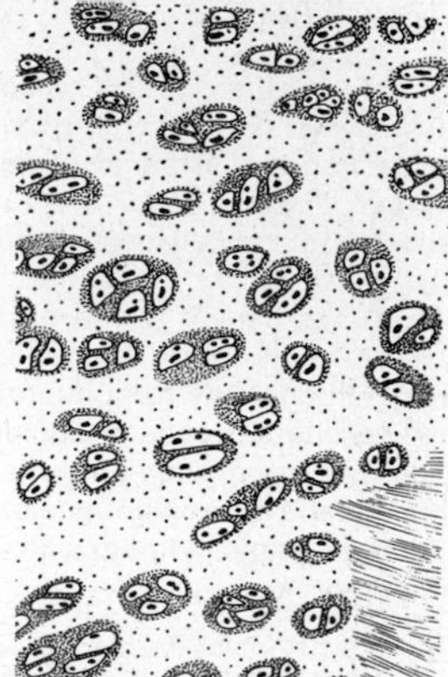

A Hyaline cartilage (rib cartilage). Approximately X 150.

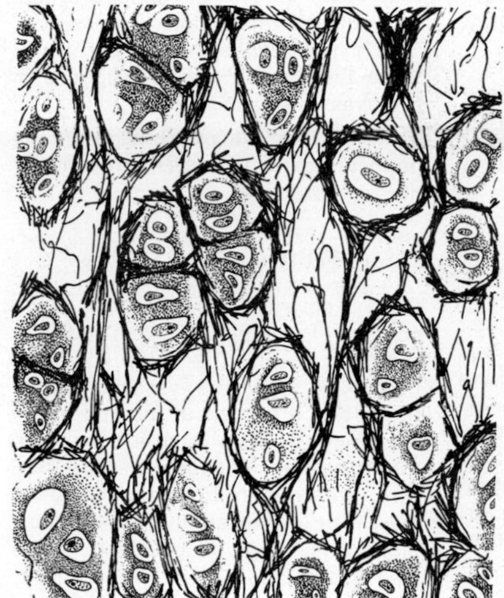

B Elastic cartilage (ear cartilage). Approximately X 150.

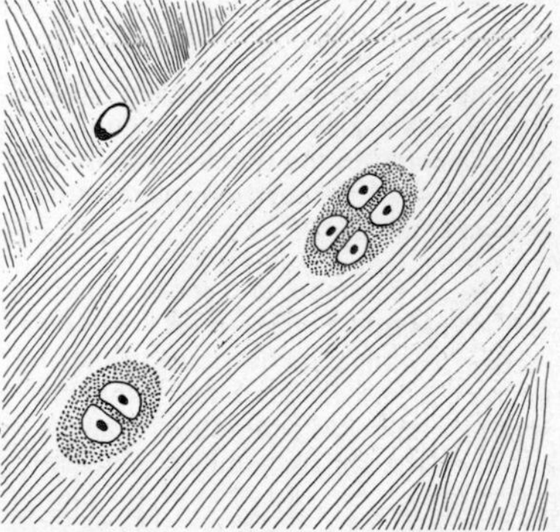

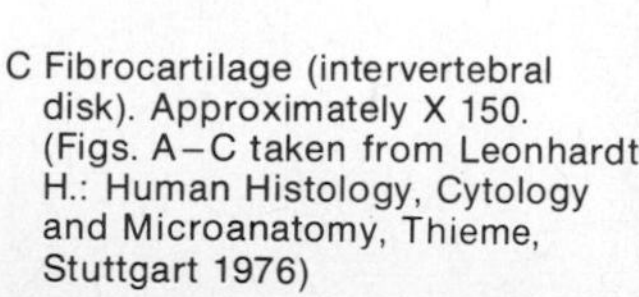

C Fibrocartilage (intervertebral disk). Approximately X 150. (Figs. A–C taken from Leonhardt, H.: Human Histology, Cytology and Microanatomy, Thieme, Stuttgart 1976)

Bone (A–C)

Osseous tissue consists of bone cells, *osteocytes*, *interstitial substance*, *collagen fibrils*, a *cement substance* and certain *mineral salts*. The interstitial substance and collagenous fibrils form the intercellular substance, *osteoid*. The fibrils belong to the organic part and the salts to the inorganic component of bone. The most important salts are calcium phosphate, calcium carbonate and magnesium phosphate. In addition there are compounds of calcium, potassium and sodium with chlorine and fluorine.

The salts determine the hardness and stability of bone. Therefore, 'decalcified bone' becomes pliable. A too low calcium content may result from lack of vitamins or hormonal disturbances. Vitamin deficiency may be due, for instance, to absence of UV irradiation on the body, with consequent failure to convert pro-vitamins to vitamin D. Inadequate calcification leads to softening of bone, e.g., in rickets.

The stability of bone is determined not only by its organic but also by its inorganic components. If there is inadequate organic material, the elasticity of the bone is lost. Bones then cannot resist stress and become brittle. The organic constituents may be destroyed artificially by incineration.

On the basis of the fiber arrangement, it is possible to distinguish two types of bone: **woven**-fibered and **lamellar** bone. Woven-fibered bone resembles in its structure ossified connective tissue and in man is usually found only during development. In the adult it occurs in the capsule of the labyrinth and near the cranial sutures.

The more common and more important **lamellar bone** (**A–B**) shows marked stratification due to its layers of interstitial substance called lamellae (**1**). These lamellae alternate with layers of bone cells (**2**). The lamellar arrangement takes place around the vascular canals (**3**). A vascular canal together with its lamellae is called an *osteon* or *haversian system* (**A**). Between the osteons are *intermediate lamellae* (**4**) consisting of former osteons. The vascular canals of the osteons communicate by smaller oblique canals, *Volkmann's canals* (**5**). The structure and arrangement of osteons depends upon the stresses on the bones and changes in stress result in a reconstruction of the osteons. Remodelling of osteons is also macroscopically observable. Particular notice should be taken, for example, of the *trajectories* within the femur since they are formed in response to the stresses exerted on it.

Bone receives its nutrients from the periosteum and the bone marrow via the nutrient foramina.

Periosteum

Bone is covered by periosteum, which consists of an external *fibrous* and deep *cambium* layer. The latter contains numerous cells and vessels. Osteoblasts which regress at the end of development but can reappear any time during healing, for example after a fracture, are formed from the cambium layer. The periosteum contains many blood and lymph vessels and nerves (see also p. 20).

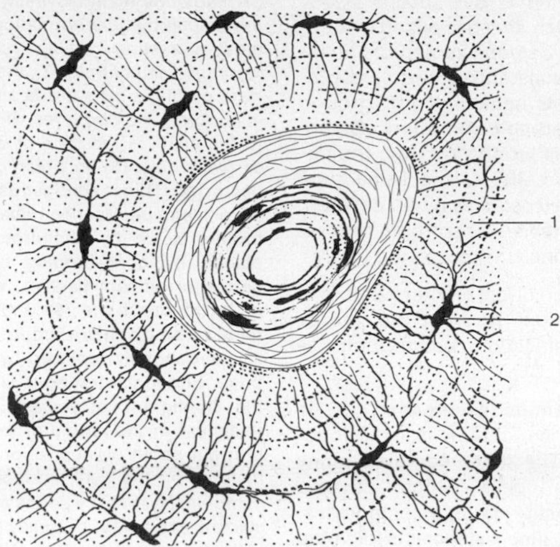

A Haversian system. Approximately X 400. In the center a haversian vessel with perivascular connective tissue.

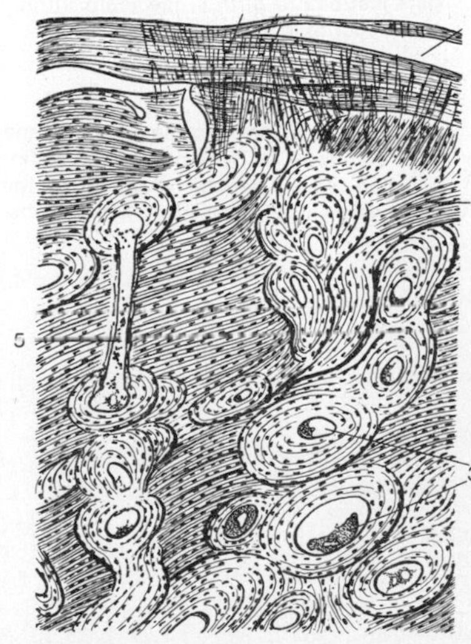

B
Cross section through the compact part of the diaphysis of a growing cancellous bone. Approximately X 50. Woven bone is being replaced by lamellar bone. (Figs. A and B are taken from Leonhardt, H.: Human Histology, Cytology and Microanatomy, Thieme, Stuttgart 1976)

Development of Bone (A–C)

Bone formation is due to the *osteoblasts* (**1**) which are specialized mesenchymal cells. Osteoblasts secrete an intercellular substance, the *osteoid*, which consists initially of soft ground substance and collagen fibers. Osteoblasts develop into *osteocytes*, the definitive bone cells. At the same time multinucleated *osteoclasts* (**2**) develop, cells connected with resorbing and remodelling bone.

We distinguish direct or intermembranous ossification (**A**) from indirect or chondral ossification (substitution ossification) (**B, C**).

Intermembranous ossification (**A**) is the development of bone from connective tissue. The latter contains many mesenchymal cells which develop via osteoblasts (**1**) into osteocytes. At the same time osteoclasts develop and collagen fibers also appear. The original bone is fibrous and it is subsequently remodelled into lamellar bone. The skull cap, the facial bones and the clavicles develop as membranous bones.

Preformed cartilaginous skeletal parts are necessary for **chondral ossification** (**B, C**) when they become replaced by bone. Growth is possible only as long as cartilage still remains. The prerequisites for replacement bone formation are *chondroclasts*, differentiated connective tissue cells, which remove cartilage and enable the osteoblasts to form bone. Two types of replacement bone formation are recognized – *endochondral* (**C**) and *perichondral*.

Endochondral ossification (**3**) begins within cartilage, and occurs near the epiphyses. Perichondral ossification (**4**), which originates in the perichondrium (**5**), is confined to the diaphysis. The *epiphysial disk* (growth plate) (**6**), which is necessary for growth in length, forms a layer between the epiphysis and the diaphysis. Within the epiphysial cartilage, the processes of ossification occur in separate zones. First, in the epiphysis is the *zone of the capping*, hyaline cartilaginous material which has not been influenced by bone formation. Next to this area of 'resting cartilage' is the *zone of cartilage cell columns* (**7**), the growth zone. Here cartilage cells divide and so increase in number. The next layer, which lies nearer to the shaft, is the *zone of large vesicular cartilage cells* (**8**), in which calcification is occurring. This is contiguous with the *zone of cartilage destruction*, where cartilage is broken down by chondroclasts and replaced by bone-forming osteoblasts. A cartilage remnant persists, which enables endochondral bone (**9**) and perichondral bone to be distinguished in the diaphysis. It is secondarily replaced by perichondral bone. Endochondral bone is destroyed by the immigrant osteoclasts. Increase in thickness in the region of the diaphysis is brought about by deposition of new bony material on the outer surface beneath the cambium layer of the periosteum. The *bone marrow cavity* (**10**) becomes larger as a result of bone destruction. All growth processes are regulated by hormones.

The bony anlagen in the epiphyses first appear after birth, except for those in the distal femoral epiphysis and the proximal tibial epiphysis. In both of these epiphyses, and in the cuboid bone, osteogenesis begins just before birth in the tenth intrauterine month (a sign of maturity).

Practical Point

Clinically, in addition to the epiphysis and the diaphysis, a *'metaphysis'* is distinguished, which denotes that part of the diaphysis which lies adjacent to the epiphysial disk.

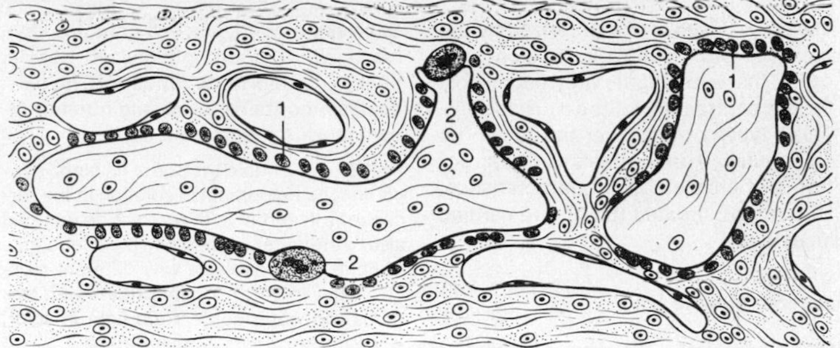

A Intramembranous ossification

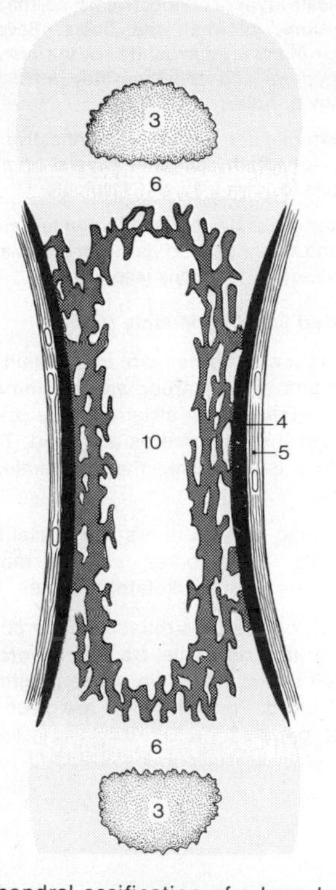

B
Chondral ossification of a long bone (diagram). Endochondral ossification in the epiphyses and perichondral ossification in the diaphysis.

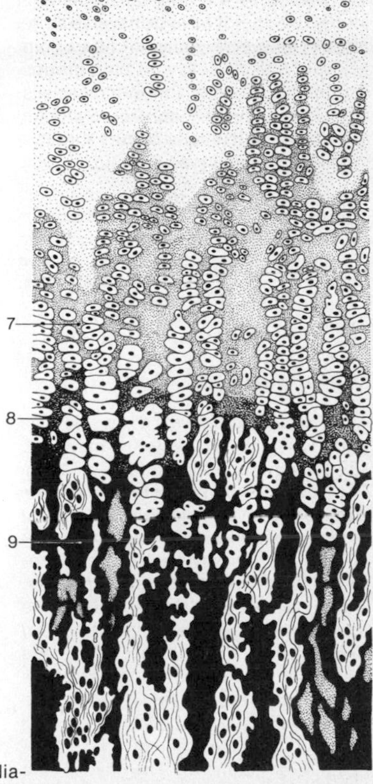

C Ossification in the region of the epiphysial disk cartilage.

Muscle (A–D)

Muscular tissue is characterized by the presence of myofibrils in its elongated cells. These myofibrils are responsible for the contractility of the muscle cells. Three types of muscular tissue can be distinguished on the basis of fine structure and physiological characteristics: smooth (**A**), striated (**B, D**) and cardiac muscle (**C**).

Smooth Muscle (A)

Smooth muscle consists of spindle-shaped cells 40–200 μm long and 4–20 μm thick, with a central nucleus. The myofibrils are difficult to demonstrate and do not have transverse striations. Transverse reticular fibers join adjacent muscle cells and bind groups into functional units. Smooth muscle is not under voluntary control. Synaptic association with axons occurs through the plasmalemma (see Vol. 3).

Hormonal influences may cause smooth muscle to increase in length and to proliferate, i.e., there may be not only an increase in the size of the cells, but cells may also be newly formed. An example is the uterus, the muscle fibers of which may reach a length of 800 μm.

Striated Muscle (B)

Striated muscle consists of muscle cells (muscle fibers) which may be 10–100 μm thick and up to 15 cm long. The nuclei lie immediately beneath the surface of the cells in the direction of the long axis of the muscle fibers. The myofibrils are easily visible and are responsible for the longitudinal striations. The transverse striations are due to the periodic alternation of smaller, lighter, singly refractile (isotropic) 'I' bands and wider, darker, birefringent, anisotropic 'A (Q)' bands. The A bands contain a middle disk (M) and the 'I' bands show a delicate, anisotropic intermediate striation (Z). The myofibrillar section which lies between two Z bands is called a **sarcomere**.

Each skeletal muscle cell contains several nuclei. The strength of each muscle fiber is related to its function. The sarcoplasm contains a variable number of mitochondria (sarcosomes).

The color of a muscle is due to its blood supply and the myoglobin in solution in the sarcoplasm. In addition, the color is determined also by the water content and the abundance of fibrils. This explains why different muscles differ in color. Thinner fibers with less fibrils and water content are light in color, while thicker fibers appear darker.

The *sarcolemma* invests individual muscle fibers as a connective tissue sheath. There is a delicate layer of connective tissue, the *endomysium*, between the fibers. Several muscle fibers are surrounded by the *internal perimysium* and together they form the primary bundle.

The *external perimysium* is a connective tissue layer which combines several primary bundles to form a muscle fascicule.

Striated skeletal muscles are voluntary muscles and are innervated via motor end-plates or myoneural junctions (see Vol. 3).

Striated Cardiac Muscle (C)

The muscle fibers, which contain a large amount of sarcoplasm, form networks. Transverse striations are present, but the sarcomeres are short. The 'I' band is narrower than in skeletal muscle.

In cardiac muscle fibers the nuclei lie centrally. *Sarcosomes* are far more numerous than in skeletal muscle.

In addition, cardiac muscle tissue contains highly refractile, transverse *intercalated disks*, which lie at the position of a Z band. Further details are given in Vol. 2, page 14.

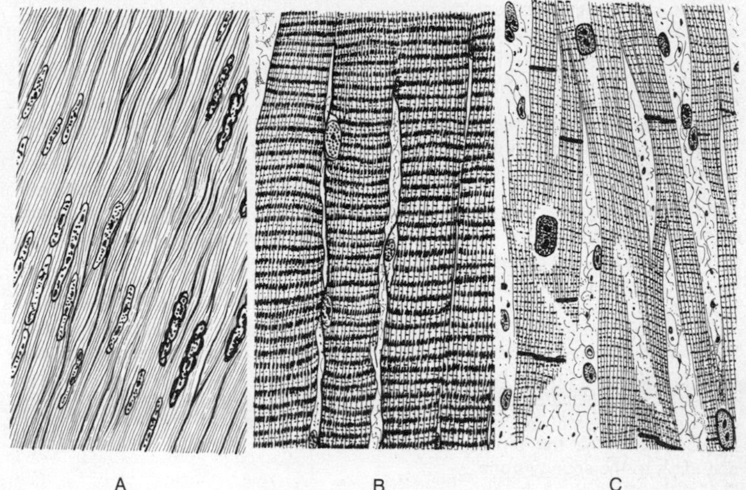

Longitudinal section of smooth muscle (A), striated muscle (B) and cardiac muscle (C). Approximately X 400.

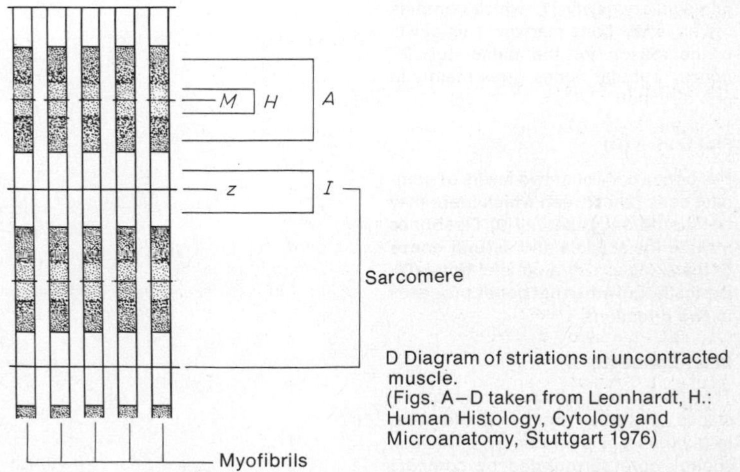

D Diagram of striations in uncontracted muscle.
(Figs. A–D taken from Leonhardt, H.: Human Histology, Cytology and Microanatomy, Stuttgart 1976)

The bones form the bony **skeleton**, and with the joints, they represent the passive locomotor system which is controlled by the active locomotor apparatus, the musculature. The different shapes of bones are dependent on their function and their position in the body. Macroscopically two differently constructed portions can be distinguished. A rather dense compact or cortical bone is generally observed on the surface. Within the short and flat bones and in the epiphyses of the long bones, there is a sponge-like meshwork formed of individual bony *trabeculae, cancellous* or *spongy bone*, *'substantia spongiosa'*. Between the meshes is the bone marrow or medulla. In the flat bones of the skull, the compact material is called the *external* and *internal laminae* and, in between them, is the *diploë*, corresponding to the spongy bone.

Long Bones (A–C)

A long bone as, for instance, the humerus (**A**), consists of a *body* and two *ends*. In the center of the shaft (body) of a long bone (**B, C**) is the bone marrow or *medullary cavity* (**1**), which contains red or yellow bone marrow. This cavity is the reason for the name 'tubular bones'. Tubular bones grow mainly in one direction.

Flat Bones (D)

Flat bones consist of two layers of compact bone (**2**) between which there may be found spongy material (**3**). Flat bones include the scapula and several bones of the skull, e. g., the parietal bone (**D**). Basically, growth in flat bones proceeds in two directions.

Short Bones (E)

The short bones, which include, for instance, the small bones of the wrist (e.g., the capitate bone [**E**]), have a spongy core surrounded by compact bone. Their growth may proceed in all three directions.

Pneumatic Bones (F)

These bones contain air-filled cavities lined by mucous membrane. They are found in the skull (ethmoid, sphenoid, maxilla [**F**], etc.).

Each bone is covered by *periosteum* and, if there is a bone marrow cavity, this is lined by the *endosteum*. Normally the periosteum and endosteum are richly innervated, and these nerves are responsible for the pain which follows a blow on a bone. Bone receives its blood supply through nutrient foramina, through which nerves can also enter. Some bones have canals which also serve for the passage of vessels, usually only veins; in these cases they are called emissaries. They are found, for example, in the vault of the skull.

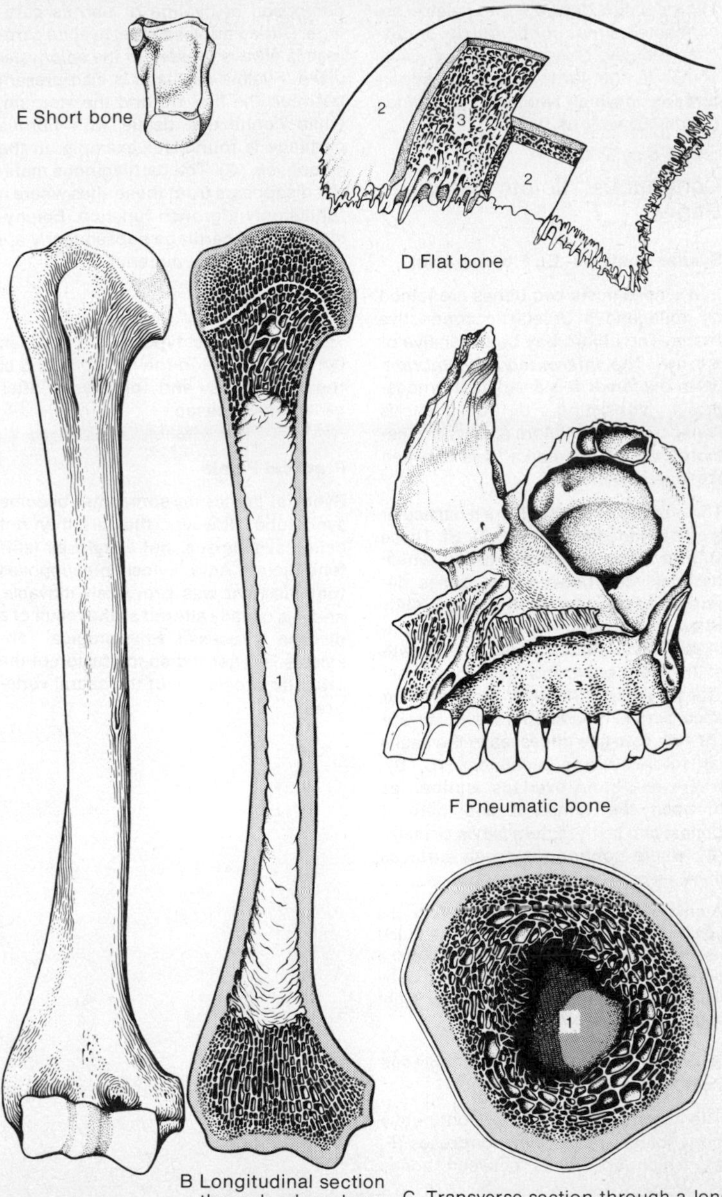

E Short bone

D Flat bone

F Pneumatic bone

A Long bone

B Longitudinal section through a long bone

C Transverse section through a long bone

The individual bones of the skeleton are connected either *continuously* or *discontinuously.* Continuous bony joints comprise the large group of **synarthroses**, in which two bones are joined directly by various tissues.

Continuous Joints Between Bones

Syndesmosis (A–E), Fibrous Joint

In a syndesmosis two bones are joined by collagenous or elastic connective tissue. The union may be expansive or narrow. The *interosseous membrane* (**A**) in the forearm is a very taut syndesmosis consisting of collagenous connective tissue. More elastic syndesmoses are the *ligamenta flava* between the vertebral arches.

The **sutures of the skull** are a particular type of syndesmosis (**B, C, D, E**). These sutures retain connective tissue, which has persisted between the bones developing from connective tissue. Only when the connective tissue has completely disappeared, does the growth of the skull cease, and the sutures fuse. The sutures of the skull are classified according to their shape: *sutura serrata* (**B**) with saw-like edges, as in the sagittal suture; *sutura squamosa* (**C, D**), where one bone overlaps another as between the temporal and parietal bones; and lastly, *sutura laevis* or *plana* (**E**), where continuous rough surfaces meet as between the nasal bones.

A specialized type of syndesmosis is the *gomphosis*, a peg-and-socket joint found in the fixation of the teeth in the alveoli of the jaw. Here the teeth are joined to the jaw by connective tissue, which allows a slight degree of displacement.

Synchondrosis (F, G), Cartilaginous Joint

The second large group of continuous bony joints are the synchondroses (**F, 2**), which are joints between bones composed of hyaline or fibrous cartilage. During adolescence, hyaline cartilage is always present in the *epiphysial disks*. Hyaline cartilage is also present between the first rib and the sternum, while connective tissue with fibrous cartilage is found, for example, in the *symphysis* (**G**). The cartilaginous material disappears from those sites where it fulfills only a growth function. Epiphysial disks of cartilage subsequently are replaced by bony material.

Synostosis (H)

This is the firmest type of joint between bony parts, e. g., in the hip bone and at the epiphyses and diaphyses after growth has ceased.

Practical Points

Synovial joints may sometimes become synostotic. However, they are then not called synostoses, but *ankyloses* (stiffened joint). An ankylosis presupposes that the joint was previously movable, and it is usually altered as the result of a disease process. Physiological ankylosis is regarded as the fusion of the articular processes of the sacral vertebrae.

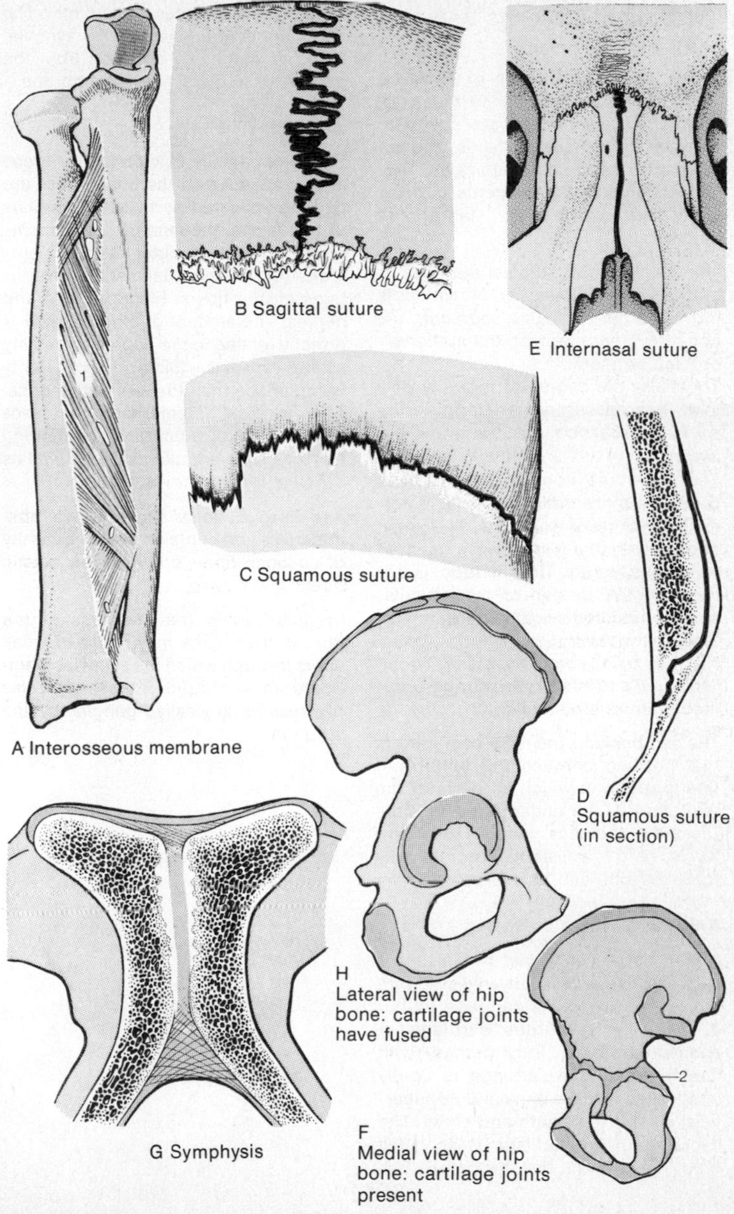

A Interosseous membrane

B Sagittal suture

C Squamous suture

D Squamous suture (in section)

E Internasal suture

F Medial view of hip bone: cartilage joints present

G Symphysis

H Lateral view of hip bone: cartilage joints have fused

Discontinuous Joints Between Bones (A–D)

These joints, **diarthroses** or **synovial joints**, consist of *articular surfaces* (**1**), an *articular capsule* (**2**), a *joint cavity* (**3**) between the articular surfaces, and according to need some *additional features* (strengthening ligaments, intercalated disks, articular lips [labra] and bursae).

In a joint with two articular surfaces or bodies, that articular body which is moved is the *moveable segment;* the one at comparative rest, the stationary or fixed segment.
To assess the degree of mobility of a joint, it is necessary to determine the *angle of excursion,* i. e. the angle between its initial and final positions. The larger the number of axes (see p. 28) the more difficult it is to determine the angle of excursion. The angle of excursion of a joint may be reduced by various factors. They include, in addition to the tension of the articular capsule, additional ligaments which restrict movement (*ligamentous limitation*, see p. 26), bony processes *(bony limitation)* and limiting surrounding soft tissues *(soft tissue limitation)*.

The *mid-position* (neutral) of a joint is that position between the initial and final position in which all parts of the joint capsule are under equal tension. Disease processes within the joint cavity (e. g., effusion) automatically force the joint into its mid-position.

Articular Surfaces or Bodies

A joint possesses at leat two articular surfaces. They are usually invested with or covered by hyaline cartilage (**4**) but occasionally by fibrous cartilage or connective tissue interspersed with fibrocartilage. The cartilage is tightly interlocked with the bone and its superficial surface is smooth and shiny. The thickness of the cartilage layer varies from 0.2–0.5 mm; but the patella has some very thick areas, up to 6 mm. The cartillage is nourished via the synovial fluid, as well as by diffusion from the capillaries in the synovial membrane.

Joint Capsule

The joint capsule may be taut or loose and is attached to the bones near the cartilage-covered surfaces. It consists of two layers, the inner *synovial membrane* (**5**) and an outer *fibrous membrane* (**6**). The synovial membrane contains elastic fibers, blood vessels and nerves. The amount of blood supply is directly related to the degree of activity so that very active joints are more richly vascularized than the less active ones. The synovial membrane possesses inward-facing processes containing fat, the *plicae articulares* (**7**), as well as synovial folds, *synovial villi.*

The fibrous membrane is of variable thickness and contains a large quantity of collagen fibers and very few elastic ones.

Irregularities in the thickness of the fibrous membrane may result in weak spots through which the synovial membrane may protrude; these cyst-like protrusions are called *ganglia* by the surgeon.

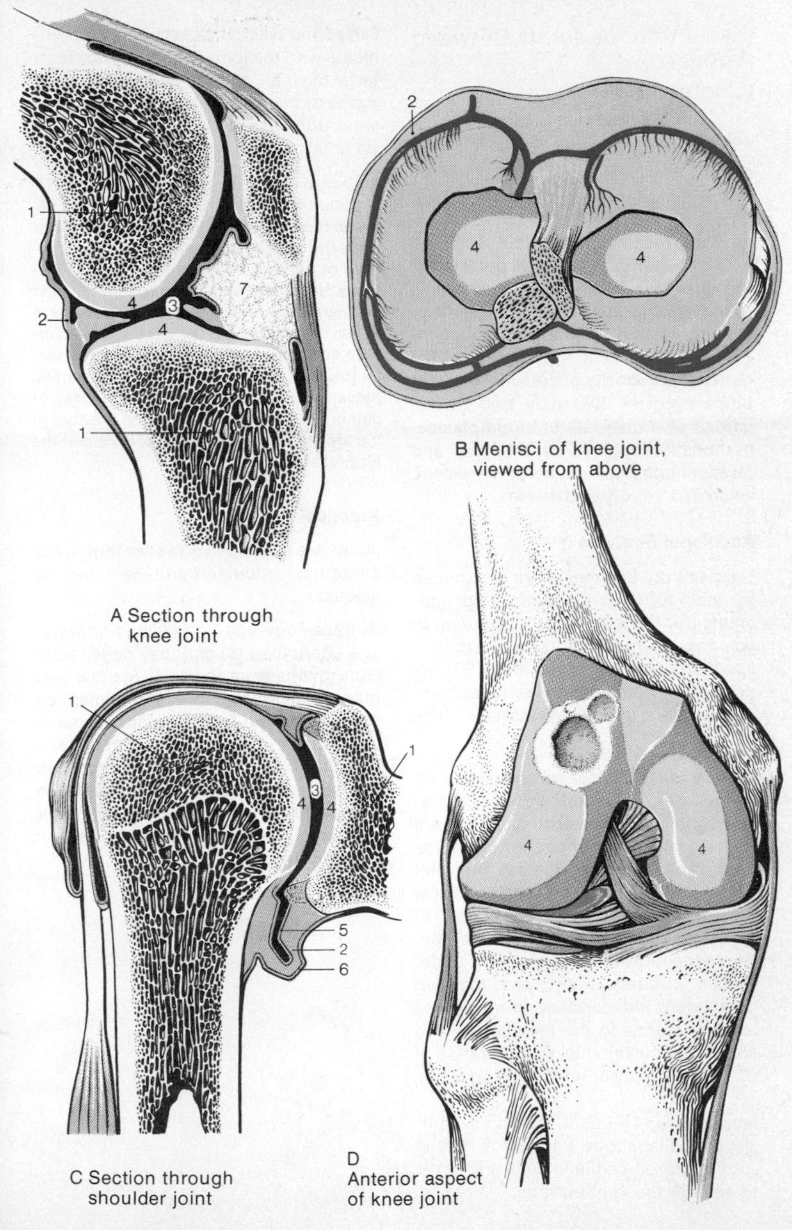

A Section through knee joint

B Menisci of knee joint, viewed from above

C Section through shoulder joint

D
Anterior aspect of knee joint

Discontinuous Joints Between Bones (Continued A–D)

Joint Cavity (1)

A joint cavity is a cleft-like capillary space which contains *synovial fluid*. This is a clear, viscous, mucin-containing fluid resembling albumin. The fluid acts as a lubricant and aids nutrition of the articular cartilage. Its viscosity, which is determined by its content of hyaluronic acid is temperature dependent – the lower the temperature, the higher the viscosity of the synovial fluid. Since synovial fluid may also be regarded as a dialysate of blood plasma, its constitution, i.e., its chemical and physical features, can be of diagnostic value in a variety of diseases.

Additional Features

Ligaments (**2**). Ligaments are designated by their function as *reinforcing ligaments* (for the joint capsule), *guiding ligaments* (in movements) or *restrictive ligaments* (to restrict movements). According to their position we speak of *intracapsular* and *extracapsular* ligaments.

Articular disks or menisci articulares (**3**) consist of collagenous connective tissue containing fibrocartilage. They are usually in close connection with the joint capsule. A disk divides the joint cavity completely, but a meniscus only partly. They affect the direction of movement, ensure good contact between the moving parts and may, under certain circumstances, produce two completely independent joint spaces as for instance in the mandibular and sternoclavicular joints. Regeneration of disks after injury or removal is possible.

Articular lips (**4**). Labra articularia consist of collagenous connective tissue with scattered cartilage cells and serve to enlarge the joint surface.

Bursae and **synovial pockets** may communicate with the joint cavity (**5**). They form large or small, thin-walled sacs lined by synovial membrane, which represent a weak point in a joint, but which produce an enlargement of the joint space.

There are various forces that act on the two articular surfaces and maintain contact between them. Firstly, there are the muscles that span the joint and guarantee a certain degree of contact between the articular surfaces. Next, there may be accessory capsular ligaments to increase the degree of contact. In addition, there is a certain degree of surface adhesion, and, as the most important factor, atmospheric pressure. Atmospheric pressure holds the articular surfaces together with a force equal to the product of the area of the smaller joint surface and the air pressure.

Practical Points

Joints are subject to age alterations; the avascular articular cartilage loses its elasticity.

Surfaces covered by cartilage undergo age alterations (**6**) and may degenerate Outgrowths from the cartilage margins may occur, which are sometimes invaded by bone-forming cells. In such instances the cartilage becomes ossified and restricts joint mobility. Such processes may affect small joints as well as large ones, and they may occur in young people if the joints in question are overstressed.

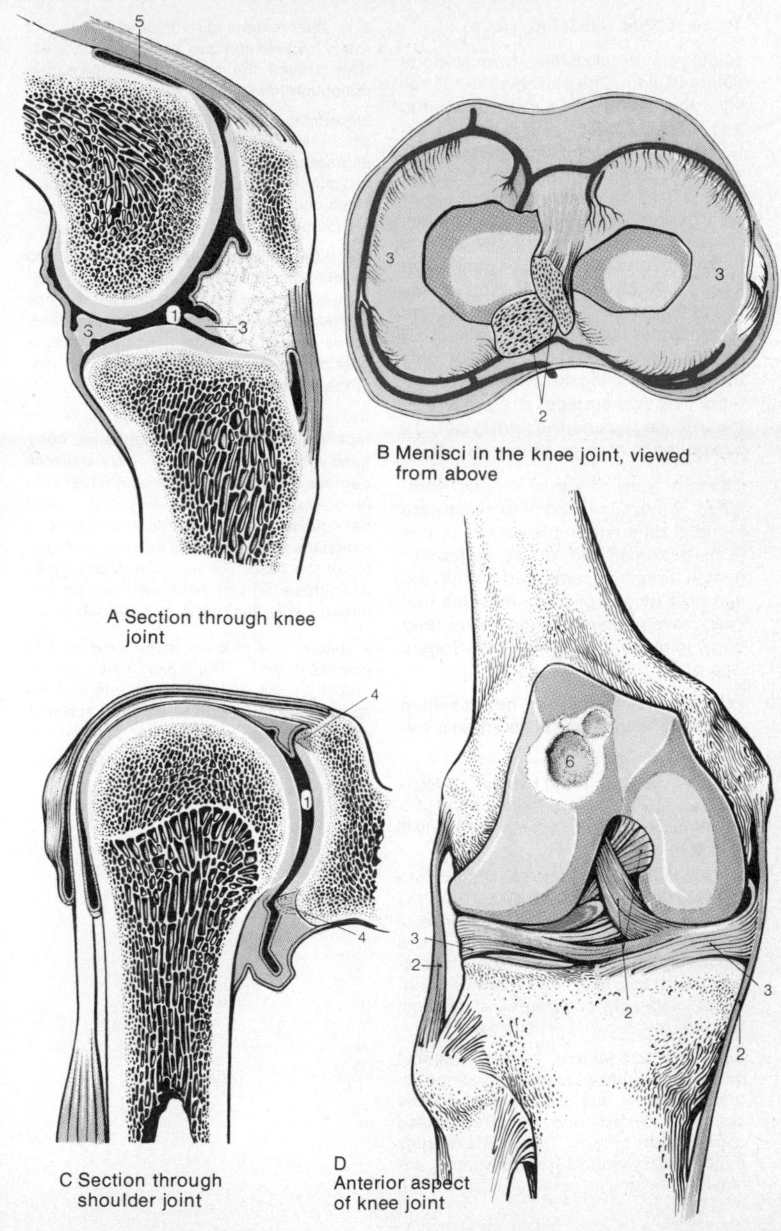

A Section through knee joint

B Menisci in the knee joint, viewed from above

C Section through shoulder joint

D Anterior aspect of knee joint

Types of Synovial Joints (A–F)

Joints may be classified from various points of view. One classification is related to the **axes** and subdivides joints into monaxial, biaxial and multiaxial articulations. A second classification divides the joints according to their **degrees of freedom** which indicate the mobility of articular surfaces against each other. Joints are therefore divided into those with one, two or three degrees of freedom. Another classification makes use of the **number of articular surfaces** and so separates simple from compound joints. A *simple joint* consists of only two surfaces lying in one capsule. If more than two surfaces are present in the articular capsule, the joint is called a *compound joint (e. g., elbow joint* **B**]).

Different types of joints may be combined. Joints combined of necessity are found at different points on two bones (e. g., proximal and distal radioulnar joints). Forcibly combined joints are activated by one or more muscles that span several joints, e. g., hand and finger joints by the flexors of the fingers (see p. 78).

Furthermore, joints may be classified according to the **shape of the articular surfaces:**

A *plane joint*, a joint with two flat surfaces possesses two degrees of freedom, and gliding movements are possible (e. g., the small vertebral joints).

A *hinge joint or ginglymus* (**A**) consists of a convex and a concave articular surface. The concave articular surface often has a ledge-shaped elevation which fits into a groove of the convex one. Tense lateral ligaments (**1**) help to fix the joint more firmly. Hinge joints have one degree of freedom (e. g., the humeroulnar articulation, [**B**]).

A *pivot or trochoid joint* includes peg and rotary joints. Both have one axis and one degree of freedom, and both have one convex cylindrical surface and a corresponding concave joint surface. The joint axis runs through the cylindrical surface which is enlarged by ligaments (annular ligament [**2**], e. g., the proximal radioulnar joint [**B**]). In a rotary joint the concave articular surface rotates around the convex (e. g., the distal radioulnar joint).

Ellipsoidal joints have a convex and a concave elliptical joint surface. They have two degrees of freedom and are multiaxial, with two principal axes. When the movements are combined, a circumduction is possible, e. g., the radiocarpal joint.

A *saddle or sellar joint* (**C**) consits of two saddle-shaped articular surfaces each having a convex and a concave curvature. It has two degrees of freedom and two main axes, but is in fact multiaxial. Circumduction is possibile (e. g., the carpometacarpal joint of the thumb [**D**]).

Ball-and-socket or *spheroidal joints* (**E**) are multiaxial and consist of a globular bony head within a cup or socket. There are three degrees of freedom and three principal axes (e. g., shoulder joint [**F**]). A special type of ball-and-socket joint is the *enarthrosis* in which the socket extends beyond the equator of the head. The hip joint is usually an enarthrosis which, however, has an enlarged cavity due to the articular labrum.

A special type of joints is the fixed joint or *amphiarthrosis*. This has very limited mobility since both the ligaments and the capsule are taut and the articular surfaces are rough, e. g., the sacroiliac joint.

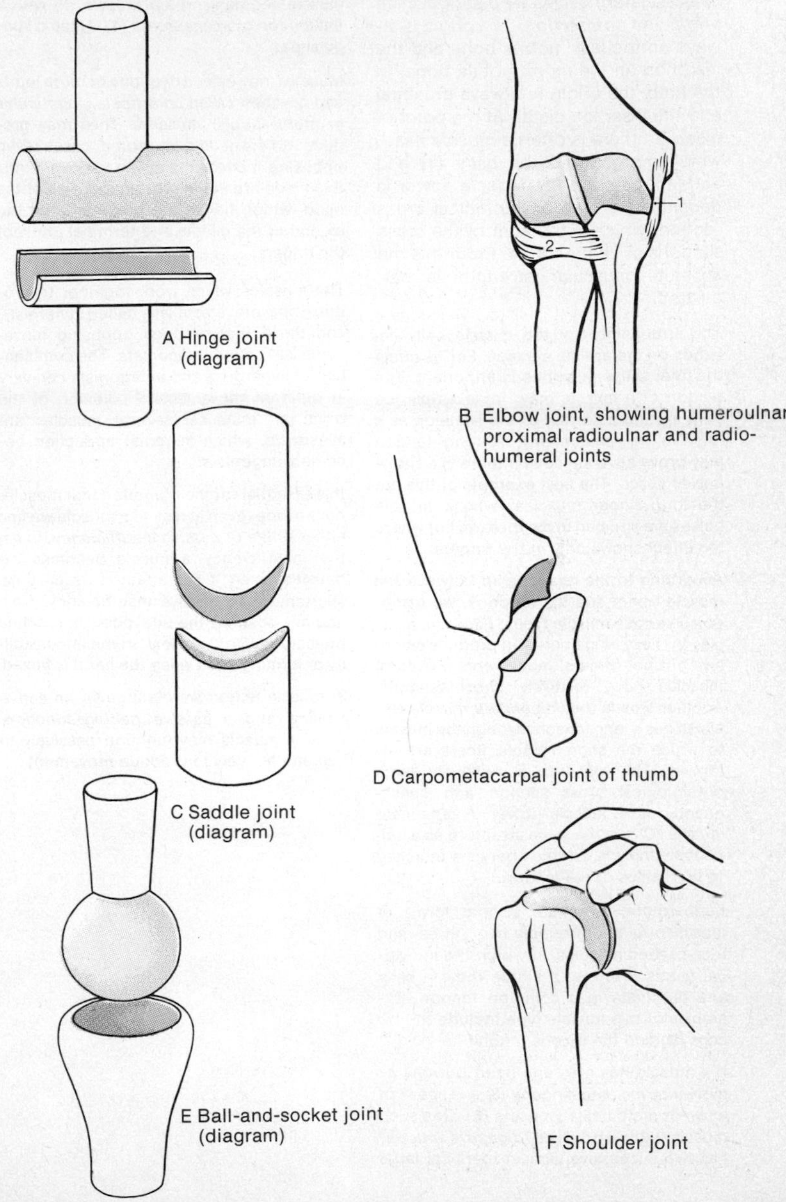

A Hinge joint (diagram)

B Elbow joint, showing humeroulnar, proximal radioulnar and radiohumeral joints

C Saddle joint (diagram)

D Carpometacarpal joint of thumb

E Ball-and-socket joint (diagram)

F Shoulder joint

In all skeletal muscles we distinguish an *origin* and an *insertion.* The origin is always on the less mobile bone and the insertion on the more mobile bone. In the limb, the origin is always proximal and the insertion distal. At the point of insertion there is often a *muscle head,* which merges into the *belly* (**1**) and ends in a *tendon* (**2**). Muscle power is dependent on the physiological cross section, which is the sum of the cross sections of all the fibers. From this the absolute muscular strength is calculated.

The arrangement of the muscle belly depends on the available space. For its effect the final active positions is important. The tendon of a muscle may, for example, be bent around a portion of the skeleton as a fulcrum *(hypomochlion).* A long tendon may prove advantageous if there is a shortage of space. The best example of this are the long finger muscles, whose muscle bellies are situated in the forearm but where the effect shows only in the fingers.

According to the relationship between the muscle fibers and the tendons, we distinguish various muscle types: *Fusiform muscles* (**A**) have long fibers and produce extensive but not forceful movements. Fusiform muscles have relatively short tendons. Another type is the *unipennate muscle* (**B**), which has a long tendon through the muscle to which the short muscle fibers are attached. This ensures a relatively large physiological cross section and consequently more muscle power. A *bipennate muscle* (**C**) has the same structure as a unipennate muscle, but the fibers are attached to both sides of the tendon.

Furthermore, there are several forms of muscle origin, for example two-, three- and four-headed muscles, in which the individual heads fuse into a single muscle belly and terminate in a common tendon. Examples of this muscle type include the biceps (**D**) and the triceps brachii.

If a muscle has only one head but one or more *intermediate tendons* (**3**), we speak of a two or more bellied muscle (**E**). One such muscle with two bellies *(digastric muscle)* has two successive, almost identical large muscle segments. A *flat muscle* (**F**) with a flat tendon or *aponeurosis* (**4**) is also distinguished.

Muscles may extend over one or more joints and are then called *uniarticular, biarticular* or *multiarticular* muscles. They may produce different and in some cases even opposing movements at the various joints. Examples are the interossei muscles of the hand, which flex at the proximal joint but extend at the middle and terminal joints of the fingers.

The muscles which work together to produce one movement are called *synergists,* and those that produce opposing movements are called *antagonists.* The combination of synergists and antagonists can vary in different movements. In flexion of the wrist for instance, several muscles are synergists, which in radial abduction become antagonists.

It is essential for their function that muscles have a *tone*, even at rest. In a muscle we find either *active* or *passive insufficiency*. In active insufficiency, a muscle becomes exhausted when it has attained its maximal shortening. In passive insufficiency, from another position the end point is reached prematurely, for example, in the impossibility of forming a fist when the hand is flexed.

In muscle action we distinguish an *active moving* and a *passive halting function.* Thus, a muscle may function passively to halt and actively to produce movement.

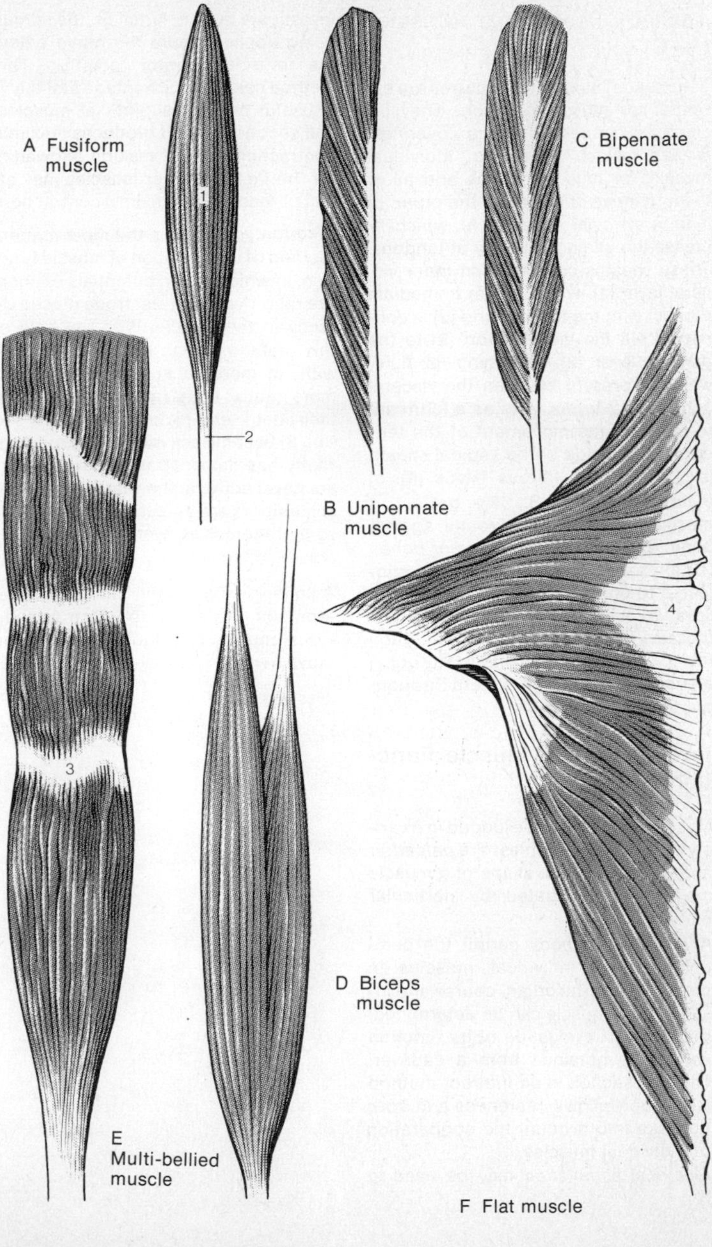

A Fusiform muscle

1

2

B Unipennate muscle

C Bipennate muscle

3

E Multi-bellied muscle

D Biceps muscle

4

F Flat muscle

Auxiliary Features of Muscles (A–C)

A number of auxiliary structures are essential for muscle function. They include: a) connective tissue coverings, *fascias*, which surround individual muscles or muscle groups and allow them to move one against the other. b) *tendon synovial sheaths (***A**), which increase the gliding capacity of tendons. These sheaths consist of an inner visceral layer (**1**), which lies in immediate contact with the tendon, and (**2**) is connected via the mesotendon (**3**) to the parietal layer (**2**). The synovial fluid, which is present between the visceral and parietal layers, acts as a lubricant to enhance the movement of the tendon. The outside of the vaginal sheath is covered by a fibrous tissue (**4**). c) *Synovial bursae* (**B**, [**5**]) protect a muscle where it lies directly against bone. d) *Sesamoid cartilages or bones* (**C**) are found where tendons are subjected to pressure. e) *Fatty tissue, corpora adiposa,* lie between individual muscles and may reduce friction. Such fatty bodies (e. g., the axillary fatty body) are found in variable numbers throughout the body.

Investigation of Muscle Function

Muscle function can be judged in a variety of ways. The simplest are *palpation* and *inspection*. The shape of a muscle may be demonstrated by particular movements.

Anatomical methods permit the demonstration of individual muscles in preparations. The origin, course and insertion of a muscle can be determined, but an exact evaluation of its function cannot be obtained from a cadaver. Thus, dissection is an indirect method which only allows inferences and does not take into account the cooperation of individual muscles.

Electrical stimulation may be used to investigate muscle function, the stimuli being applied where the nerve enters the muscle ('motor point'). This method has the disadvantage first that it is useful only for superficial muscles. and secondly, that it produces maximal contraction without making allowance for the fact that other muscles may affect or reduce this maximal contraction.

Electromyography is the most modern method of investigation of muscle function, in which action potentials of fibers are recorded by an electrode placed directly in the muscle. With the help of this method, it has been shown that, with an increase in effort, more and more motor units (muscle fibers with their motor end plates and nerves, see Vol. 3) become activated. Electromyography has demonstrated that all fibers are never active at the same time. While some fibers are at rest, others contract so that there is an even increase or decrease in tension.

A limiting factor is the difficulty in determining the extent to which an individual muscle contributes to any given movement.

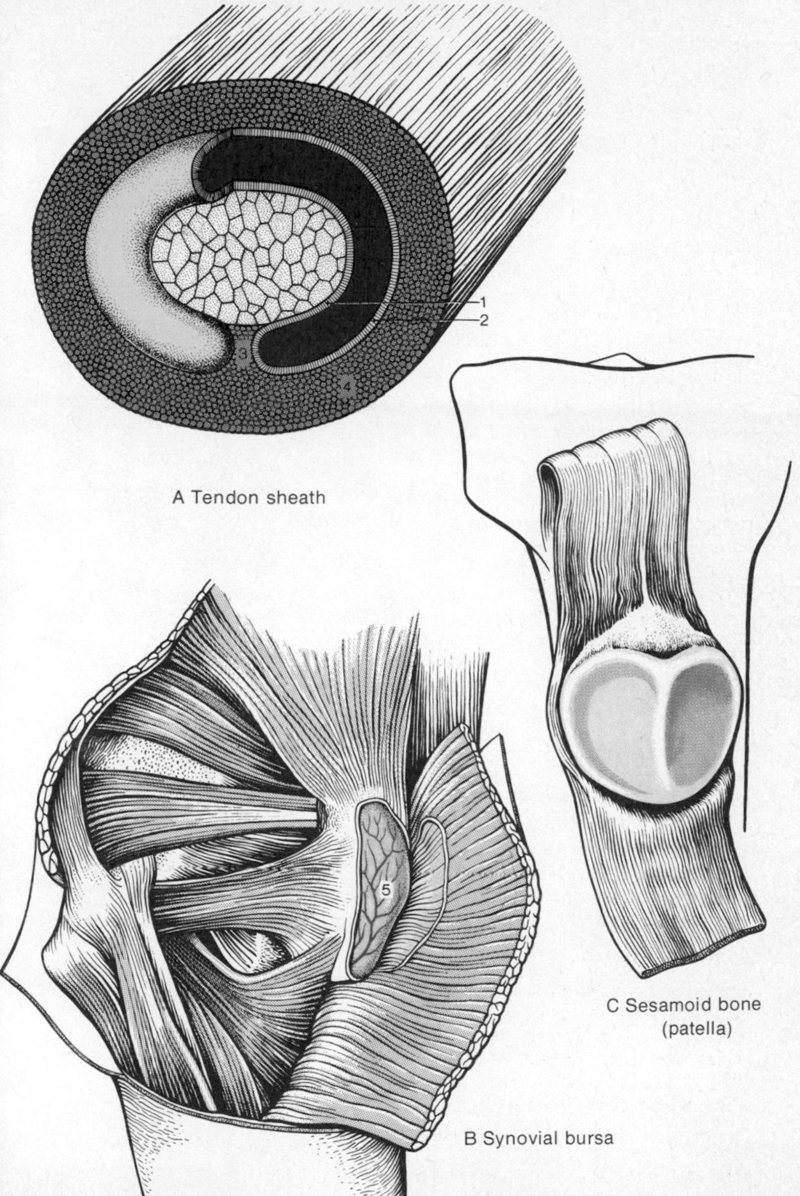

A Tendon sheath

C Sesamoid bone (patella)

B Synovial bursa

Systematic Anatomy of the Locomotor Apparatus

The **vertebral column** forms the basic structure of the trunk. It consists of 33–34 *vertebrae* and *intervertebral disks*. The vertebrae are divided into 7 *cervical*, 12 *thoracic*, 5 *lumbar*, 5 *sacral* and 4–5 *coccygeal vertebrae.* The sacral vertebrae fuse to form the *sacrum* and the coccygeal vertebrae fuse to form the *coccyx*.

Cervical Vertebrae (A–F)

The first vertebra, the **atlas**, the second, the **axis** and the seventh, the **vertebra prominens**, are distinguished from the rest of the cervical vertebrae. There are only small differences between the 3rd–6th cervical vertebrae (**A, D, E**). The *vertebral body* (**1**) lies immediately behind the *vertebral arch* (**2**). Each vertebral arch has an anterior part, the *pedicle* (**3**), and a posterior part, the *lamina* (**4**). At the point of transition between the two parts, the *superior articular process* (**5**) and the *inferior articular process* (**6**) project cranially or caudally. There is a narrow indentation between the body and the superior articular process, the *incisura vertebralis superior* (**7**). A broader *incisura vertebralis inferior* (**8**) is present between the body and the inferior articular process. The articular processes have *articular surfaces* (**9**), the superior facing dorsally and the inferior facing ventrally. From the median convergence (juncture) of the laminae, a spinous process (**10**) projects dorsally and is bifurcated at the tip in the 3rd–6th cervical vertebrae. Between the body and the arch of the cervical vertebrae lies a relatively large *vertebral foramen* (**11**). The *transverse processes* (**12**) extend laterally.

Each transverse process develops from the anlage of a vertebra and a rib (see p. 52). The rib anlage is incompletely fused with the vertebral anlage so that the *foramen transversarium* (**13**) develops. The transverse process also has an *anterior tubercle* (**14**) and a *posterior tubercle* (**15**); between them we find a groove, the *sulcus for the spinal nerve* (**16**).

The anterior tubercle of the 6th cervical vertebra (**D**) can be very large and is designated as the *carotid tubercle* (**17**). On the upper articular surface of the body of the 3rd–7th cervical vertebrae there are laterally two protuberances, the *processi uncinati* (**18**, see p. 58).

The 7th cervical vertebra (**C**) has a particularly large spinous process, which is usually the highest palpable spinous process of the vertebral column; it is therefore called the *vertebra prominens.*

Variants

If the transverse process of the 7th cervical vertebra (**F**) is incomplete and the rib anlage remains independent, a **cervical rib** (**19**) results. Cervical ribs are usually bilateral, but if unilateral, they are more common on the left than on the right. The transverse foramen is often bisected in various vertebrae. The 7th vertebra usually lacks an anterior tubercle.

Practical Points

The presence of a cervical rib may cause a triad of disorders.

1 Pain due to distortion of vessels.
2 Pains related to the brachial plexus (sensory disturbances, especially of the ulnar nerve).
3 Palpable abnormalities in the greater supraclavicular fossa.

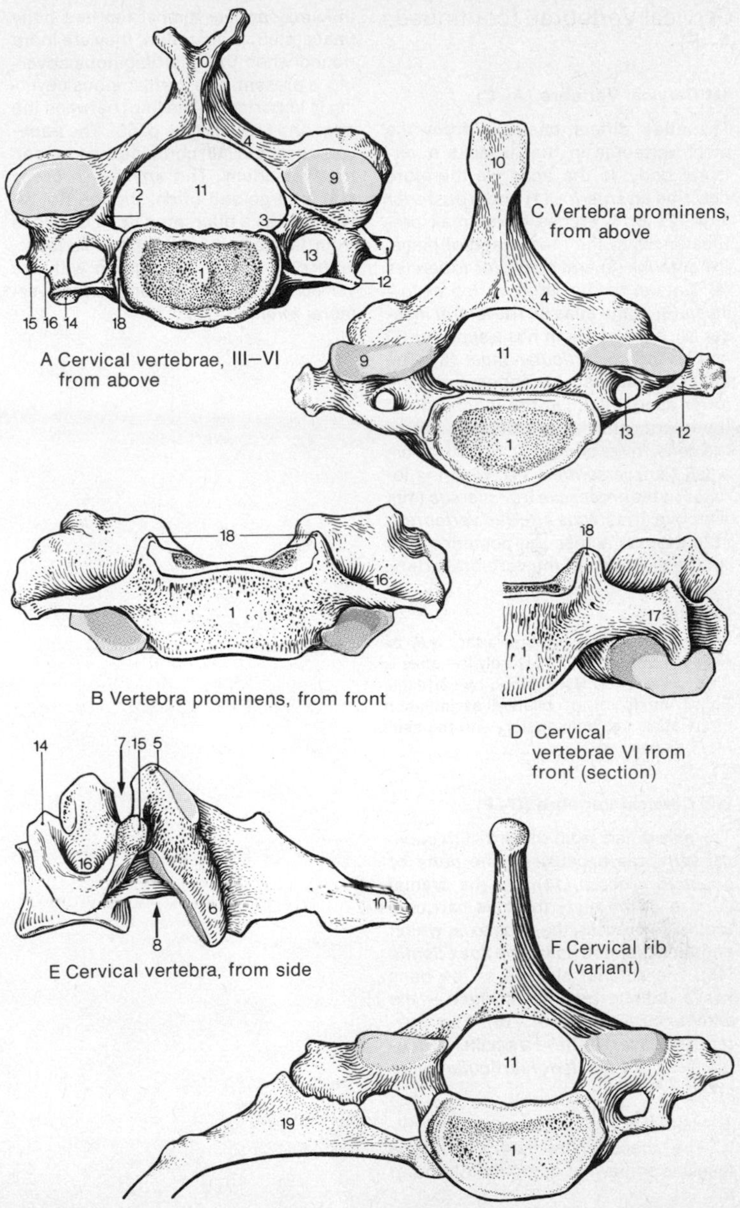

A Cervical vertebrae, III–VI from above

C Vertebra prominens, from above

B Vertebra prominens, from front

D Cervical vertebrae VI from front (section)

E Cervical vertebra, from side

F Cervical rib (variant)

Cervical Vertebrae (continued, A–F)

1st Cervical Vertebra (A–C)

The **atlas** differs basically from the other vertebrae in that it lacks a vertebral body. In the atlas we therefore describe an *anterior* (**1**) and a *posterior arch* (**2**). Both arches have small protuberances in the mediosagittal plane, the *anterior* (**3**) and *posterior tubercles* (**4**). Lateral to the large *vertebral foramen* (**5**) of the atlas lie the *lateral masses* (**6**), each of which has a *superior* (**7**) and an *inferior articular facet* (**8**). The upper articular facet is concave and the lower almost flat. On the inner side of the anterior arch is the articular facet for the dens, *fovea dentis* (**9**). From the *foramen transversarium* (**11**), which is located in the *processus transversus* (**10**), a groove, the *sulcus arteriae vertebralis* (**12**), extends across the posterior arch for the reception of the vertebral artery.

Variants

The sulcus for the vertebral artery may be replaced by a *canal* (**13**). Rarely the atlas is divided into two halves joined by cartilage. Equally rarely uni- or bilateral assimilation of the atlas, i.e., bony fusion with the skull may be observed.

2nd Cervical Vertebra (D–F)

The **axis** differs from the 3rd–6th cervical vertebrae because of the *dens* or *odontoid process* (**14**). On the cranial surface of the body the axis carries a tooth-like process, the *dens axis*, which ends in a rounded point, the *apex dentis* (**15**). The anterior surface of the dens has a definite articular surface – the *anterior articular facet* (**16**). The posterior surface may have a smaller articular facet, the *posterior articular facet* (**17**).

The lateral articular facets slope laterally. The shape of the lateral articular facets is somewhat complex. Although they may appear almost flat in a bony (macerated) preparation, they are more ridged when their cartilaginous covering is present. The cartilaginous covering is important in the joint between the atlas and the axis (see p. 60). The *transverse process* (**18**) contains the foramen transversarium. The *spinous process* (**19**) is large and often, though not always, it has a bifurcated tip. It develops from the joined parts of the *vertebral arch* (**20**), which in common with the *vertebral body* (**21**), encompass the *vertebral foramen* (**22**).

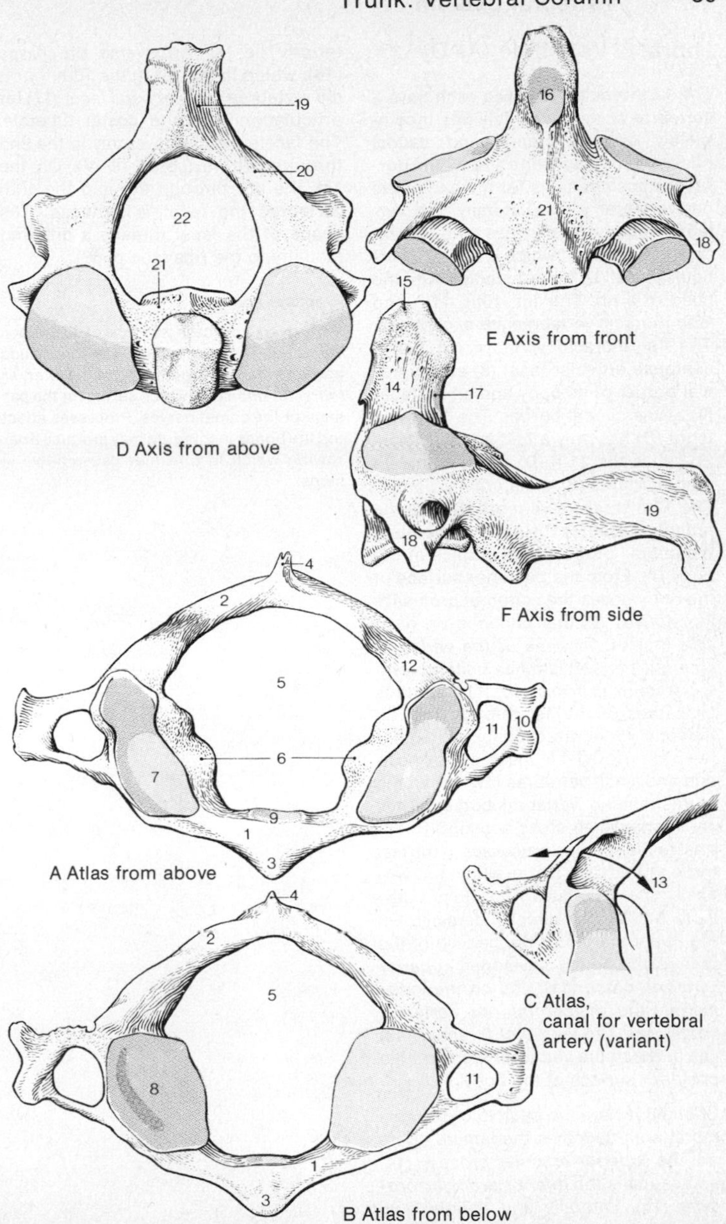

D Axis from above

E Axis from front

F Axis from side

A Atlas from above

C Atlas, canal for vertebral artery (variant)

B Atlas from below

Thoracic Vertebrae (A–D)

The 12 **thoracic vertebrae** each have a *vertebral body* (**1**), which has incompletely ossified cranial and caudal plates of compact bone and on the dorsal surface openings for the exit of the basivertebral veins. Laterally, the vertebral body usually has two *costal facets* (**2**), each of which is half of an articular facet (**D**) for articulation with the head of a rib. The 1st, 10th, 11th and 12th thoracic vertebrae are exceptions. The 1st thoracic vertebra (**D**) has a complete articular facet (**3**) at the cranial border of its body and a half facet (**4**) at the caudal border. The 10th vertebra (**D**) has only a half articular facet (**5**), while the 11th (**D**) has a complete articular facet (**6**) at its cranial border. The 12th thoracic vertebra (**D**) has the articular facet for the head of the rib in the middle of the lateral surface of the body (**7**). From the posterior surface of the body arises the *vertebral arch* with its *pedicles* (**8**) that continue on each side into the *laminae of the vertebral arch* (**9**). The two laminae unite to form the *spinous process* (**10**). The spinous processes of the 1st through the 9th thoracic vertebrae overlap each other like roof tiles, so that their tips lie one to one and a half vertebrae lower than the corresponding vertebral bodies. They are triangular in cross section in contrast to the spinous processes of the last three thoracic vertebrae which are vertically oriented plates. They do not descend but extend directly dorsally. On the upper margin of the pedicle of the arch is the poorly developed *superior vertebral notch* (**11**), and on the lower margin the deeper *inferior vertebral notch* (**12**). The *vertebral foramen* (**13**) lies between the vertebral arch and the posterior surface of the body.

Cranially, where the pedicle of the vertebral arch becomes the lamina, there are the *superior articular process* (**14**) and caudally the *inferior articular process* (**15**). Laterally and a little posteriorly lie *the transverse processes* (**16**), which in the 1st to the 10th thoracic vertebrae carry a *costal facet* (**17**) for articulation with the costal tubercle. The facets are concave only in the 2nd through 5th vertebrae (II–V). On the 1st, the 6th through 9th and the 10th vertebrae the facet is flattened. The shape of the facet imparts a differing mobility to the ribs (see p. 68).

Practical Points

A transverse process is typical of all thoracic vertebrae. The vertebral notches, one caudal and one cranial, together form the *intervertebral foramen* (**18**) which serves for the passage of the spinal nerves. Processes affecting the bones in this area may produce a narrowing which in turn may cause nerve lesions.

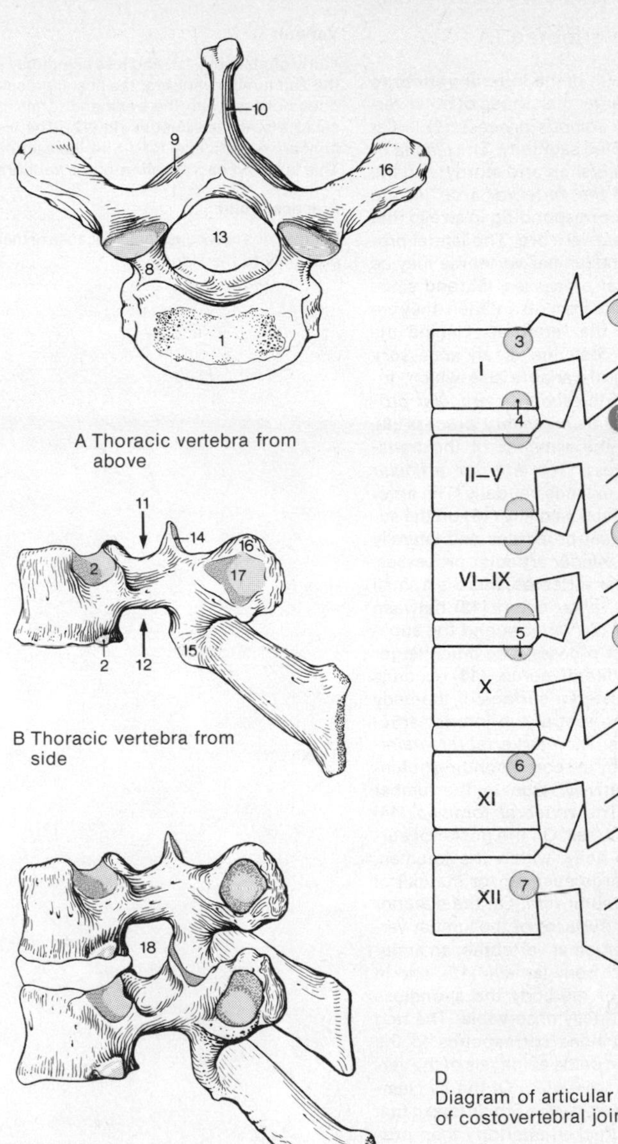

A Thoracic vertebra from above

B Thoracic vertebra from side

C
Two thoracic vertebrae from side

D
Diagram of articular facets of costovertebral joints

Lumbar Vertebrae (A–C)

The *bodies* (**1**) of the **lumbar vertebrae** are much larger than those of other vertebrae. The *spinous process* (**2**) is flat and is directed sagittally. The *lamina of the arch* (**3**) is short and sturdy, and the *pedicles of the vertebral arch* (**4**) are very thick, corresponding in size to that of the lumbar vertebra. The lateral processes of the lumbar vertebrae may be called *costal processes* (**5**), and since they originate from rib anlagen, they are fused with the vertebrae. Behind the processus costarius is an *accessory process* (**6**) of variable size which, together with the *superior articular process* (**7**) and its *mamillary process* (**8**), represents the remnant of the *transverse process.* The *inferior articular process* (**9**) extends caudally. The articular facets face medially (**10**) on the superior articular processes and laterally (**11**) on the inferior articular processes. As in all other vertebrae, there is a small *superior vertebral notch* (**12**) between the body of the vertebra and the superior articular process. The much larger *inferior vertebral notch* (**13**) extends from the posterior surface of the body as far as the root of the inferior articular process. The *intervertebral foramina,* formed by the corresponding notches, are relatively large in the lumbar vertebrae. The *vertebral foramen* (**14**) is relatively small. On the posterior surface of the body, within the foramen, there is a large opening for the exit of the basivertebral vein. On the superior and inferior surfaces of the lumbar vertebrae, as on other vertebrae, an annular, compact bony lamella (**15**), and in the center of the body the spongiosa (**16**) are distinctly observable. The ring of compact bone corresponds to the bony portion of the epiphysis of the vertebral body (see p. 52). Of the five lumbar vertebrae only the 5th differs in that its body is thicker anteriorly than posteriorly.

Variants

Fairly often in the 1st, and less commonly in the 2nd lumbar vertebra, the costal process does not fuse with the bone and forms instead a so-called **lumbar rib** (**17**). The last lumbar vertebra may fuse with the sacrum. This is called **sacralization** of the vertebra.

Practical Point

Lumbar ribs may cause pain because of their proximity to the kidney.

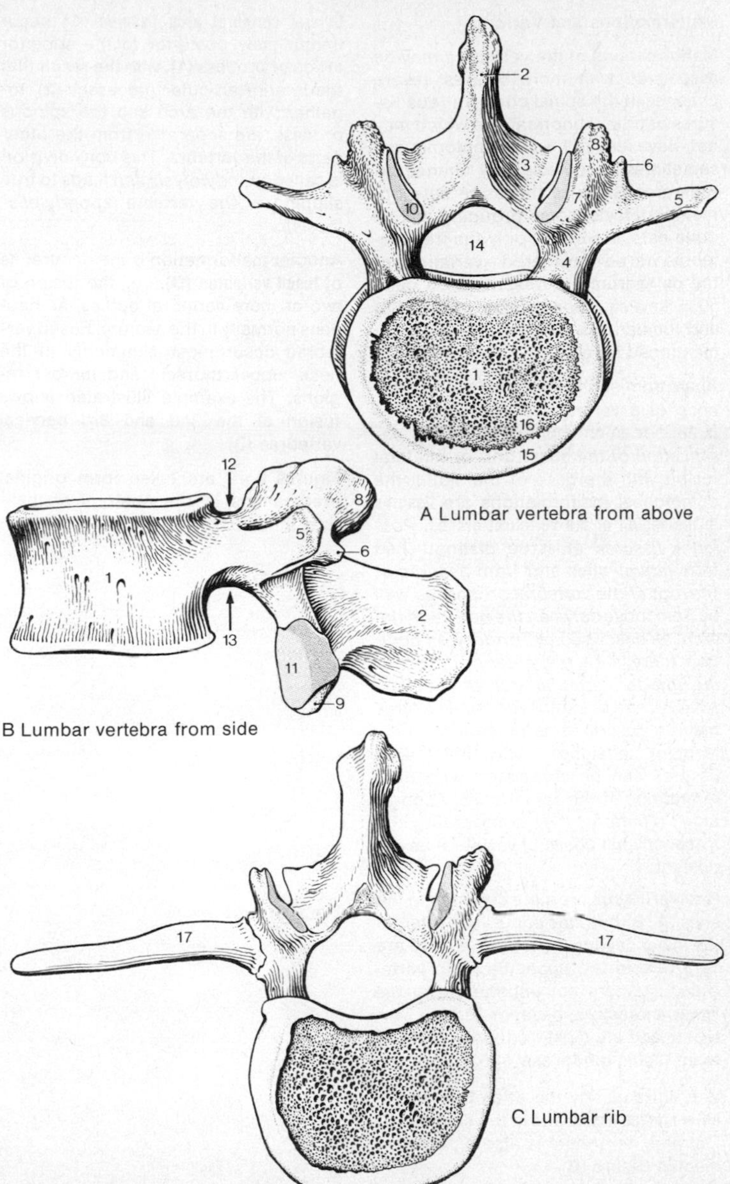

A Lumbar vertebra from above

B Lumbar vertebra from side

C Lumbar rib

Malformations and Variants

Malformations of the vertebrae may be associated with more or less severe changes in the spinal cord. Various fissures or other abnormalities which may not have caused any symptoms can sometimes be detected by chance on radiographs. Since these are developmental defects, some grouping will be done here. Moreover, only the free vertebrae will be considered – variations of the os sacrum are described on page 50. Likewise, cervical ribs (see p. 36) and lumbar ribs (see p. 42) will not be mentioned here.

Apart from such variations as the presence of a *vertebral artery canal* (see p. 36), or such malformations as *assimilation of the atlas* (uni- or bilateral fusion with the base of the skull), the commonest malformations are **fissures in the region of the vertebral arches.** *Posterior fissures* must be distinguished from *lateral* ones and from *fissures at the root of the vertebral arches,* as well as from those *between the body and the arch*, as described by *Töndury.* In addition, there is the rare *anterior fissure of the anterior vertebral arch of the atlas*. Anterior and posterior vertebral fissures may be described as median fissures. Median posterior vertebral arch fissures can be associated with malformations of the spinal cord. According to *Töndury*, they arise during the mesenchymal phase of vertebral development.

Posterior fissures are quite common in the atlas (**A, B**) but they occur less often in the lower cervical vertebrae (**E**) and are very rare in the upper thoracic vertebrae. They are not uncommon in the lower thoracic and upper lumbar vertebrae and are most frequent in the sacrum (spina bifida, see p. 50).

Very infrequently the atlas has an **anterior median fissure** and in the example illustrated here there is also a posterior median fissure (**B**).

Lateral vertebral arch fissures (**C**) occur immediately posterior to the superior articular process (**1**), with the result that the inferior articular processes (**2**), together with the arch and the spinous process, are separated from the other parts of the vertebra. This bony division is called *spondylolysis* and leads to true slipping of the vertebra *(spondylolisthesis).*

Another malformation is the occurence of **fused vertebrae** (**D**), i.e., the fusion of two or more vertebral bodies, as happens normally in the sacrum. Fused vertebrae occur most commonly in the neck, upper thoracic and lumbar regions. The example illustrated shows fusion of the 2nd and 3rd cervical vertebrae (**D**).

Figures **A–E** are taken form original preparations in the Anatomical Institute, Innsbruck.

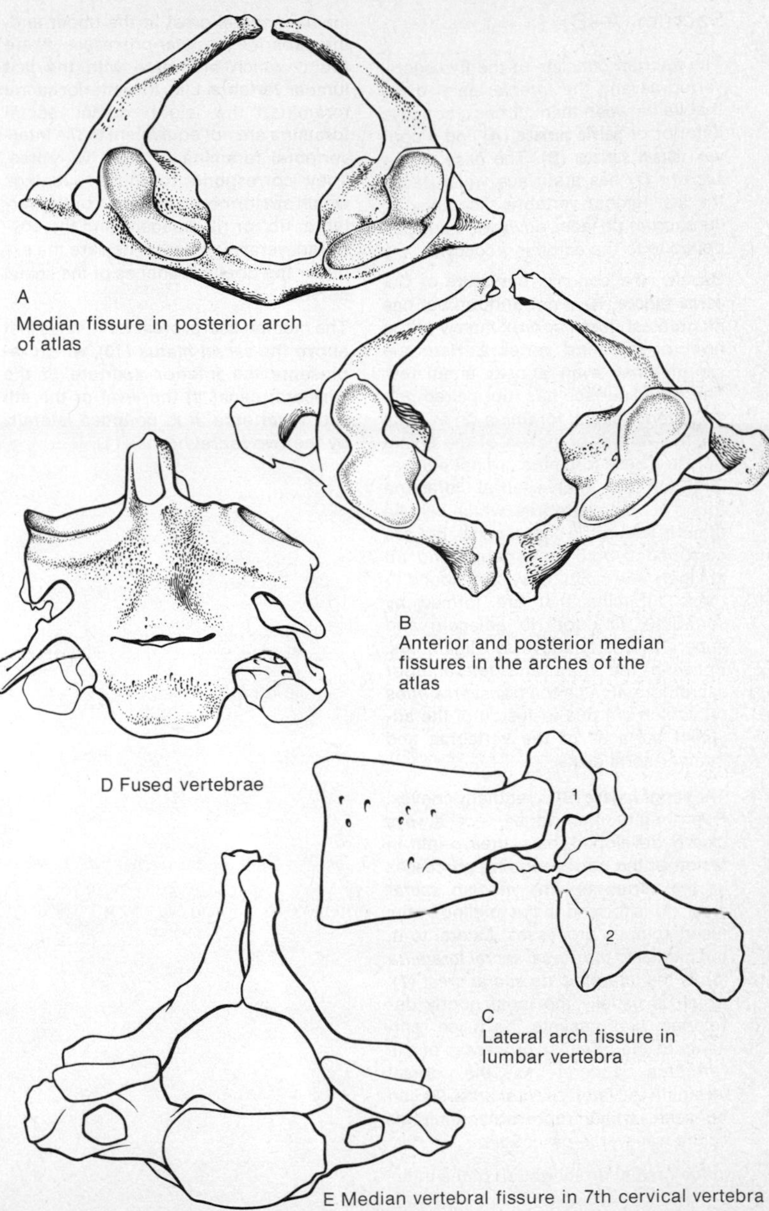

A
Median fissure in posterior arch of atlas

B
Anterior and posterior median fissures in the arches of the atlas

D Fused vertebrae

C
Lateral arch fissure in lumbar vertebra

E Median vertebral fissure in 7th cervical vertebra

Sacrum (A–B)

The **sacrum** consists of the five sacral vertebrae and the intervertebral disks that lie between them. It has a concave anterior or **pelvic surface** (**A**) and a convex **dorsal surface** (**B**). The *base of the sacrum* (**1**) has a surface which faces the last lumbar vertebra. The *apex of the sacrum* (**2**) faces downward and lies opposite to the adjoining coccyx.

Usually, the concave curvature of the **pelvic surface** (**H**) is not uniform but has its greatest depth approximately at the level of the third vertebra. Here the sacrum may even appear angulated. The pelvic surface has four paired pelvic *anterior sacral foramina* (**3**) as exits for the ventral branches of the spinal nerves. These foramina are not equivalent to the intervertebral foramina found in other vertebrae, which here lie directly within the sacral canal, but are surrounded both by vertebral and rib anlagen (see p. 52). They correspond to those foramina that are formed by vertebrae, ribs (or rib anlagen) and superior costotransverse ligaments. Between the right and left anterior sacral foramina lie the *transverse lines* (**4**), which are due to fusion of the adjacent surfaces of the vertebrae and intervertebral disks.

The **dorsal surface** (**B**) is regularly convex. Five longitudinal ridges, not always clearly developed, have their origin in fusion of the corresponding processes of the vertebrae. The *median sacral crest* (**5**) is formed in the midline by the fused spinous processes. Lateral to it, but medial to the *dorsal sacral foramina* (**6**), is the *intermediate sacral crest* (**7**), which is usually the most poorly developed. It represents the fused remnants of the articular processes of the vertebrae. Lateral to the dorsal foramina the *lateral sacral crest* (**8**) can be seen, which represents remnants of the transverse processes.

In the cranial prolongation of the intermediate sacral crest at the upper end, the *superior articular processes* (**9**) are found which articulate with the last lumbar vertebra. Like the anterior sacral foramina, the eight dorsal sacral foramina are not equivalent to the intervertebral foramina of other vertebrae. They correspond to those openings which are formed in common by the vertebra, rib (or rib anlagen) and the costotransverse ligament. They are the exits for the dorsal branches of the spinal nerves.

The median sacral crest terminates just above the *sacral hiatus* (**10**), which represents the inferior aperture of the vertebral canal at the level of the 4th sacral vertebra. It is bounded laterally by the two *sacral horns* (**11**).

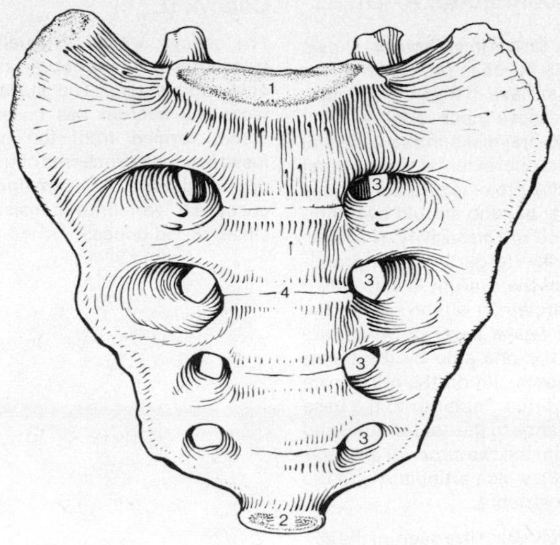

A Sacrum from front

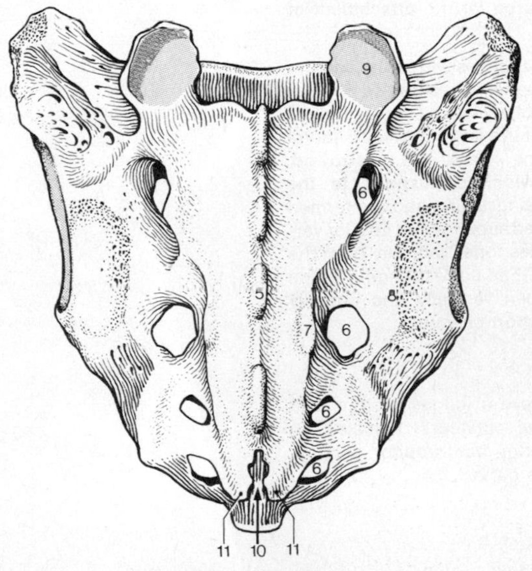

B Sacrum from back

Sacrum (continued, A–D)

A view of the **sacrum from above** (**A**) shows in the middle the *base* (**1**), which forms the contact surface of the intervertebral disk with the last lumbar vertebra. Of all the intervertebral disks in the vertebral column, this one extends the furthest forward. It also projects furthest into the pelvis (see p. 62) and should by definition be called the **promontory**. However, in present day usage the most prominent point of the sacrum is also called the promontory. On either side of the base lie the *lateral parts* (**2**) which are formed on the one side by the transverse processes and on the other from rudiments of ribs. Posterior to the base lies the entrance to the sacral canal and lateral to it are the two *superior articular processes* (**3**), which articulate with the last lumbar vertebra.

In a **lateral** view (**B**) of the sacrum the *auricular surface* (**4**) for the articulation with the hip bone can be seen. Posterior to it lies the *sacral tuberosity* (**5**), a roughened area for the attachment of ligaments.

The *sacral canal* lies within the sacrum and, corresponding in shape to the sacrum, is irregularly curved and of uneven width. About the level of the 3rd sacral vertebra the canal is narrowed. Channels, which correspond to the intervertebral foramina and are formed from the fused superior and inferior vertebral notches, open laterally from the sacral canal. The corresponding sacral foramina open ventrally and dorsally from these short channels.

Sex Differences

Males (**D**) have a longer sacrum with more marked curvature. Females (**C**) have a shorter but broader sacrum, which is less curved.

Coccyx (E, F)

The coccyx, which is usually formed from three to four vertebrae, is normally only rudimentary. The surface which faces the sacrum has *cornua* (**6**) or *horns*, formed from the completely fused articular processes of the 1st coccygeal vertebra. The remainder of the coccygeal vertebrae consist only of small, round bones.

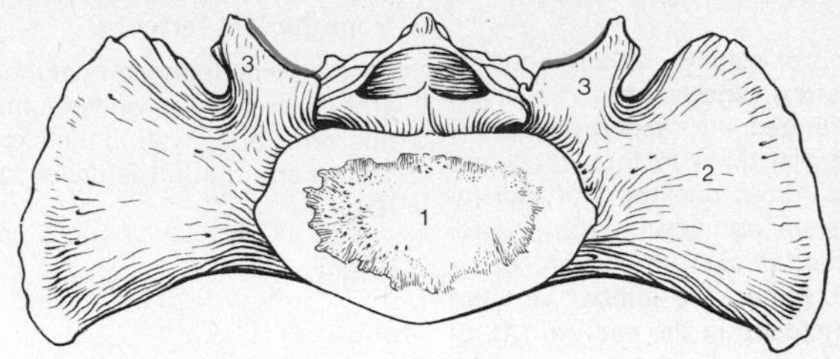

A Superior view of sacrum

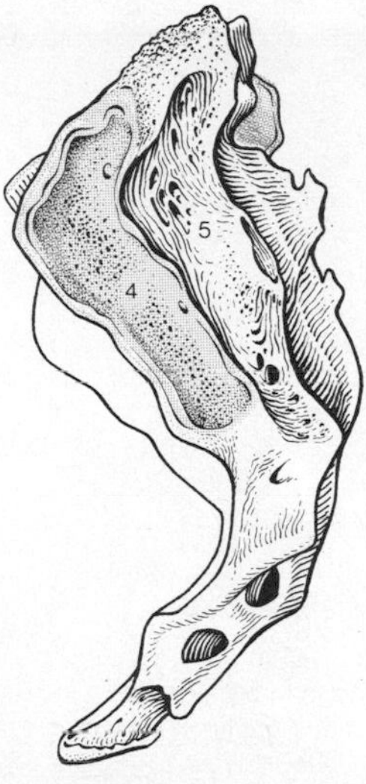

B Lateral view of sacrum

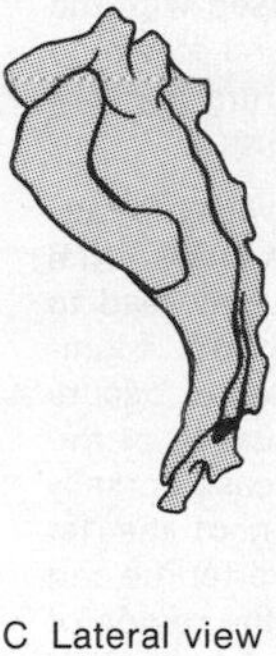

C Lateral view of a female sacrum

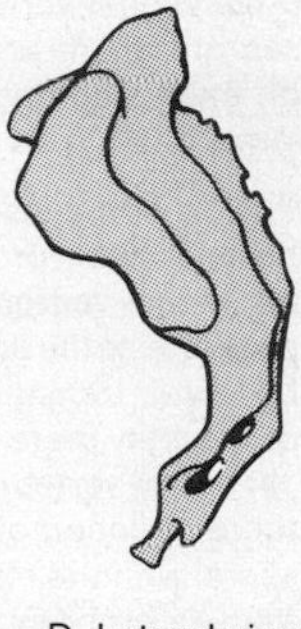

D Lateral view of a male sacrum

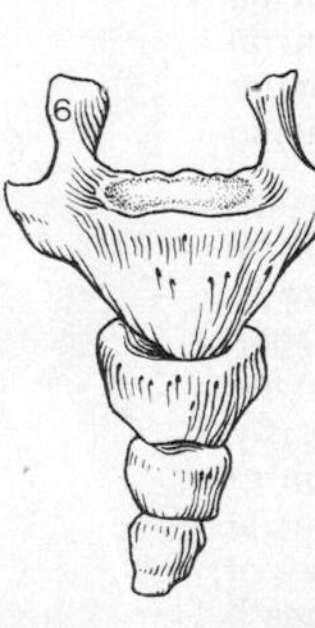

E Anterior view of coccyx

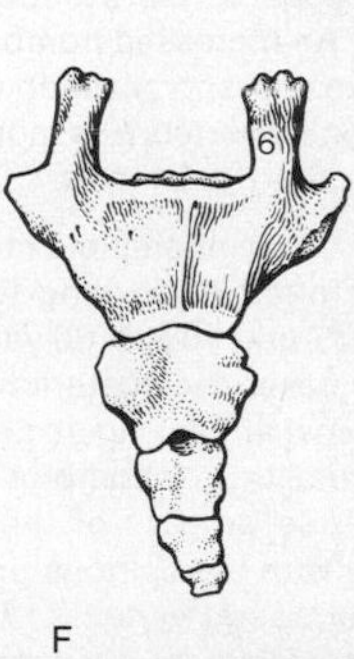

F Posterior view of coccyx

Variations in the Sacral Region (A–D)

The vertebral column usually consists of **24 presacral vertebrae**, the remainder being arranged into five fused sacral vertebrae and three to four coccygeal vertebrae. About one third of individuals have an additional sacral vertebra, so that the sacrum consists of six vertebrae. Either one lumbar vertebra may be included in the sacrum (**A**), or the 1st coccygeal vertebra may be fused with it (**B**). Situation (**A**) is called **sacralization of a lumbar vertebra**, and (**B**) is called **sacralization of the coccyx** or a **coccygeal vertebra**. If either a lumbar or a coccygeal vertebra is fused with the sacrum, there are five sacral foramina on each side and the sacrum appears larger than in its typical form.

Fusion of the last lumbar vertebra may be unilateral, producing a **lumbo-sacral transitional vertebra**, which may lead to scoliosis of the spine (see p. 62). A lumbosacral transitional vertebra occurs also when there is **lumbalization** of the 1st sacral vertebra. In this case dorsally there is incomplete fusion of the 1st sacral with the rest of the vertebrae and there is no bony union in the region of the lateral parts, i. e., in those areas that originated from remnants of ribs.

It should be noted that when lumbalization of a sacral vertebra occurs, there may nevertheless be five vertebrae if the 1st coccygeal vertebra is fused with the sacrum. An increased number of sacral vertebrae, i. e., sacralization of a lumbar or coccygeal vertebra, is more common in males than in females.

Quite often an incomplete medial sacral crest is found (according to *Hintze* in 44% at 15 and 10% at 50 years of age). In these cases the posterior wall of the sacral canal appears to be defective (**C**). Apart from this, incomplete fusion of the spinous process of the 1st sacral vertebra with the spinous processes of the other sacral vertebrae produces a vertebral arch in the 1st sacral segment and so the medial sacral crest starts from the 2nd vertebra.

Lastly, sometimes none of the vertebral arches are fused, so that there is no posterior bony wall in the sacral canal. This malformation is called **spina bifida** (**D**).

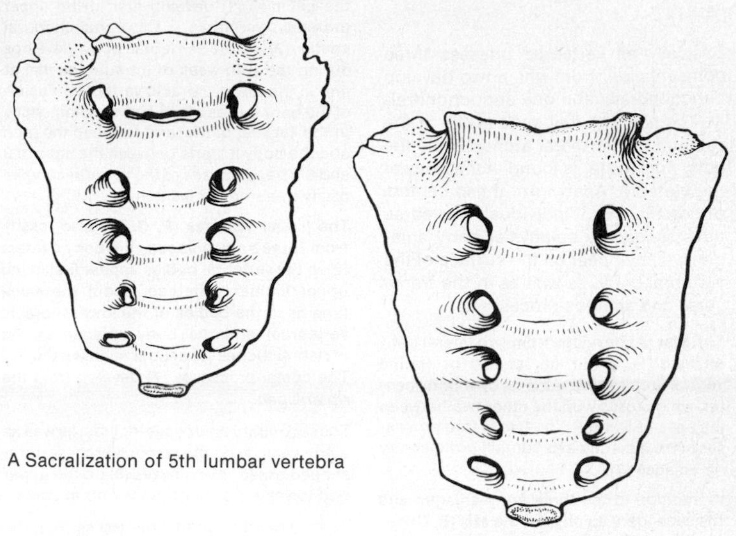

A Sacralization of 5th lumbar vertebra

B Sacralization of 1st coccygeal vertebra

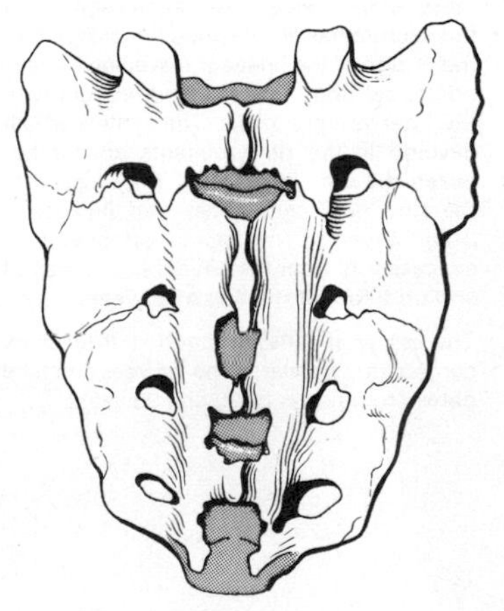

C Incomplete medial sacral crest

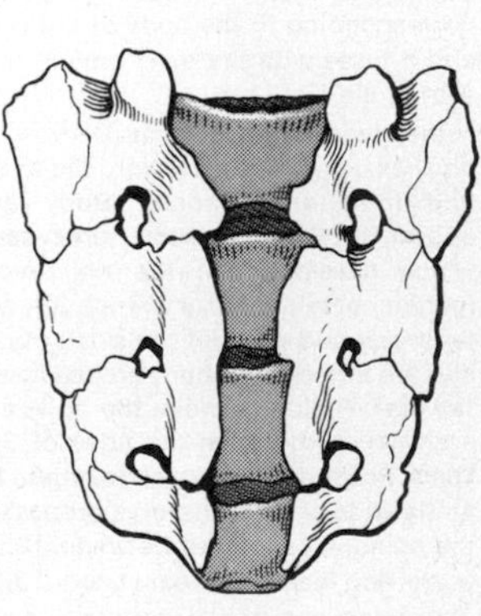

D Spina bifida

Ossification of the Vertebrae (A–I)

Basically all vertebrae possess three *bony anlagen,* from which two develop perichondrally and one endochondrally. The perichondral cuffs (**1**) lie at the roots of the vertebral arches while the bony nucleus (**2**) is found in the body of the vertebra. Apart form these centers of ossification, individual vertebrae have secondary epiphysial bony anlagen which appear on the surface of the vertebral body, as well as in the transverse and spinous processes.

The **atlas** (**A**) develops from two lateral bony anlagen (**1**), but in the 1st year of life the ventral arch may develop its own bony center, which fuses with the other two between the ages of 5 and 9. The transverse processes of the atlas and axis contain rudimentary rib anlagen (**3**).

In addition to the three bony anlagen and the secondary epiphyses, the **axis** (**B, C**) has further ossification centers. The dens (**4**) is usually considered to arise from the bony anlage of the body of the atlas, although, according to another theory (Ludwig), it is formed from the so-called dental processes. Relatively late a bony center *(ossiculum terminale)* develops in the *apex of the dens* (**5**), corresponding to the body of the proatlas, and it fuses with the dens only in the 25th year of life.

In the other **cervical vertebrae** (**D**) *three typical bony anlagen* develop toward the end of the 2nd intrauterine month. Bony anlagen appear in the transverse processes (**6**), which develop from the rib precursors (parietal bars), and from which the anterior tubercles and parts of the posterior tubercles are formed. The bony arches fuse in the 1st year. Fusion between the body and the arch occurs between the ages of 3 and 6 years. *Secondary epiphysial anlagen* appear at the ends of the transverse processes and the spinous processes between 12 and 14 years, and fuse with them at about 20 years. The *epiphyses of the vertebral bodies,* a cranial and a caudal cartilaginous plate, ossify from the 8th year onward in ring form (annular epiphysis) and fuse with the body from about the age of 18.

In the **thoracic region** (**E**) the bony anlagen of the pedicles (**1**) develop first in the upper thoracic vertebrae. The endochondral center (**2**) of the vertebral body develops during the 10th week of intrauterine life, at first in the lower thoracic vertebrae. Fusion of the bony halves of the arches commences in the 1st year of life, and between the arch and the body it starts between the ages of 3 and 6. The *epiphyses of the vertebral bodies* ossify in a ringlike fashion.

The **lumbar vertebrae** (**F, G, K**), also, ossify from three *bony anlagen;* the bony centers (**2**) in the vertebral bodies appear first in the upper lumbar vertebrae (about the same time as in the bodies of the lower thoracic vertebrae) and the bony anlagen in the vertebral arches (**1**) appear somewhat later. The costal processes (**7**) develop from the *rib anlagen.*

The *secondary epiphyses* include, as well as a bony anlage on the spinous process, ring-shaped osseous epiphyses (**8**) on the upper and lower surfaces of the vertebral bodies.

In each of its segments the **sacrum** (**H, I**) develops, like the rest of the vertebrae, from three *bony anlagen*, and in addition from a *rib anlage* (**9**) in the region of the lateral mass on each side. Thus, each segment of the sacrum has *five ossification anlagen.* In the region of the lineae transversae there is additional bony fusion of the margin with the intervertebral disks. The centers which develop in the rib rudiments appear between the 5th–7th month. They fuse with the other bony centers between the ages of 2 and 5 years. The sacral vertebrae fuse successively from the caudal to the cranial end up to about the age of 25 years.

The **coccygeal vertebrae** develop from bony centers that appear in the 1st year and fuse between the ages of 20 and 30 years.

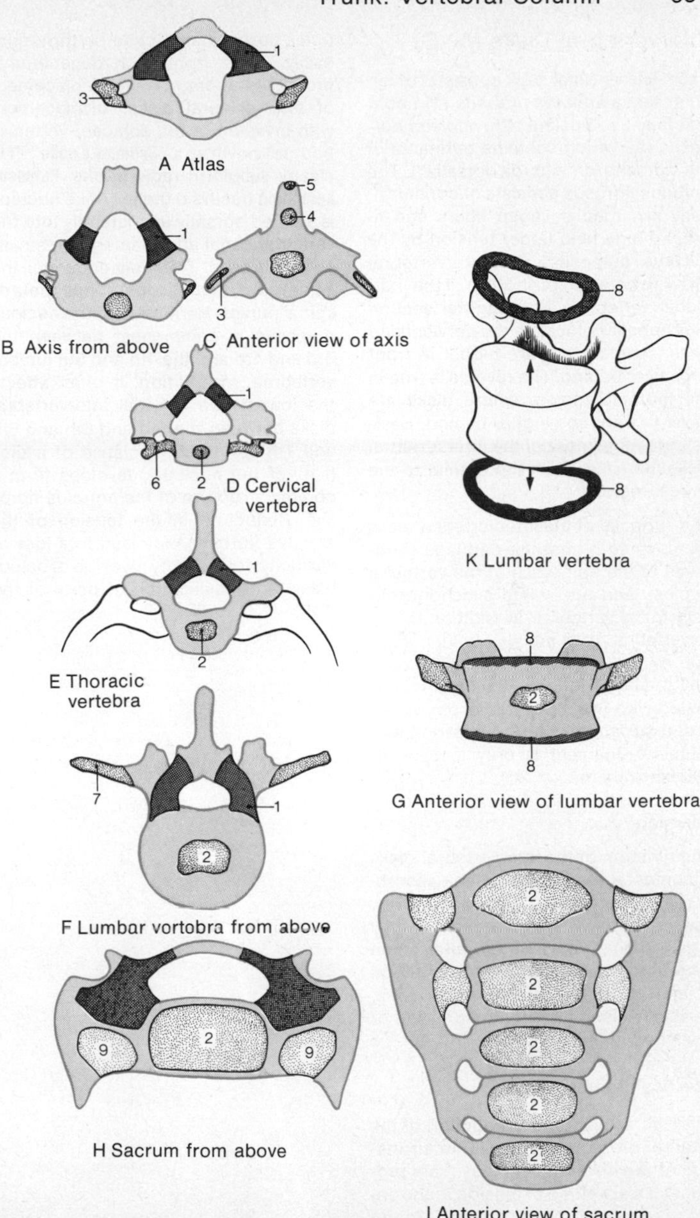
1
3
A Atlas
5
4
1
3
B Axis from above
C Anterior view of axis
1
6
2
D Cervical vertebra
1
2
E Thoracic vertebra
7
1
2
F Lumbar vortobra from above
8
8
K Lumbar vertebra
8
2
8
G Anterior view of lumbar vertebra
9
2
9
H Sacrum from above
2
2
2
2
2
I Anterior view of sacrum

Intervertebral Disks (A–D)

Each **intervertebral disk** consists of an outer tense *annulus fibrosus* (**1**) and a soft jelly-like nucleus, the *nucleus pulposus* (**2**), which contains remnants of the notochord ("chorda dorsalis"). The annulus fibrosus consists of concentrically arranged collagen fibers and fibrocartilage held under tension by the nucleus pulposus. The intervertebral disks lie between the bodies of the individual vertebrae. In a sagittal section they appear conical. In the cervical and lumbar region they are higher in front and lower behind. The reverse is true in the thoracic region, where disks are lower in front and higher behind. Basically, the thickness of the intervertebral disks increases from the cranial to the caudal region.

The surfaces of the intervertebral disks are covered by hyaline cartilage (remnants of the epiphyses of the vertebral bodies), and are united synchondrotically to the vertebrae. In addition, the intervertebral disks are also held in position by the longitudinal ligaments (**3**). The posterior longitudinal ligament is united with the disks (see p. 56) over a broad surface, while the anterior longitudinal ligament is only loosely attached to them.

Function

The function of the intervertebral disks is comparable to that of shock absorbers in automobiles. Loading compresses them and when it is released, they regain their original shape after some time. In movements within the vertebral column (**C, D**) the intervertebral disks, as elastic elements, are compressed or stretched unilaterally.

Practical Points

With increasing age, a reduction of the internal pressure may result in shrinkage of the nucleus pulposus. This produces a slackening of tension in the annulus fibrosus and it can be torn more easily. Apart from such degenerative processes, there may be displacement of intervertebral disks. Displacement with invasion of the adjacent vertebral body is known as a "**Schmorl's node**". It is clearly visible in radiographs. **Pulposus herniation** occurs if the jelly-like nucleus is pushed dorsally and laterally into the vertebral canal after damage to the annulus fibrosus. This may endanger the spinal cord, or individual spinal roots or spinal nerves. Herniation of the nucleus pulposus is commonest between the 3rd and 4th and the 4th and 5th lumbar vertebrae. In addition, it often affects the lowest two cervical intervertebral disks between the 5th and 6th and 6th and 7th vertebrae. Prolapse of a disk (i. e., of the nucleus) develops from a complete rupture of the annulus fibrosus. Reduction in the tension of the annulus fibrosus may lead to a loss of elasticity, followed by invasion of osteoblasts and ossification of parts of the disk.

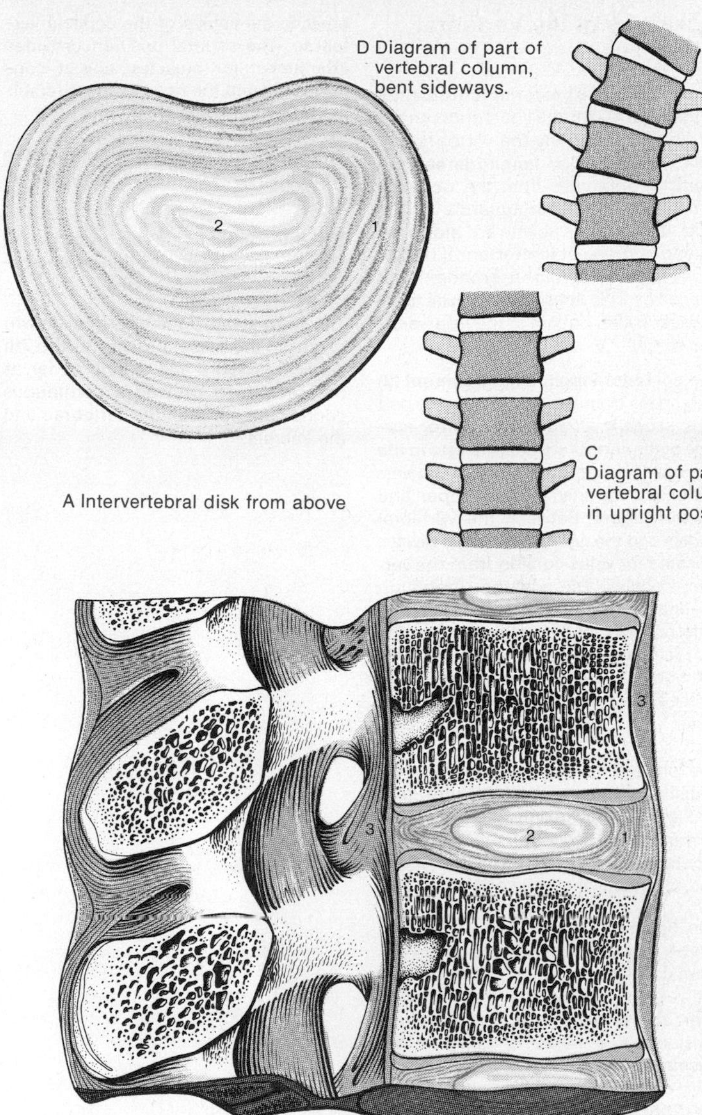

D Diagram of part of vertebral column, bent sideways.

A Intervertebral disk from above

C Diagram of part of vertebral column in upright position

B Median sagittal section

Ligaments of the Vertebral Column (A–D)

The **anterior and posterior longitudinal ligaments (A–C):** the ligaments run anteriorly or posteriorly the vertebral bodies. The **anterior longitudinal ligament** (**1**) originates from the occipital bone, or the anterior tubercle of the atlas, and extends downward along the anterior surface of the vertebral bodies as far as the sacrum. It broadens out caudally and is **always firmly bound to the vertebral bodies**, but not to the intervertebral disks.

The **posterior longitudinal ligament** (**2**) also arises from the occipital bone and runs caudally along the posterior surface of the vertebral bodies to end in the sacrum. It is firmly attached to the vertebral bodies only at their upper and lower margins. Between the vertebral bodies and the ligament there is always a fissure for veins coming from the vertebral bodies. The posterior longitudinal ligament is **firmly attached to the intervertebral disks** and, particularly in the thoracic and lumbar regions, it forms rhomboid lateral fibrous extensions (**3**). These strongly secure the intervertebral disks.

The longitudinal ligaments increase the stability of the vertebral column, particularly during flexion and extension movements. They have therefore two functions, namely to restrict movement and to protect the intervertebral disks.

The **ligamenta flava** (**D4**) extend between the vertebral arches (**5**). Their chief constituent is elastic fibers, which are responsible for their yellow color. Even at rest these ligaments are under tension. During flexion of the spine they become more extended and *help the return of the vertebral column to the erect position*.

The **ligamentum nuchae** (not shown) extends from the external occipital crest to the spines of the cervical vertebrae. The sagittal position provides attachment for muscles, and it continues beyond the neck as the interspinal and supraspinal ligaments.

The **intertransverse ligaments** (**6**) are short ligaments between the transverse processes.

The **interspinal ligaments** (not shown) are also short ligaments that extend between the spinal processes.

The **supraspinal ligaments** (not shown) begin on the spinal process of the 7th cervical vertebra and extend as far as the sacrum to provide a continuous connection between the vertebrae and the sacrum.

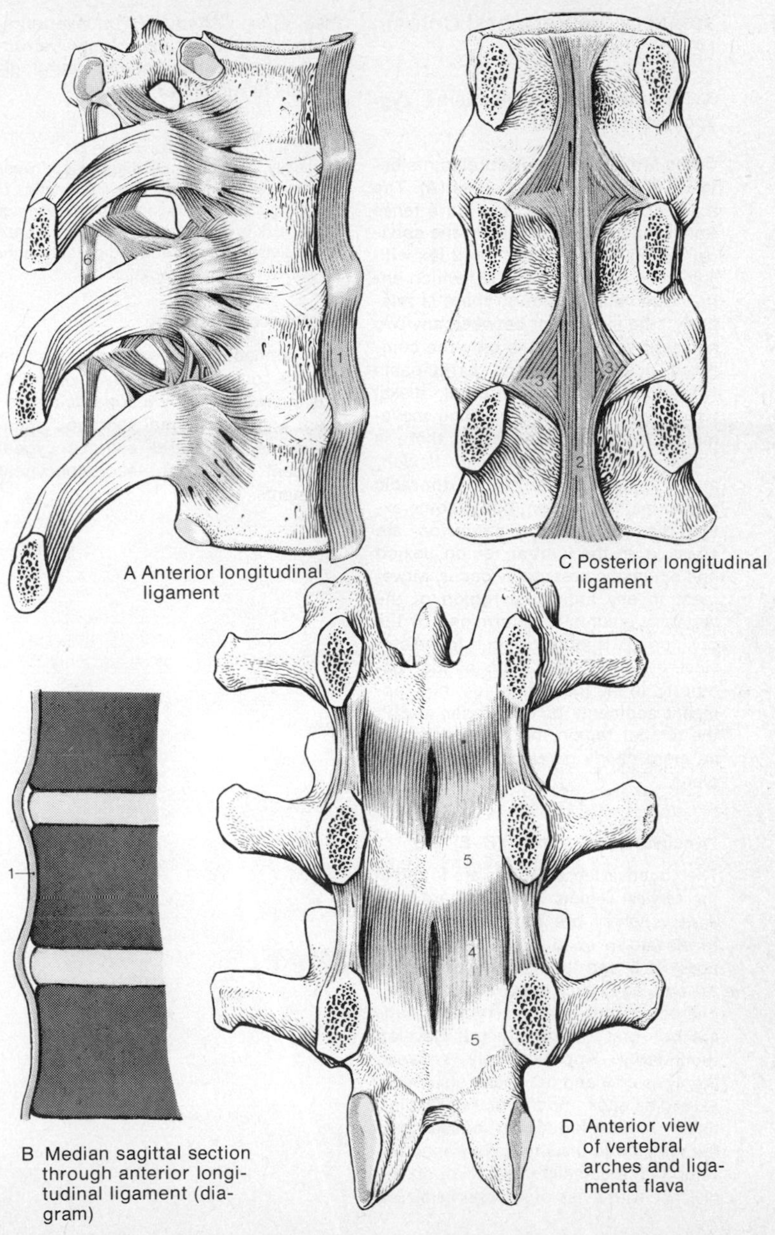

A Anterior longitudinal ligament

C Posterior longitudinal ligament

B Median sagittal section through anterior longitudinal ligament (diagram)

D Anterior view of vertebral arches and ligamenta flava

Joints of the Vertebral Column (A–E)

Joints Intervertebral Juncturae Zygapophyseales (A–B)

These are the small vertebral joints between the articular processes (**A**). The *articular capsules* become more tense from cranially to caudally. In the cervical region they are broad and lax with *meniscus-like infoldings* (**B**) which enhance mobility, although there is relatively little movement between any two adjacent vertebrae. It is only the combined action of all the participants (vertebrae and intervertebral disks) which results in corresponding movements. In the **cervical** region there is *lateral, forward,* and *backward flexion,* and a limited *rotation.* In the **thoracic** region mainly *rotation*, but to some extent also *flexion* and *extension* are possible. In the **lumbar** region flexion and extension essentially occur. Movement in any individual region of the vertebral column is determined by the position of the joint surfaces. In the cervical vertebrae they face almost anteriorly, in the thoracic spine they represent segments of a cylinder and in the lumbar region the articular facets lie more nearly parallel to the sagittal plane.

"Uncovertebral Joints" (C–E)

The "uncovertebral" joints are found in the **cervical** region. The *uncinate processes,* which are flat at first, begin to elevate in childhood. Between the ages of 5 and 10 fissures appear in the cartilage which assume an articular character; thus "uncovertebral" joints are not present initially but develop *secondarily*. Approximately between the ages of 9 and 10, these structures extend as gaps into the disks. This initially confers functional advantages, but later on in life the fissure may develop into a complete tear through the disk (**E**), with a risk of **pulposus herniation** (see p. 54). Although "uncovertebral joints" are initially physiological structures, later they may become pathological due to rupture of the disk.

Practical Points

Clinically, the differential diagnosis between "uncovertebral joints" and traumatic or pathologic changes is very difficult. Damage to the disk is most common at C 5, where it may be visible in a lateral radiograph as the so-called *"lordotic crack"*.

Sacrococcygeal Joint

The connection between the sacrum and the coccyx is often a *synovial joint.* It is strengthened by a superficial ligament and deep dorsal sacrococcygeal ligaments, a ventral sacrococcygeal ligament and lateral sacrococcygeal ligaments.

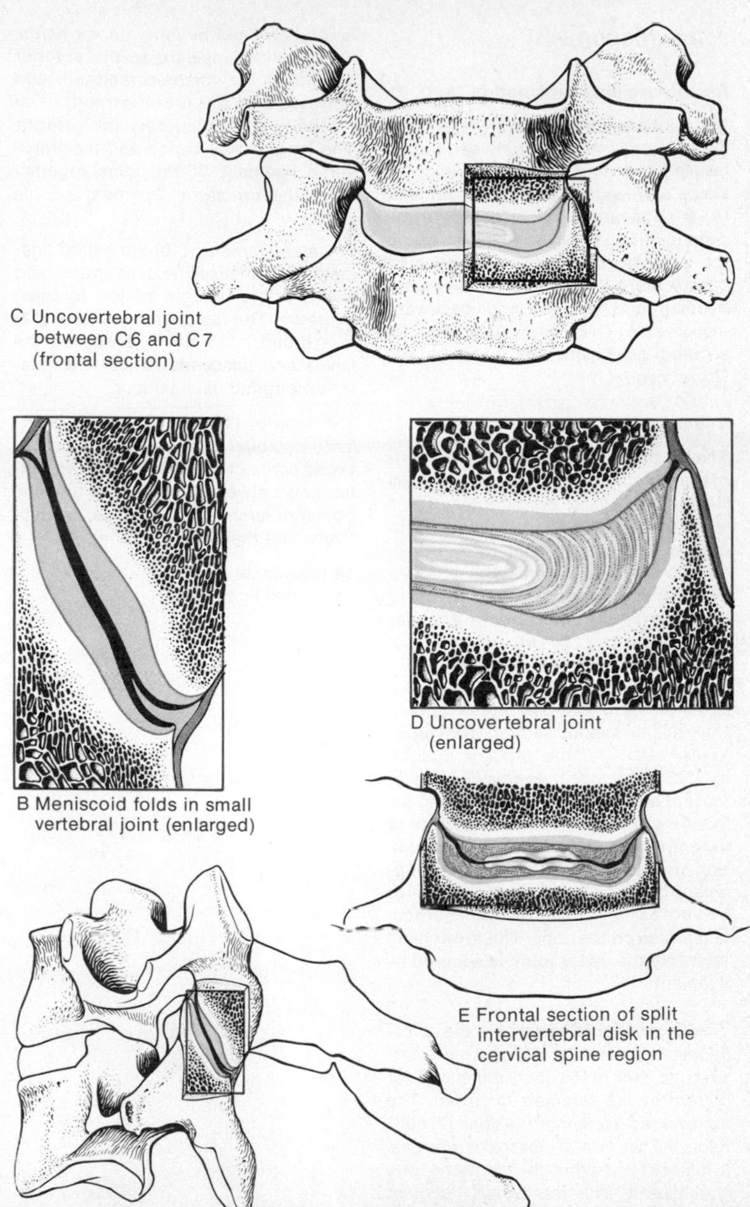

C Uncovertebral joint between C6 and C7 (frontal section)

B Meniscoid folds in small vertebral joint (enlarged)

D Uncovertebral joint (enlarged)

E Frontal section of split intervertebral disk in the cervical spine region

A Sagittal section through intervertebral joint

Joints (continued)

Atlanto-occipital Articulation (A, D, E)

The right and left **atlanto-occipital articulation** is a combined joint between the atlas and the occipital bone, which in shape corresponds to an ellipsoid joint (**A, D**). The articular surfaces are the *superior articular facets* of the atlas and the *occipital condyles* (**1**). The joint capsules are lax and permit sideways bending and forward and backward movements. This **"upper head joint"** is secured by ligaments, just like the *"lower head joint"*.

Atlanto-axial Articulation (B–E)

The so-called **"lower head joint"** consists of the conjoined **median** and **lateral atlanto-axial articulations.** Functionally it is a *rotary joint* in which movement of 26° to each side is possible from the mid-position. In the lateral joints the articular facets are the *inferior articular facets of the atlas* (**2**) and the *superior articular facets of the axis* (**3**). The incongruity of the articular surfaces is reduced by a cartilaginous covering and *meniscoid synovial folds* (**4**). The folds appear triangular in sagittal section (**C**). The articular facets of the median atlanto-axial joints include the *anterior articular facet of the dens of the axis* (**5**), and the *fovea dentis on the posterior surface of the anterior arch of the atlas* (**6**). In addition, in the region of the *transverse ligament of the atlas* (**7**), which extends behind the dens, there is another articular surface on the dens. The lower head joint, like the upper joint, is secured by ligaments.

The **ligaments of both joints** are the *apical ligament of the dens* (**8**), which extends from the apex of the dens to the anterior margin of the foramen magnum. The *transverse ligament of the atlas* (**7**) connects the two lateral masses of the atlas. It passes posterior to the dens and stabilizes it. The transverse ligament is strengthened by *longitudinal bands* (**9**) which run upward to the anterior margin of the foramen magnum and downward to the posterior surface of the body of the 2nd cervical vertebra. The longitudinal bands and the transverse ligament of the atlas together form the *cruciform ligament of the atlas.*

The *alar ligaments* (**10**) are paired ligaments that arise on the dens and ascend to the lateral margin of the foramen magnum. The *tectorial membrane* (**11**) is a broad band which arises on the clivus and descends to join the posterior longitudinal ligament.

The *anterior* (**12**) and *posterior* (**13**) *atlanto-occipital membranes* consist of broad connective tissue fiber bands extending between the anterior and the posterior arches of the atlas, respectively, and the occipital bone.

14 Ligamenta flava,
15 Nuchal ligament.

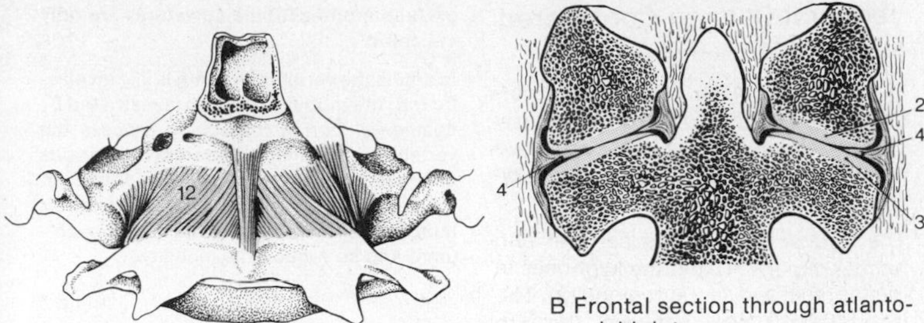

A Anterior view of atlanto-occipital joint

B Frontal section through atlanto-axial joints

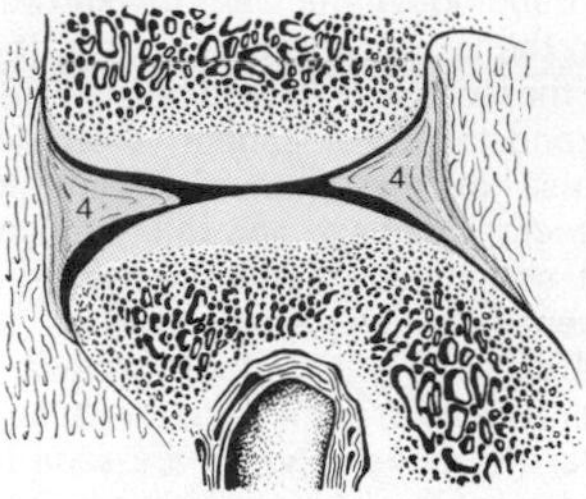

C Sagittal section through lateral atlanto-axial joint

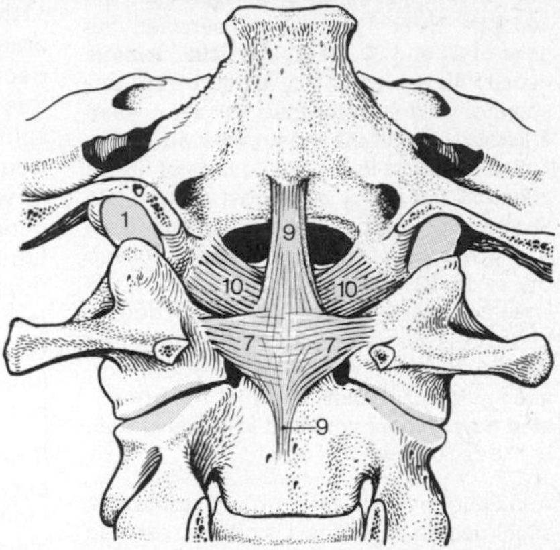

D Ligaments of "head joints"

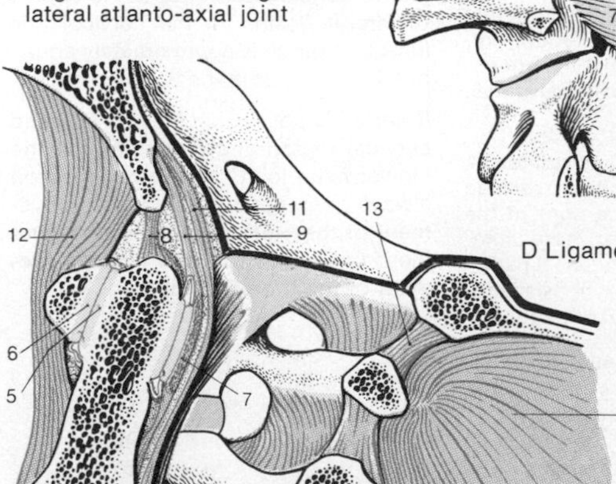

E Median sagittal section in region of "head joints"

Vertebral Column Considered as a Whole (A–H)

In the sagittal plane the vertebral column of the adult shows two anteriorly convex curvatures, **lordoses**, and two posteriorly convex curvatures, **kyphoses.**

The lordoses are in the cervical and lumbar regions (**1**) and the kyphoses in the thoracic and sacral regions (**2**). The intervertebral disk between the 5th lumbar vertebra and the sacrum is sometimes called the promontory (see p. 48).

Practical Points

The curvature in the cervical region is quite variable. Three types occur between the ages of 20 and 30 years. The **"true" lordosis** usually illustrated (**A**) is actually very uncommon. A double lordosis (**B**), also called a **lordotic bend**, is the most common and is typical of adults in the 3rd decade of life. In addition, there may be almost a complete absence of lordosis, the **attenuated form**, (**C**). Investigation of differences between the sexes has shown that true lordosis is less common in females, that double lordosis is less common in females, that double lordosis occurs with equal frequency in both sexes, and that the attenuated type is more common in females than in males (Drexler).

A lateral curvature is known as **scoliosis**. A slight degree of scoliosis is often present in radiographs, deviation to the right of the median sagittal plane being more common than to the left. The commonest pathological finding is increased kyphosis (adolescent kyphosis, kyphosis of old age).

The curvatures of the vertebral column develop as a result of the stresses of sitting and standing. Its load capacity is dependent on the degree of ossification of the vertebrae, so that the final posture (**D**) is not achieved until after puberty. The line of the center of gravity lies partly in front of and partly behind the vertebral column. In a child of ten months (**E**) the curvatures are already present, but the line of the center of gravity (**3**) lies behind the vertebral column. In infants of three months (**F**) the curvatures are only indicated.

In adults the vertebral column is like an elastic rod, the mobility of which is restricted by ligaments. During the ageing process the vertebral column undergoes various changes, so that in the elderly a reduction in the thickness of the disks produces a rather uniform kyphosis of the entire vertebral column, and so reduces its mobility.

Movements of the Vertebral Column

Forward and backward bending (flexion and extension) occur primarily in the cervical and lumbar spine. Backward bending is particularly marked between the lower cervical vertebrae, the 11th thoracic and 2nd lumbar vertebrae and the lower lumbar vertebrae. Because of the greater mobility in this region, damage and injury to the spinal column due to overstrain is more frequent here than at other levels. In forward bending (blue) and backward bending (yellow) of the cervical (**G**) and lumbar (**H**) spine changes are seen in the intervertebral disks, which are subject to considerable stress. The degree of *lateral flexion* in the cervical and lumbar regions is approximately equal, but it is greatest in the thoracic region.

Rotation is possible in the thoracic and cervical region and particularly in the "lower head joint" area. Head rotation always goes hand in hand with movement of the "lower head joint", movement of the cervical and slight movement of the thoracic spine.

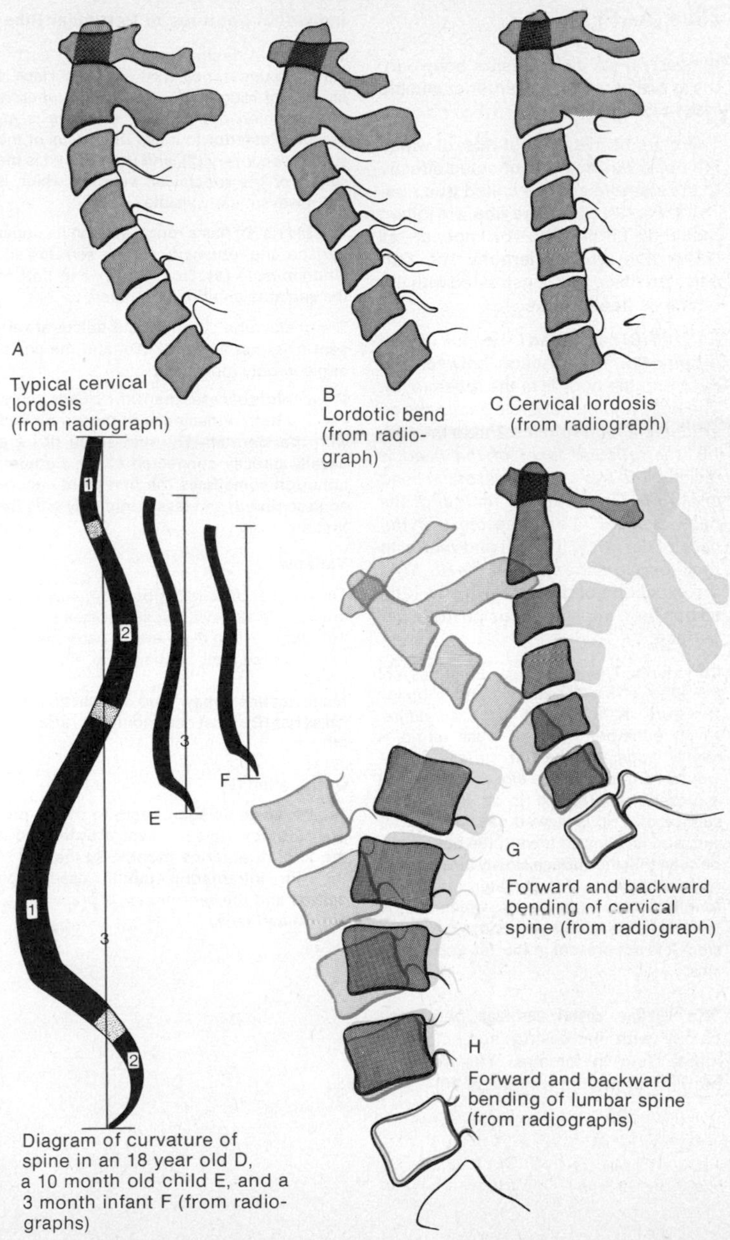

A
Typical cervical lordosis (from radiograph)

B
Lordotic bend (from radiograph)

C Cervical lordosis (from radiograph)

Diagram of curvature of spine in an 18 year old D, a 10 month old child E, and a 3 month infant F (from radiographs)

G
Forward and backward bending of cervical spine (from radiograph)

H
Forward and backward bending of lumbar spine (from radiographs)

Ribs (A–F)

In each **rib** we distinguish a bony part, the **os costale**, and at the anterior end the **costal cartilage**.

There are twelve pairs of ribs, of which the upper seven are connected directly to the sternum and are called **true ribs**. The lower five ribs, **false ribs**, are joined indirectly (8th–10th) or not at all (11th–12th) to the sternum. The 11th and 12th rib can be constrasted with the others as **floating ribs**.

Each **rib** (**C**) has a *head* (**1**) a *neck* (**2**) and a *body* (**3**). The junction between the neck and the body is at the *tubercle* (**4**). The head and the tubercle each have an *articular facet.* From the 2nd to the 10th rib, the *articular facet of the head* is divided into two by the *crest of the head of the rib.* On the upper margin of the neck of most ribs is the *crest of the neck of the rib* (**5**). Lateral and ventral to the tubercle is the *angle of the rib*. With the exception of the 1st, 11th and 12th, all ribs have a *costal sulcus* on the lower surface.

Curvatures: There are three curvatures – of the edge, of the flat surface and a torsion curvature. Although the *edge curvature*, which is the principal one in the 1st rib, is readily apparent, the *flat surface curvature* can only be seen on close inspection. It is present from the 3rd rib on. If the upper surface of a rib is viewed near its anterior end, and is followed toward the back it will be seen that the surface slowly turns dorsally. In addition to this curvature, there is a longitudinal twist in the rib, which is most marked in the middle ribs and is called *torsion*. It is not present in the 1st, 2nd or 12th ribs.

The **hyaline costal cartilage** begins to calcify with increasing age, more in males than in females. This reduces mobility of the thorax (see p. 70).

Individual Features of Particular Ribs

The **1st rib** (**A**) is small and flattended. On the inner circumference of its cranial surface is an area of roughness, the *scalene tubercle* (**6**), to which the anterior scalenus is attached. Posterior to it lies the *sulcus of the subclavian artery* (**7**), and in front of it is the *sulcus of the subclavian* vein (**8**), which is not always clearly visible.

The **2nd rib** (**B**) has a rough area on its upper surface, the *tuberosity for the serratus anterior muscle* (**9**), from which one part of the serratus anterior originates.

The costal tubercle and costal sulcus are absent from **ribs 11 and 12** (**D**), and the costal angle is only indicated.

In two thirds of cases the 10th rib ends freely, i.e., it is not connected with the 9th rib and with the sternum. The first seven ribs are usually directly connected to the sternum, although sometimes the first eight may be so associated, and less commonly only the first six.

Variants

The number of pairs of ribs is variable. There are usually 12 pairs, but sometimes 11 or 13 are found. When there are 13 pairs, cervical (see p. 36) or lumbar ribs (see p. 42) may be present.
Malformations may lead to **fenestrated** or **forked ribs** (**E**). Most commonly they affect the 4th rib.

Ossification (F)

The cartilage anlagen begin to ossify, progressing from dorsal to ventral by the end of the 2nd intrauterine month. By the end of the 4th intrauterine month ossification ceases and the ventral part is preserved as the rib cartilage.

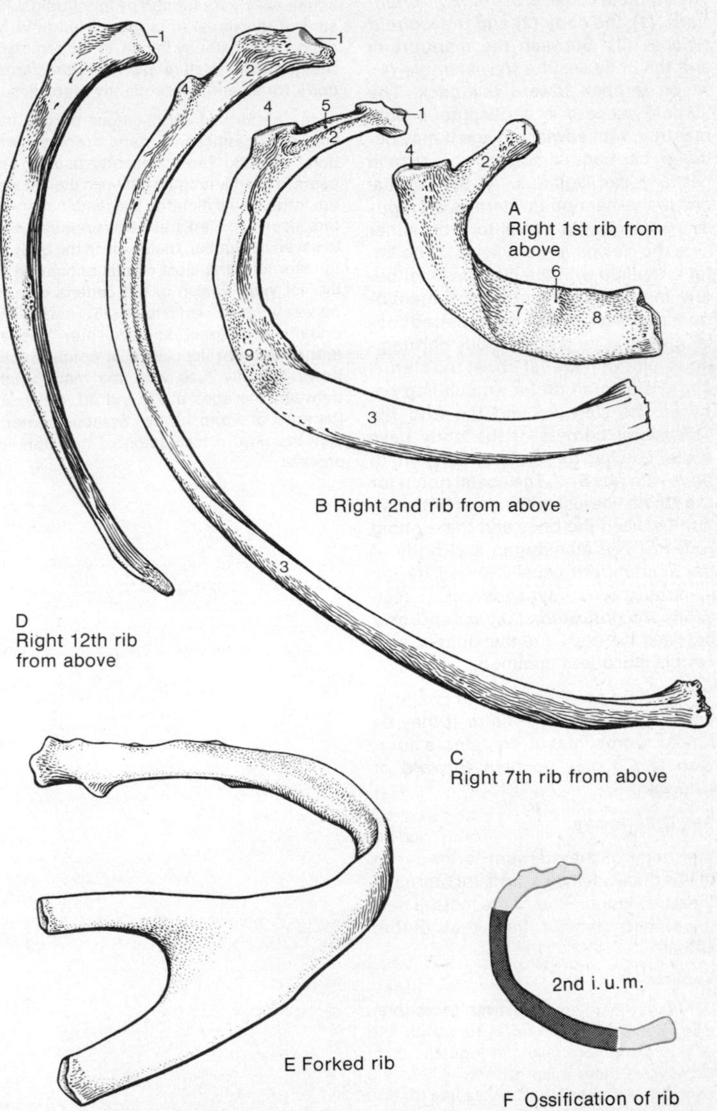

A Right 1st rib from above

B Right 2nd rib from above

C Right 7th rib from above

D Right 12th rib from above

E Forked rib

F Ossification of rib

Sternum (A–F)

The **sternum** consists of the *manubrium sterni* (**1**), the *body* (**2**) and the *xiphoid process* (**3**). Between the manubrium and the body lies the *sternal angle* (**4**), which is open toward the back. The xiphoid process is cartilaginous until maturity; with advancing age it may become ossified completely or remain partially cartilaginous. At the cranial end of the manubrium sterni is the *jugular notch* (**5**) and lateral to it on either side the *clavicular notches* (**6**). The latter articulate with the clavicle. Just below the clavicular notch, the manubrium again has an additional paired *costal notch* (**7**) for a continuous cartilaginous joint with the 1st rib. At the sternal angle is a *notch* (**8**) for articulation between the sternum and the 2nd rib. The lateral borders of the body have costal notches for continuous connections with ribs 3–7. The costal notch for the 7th rib lies just at the point of transition between the body and the xiphoid process. The manubrium and body of the sternum are usually joined by the *manubriosternal synchondrosis* (see p. 68). A *xiphosternal synchondrosis* between the body and the xiphoid process is much less common.

The xiphoid process varies in shape. It may consist of one piece or it may be forked. Sometimes it contains a foramen and it may be bent forward or backward.

Sex Differences

The body of the sternum is longer in males than in females, and, for sterna of the same length, that of the male is narrower and slimmer than that of the female.

Variants

Very rarely there are **suprasternal bones** (**A 9**), also called the episternum, at the cranial end of the manubrium near the jugular notch. Sometimes there is an opening within the sternum, a **congenital sternal fissure** (**D 10**), which arises during development.

Ossification (F)

The sternum develops from *paired sternal bands* which are formed by longitudinal fusion of individual rib anlagen, followed by fusion of the sternal bands. In the region of the jugular notch a *paired suprasternal body* forms and subsequently regresses.

In the preformed cartilaginous part of the sternum, ossification starts from several bony centers. The first center usually appears in the manubrium between the 3rd and 6th intrauterine months. The remaining centers, usually paired, but partly unpaired, five to seven in number, then arise in the body of the sternum, the most caudal appearing in the 1st year. Fusion of the centers occurs between the ages of 6 to 20 (25) years. Secondary epiphyseal anlagen may appear in the region of the clavicular notch which, however, only fuse with the manubrium between the ages of 25 and 30. Between the ages of 5 and 10, two osseous centers may develop in the region of the xiphoid process.

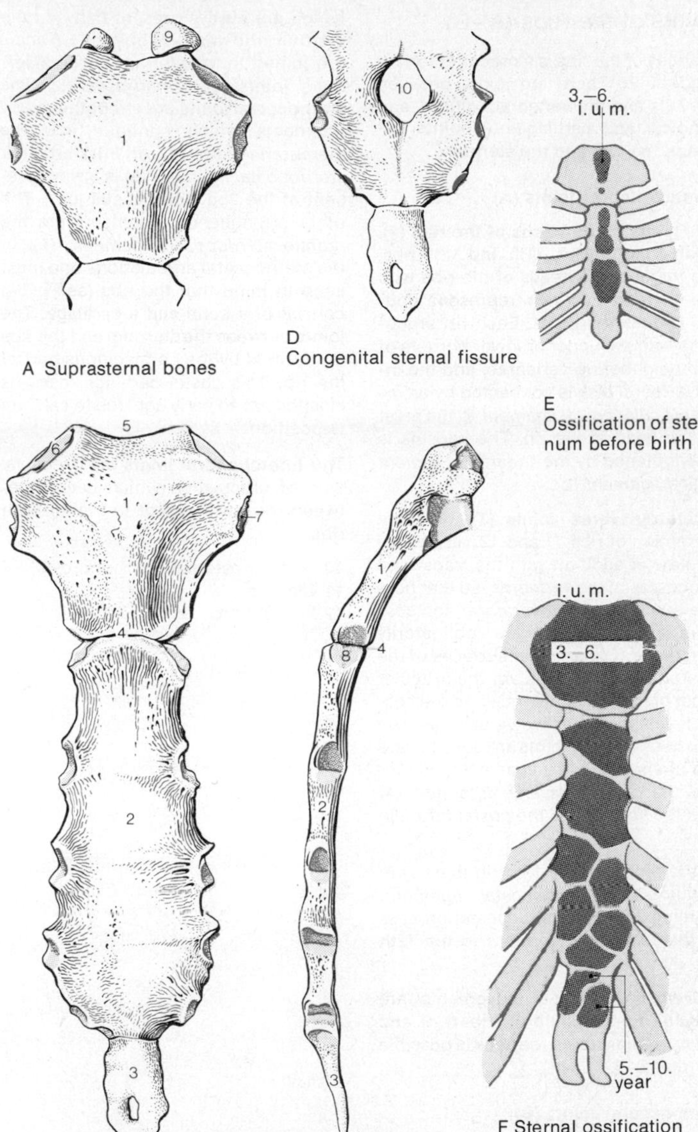

A Suprasternal bones

B
Sternum from front

C
Sternum from side

D
Congenital sternal fissure

E
Ossification of sternum before birth

F Sternal ossification between ages of 5 and 10 years

Joints of the Ribs (A–B)

Mobility of the ribs is a precondition for respiration. There are joints between the ribs and the vertebral column, and synovial and cartilaginous joints between the ribs and the sternum.

Costovertebral Joints (A)

The **joints of the heads of the ribs** (**1**). Apart from the 1st, 11th and 12th ribs, the joints of the heads of the ribs with the vertebral column represent double-chambered joints. Each rib articulates with the upper or lower borders of two neighboring vertebrae, and the intervertebral disk is connected by an *intra-articular costal ligament* to the crest of the head of the rib. The capsule is strengthened by the *superficial radiate costal ligament* (**2**).

Costotransverse Joints (3). With the exception of ribs 11 and 12, all ribs articulate in addition with the transverse processes of the vertebrae, so that here the two joints, *costovertebral* and *costotransverse joints*, are obligatorily combined. The articular surfaces of the costotransverse joints are the articular facet of the costal tubercle and the costal fovea of the transverse process. The capsules of these joints are delicate and are strengthened by ligaments, including the *costotransverse ligament* (**4**) and the *ligament of the costal tubercle* (**5**).

In the region of the 12th rib there is in addition the *lumbocostal ligament*, which extends from the costal process of the 1st lumbar vertebra to the 12th rib.

Movements: Sliding movements are possible for the 1st rib and ribs 6–9, and rotary motion about the neck is possible for ribs 2–5.

Sternocostal Joints (B)

Only some of the junctions between the ribs and the sternum are synovial joints which are always present between the sternum and ribs 2–5, but ribs 1, 6 and 7 are joined to the sternum by *cartilaginous joints, synchondroses* (**6**). The sternocostal joints are strengthened by ligaments which continue into the *membrana sterni* (**7**). An intra-articular *sternocostal ligament* (**8**) is always present at the 2nd sternocostal joint. The other strenghening ligaments are the *radiate sternocostal ligaments* (**9**). In the sternocostal articulations one must keep in mind that the ribs (see p. 64) consist of a bone and a cartilage. The joints between the sternum and the ribs are formed by the cartilaginous part of the rib. This costal cartilage loses its elasticity at an early age due to calcium deposition.

The **interchondral joints** are a special type of articulation which occurs between the cartilages of to the 6th–9th ribs.

10 Manubriosternal synchondrosis,
11 Clavicle,
12 Xiphoid process.

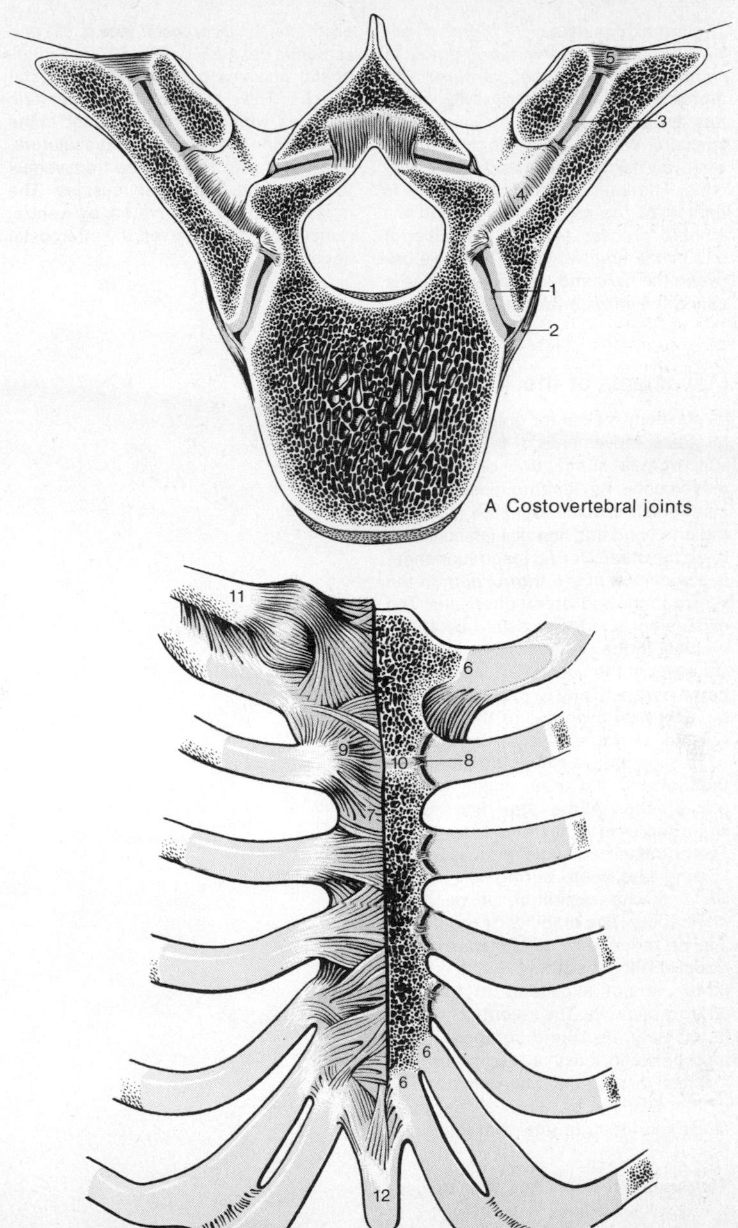

A Costovertebral joints

B Costosternal connections

The thorax consists of *12 thoracic vertebrae and their intervertebral disks, 12 pairs of ribs and the sternum*. The thorax encloses the **thoracic cavity**, which has a *superior* (**1**) and an *inferior* (**2**) *aperture*. While the superior aperture is relatively narrow, the inferior one is very wide. The inferior thoracic aperture is limited by the *costal arch* (**3**) and the *xiphoid process* (**4**) and the superior one by the first two ribs. The angle between the right and left costal arches is called the *infrasternal angle* (**5**).

Movements of the Thorax

Its elasticity makes for great resistance to stress. Movements of the thorax result from a summation of individual movements. As limiting positions we distinguish **maximal expiration** (**A, B**) on the one hand and **maximal inspiration** (**C, D**) on the other. During inspiration there is a widening of the thorax both in the ventrodorsal and lateral directions. The expansion is made possible by 1) the mobility in the costovertebral joints, 2) elasticity of the costal cartilages which permit twisting, and 3) to a slight extent by increased kyphosis of the thoracic column. During expiration the ribs are depressed, thus diminishing the size of the thorax in the ventrodorsal and lateral direction. At the same time there is some decrease in the thoracic kyphosis. The infrasternal angle increases, becoming less acute during inspiration, while during expiration it becomes more acute. The mobility of the thorax may be reduced by calcification of the costal cartilages so that the shape of the thorax is not expanded to the respiratory capacity. The essential factor is its mobility, i.e., the difference in volume between maximal expiration and maximal inspiration. Disorders not only of the cartilage but also of the joints cause reduction of total thoracic function.

The **forces which move the thorax** are generated by the *intercostal* (see p. 82) and *scalenus muscles* (see p. 80). The intercostal muscles occupy the intercostal spaces. They are primitive metameric muscles, which must be included in the autochthonous thoracic musculature. The latter also include the transversus thoracis and subcostal muscles. The musculature is innervated by ventral rami of the spinal nerves, the intercostal nerves.

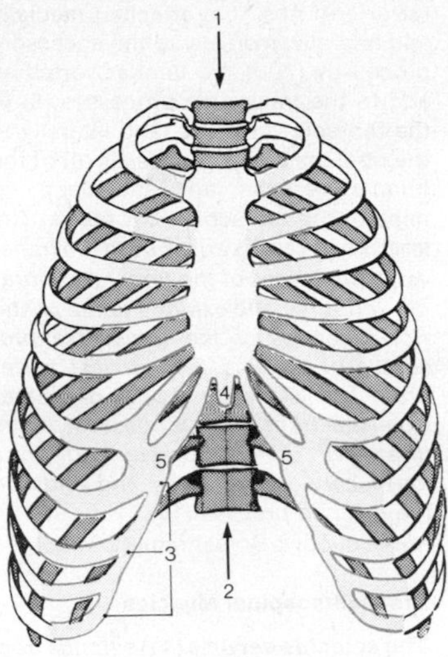

A Thorax – expiratory position from front

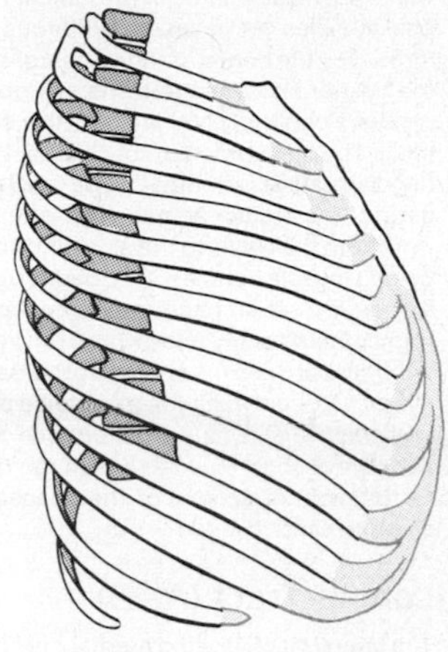

B Thorax – expiratory position from side

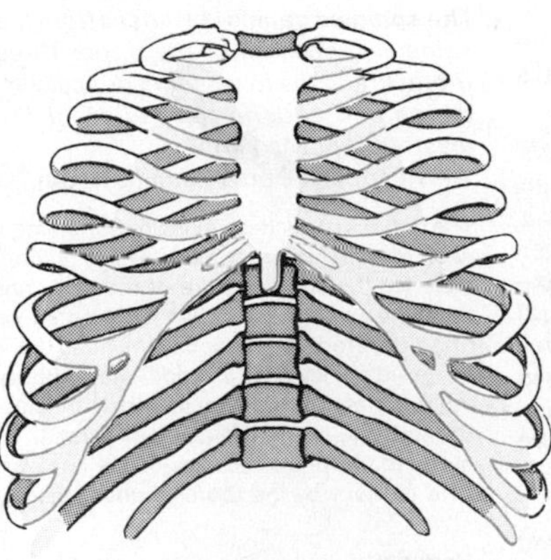

C Thorax – inspiratory position from front

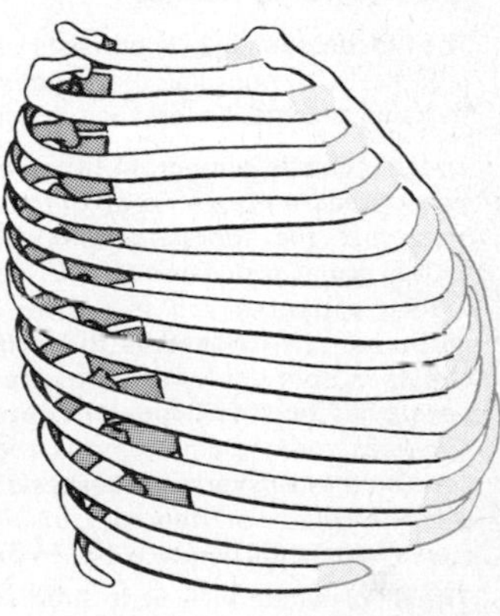

D Thorax – inspiratory position from side

This group includes *all the muscles innervated by the dorsal rami of the spinal nerves*. Together they are called the **erector spinae**. In the living body there are two longitudinal columns lateral to the spinous processes, which are most marked in the lumbar region. The muscles lie in an osteofibrous canal formed by the bones of the vertebral arches, the costal processes and the spinous processes. Posteriorly and laterally this canal is limited by the thoracolumbar fascia. We distinguish **lateral superficial** from **medial deep tracts** of the erector spinae. The lateral tract runs from the pelvis to the skull and consists of long muscle bundles. The medial tract has a *straight* and an *oblique component*. The former includes muscles which run vertically, either between the spinous processes (*interspinal*) or betwenn the transverse processes (*intertransversal*). The oblique system consists of short muscles which run oblique to the main directions of the space *(transversospinal).*

Lateral Tract (A–B)

The lateral tract, like the medial one, may be divided into *intertransverse* and *transversospinal* muscle groups.

Intertransverse Muscles

The **iliocostalis** (**1, 2, 3**) consists of the iliocostalis lumborum, the iliocostalis thoracis and the iliocostalis cervicis.

The **iliocostalis lumborum** (**1**) *extends from the sacrum, external lip of the iliac crest and the thoracolumbar fascia to the costal processes of the upper lumbar vertebrae and the lower six–nine ribs.* The **iliocostalis thoracis** (**2**) *stretches from the lower six to the upper six ribs,* and the **iliocostalis cervicis** (**3**) *arises from the 6th–3rd ribs and inserts on the transverse processes of the 6th–4th cervical vertebrae.*
Nerve supply: Dorsal rami (C4–L3).

The **longissimus** (**4, 5, 6**) is subdivided into the longissimus thoracis (**4**) and cervicis (**5**) and the longissimus capitis (**6**). The **longissimus thoracis** *arises from the sacrum, the spinous processes of the lumbar vertebrae* and the *transverse processes of the lower thoracic vertebrae and extends to the 1st or 2nd ribs.* It is attached medially and laterally; medially to the accessory processes (**7**) of the lumbar vertebrae and to the transverse processes (**8**) of the thoracic vertebrae, and laterally to the ribs, the costal processes (**9**) of the lumbar vertebra and the deep lamina of the thoracolumbar fascia. The **longissimus cervicis** *arises from the transverse processes of the upper six thoracic vertebrae* and *extends to the posterior tubercles of the transverse processes of the 2nd–5th cervical vertebrae.* The **longissimus capitis** originates *from the transverse processes of the three–five upper thoracic and three lower cervical vertebrae and ends on the mastoid process* (**10**).
Nerve supply: Dorsal rami (C2–L5)

Transversospinal Muscles

The **splenius cervicis** (**11**) *extends from the spinous processes of the 3rd to 6th thoracic vertebrae to the transverse processes of the 1st and 2nd cervical vertebra.*

The **splenius capitis** (**12**) *arises from the spinous processes of the upper three thoracic and the lower four cervical vertebrae and ends in the region of the mastoid process* (**10**).
Nerve supply: Dorsal rami (C1–C8).

The actions of all these muscles supplement each other. The first two are largely responsible for the erect posture of the body and then the two splenii, when contracted on one side, produce rotation of the head to the same side. They have an additional supporting function for the other instrinsic muscles of the back. In the thoracic and lumbar regions the intrinsic muscles of the back are held in place by the thoracolumbar fascia.

Variants

Variations in the number of muscle slips is common. I–XII = 1st–12th ribs.

The levatores costarum are described on page 78.

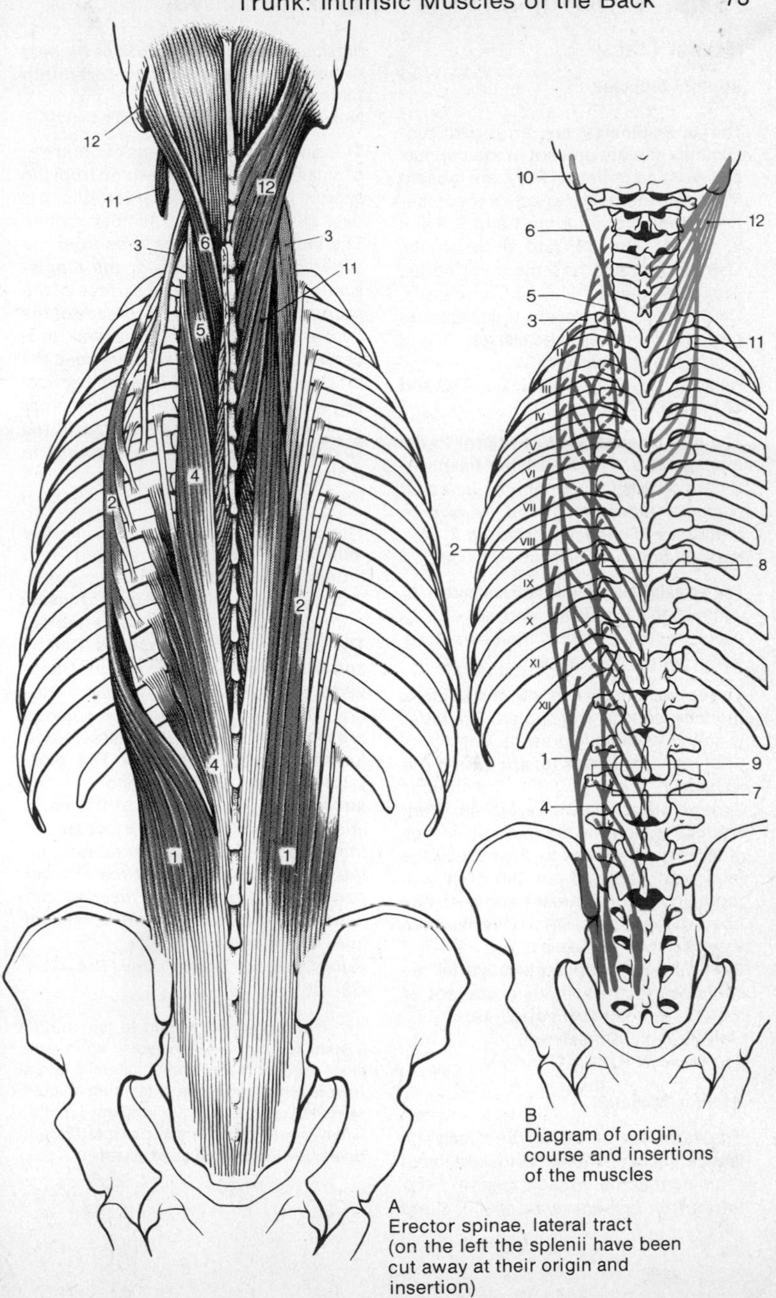

A
Erector spinae, lateral tract
(on the left the splenii have been cut away at their origin and insertion)

B
Diagram of origin, course and insertions of the muscles

Medial Tract

Straight Muscles

The **interspinales** are arranged segmentally and are present in the cervical and lumbar regions. They are absent from the thoracic region, except between thoracic vertebrae 1 and 2, 2 and 3, and 11 and 12, and between the 12th thoracic and 1st lumbar vertebrae. *They link adjacent spinous processes.* On either side there are **6 interspinales cervicis (1)**, **4 interspinales thoracis (2)** and **5 interspinales lumborum (3)**.
Nerve supply: Dorsal rami (C1–Th3 and Th11–L5).

The **intertransversarii** lie lateral to the interspinales. The **6 posterior intertransversarii cervicis (4)** connect *the adjacent posterior tubercles of the transverse processes of cervical vertebrae 2–7.*
Nerve supply: Dorsal rami (C1–C6).

The **4 medial intertransversarii lumborum (5)** connect the *mamillary and accessory processes of adjacent lumbar vertebrae.*
Nerve supply: Dorsal rami (L1–L4).

The **spinalis** is divided into the spinalis thoracis, cervicis and capitis. The latter is only occasionally present. The fibers of the **spinalis thoracis (6)** *arise from the spinous processes of the 3rd lumbar through 10th thoracic vertebrae. They are inserted on the spinous processes of thoracic vertebrae 8–2* whereby the innermost fibers, (from the 10th–8th thoracic vertebrae) are the shortest. The fibers of the **spinalis cervicis (7)** *arise from the spinous processes of the 2nd thoracic through 6th cervical vertebrae and insert on the spinous processes of the 4th–2nd cervical vertebrae.*
Nerve supply: Dorsal rami (C2–Th10).

Oblique Muscles

The **rotatores breves (8)** and **longi (9) thoracis** (cervicis, lumborum) are most prominent in the thoracic region. *Each arises from a transverse process and runs to the next, or next but one highest spinous process* where it is inserted into the base.
Nerve supply: Dorsal rami (Th1–Th11).

The **multifidus (10)** consists of a number of small fasciculi which extend from the sacrum to the 2nd cervical vertebra. It is best developed in the lumbar region. The individual fascicles *arise from the superficial aponeurosis of the longissimus muscle, the dorsal surface of the sacrum, the mamillary processes of the lumbar vertebrae, the transverse processes of the thoracic vertebrae and the articular processes of 7th–4th cervical vertebrae.* The muscle bundles cross 2–4 vertebrae and are *inserted in the spinous processes of the appropriate higher vertebrae.*
Nerve supply: Dorsal rami (C3–S4).

The **semispinalis**, which overlies the multifidus laterally, is divided into thoracic, cervical and cephalic ("capitis") parts. Individual muscle bundles cross five or more vertebrae. The fibers of the **semispinalis thoracis** and **cervicis (11)** *arise from the transverse processes of all thoracic vertebrae. They are inserted in the spinous processes of the upper 6 thoracic and lower 4 cervical vertebrae.* The **semispinalis capitis (12)**, which is one of the strongest of the muscles of the neck, *arises from the transverse processes of the upper 4–7 thoracic vertebrae and the articular processes of the 5 lower cervical vertebrae. It is inserted between the superior and inferior nuchal lines of the skull.*
Nerve supply: Dorsal rami (Th4–Th6, C3–C6 and C1–C5).

The muscles which belong to the straight system function as extensors when both sides are innervated and unilaterally lateral flexors when only one side is innervated. Muscles of the oblique system function when unilaterally innervated as rotators, and bilaterally innervated as extensors.

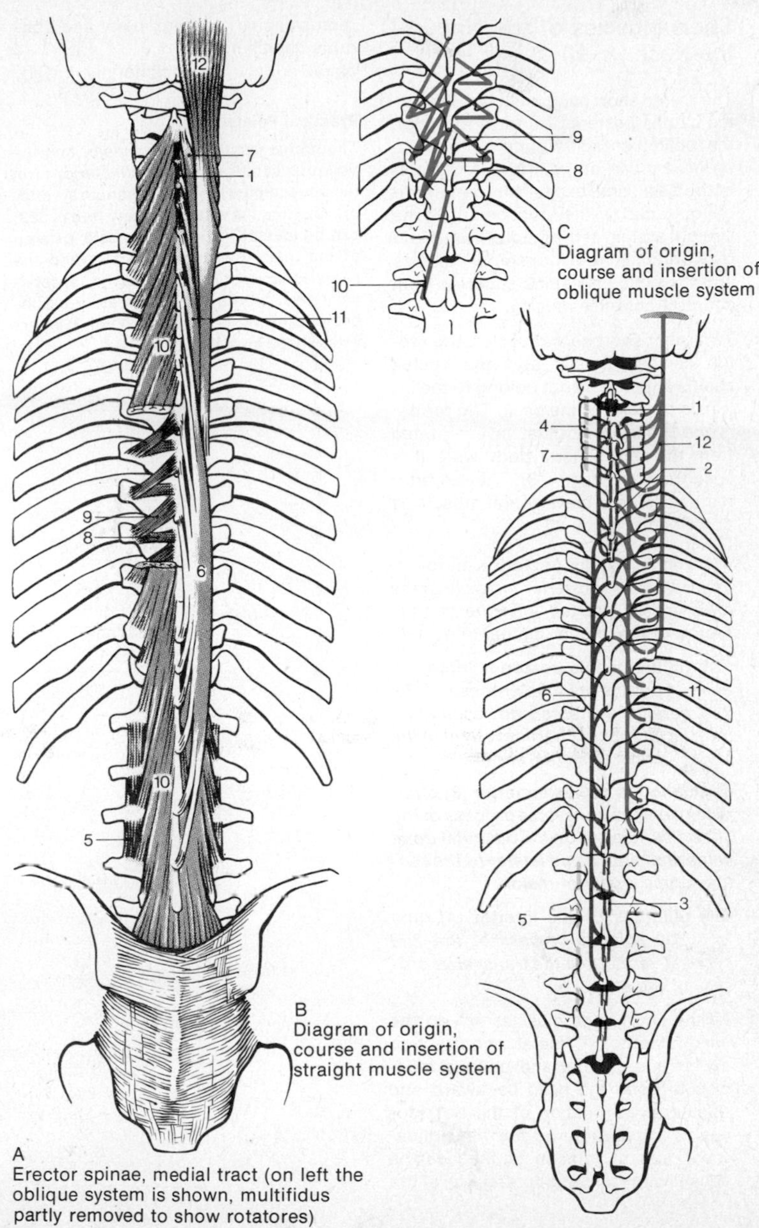

A
Erector spinae, medial tract (on left the oblique system is shown, multifidus partly removed to show rotatores)

B
Diagram of origin, course and insertion of straight muscle system

C
Diagram of origin, course and insertion of oblique muscle system

Short Muscles of the Nape of the Neck (A–B)

The paired short nape muscles, the rectus capitis posterior minor and major, the obliquus capitis superior and inferior, are part of the intrinsic muscles of the back, and, except for the inferior obliquus capitis, they, too, belong to the straight system of the medial tract. Both recti originate from interspinal muscles and the obliquus capitis superior from an intertransverse muscle.

Two other short neck muscles, the rectus capitis lateralis and the rectus capitis anterior, do not belong to the intrinsic muscles of the back. The former is one of the muscles that have migrated from the ventrolateral body wall: it is described on page 78. The anterior rectus capitis, a prevertebral muscle, is described on page 80.

The **rectus capitis posterior minor** (**1**) *arises from the posterior tubercle of the atlas and is inserted into the midline region of the inferior nuchal line.*

The **rectus capitis posterior major** (**2**) *arises from the spinous process of the 2nd cervical vertebra and is inserted into the inferior nuchal line lateral to the rectus capitis posterior minor.*

The **obliquus capitis superior** (**3**) *originates from the transverse process of the atlas. It is inserted on the occipital bone somewhat above and lateral to the rectus capitis posterior major.*

The **obliquus capitis inferior** (**4**) *runs from the spinous process of the 2nd cervical vertebra to the transverse process of the atlas.*

All the short nape muscles act on the head joints. Bilateral contraction causes the straight and oblique muscles to bend the head backward and unilateral contraction of the obliquus capitis superior turns the head sideways. Lateral rotation of the head is caused by synergistic contraction of the rectus capitis posterior major and obliquus capitis inferior.
Nerve supply: Suboccipital nerve (C1).

Practical Points

The rectus capitis posterior major and the obliquus capitis superior and inferior form the **suboccipital triangle** (trigonum a. vertebralis). Here the vertebral artery (see p. 332) can be located, lying on the posterior arch of the atlas. Between the artery and the posterior arch of the atlas lies the 1st cervical nerve, whose dorsal ramus, the suboccipital nerve, (see p. 332 and Vol. 3) innervates these muscles.

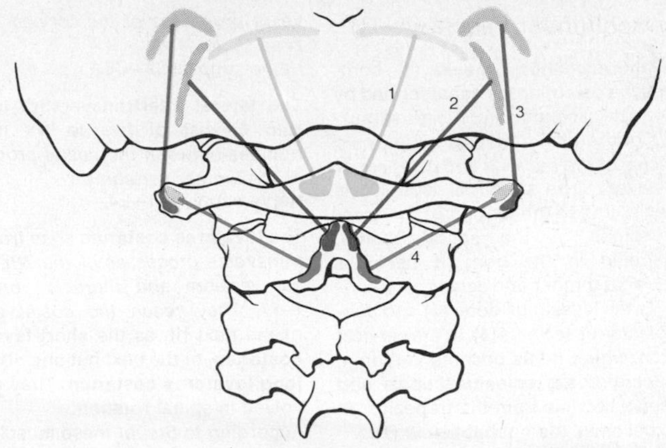

B Diagram of origin, course and insertions of the muscles

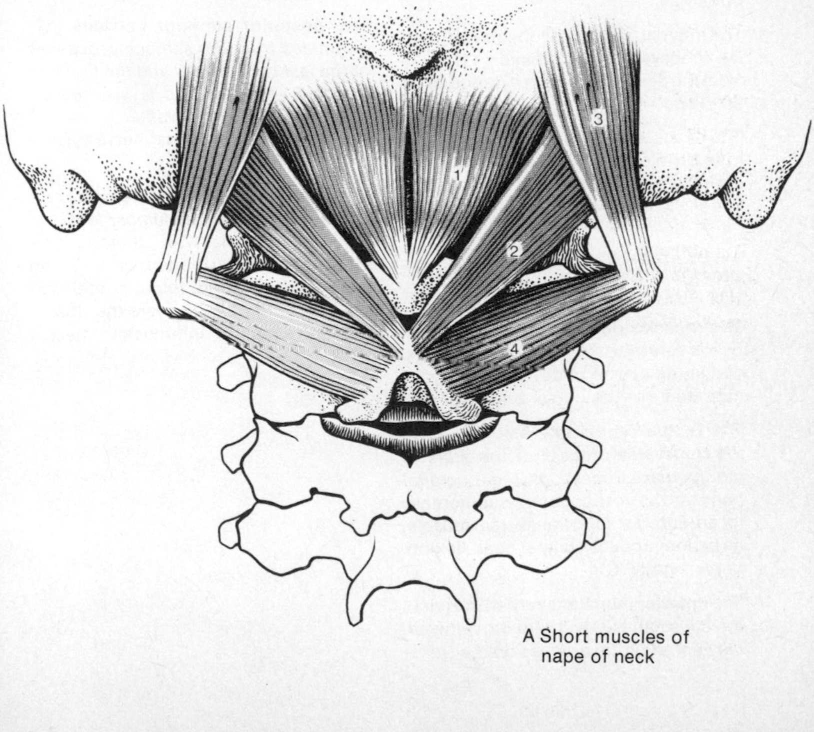

A Short muscles of nape of neck

Thoracolumbar Fascia (A–B)

The **thoracolumbar fascia** (**1**) completes the osteofibrous canal formed by the vertebral column and the dorsal surfaces of the ribs. *It invests all intrinsic muscles of the back* (**2**) *and consists of two layers.* The **superficial layer** (**3**) is firmly bound to the tendon of the erector spinae in the sacral region. Ascending in the body it becomes somewhat thinner and serves as an origin for the latissimus dorsi (**4**) and posterior inferior serratus (**5**). In the cervical region, where it has become very thin, it separates the splenius capitis and splenius cervicis from the trapezius (**6**) and becomes the nuchal fascia (**7**).

The **deep layer** (**8**) arises from the costal processes (**9**) of the lumbar vertebrae and separates the intrinsic back muscles (**2**) from those of the ventrolateral body wall.

The internal abdominal oblique (**10**) and the transversus abdominis (**11**) arise from the deep layer which extends as far as the ilac crest.

The nuchal fascia (**7**) continues laterally forward into the superficial cervical fascia (see p. 316). The nuchal ligament lies in the midline of the nuchal fascia.

Migrant Ventrolateral Muscles (A–B)

The muscles described are innervated by the ventral rami of the spinal nerves, and in the course of development have migrated into the dorsal body wall.

The **rectus capitis lateralis** *runs from the transverse process of the atlas to the jugular process of the occipital bone* and corresponds developmentally to an anterior intertransverse muscle. Its action produces lateral head flexion.
Nerve supply: C1.

The **anterior intertransversarii cervicis** are six small bundles running *between the ventral protuberances on the transverse processes of the cervical vertebrae.*
Nerve supply: C2–C6.

The **lateral intertransversarii lumborum** consist of five to six muscle bundles *between the costal processes of the lumbar vertebrae.*
Nerve supply: L1–L4.

The **levatores costarum** *arise from the transverse processes of the 7th cervical vertebra and thoracic vertebrae 1–11. They reach the costal angles* of the next rib as the **short levatores costarum**, or the next but one rib as the **long levatores costarum**. They are involved in spinal rotation.
According to *Steubl* these muscles are innervated by the dorsal rami of the spinal nerves and so belong to the lateral tract of the intrinsic back muscles.
Nerve supply: Dorsal rami of the spinal nerves!

The **posterior superior serratus** (**12**) *originates from the spinous processes of the last two cervical and the first two thoracic vertebrae and is inserted on ribs 2–5, which it elevates.*
Nerve supply: Intercostal nerves (Th1–Th4).

The **posterior inferior serratus** (**5**) *arises from the thoracolumbar fascia* in the region of the 12th thoracic vertebra and lumbar vertebrae 1–3 and *usually extends* with four digitations *to the 12th–9th ribs.* It lowers the ribs.
Nerve supply: Intercostal nerves (Th9–Th12).

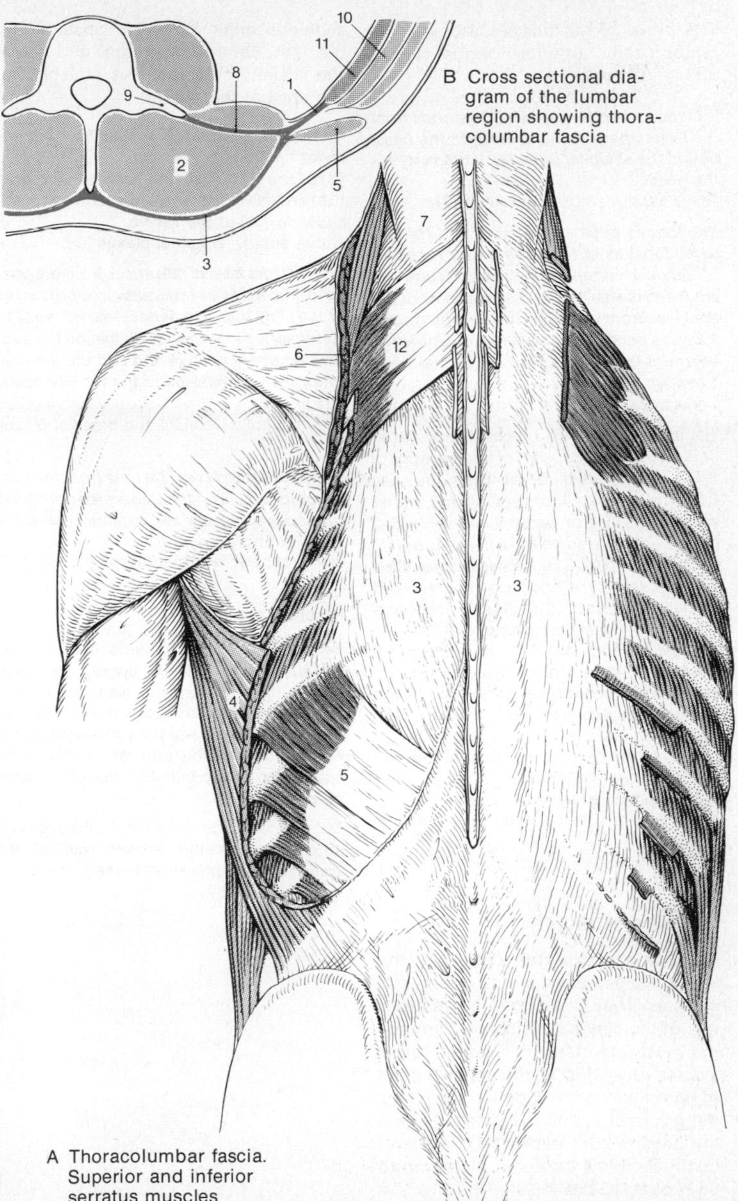

B Cross sectional diagram of the lumbar region showing thoracolumbar fascia

A Thoracolumbar fascia. Superior and inferior serratus muscles

Prevertebral Muscles (A–B)

The prevertebral muscles include the rectus capitis anterior, longus capitis and longus colli.

The **rectus capitis anterior** (**1**) *extends from the lateral mass of the atlas* (**2**) *to the basal part of the occipital bone* (**3**). It helps to flex the head.
Nerve supply: Cervical plexus (C 1).

The **longus capitis** (**4**) *arises from the anterior tuberles of the transverse processes of cervical vertebrae 3–6* (**5**). It runs upward and is *attached to the basal part of the occipital bone* (**6**). The two longi capitis muscles bend the head forward. Unilateral action of the muscle helps to tilt the head sideways.
Nerve supply: Cervical plexus (C 1–C 4).

The **longus colli** (**7**) is roughly triangular in shape because it consists of three groups of fibers. The **superior oblique fibers** (**8**) *arise from the anterior tubercles on the transverse processes of cervical vertebrae 5–2* (**9**) *and are inserted on the anterior tubercle of the atlas* (**10**). The **inferior oblique fibers** (**11**) *run from the bodies of the 1st–3rd thoracic vertebrae* (**12**) *to the anterior tubercle on the transverse process of the 6th cervical vertebra* (**13**). The **medial fibers** (**14**) *extend from the bodies of the upper thoracic and lower cervical vertebrae* (**15**) *to the bodies of the upper cervical vertebrae* (**16**). Unilateral contraction of the muscle bends and turns the cervical vertebral column to the side. Together, both longi colli muscles bend the cervical spine forward.
Nerve supply: Cervical and brachial plexus (C 2–C 8).

Scalene Muscles

The **scalene muscles** represent the cranial continuation of the intercostal muscles. They arise from the vestigial ribs of the cervical vertebrae. They are the most important muscles for quiet inspiration as they lift the first two pairs of ribs and thus the superior part of the thorax. Their action is increased when the head is bent backward. Unilateral contraction tilts the cervical column to one side. Occasionally there is a scalenus minimus which arises from the 7th cervical vertebra and joins the scalenus medius. It is attached to the apex of the pleura.

The **scalenus anterior** (**17**) *arises from the anterior tubercles of the transverse processes* (**3**) *of the (3rd) 4th–6th cervical vertebrae* (**18**) and is *inserted on the anterior scalene tubercle* (**19**) *of the 1st rib.*
Nerve supply: Brachial plexus (C 5–C 7).

The **scalenus medius** (**20**) *arises from the posterior tubercles of the transverse processes of the (1st) 2nd–7th cervical vertebrae* (**21**). It is *inserted into the 1st rib behind the subclavian artery groove and into the external intercostal membrane of the 1st intercostal space* (**22**).
Nerve supply: Cervical and brachial plexus (C 4–C 8).

The **scalenus posterior** (**23**) *runs from the posterior tubercles on the transverse processes of the 5th–7th cervical vertebrae* (**24**) *to the 2nd (3rd) rib* (**25**).
Nerve supply: Brachial plexus (C 7–C 8).

Practical Points

Between the scalenus anterior and scalenus medius lies the **scalene opening** (**26**), also called the "posterior scalene aperture," through which pass the brachial plexus (see p. 346 and Vol. 3) and the subclavian artery. Retroversion of the arm may occlude the subclavian artery between the rib and the clavicle.

Together with the longus colli, the scalenus anterior forms the medial wall of the **scalenovertebral triangle** (**27**; see p. 352).

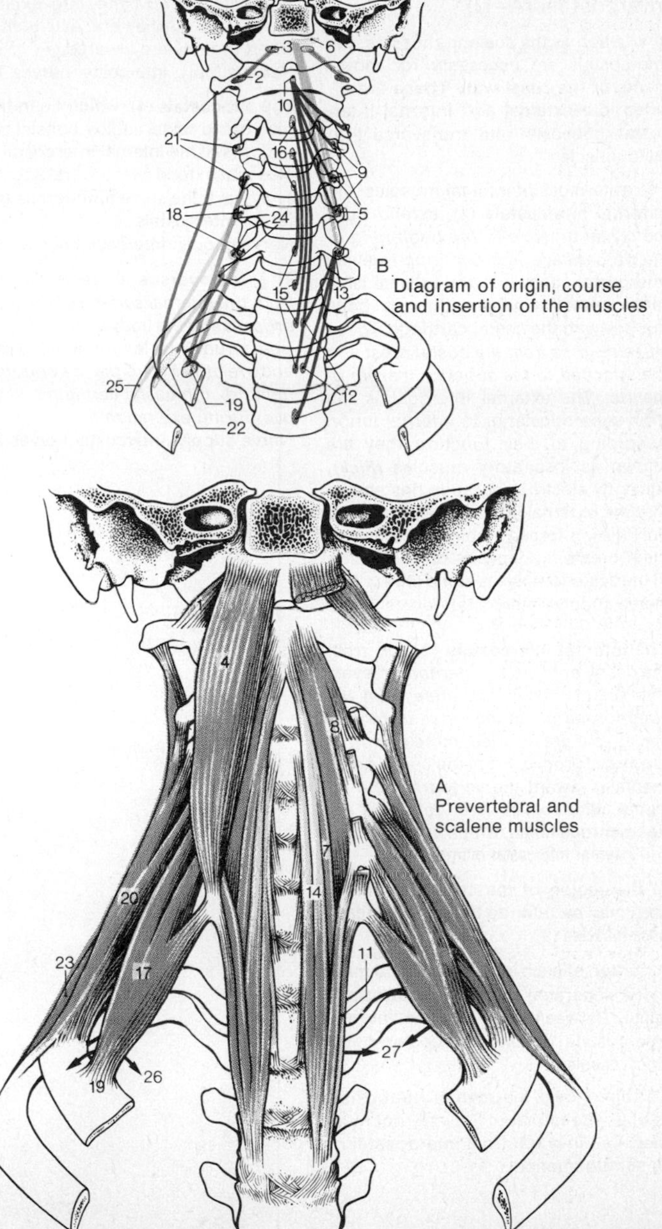

B
Diagram of origin, course and insertion of the muscles

A
Prevertebral and scalene muscles

Intercostals (A–D)

In addition to the scalene muscles, the intercostals are necessary for movements of the chest wall. These are divided into external and internal intercostal, subcostal and transverse thoracic muscles.

The outermost intercostal muscles, the **external intercostals** (**1**), *extend from the costal tubercle to the beginning of the rib cartilage* and continue in every intercostal space into the **external intercostal membrane** where the rib bone merges with the costal cartilage. *These muscles arise from the costal crest and are attached to the superior margin of the rib.* The external intercostals run from superoposterior to inferoanterior. According to their function they are known as inspiratory muscles *(Fick)*. Recently electromyography has shown that the external intercostals are active only during forced inspiration and that quiet breathing depends on the action of the scalene muscles alone (see p. 80).
Nerve supply: Intercostal nerves 1–11.

The **internal intercostals** (**2**) *run from the costal angle to the sternum* in every intercostal space. *They arise from the superior margin of the inner surface of the rib and are inserted in the region of the costal groove.* From the costal angle medially toward the vertebrae, the internal intercostals are replaced by ligamentous fibers, which are known as the **internal intercostal membrane.**

In the region of the costal cartilages they may be referred to as **intercartilaginous muscles** (**3**).

A portion of each inner intercostal muscle is separated off as the **intercostales intimi.** Between them and the internal intercostals lie the intercostal nerve and vessels.

The direction of the internal intercostals is opposite to that of the external muscles, i.e., they run from inferoposterior to superoanterior.

According to *Fick* they are expiratory muscles, i. e., they are activated only when the ribs are lowered.
Nerve supply: Intercostal nerves 1–11.

The **subcostals** (**4**), which lie in the region of the costal angles, consist mainly of fibers of the internal intercostal muscles that extend over several segments. They have the same function as the internal intercostals.
Nerve supply: Intercostal nerves 4–11.

The **transversus thoracis** (**5**) *arises from the internal surface of the xiphoid process and the body of the sternum*. Its fibers run in a laterocranial direction and *are attached to the lower border of the 2nd–6th costal cartilages. It is active during expiration.*
Nerve supply: Intercostal nerves 2–6.

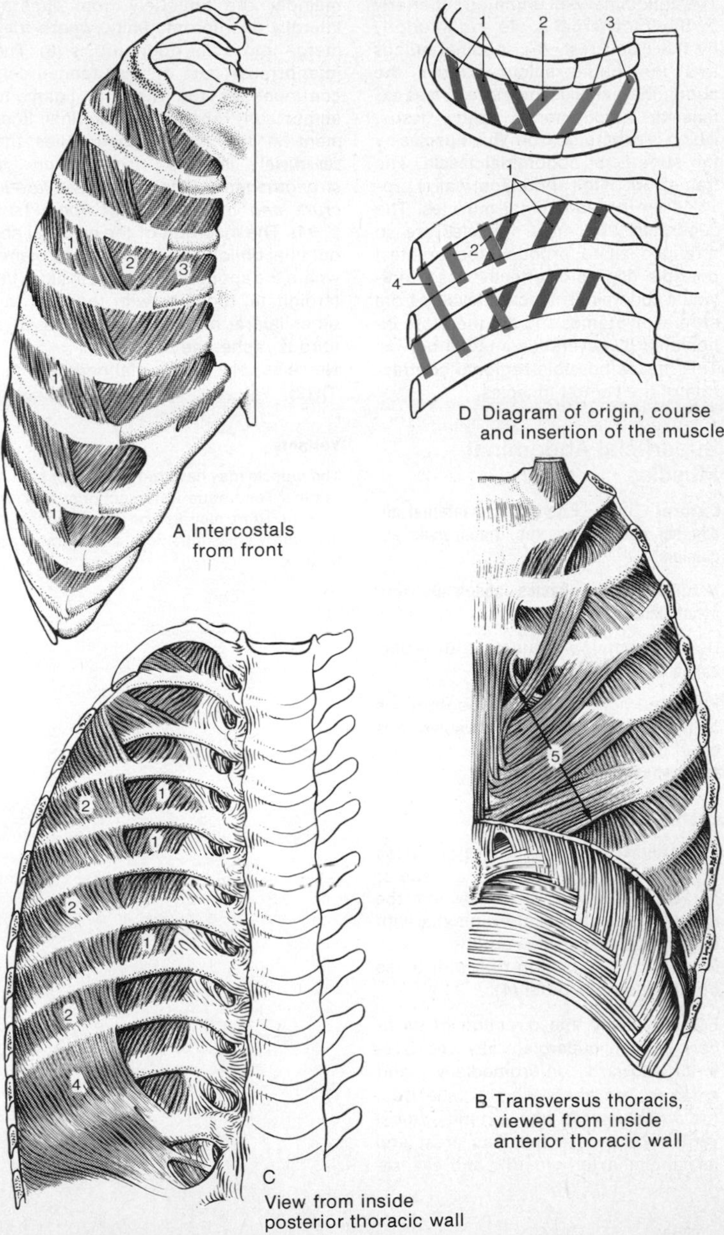

A Intercostals from front

D Diagram of origin, course and insertion of the muscles

B Transversus thoracis, viewed from inside anterior thoracic wall

C View from inside posterior thoracic wall

The abdominal wall is limited superiorly by the infrasternal angle and inferiorly by the iliac crest, the inguinal sulcus and the pubic sulcus. Under the abdominal skin lies the more or less extensive subcutaneous fatty tissue, which is separated from the muscles by the superficial abdominal fascia. The framework of the abdominal wall is provided by the abdominal muscles. The superficial abdominal muscles are so arranged as to produce the greatest possible degree of effectiveness. Individual abdominal muscles develop from several myotomes and are therefore innervated by several segmental nerves. This makes possible regional contraction of the ventral muscles.

Superficial Abdominal Muscles

Lateral Group: External and **internal abdominal oblique muscles, transversus abdominis.**

Medial Group: Rectus abdominis and **pyramidalis.**

Deep Abdominal Muscles: Quadratus lumborum and **psoas major.**

Flattened ligaments, the aponeuroses of the lateral abdominal muscles, enclose the rectus abdominis to form the **rectus sheath** (see p. 88).

Lateral Group (A–B)

The **external abdominal oblique** (**1**) *arises with eight slips on the outer surface of the 5th–12th ribs* (**2**). Between the 5th–(8th) 9th ribs it interdigitates with the slips of the serratus anterior (**3**) and between the 10th–12th ribs with those of the latissimus dorsi (**4**).

Fundamentally, the direction of its fibers is from superolaterally and posterior toward inferomedially and anterior. The fibers which come from the three lowest ribs extend almost vertically down to the iliac crest and its labium externum (**5**), and the remainder run obliquely from superolaterally to inferomedially, where they merge into a flat aponeurosis (**6**). The inferiormost part of the aponeurosis continues as the inguinal ligament. Immediately above the inguinal ligament in the medial region lies the **superficial inguinal ring**, which is *strengthened by the medial and lateral crura and the intercrural fibers* (see p. 94). The insertion of the external abdominal oblique is in the median plane, where the aponeuroses of both sides interdigitate, together with those of the other lateral abdominal muscles, in a fibrous raphe, the **linea alba**.

Nerve supply: Intercostal nerves (Th5–Th12).

Variants

The muscle may have more or fewer slips of origin. Tendinous intersections may be present. There may also be connections with the nearby latissimus dorsi and serratus anterior.

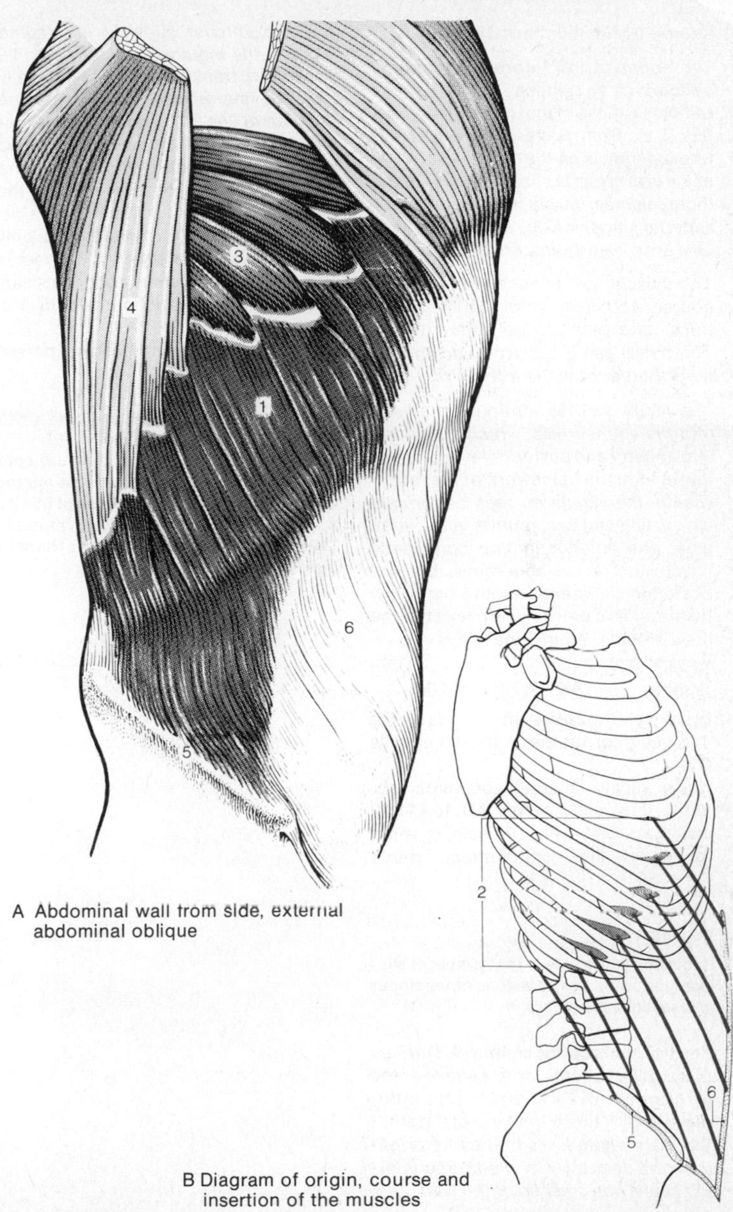

A Abdominal wall from side, external abdominal oblique

B Diagram of origin, course and insertion of the muscles

Lateral Group (continued) (A–B)

The *origin* of the **internal abdominal oblique (A 1)**, whose fibers ascend rather like those of the internal intercostals, i. e., from posteroinferior to anterosuperior, *is on the intermediate line of the iliac crest* (**2**), *the deep layer of the thoracolumbar fascia and the anterior superior iliac spine* (**3**). Some fibers may also arise from the *inguinal ligament* (**4**).

The muscle has an ascending fan-like course. Accordingly, toward the insertions, **three parts** can be differentiated. The **cranial part** *is inserted into the inferior border of the last three ribs* (**5**).

The **middle part** (**6**) *continues medially into the aponeurosis, which is divided into anterior and posterior layers.* These layers form the framework of the *rectus sheath, the vagina m. recti abdominis* (see p. 88), and they reunite in the linea alba. The anterior lamina completely covers the rectus abdominis, but the posterior lamina ends about 5 cm below the navel as a cranially convex line, the *linea arcuata*. As this margin is not always sharply defined it is more correct to speak of an *area arcuata (Lanz).*

In the male the **caudal part** extends on the spermatic cord as the cremaster muscle (**7**).
Nerve supply: Internal abdominal oblique: intercostal nerves (Th 10–Th 12 and L1). Cremaster muscle: genital ramus of the genitofemoral nerve (L1–L2).

Variants

Reduction or increase in the number of slips inserting on the ribs as well as of tendinous intersections may occur.

The **transversus abdominis (A 8)** *arises by six slips from the inner surface of the cartilage of ribs 7–12* (**9**); its slips interdigitate with those of the costal part of the diaphragm. *It also takes its origin from the deep layer of the thoracolumbar fascia, the inner lip of the iliac crest* (**10**), *the anterior superior iliac spine* (**11**) *and the inguinal ligament* (**12**). Its fibers run transversely to a medially concave line which is known as the *"semilunar line"*. The aponeurosis begins at this line. It is cranial to the linea or area arcuata and participates in the formation of the posterior layer of the rectus sheath. Caudal to the area arcuata (see above) the aponeurosis only forms the anterior layer of the rectus sheath. The transversus abdominis participates via its aponeurosis in the linea alba.
Nerve supply: Intercostal nerves (Th7–Th12 and L1).

Variants

The transversus abdominis may fuse completely in its lower region with the internal abdominal oblique, and because of this it is sometimes called the *"complex muscle"*. There are reports in the literature of its complete absence.

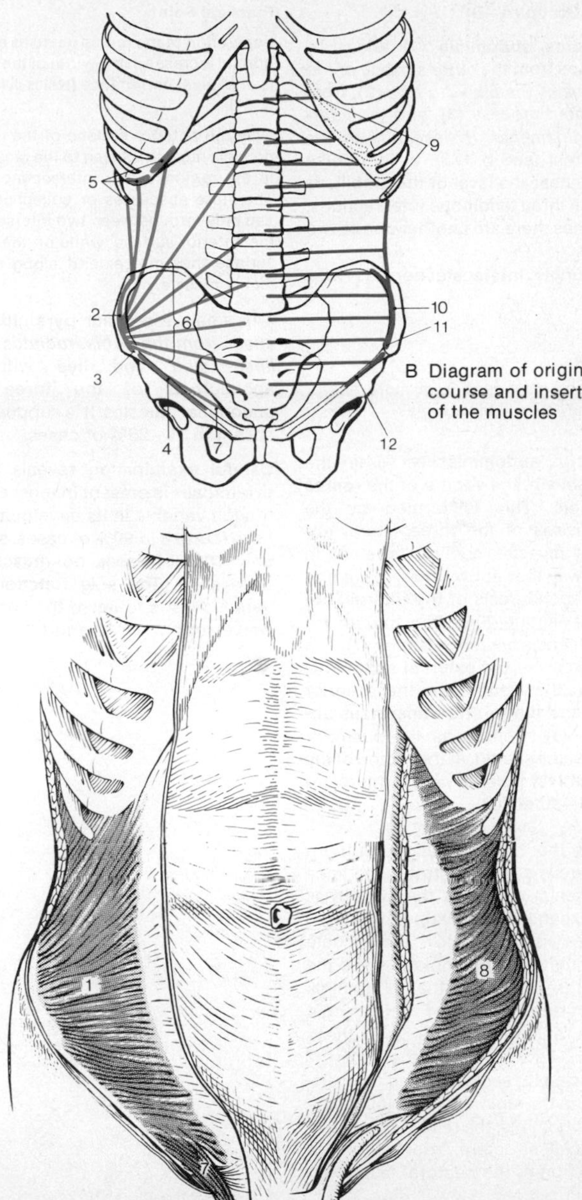

B Diagram of origin, course and insertion of the muscles

A Abdominal wall from front, internal abdominal oblique and transversus abdominis

Medial Group (A–D)

The **rectus abdominis** (**1**) arises by three slips from the *outer surface of the cartilages of the 5th–7th ribs* (**2**), from the *xiphoid process* (**3**), and the *intervening ligaments. It descends to the pubic crest* (see p. 173). In its course down to near the level of the umbilicus there are three tendinous intersections, sometimes there are another one or two below it.
Nerve supply: Intercostal nerves (Th 5–Th 12).

Variants:

The muscle may arise from more ribs or, rarely, may be entirely absent.

The rectus abdominis lies within the rectus sheath, the **vagina** of the **rectus abdominis**. This is formed by the aponeuroses of the three lateral abdominal muscles coming together in such a way that above the *arcuate line* (**4**) the aponeurosis of the internal abdominal oblique (**5**) divides into an *anterior* (**6**) and a *posterior lamina* (**7**). The aponeurosis of the external abdominal oblique (**8**) strengthens the anterior lamina and that of the transversus abdominis (**9**) strengthens the posterior lamina of the sheath. In the region of the **linea alba** (**10**) there is partial intertwining of the fibers (**B**).

Between the individual aponeurotic fibers there is a fatty infiltrate. The linea alba extends as far as the symphysis and is expanded at the superior margin of the pelvis (**11**). Below the arcuate line the rectus is incomplete, since the aponeuroses of all the abdominal muscles run in front of both rectus muscles, and the inner side of these muscles is covered only by the transversalis fascia (**12**; see p. 90) and the peritoneum. In the region of the origin of the rectus abdominis, the rectus sheath is a thin fascial structure, representing a continuation of the pectoral fascia.

Practical Points

Separation of the rectus muscles and an abnormal increase in the width of the linea alba is of clinical importance (**rectus diastasis**; see p. 94).

Only the anterior surface of the rectus abdominis muscle is fused to the rectus sheath in the region of the intersecting tendons. Therefore abscesses or collections of pus can only form between two intersections on the anterior surface, while on the posterior surface they may extend along the entire rectus muscle.

The small, triangular **pyramidalis** (**13**) *arises from the pubis, radiates into the linea alba* and lies within the aponeurosis of the three lateral abdominal muscles. It is supposed to be absent in 16–25% of cases.

Careful examination reveals that the pyramidalis is present in most cases, although variable in its development. We have found it in 90% of cases, so that in only 10% of cases no muscle fibers were seen. The sole function of the pyramidalis is to tense the linea alba.
Nerve supply: Th 12 and L 1.

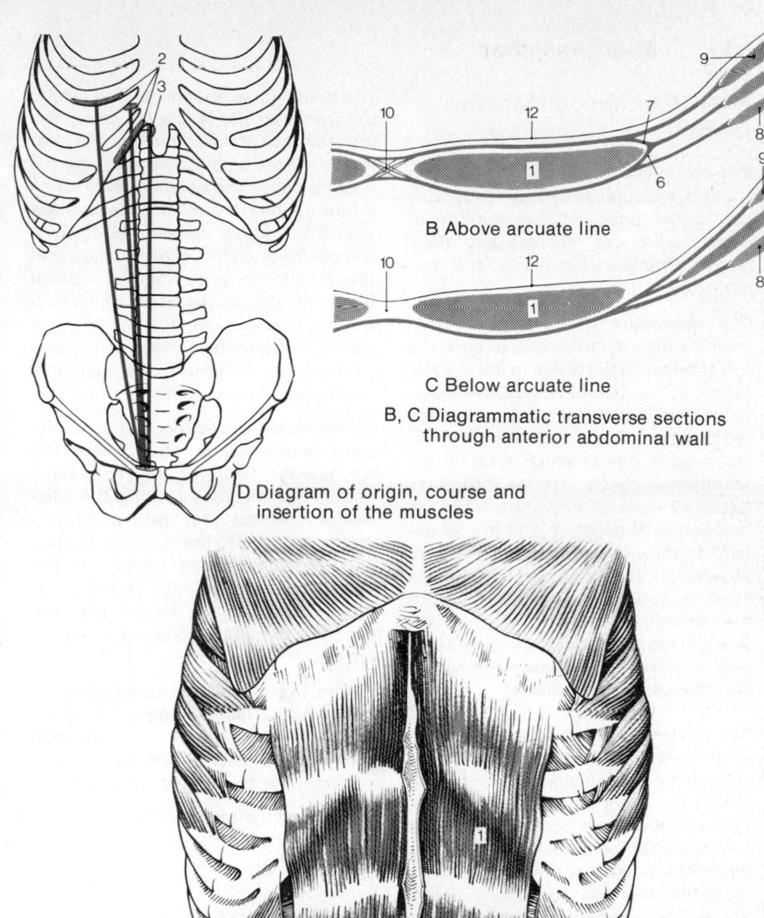

B Above arcuate line

C Below arcuate line

B, C Diagrammatic transverse sections through anterior abdominal wall

D Diagram of origin, course and insertion of the muscles

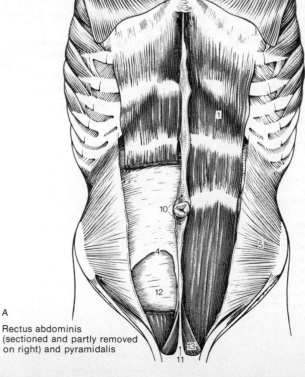

A

Rectus abdominis (sectioned and partly removed on right) and pyramidalis

Fasciae of Abdominal Wall (A–B)

The abdominal wall can be divided into the *skin, subcutaneous fatty tissue with connective tissue lamellae, superficial abdominal fascia muscles and their fasciae, transversalis fascia and the peritoneum.*

The **connective tissue lamellae** that traverse the subcutaneous fatty tissue are arranged in flat layers in the inferior region of the abdominal wall, the inguinal region. In medical practice this has led to them being referred to as separate fasciae, one of which is called the **subcutaneous fascia** (**1**) or **"Camper's fascia"**. This is of importance for the surgeon as between it (and it may extend to the upper thigh) and the true superficial abdominal fascia lie the larger, subcutaneous vessels. A part of the connective tissue lamella, which extends in the direction of the genital organ is called the **suspensory ligament of the penis** (**2**) or of the **clitoris.**

The **superficial abdominal fascia** (**3**) is a thin layer, strengthened only in the region of the linea alba (see p. 94), which covers the entire muscles of the anterior wall and their aponeuroses. The medial part of the fascia continues into the **fundiform ligament of the penis** (**4**) or the **clitoris** which contains many elastic fibers. This ligament divides into two crura to surround the corpus cavernosum of the penis.

In the region of he superficial inguinal ring the fascia fuses with the extension of the aponeurosis of the external abdominal oblique to form the **external spermatic fascia** (**5**), which provides the outer covering of the spermatic cord. With the aponeurosis of the external abdominal oblique it is more firmly bound also in the region of the inguinal ligament and then continues in the **fascia of the thigh** (**6**).

The inner, loose abdominal wall fascia, the **transversalis fascia** (**7**), covers the inner surface of the abdominal muscles. It is taut in the umbilical region, where it may be called the **umbilical fascia** (**8**). Inferiorly the transversalis fascia fuses with the inguinal ligament (**9**) to form the posterior wall of the inguinal canal (see p. 94). It extends from the inguinal ligament into the **iliac fascia**, which covers the iliac muscle (**10**). Superiorly it covers the inferior surface of the diaphragm and posteriorly the quadratus lumborum and psoas major.

In the region of the inguinal canal the transversalis fascia, strengthened by aponeurotic fibers of the transversus abdominis, thickens to form the **interfoveolar ligament** (**11**), (see p. 96). Attached medially to the rectus abdominis (**12**) the transversalis fascia and the transversus abdominis extend as a band, known as the **inguinal falx** (**13**), which is connected to the inguinal ligament.

Lateral to the interfoveolar ligament the transversalis fascia evaginates at the deep inguinal ring (**14**) to form the **internal spermatic fascia.** Below the inguinal ligament lies the femoral canal (**15**).

16 Cord of the umbilical artery
17 Urachal cord.

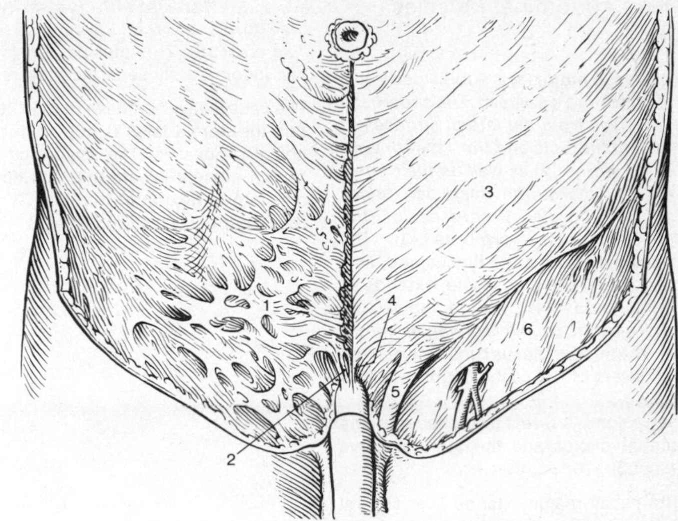

A Right, superficial connective tissue lamellae; left, external superficial abdominal fascia

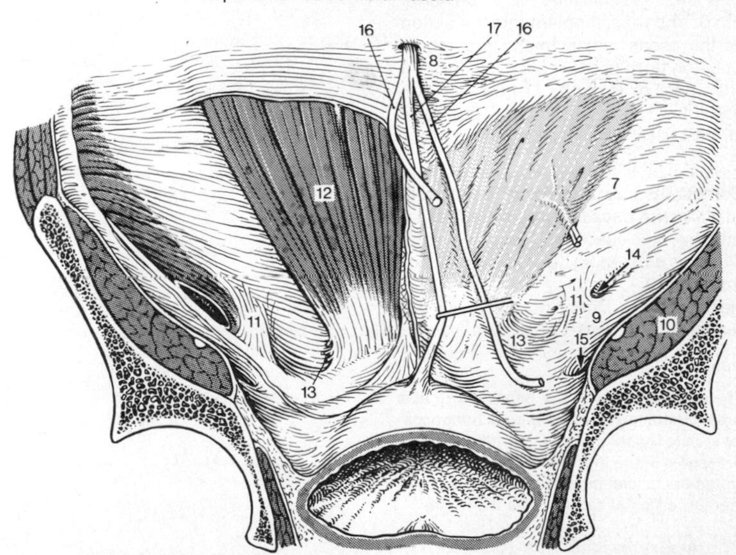

B Anterior abdominal wall from inside with transversalis fascia on right

Deep Abdominal Muscles (A–B)

The **psoas major** (**1**) is subdivided into a **superficial** and a **deep part.** *The superficial part arises from the lateral surfaces of the 12th thoracic and the 1st–4th lumbar vertebrae (***2***) as well as their intervertebral disks. The deep part arises from the costal processes of the 1st–5th lumbar vertebrae* (**3**). The psoas major joins the iliacus and, surrounded by the iliac fascia, extends as the **iliopsoas** (**4**) through the lacuna musculorum to the *trochanter minor* (**5**). The lumbar plexus runs between the two layers of the psoas major (see also p. 222).
Nerve supply: Direct branches from the lumbar plexus and the femoral nerve (L1–L3).

The psoas major extends over several joints and is capable of considerable elevation of the leg. The iliacus muscle (see p. 222), with which it joins to form the iliopsoas muscle, is a powerful flexor and thus supplements the action of the psoas major. In the recumbent position both psoas muscles help to lift the upper or lower half of the body. In addition, the psoas major can give slight assistance in lateral flexion of the vertebral column.

Sometimes a **psoas minor** is found, split off from *the psoas major*, which enters into the iliac fascia and *inserts on the iliopubic eminence.* It acts as a tensor of the fascia.
Nerve supply: Direct branch from the lumbar plexus (L1–L3).

Practical Points

The fascia surrounds the psoas major as a tube, stretching from the medial lumbocostal arch to the thigh. Thus, any inflammatory processes in the thoracic region can extend within the fascial tube to appear as wandering abscesses as far down as the thigh.

The **quadratus lumborum** (**6**) *extends to the 12th rib* (**7**) *and to the costal processes of the 1st–3rd (4th) lumbar vertebrae* (**8**). *It arises from the inner lip of the iliac crest* (**9**). This muscle consists of two incompletely separated layers.

The ventral layer reaches to the 12th rib and the dorsal layer is attached to the costal processes. The quadratus lumborum muscle lowers the 12th rib and aids lateral flexion of the body.
Nerve supply: Th12 and L1–L3.

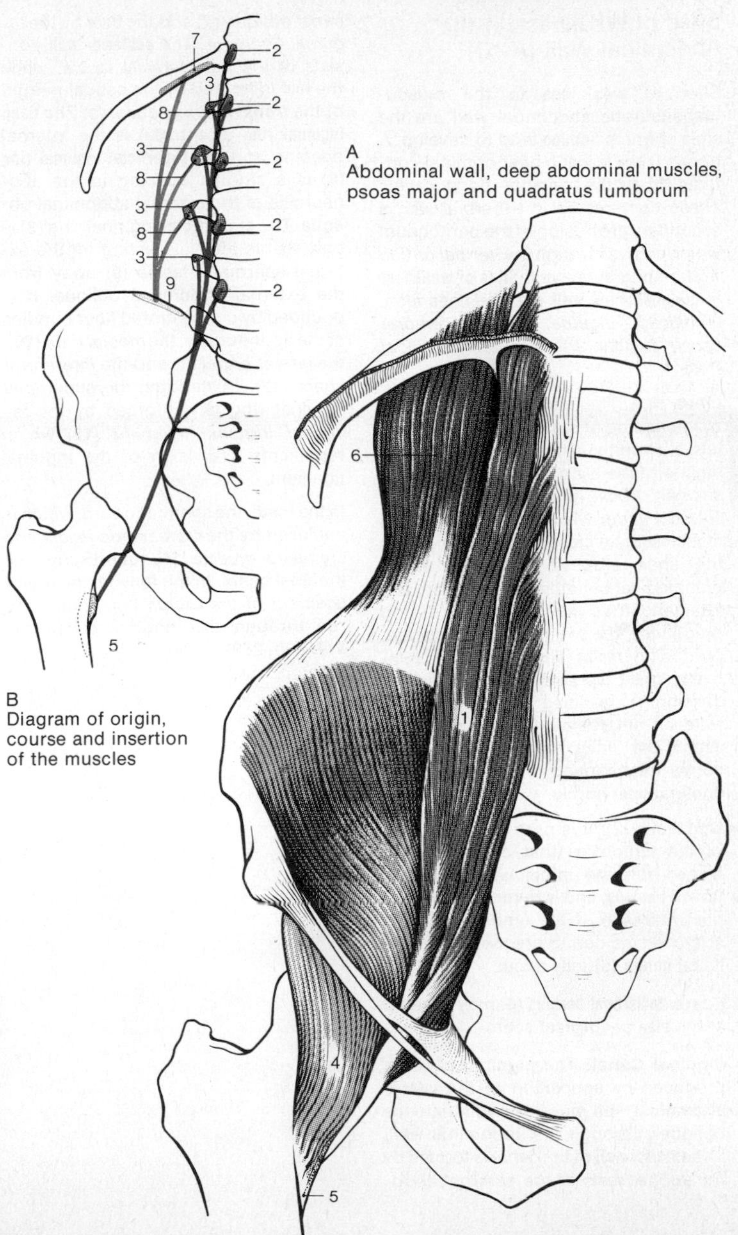

A
Abdominal wall, deep abdominal muscles, psoas major and quadratus lumborum

B
Diagram of origin, course and insertion of the muscles

Sites of Weakness in the Abdominal Wall (A–D)

Sites of weakness in the musculoaponeurotic abdominal wall are the sites at which **hernias** tend to develop. A hernia is the escape of abdominal contents from the original body cavity. These contents lie in a *hernial sac*, a secondary protrusion of the peritoneum which comes through the *hernial orifice* in the abdominal wall. **Sites of weakness in the abdominal wall** are: the *linea alba, umbilicus, inguinal region, femoral canal, lumbar triangle* and *surgical scars.*

Linea alba: The linea alba (**1**) is formed by interlacing of the aponeuroses of the lateral abdominal muscles and is a tendinous raphe lying between the rectus sheaths. Above the umbilicus (**2**) it is 1–2 cm wide, while below it the recti muscles (**3**) lie closer to each other and the linea alba is narrower. Under pathological conditions when there is a fat pendulous abdomen, or during pregnancy, the two recti may separate, producing **rectus diastasis (A)**. A relatively small **epigastric hernia** (**4**) may develop in the linea alba. It develops from an enlargement of a small hole within the linea alba. An epigastric hernia may expand into a ventral abdominal wall hernia.

Umbilicus (**2**): It is produced by fusion of the structures that originally protruded from the umbilicus with the adjacent tissues, and is reinforced by connective tissue. If the umbilical ring is stretched, as during pregnancy, an **umbilical hernia** (**5**) may occur.

Scars: Incisional hernias (**6**) may develop at the site of surgical scars.

Inguinal Canal: The inguinal canal is produced by apposition of the lateral abdominal wall muscles and it extends obliquely through the abdominal wall. The **anterior wall** of the canal is formed by the *aponeurosis of the external abdominal oblique* (**7**) and the **floor** by the *inguinal ligament*. The **posterior wall** consists of the *transversalis fascia*, while the **roof** is formed by the caudal margin of the *transversus abdominis*. The **deep inguinal ring** (see p. 96) is the internal opening and the **superficial inguinal ring** (**8**) is a slit-like opening in the aponeurosis of the external abdominal oblique. The superficial inguinal ring (**8**) is only visible after dissecting off the external spermatic fascia (**9**) away from the external abdominal oblique. It is bounded by concentrated fiber bundles of the aponeurosis, the *medial crus* (**10**), the *lateral crus* (**11**) and the *intercrural fibers* (**12**). Posteriorly, the superficial inguinal ring is reinforced by the *reflected inguinal ligament* (**13**) which represents a division of the inguinal ligament.

In the male, the spermatic cord, which is enclosed by the *cremasteric fascia* and *cremaster muscle* (**14**), runs through the inguinal canal. In the female, the *round ligament of the uterus* and lymphatics run through the inguinal canal (see Vol. 2, p. 288).

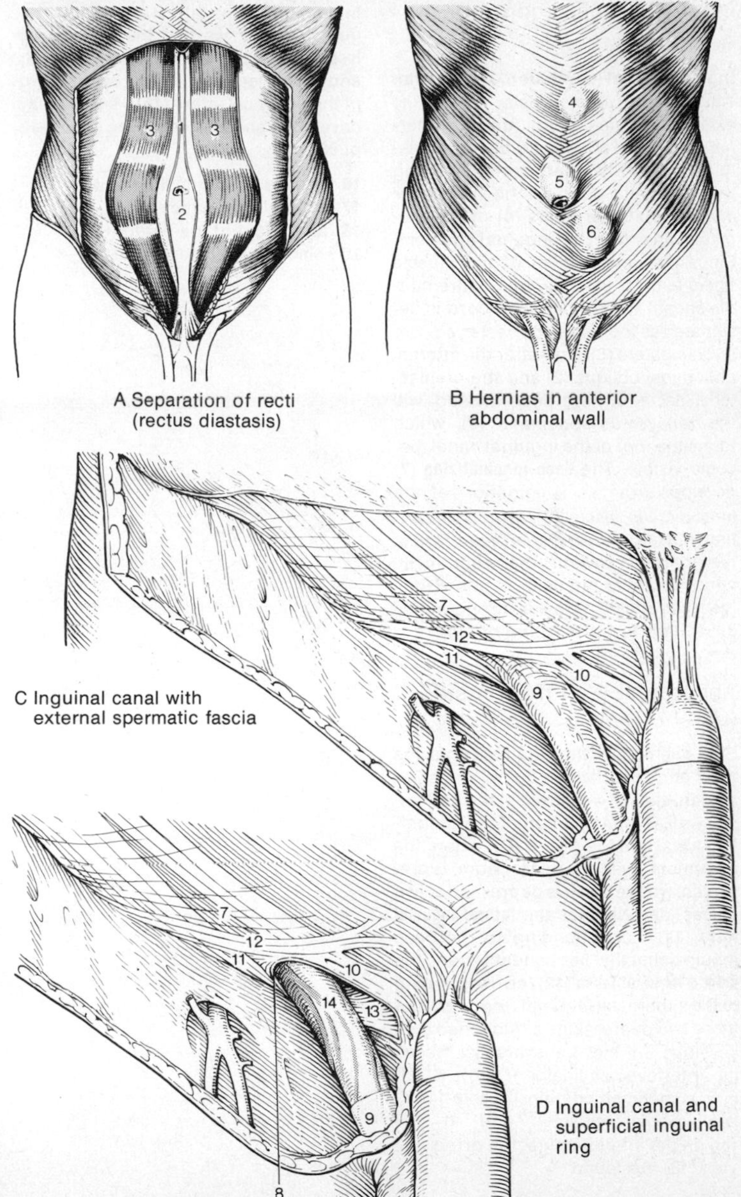

A Separation of recti (rectus diastasis)

B Hernias in anterior abdominal wall

C Inguinal canal with external spermatic fascia

D Inguinal canal and superficial inguinal ring

Inguinal Canal (continued, A–B).

Inguinal Canal (continued, A–B). After splitting the *aponeurosis* (**1**) of the external abdominal oblique, the internal abdominal oblique (**2**) becomes visible. Some of its fibers continue along the spermatic cord as the *cremaster muscle* (**3**). Other fibers (**4**) of the cremaster arise from the inguinal ligament. Since the development of the muscle fibers is quite variable, this entire middle sheath of the spermatic cord is designated as the *fascia cremasterica cum m. cremastere* (**5**). Only after the internal abdominal oblique (**2**) and the cremasteric fascia (**5**) have been incised, will the *transversus abdominis* (**6**), which forms the roof of the inguinal canal, become visible. The **deep inguinal ring** (**7**) develops from an evagination of the *transversalis fascia* (**8**), which is continued as the *internal spermatic fascia,* the innermost covering of the spermatic cord. Medial to the deep inguinal ring, the transversalis fascia is strengthened by the *interfoveolar ligament* (**10**).

Abdominal Wall from Inside (C)

Both openings of the inguinal canal, the deep and superficial inguinal rings, represent sites of weakness in the abdominal wall. By examination of the abdominal wall from the inside (**C**), where the innermost layer, the peritoneum, is preserved, we see that it is depressed in two places, described as the **lateral inguinal fossa** (**11**), corresponding to the deep inguinal ring that lies beneath it, and the **medial inguinal fossa** (**12**), corresponding to the superficial inguinal ring. Between these two depressions a thickened area develops in the transversalis fascia, the interfoveolar ligament (**10**), which may sometimes contain muscle fibers (interfoveolar muscle), and in this region the inferior epigastric artery and vein (**13**) are found.

In addition to the lateral and medial inguinal fossae, we find the **supravesical fossa** (**14**) which is medial to the latter and separated from it only by the cord of the umbilical artery (**15**). Hernias may develop at any of these three sites (see p. 98).

16 Reflected inguinal ligament,
17 External spermatic fascia,
18 Cut margin of the peritoneum,
19 Femoral canal (see p. 98).

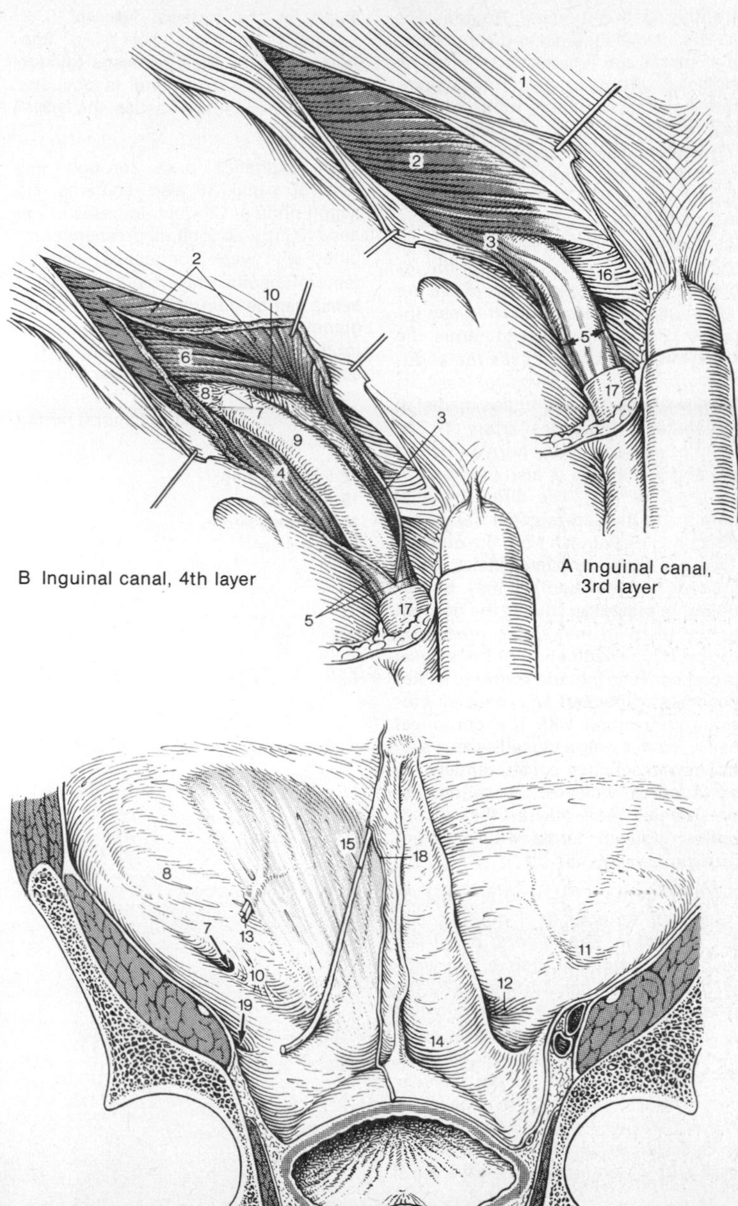

A Inguinal canal, 3rd layer

B Inguinal canal, 4th layer

C Abdominal wall from within, transversalis fascia on left, peritoneum on right

Hernias in the Inguinal Region: The lateral, medial inguinal and supravesicular fossae are regions of minimal resistance. Under certain circumstances they become stretched, bulge out and **inguinal hernias** may occur. Two types of inguinal hernias are distinguished – direct and indirect – and *both traverse the superficial inguinal ring*. The **direct inguinal hernia** (**1**) *has its hernial orifice in the medial inguinal fossa.* An **indirect inguinal hernia** (**2**) *passes through the inguinal canal.* It uses as *points of exit the lateral inguinal fossa* and *the deep inguinal ring*. Another type of hernia, the **supravesical hernia** (**3**), *leaves the abdomen through the supravesical fossa;* its hernial orifice, therefore, lies medial to the obliterated umbilical artery (**4**). The point of passage of this hernia through the abdominal wall is also the superficial inguinal ring. The direct inguinal hernia and the supravesical hernia are difficult to distinguish from the outside. They are always **acquired hernias**, while indirect inguinal hernias may be acquired or **congenital**. During the descent of the testis in males, the *processus vaginalis,* an evagination of the serosa, is carried along into the scrotum. It later becomes obliterated and loses all previous connection with the peritoneal cavity, so that only a closed serous sac, the cavum serosum scroti, remains. In some cases, however, a connection persists and there may be then a congenital inguinal hernia with a patent processus vaginalis.

Femoral Canal: The femoral canal (**5**) represents an additional possible site for herniation. *The femoral canal lies below to the inguinal ligament* (**6**), *within the vascular compartment* (**7**), the medial femoral aperture. Laterally this is separated from the *muscular compartment* (**8**) by the *iliopectineal arch* (**9**). In the medial part of the *vascular compartment,* medial to the large femoral vessels, lies the femoral canal (**5**). It is **bordered medially** by the **lacunar ligament** (**10**), which merges with the **dorsal border** of the **pectineal ligament** (i. e., Cooper's ligament) across a ligamentous arch, the processus falciformis lacunaris. The canal is occupied by loose connective tissues, the **femoral septum** (**11**).

The lymphatics pass through this femoral canal. It also contains the lymph node of Cloquet. In cases of excessive intra-abdominal pressure combined with weak connective tissue, a femoral hernia may result. A **femoral hernia** can be differentiated from an inguinal hernia by its position in relation to the inguinal ligament and to the scrotum or the labium majus. Only an inguinal hernia can reach the scrotum or labia majora, while a femoral hernia appears in the thigh.

12 Femoral vein,
13 Femoral artery,
14 Femoral nerve,
15 Iliopsoas.

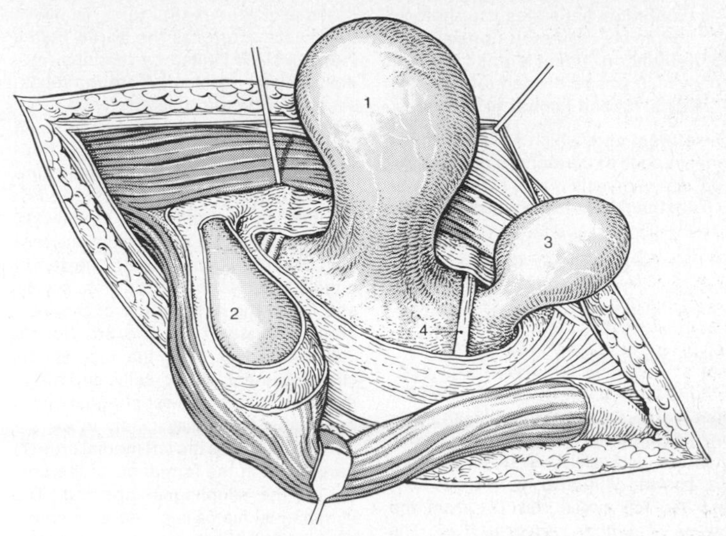

A Hernias in inguinal region; superficial layers of abdominal wall transected

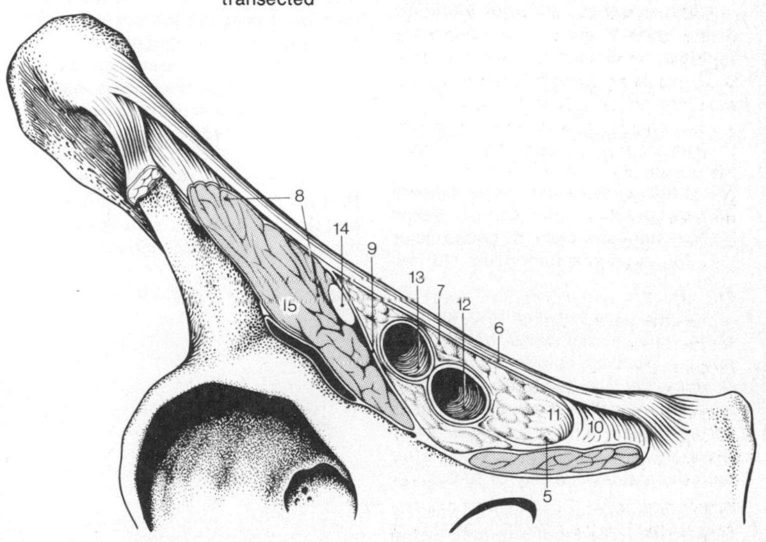

B Muscular and vascular compartments with femoral canal

The **diaphragm** separates the thoracic and abdominal cavities. It consists of a **central tendon** (**1**) and a muscular portion, which can be divided into **sternal** (**2**), **costal** (**3**) and **lumbar** (**4**) **parts.**

The sternal part, which arises from the inner surface of the xiphoid process (**5**), consists of muscle that is rather lighter in color than the rest and which radiates into the central tendon.

The **costal part** arises from the inner surfaces of the cartilage of ribs 7–12 by means of individual slips which alternate with the slips of origin of the transversus abdominis.

The **lumbar part** (**4**) has a medial and a lateral crus and occasionally an intermediate crus splits off from the medial crus. The **right medial crus** (**6**) *arises from the bodies of lumbar vertebrae 1–4, and the* **left medial crus** (**7**) *from the bodies of lumbar vertebrae 1–3.* The **lateral crus** (**8**) *originates from two arches,* formed by the *medial arcuate ligament* (**9**); Psoas arcade or medial lumbocostal arch), and *the lateral arcuate ligament* (**10**; quadratus arcade or lateral lumbocostal arch).

The psoas arcade extends from the lateral surface of 1st (2nd) lumbar vertebral bodies to the costal process (**11**) *of the 1st lumbar vertebra.*

The lateral arcuate ligament extends from this process to the 12th rib. Below these tendinous arches the psoas major (**12**) and quadratus lumborum (**13**) are visible.

There are gaps between the lumbar, costal and sternal parts of the diaphragm which are points of minimal resistance. Between the lumbar and costal components lies the **lumbocostal or vertebrocostal trigone** (**14**), and between the sternal and costal parts is the **sternocostal trigone** (**15**) or hiatus.

The double-domed diaphragm, which is slightly depressed in the middle by the heart, is pierced by openings for the passage of various structures. Between the medial crura lies the **aortic hiatus** (**16**), which is limited by tendons (median arcuate ligament). Through it passes the aorta and posteriorly to it the thoracic duct. The right medial crus (**6**) consists in reality of three muscle bundles, of which that arising from the lumbar vertebrae is the largest and it reaches the central tendon directly (**1**). A 2nd bundle (**17**) arises from the median arcuate ligament (**18**), the tendinous border of the aortic hiatus (**16**), and forms the right border of the **esophageal hiatus** (**19**). The 3rd bundle (**20**) also arises from the median arcuate ligament, but dorsally, and forms the left border of the esophageal opening as the "**hiatus sling**". Only in exceptional cases does the left medial crus (**7**) participate in the formation of the border of the esophageal opening. The esophageal hiatus is bordered by muscle, and through it pass the esophagus and the anterior and posterior vagal trunks. The **foramen for the vena cava** (**21**) lies in the central tendon, and through it pass the inferior vena cava and a branch of the right phrenic nerve. The greater and lesser splanchnic nerves, on the right the azygos vein and on the left the hemiazygos vein, pass through unnamed openings in the medial crus, or between it and the intermediate crus if present. The sympathetic trunk runs between the intermediate and lateral crura. The superior epigastric artery runs through the sternocostal trigone.

Nerve supply: Phrenic nerves ([C3], C4 [C5]).

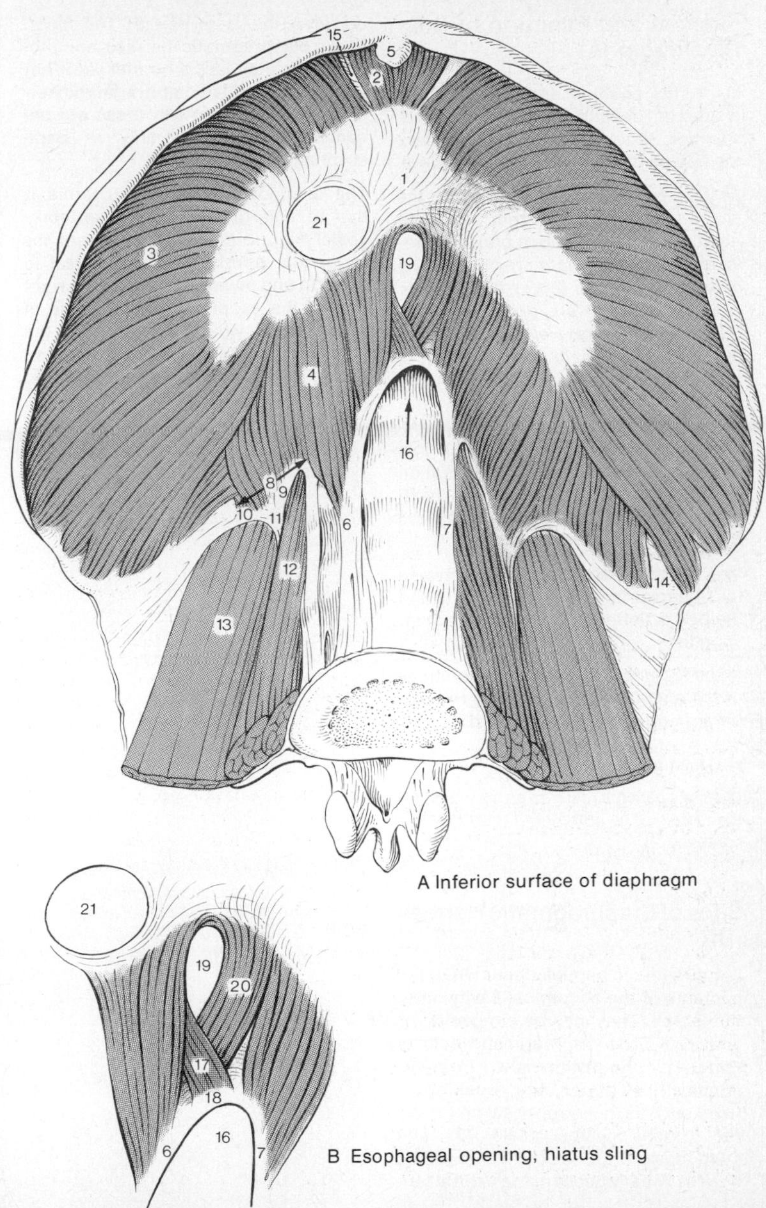

A Inferior surface of diaphragm

B Esophageal opening, hiatus sling

Position and Function of the Diaphragm (A)

In life the position and shape of the diaphragm depend on the phases of respiration, the position of the body and the degree of distension of the viscera.

As the principal respiratory muscle, the shape of the diaphragm changes greatly during the various phases of respiration. *In the upright position during maximal expiration* (blue), *both domes of the diaphragm are projected upon the anterior thoracic wall, on the right at the level of the 4th rib and on the left at the 5th intercostal space. During maximal inspiration* (red) *the diaphragm descends by one to two intercostal spaces.* The sternal part and its origin act as a fixed point. During expiration the muscle fibers rise and during maximal inspiration they descend toward the center of the tendon.

The **costodiaphragmatic recess** between the upper surface of the diaphragm and the ribs is flattened during maximal inspiration.

In the recumbent position convolutions of the abdominal viscera push the diaphragm upward and backward.

Practical Points

Dyspneic patients prefer to sit and so relieve the thorax of the pressure of the abdominal contents.

Sites of Diaphragmatic Hernias (B)

Diaphragmatic hernias occur when the contents of the abdominal cavity enter the thorax. They may be congenital or acquired. True diaphragmatic defects (blue) must be distinguished from enlargement of pre-existing weak spots (red), such as the esophageal hiatus (**1**), the trigona lumbocostale (**2**) and sternocostale (**3**). True diaphragmatic hernias usually occur in the central tendon (**4**) or the costal part (**5**). The majority of diaphragmatic hernias are prolapses, as they lack a hernial sac. They are known as **false diaphragmatic hernias**. **True hernias** with a sac are uncommon and occur only as paraesophageal hernias.

The commonest congenital hernia is due to enlargement of the vertebrocostal trigone (**2**). Another type of the congenital hernia is **paraesophageal** in position and always occurs on the right side of the esophagus. It is a type of **hiatus hernia**, which, however, in the great majority of cases is an acquired sliding hernia. Sliding hernias have no hernial sac and develop through enlargement of the esophageal hiatus (**1**).

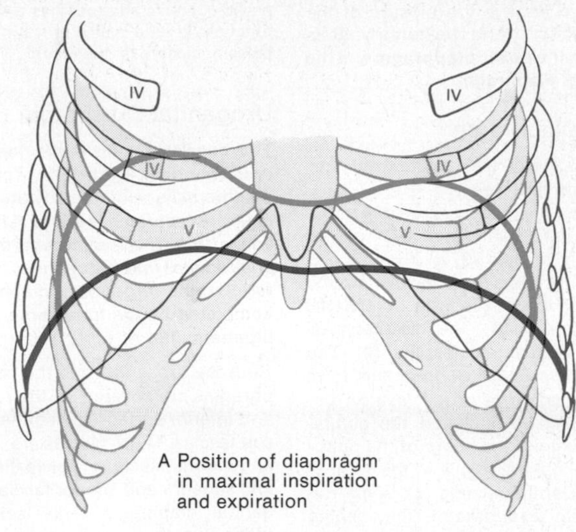

A Position of diaphragm in maximal inspiration and expiration

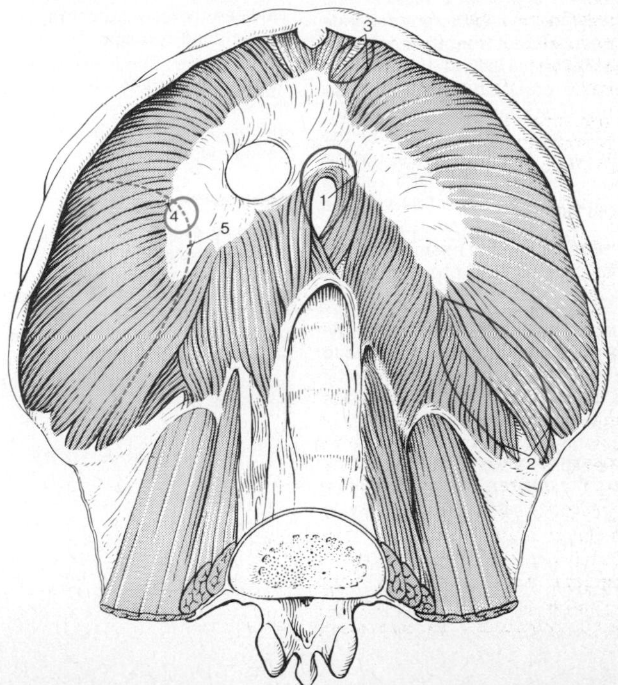

B Sites of occurrence of diaphragmatic hernias

The pelvic floor is the closure of the trunk inferiorly and posteriorly. It is formed by the **pelvic diaphragm** and the **urogenital diaphragm.**

Pelvic Diaphragm

This consists of the **levator ani** and **coccygeus muscles**.

The **levator ani** (**1**) *arises from the pubic bone* (**2**), *the tendinous arch of the levator ani muscle* (**3**) *and the ischial spine* (**4**). Its fibers are divisible into the **puborectalis muscle** (**5**), with its **prerectal (or anterior) fibers**, the **pubococcygeal** and the **iliococcygeal muscles** (**7**). The medial fibers of the puborectalis form the so-called *crura of the levator*, between which is enclosed the *genital hiatus*. Some of the fibers of the puborectalis end pararectally in the sphincter ani externus muscle (**8**), some run on to form a retrorectal sling behind the rectum. The prerectal fibers extend into the perineum and thereby separate the urogenital tract from the anal tract. The genital hiatus is limited laterally by the levator crura and posteriorly by these prerectal fibers. Through the genital hiatus pass the urethra and the genital canal (vagina), while behind the prerectal fibers only the rectum (anal canal) passes. The fibers of the pubococcygeal muscle laterally extend onto the anococcygeal ligament (**9**) and insert on this or directly onto the coccyx (**10**).

The genital hiatus is narrower in the male and broader in the female. Due to the width of the aperture of the genital hiatus a 2nd closure mechanism – the urogenital diaphragm – is essential.

The **coccygeal muscle** (**11**) *arises by means of a tendon from the ischial spine and ends on the coccyx.* It may be absent.

Function

The levator ani is concerned with intra-abdominal pressure. It bears the weight of the pelvic contents and thus has a supporting function. In its dynamic function it participates in closure of the rectum.

Urogenital Diaphragm (12)

This consists mainly of the **deep transversus perinei**. The posterior part of the diaphragm is reinforced by the **superficial transversus perinei** (**13**). *This arises from the ischial tuberosity* (**14**) *and radiates into the perineal body.* Anteriorly the urogenital diaphragm is completed by the **transverse perineal ligament** (**15**).

Both the urogenital and the pelvic diaphragms are covered on their superior and inferior surfaces by connective tissue fascias. These fascias are: superior and inferior fascias of pelvic diaphragm and superior and inferior fascias of urogenital diaphragm. The **ischiorectal fossa**, which is open posteriorly, lies between the pelvic diaphragm and the urogenital diaphragm.

Nerve supply: The pelvic diaphragm is usually supplied by a long branch from the sacral plexus and the urogenital diaphragm by branches from the pudendal nerve.

Practical Points

In women, overstretching of the pelvic diaphragm may cause prolapse of the internal reproductive organs. This is particularly liable to occur after childbirth. It must always be borne in mind that the levator ani muscle may be torn during parturition, with consequent damage to the pelvic diaphragm.

Further details of the pelvic floor are given in Vol. 2, pp. 292–296.

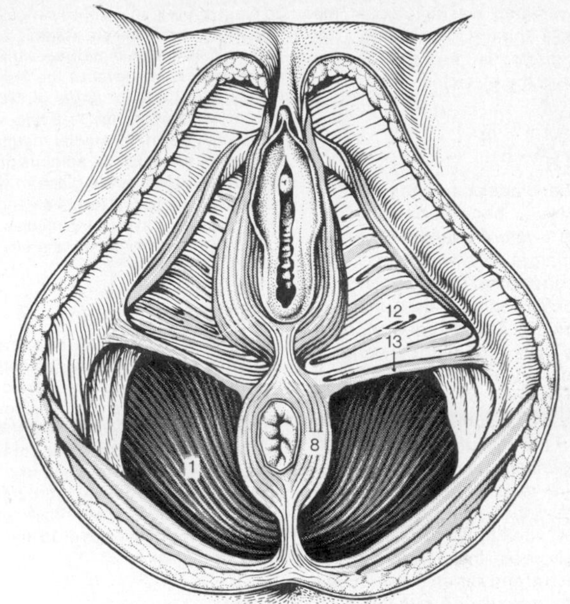

A Pelvic floor in the female,
pelvic and urogenital diaphragms

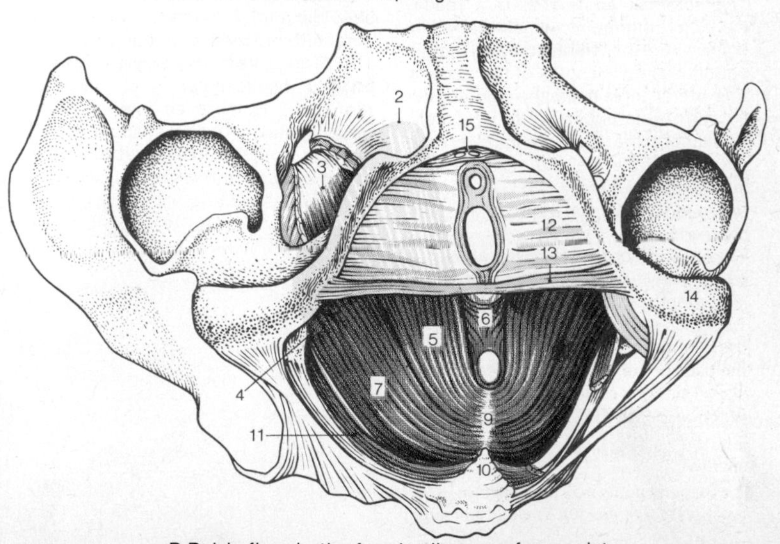

B Pelvic floor in the female, diagram of musculature

In the upper limb we distinguish the **shoulder girdle** and the **free extremity**. The shoulder girdle is formed by the scapulae and the clavicles.

Scapula (A–E)

The shoulder blade or **scapula (A–E)** is a flat, triangular bone. It has a *medial margin* (**1**), a *lateral margin* (**2**) and a *superior margin* (**3**), which are separated from each other by the *superior* (**4**) and *inferior* (**5**) *angles* and the truncate *lateral angle* (**6**). The anterior or *costal surface* is flat and slightly concave (subscapular fossa). It sometimes shows clear lines of muscle attachments. The *dorsal surface* is divided by the *spine of the scapula* (**7**) into a smaller *supraspinous fossa* (**8**) and a larger *infraspinous fossa* (**9**). The spine of the scapula has a triangular base medially, which rises laterally to terminate in a flattened process, the *acromion* (**10**). Near the lateral end lies an oval *articular facet* (**11**) for articulation with the clavicle.

The *acromial angle* (**12**) is a readily palpable bony point, which marks the place where the lateral acromial margin continues into the spine of the scapula. The lateral angle bears the *glenoid cavity* (**13**). At its upper border is a small projection, the *supraglenoid tubercle* (**14**). Below the glenoid cavity lies the *infraglenoid tubercle* (**15**). The *neck of the scapula* (**16**) is adjacent to the glenoid cavity.
The *coracoid process* (**17**) lies above the glenoid cavity. It is bent at a right angle lateroventrally and its tip is flattened. Together with the acromion it protects the joint which lies beneath it. Medial to the base of the coracoid process, on the upper margin of the scapula, lies the *scapular notch* (**18**).

Variants

The scapular notch may be transformed into a *scapular foramen* (**19**). The medial margin of the scapula is sometimes concave and the scapula is then called a **scaphoid scapula**.
The scapula lies on the thorax with the base of its spine at the level of the 3rd thoracic vertebra. The inferior angle of the scapula should lie between ribs 7–8 and, when the arm hangs down, its medial margin should be parallel to the row of spinous processes. The **scapular plane** is the plane in which the scapular plate lies. It forms an angle of 60° with the plane of symmetry (median sagittal). The glenoid cavity faces laterally and anteriorly.

Ossification

The scapula develops **(E)** from several ossification centers. In the 3rd intrauterine month a large bony center develops in the region of the supra- and infraspinous fossae and the spine of the scapula. In the 1st year of life a center develops in the coracoid process, and between the ages of 11 and 18 smaller centers appear throughout the scapula. All the centers fuse with each other, starting at the age of 16 and finishing at about the age of 22.

Ligaments of the Scapula

The **coracoacromial ligament** crosses the shoulder joint and extends between the coracoid process and the acromion. The **superior transverse scapular ligament** bridges the scapular notch. (Only in rare cases is there an inferior transverse ligament of the scapula, which extends from the margin of the spine of the scapula to the glenoid cavity.)

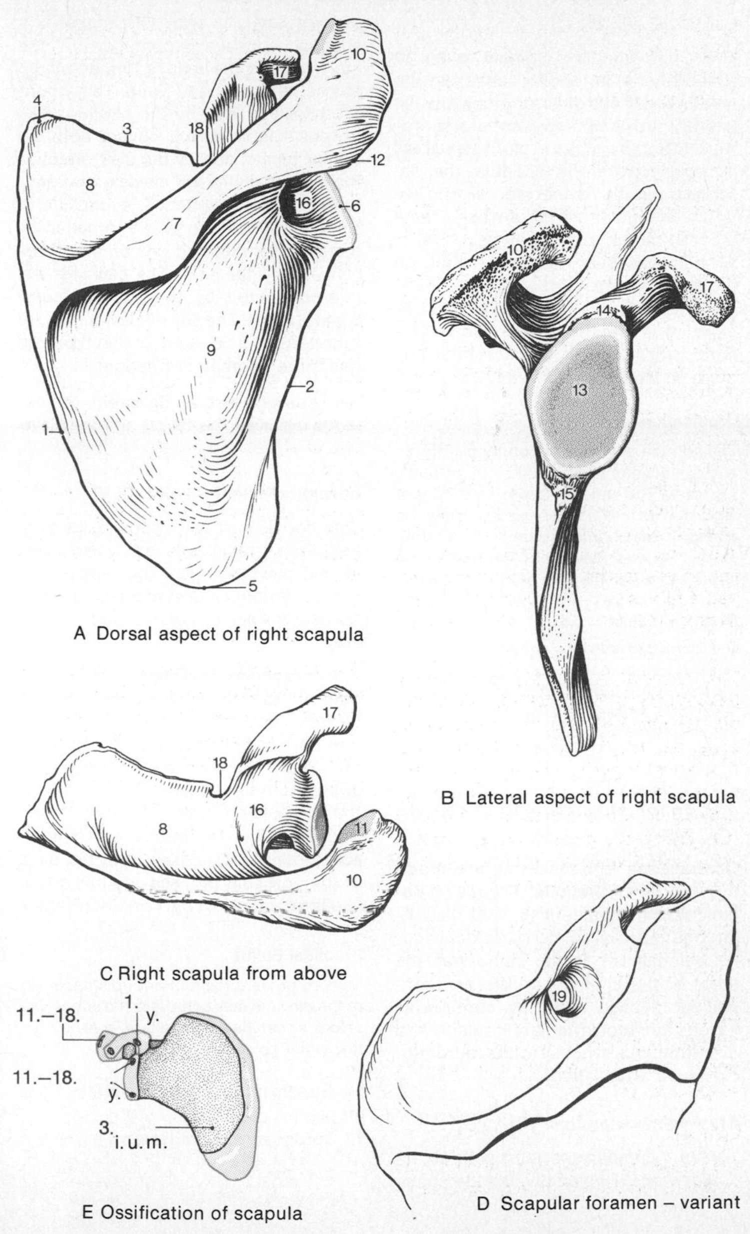

A Dorsal aspect of right scapula

B Lateral aspect of right scapula

C Right scapula from above

D Scapular foramen – variant

E Ossification of scapula

Clavicle (A, B, F)

The collar bone or **clavicle** is an S-shaped bone, anteriorly convex in the medial two thirds of its length, while the lateral third is concave anteriorly. Toward the sternum is the stout **sternal end** (**1**) and toward the scapula the flat **acromial end** (**2**). At the sternal end we find a triangular *sternal articular facet* (**3**). The *acromial articular facet* (**4**) is almost oval. Near the sternal end, on the lower surface of the clavicle, is the *impression for the costoclavicular ligament* (**5**). The prominent *conoid tubercle* (**6**) lies near the acromial end close to the *trapezoid line* (**7**).

Ossification

The clavicle develops in connective tissue, and ossification begins in the 6th intrauterine week. The ends are preformed in cartilage but an ossification center does not appear in the sternal end until 16–20 years of age. It synostoses with the rest of the clavicle between the ages of 21 and 24 years.

Practical Points

Cleidocranial dysostosis is a malformation due to maldevelopment or non-development of the connective tissue part of the clavicle. It is associated with defects of those bones of the skull that are preformed in connective tissue.

Joints of the Shoulder Girdle (C–E)

Connections with the trunk are made through a continuous fibrous (costoclavicular) ligament (**8**) and discontinuous synovial joints (sternoclavicular årticulation). In the same way the parts of the shoulder girdle are connected to each other by continuous fibrous (coracoclavicular ligament) and discontinuous synovial joints (acromioclavicular articulation).

Sternoclavicular Joint (C)

This is a complicated joint with an *articular disk* (**9**) which divides the space of joint cavity in two. The socket is a shallow concave indentation in the sternum, and the head is formed by the sternal end of the clavicle. The incongruity is adjusted by the cartilage-like fibrous tissue, which covers both articular facets, and by the disk, which is fixed cranially to the clavicle and caudally to the sternum. The capsule is slack and thick and is strengthened by the *anterior* (**10**) and *posterior sternoclavicular ligaments.* The clavicles are interconnected by the *interclavicular ligament* (**11**). The sternoclavicular loint functions as a ball-and-socket type and has three degrees of freedom.

The **costoclavicular ligament** (**8**) extends between the 1st rib and the clavicle.

Acromioclavicular Joint (D, E)

This consists of two apposing, almost flat joint surfaces covered by cartilage-like fibrous tissue (**12**). The capsule has a strengthening ligament on its superior surface, the *acromioclavicular ligament* (**13**).

The **coracoclavicular ligament** extends between the coracoid process and the clavicle. It can be divided into anterolateral and posteromedial parts. The lateral part, the **trapezoid ligament** (**14**), arises from the upper medial margin of the coracoid process and extends to the trapezoid line. The medial part, the **conoid ligament** (**15**), arises from the base of the coracoid process and has a fan-like termination on the conoid tubercle.

Practical Points

Marked posterior and inferior displacement of the clavicle may compress the subclavian artery, as can be detected by a weakening of the radial pulse.

16 Superior transverse scapular ligament,
17 Coracoacromial ligament.

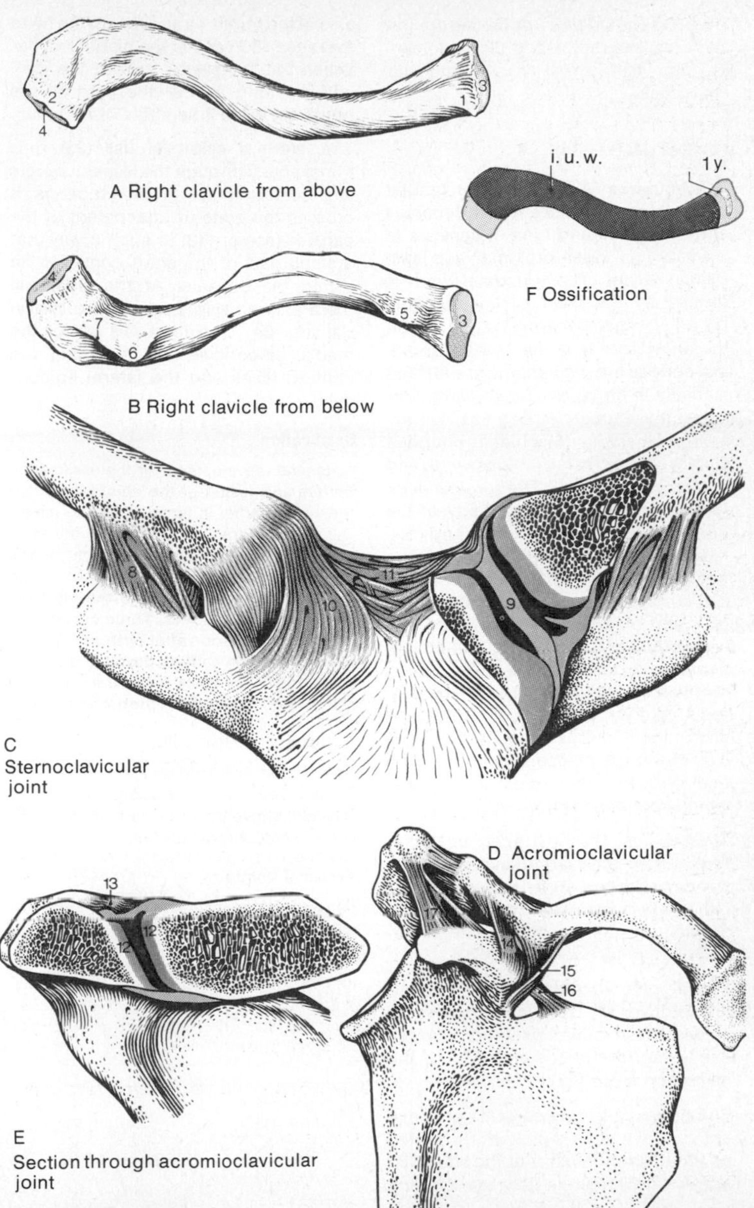

A Right clavicle from above

F Ossification

B Right clavicle from below

C Sternoclavicular joint

D Acromioclavicular joint

E Section through acromioclavicular joint

The bones of the **free upper limb** are the humerus, the radius and ulna, the carpal and metacarpal bones and the phalanges.

Humerus (A–H)

The **humerus** (**A–H**) is a long tubular bone which articulates with the scapula and the radius and ulna. It consists of the **body** and **upper** (proximal) and **lower** (distal) ends. The proximal end is formed by the *head of the humerus* (**1**), adjoining the *anatomic neck* (**2**). On the anterolateral surface of the proximal end lies the *greater tubercle* (**3**), and medially is the *lesser tubercle* (**4**). Between these tubercles begins the *intertubercular sulcus* (**5**) which is bounded distally by the *crests of the lesser* (**6**) and *greater* (**7**) *tubercles*. The *surgical neck* (**8**) lies proximally on the body of the humerus. In the middle of the body lies laterally the *deltoid tuberosity* (**9**). The body may be divided into an *anteromedial surface* (**10**) with a *medial border* (**11**), and an *anterolateral surface* (**12**) with a *lateral border* (**13**), which becomes sharpened distally. The *sulcus for the radial nerve* (**14**) lies on the posterior surface of the body. The distal end of the humerus bears on its medial side the large *medial epicondyle* (**15**) and on the lateral side the smaller *lateral epicondyle* (**16**).

The *trochlea* (**17**) and the *capitulum* (**18**) form surfaces for articulation with the bones of the forearm. The *radial fossa* (**19**) lies proximal to the capitulum, and proximal to the trochlea is the somewhat larger *coronoid fossa* (**20**).

Medial to the trochlea (**D**) there is a shallow groove, the *sulcus for the ulnar nerve* (**21**). On the posterior surface above the trochlea is a deep pit, the *olecranon fossa* (**22**).

The humerus is twisted at its proximal end, i. e., the head is posteriorly rotated at about 20° in relation to the shaft **(torsion angle)**. The angle between the long axis of the humerus and that of the head averages 130°, and at the distal end, between the transverse axis of the joint and the long axis of the body of the humerus, there is an angle of 76° to 89°.

The **proximal epiphysial line** (**23**) runs transversely through the lesser tubercle and inferior to the greater tubercle. It crosses the zone of attachment of the capsule (see p. 113) in such a way that a small part of the shaft comes to lie within the capsule. At the **distal end** there are two **epiphyses** and two **epiphysial lines** (**24**). One epiphysis carries the medial epicondyle and the other the joint surfaces and the lateral epicondyle.

Ossification

In general, development of the ossification centers and fusion of the epiphyses occur somewhat earlier in females than in males. The perichondral bone anlage in the shaft appears in the 2nd–3rd intrauterine month. The endochondral ossification centers in the epiphyses appear between the 2nd week of life and the 12th year. Three centers appear proximally soon after birth, and distally four ossification centers develop later. The distal epiphysial disks fuse during puberty and the proximal disks at the end of puberty.

Variants

Just above the medial epicondyle a *supracondylar process* is occasionally found (**25**), and above the trochlea there may be a *supratrochlear foramen* (**26**).

Practical Points

50% of fractures of the humerus occur in the shaft. There is a risk of damage to the radial nerve.

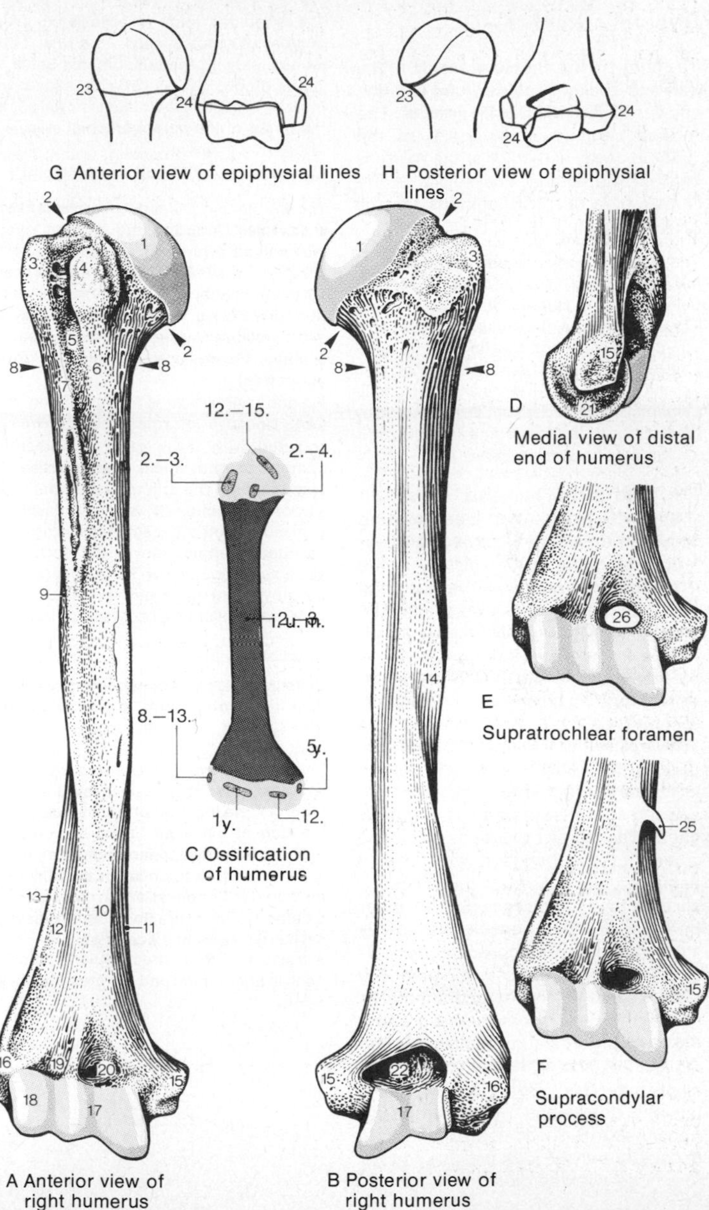

G Anterior view of epiphysial lines

H Posterior view of epiphysial lines

A Anterior view of right humerus

B Posterior view of right humerus

C Ossification of humerus

D Medial view of distal end of humerus

E Supratrochlear foramen

F Supracondylar process

Shoulder Joint (A–G)

The bony socket, the **glenoid cavity**, of the ball-and-socket **shoulder joint** is much smaller than the **head of the humerus.** The hyaline cartilage covering (**1**) of the glenoid cavity is thicker at the margins than in the center. The socket is enlarged by a fibrocartilaginous tip, the **glenoidal lip** (**2**).

The socket is perpendicular to the plane of the scapula and the position of the scapula determines the attitude of the entire joint. The surface of the glenoid cavity has an area of 6 cm^2 to withstand an atmospheric pressure of 6 kp on the joint. The upper limb weighs about 4 kg. As there are no strong ligaments, the shoulder joint is maintained by the action of the enveloping muscles. It is known as a "**muscle-dependent joint**".

The head of the humerus (**3**) is ball-shaped. Its hyaline cartilage covering begins at the anatomical neck and extends somewhat farther distally at the intertubercular sulcus. The cartilage gives the head a more oval shape. The **synovial membrane of the capsule** is attached at the glenoidal lip. It is evaginated like a sac along the long intracapsularly running biceps tendon and surrounds it as a *tubular sheath* (**4**). The **fibrous portion of the joint capsule** in the upper arm (**C**) forms a connective tissue layer across the intertubercular sulcus and converts it into an osteofibrous canal. The **articular capsule** is slack and when the arm hangs down it has a pendent pouch-like part on its medial surface, the *axillar recess* (**5**). The upper portion of the capsule is partly strengthened by the *coracohumeral ligament* (**6**) and three weak glenohumeral ligaments. The coracohumeral ligament (**6**) arises from the base of the coracoid process and radiates into the capsule, extending to the greater and lesser tubercles. When the arm is hanging in its normal anatomic position, the upper half of the head of the humerus is in contact with the joint capsule and the lower half with the glenoid cavity.

The shoulder joint is associated with a number of synovial sacs. As a rule, it communicates with the subcoracoid bursa, the subtendinous bursa of the subscapular muscle, the intertubercular synovial sac and the bursa of the coracobrachial muscle.

Movements of the Shoulder Joint

The shoulder joint has **three degrees of freedom of movement. Abduction** and **adduction** refer to movements away from the position of rest (**D**) of the head of the humerus in the scapular plane (see p. 106). Purely lateral abduction (**E**) always produces **retroversion** and slight **rotation**, while abduction from the scapular plane is anteriorly directed (frontal abduction).
Flexion **(anteversion)** is forward lifting of the arm. Because of rotary components associated with these other movements, a compound movement, **circumduction**, occurs in which the arm traces the surface of a cone. Abduction (**E**) is *always* associated with movement of the scapula; excessive associated scapular movement occurs with abduction of more than 90° (**F**), because then the movement of the joint is restricted by the coracoacromial ligament (see p. 108).

Practical Points

Dislocation is more common in the shoulder than in any other joint. If associated with a torn capsule, it usually occurs low and in front.
The palpable and visible protuberance of the shoulder joint is produced by the greater tubercle, the location of which indicates the position of the head of the humerus. The protuberance disappears when the shoulder is dislocated, as the head of the humerus is no longer in its socket. When palpating a dislocated shoulder the finger enters an empty cavity (**G**) below the acromion.
A fracture of the (intracapsular) anatomical neck is uncommon and the prognosis is very poor.

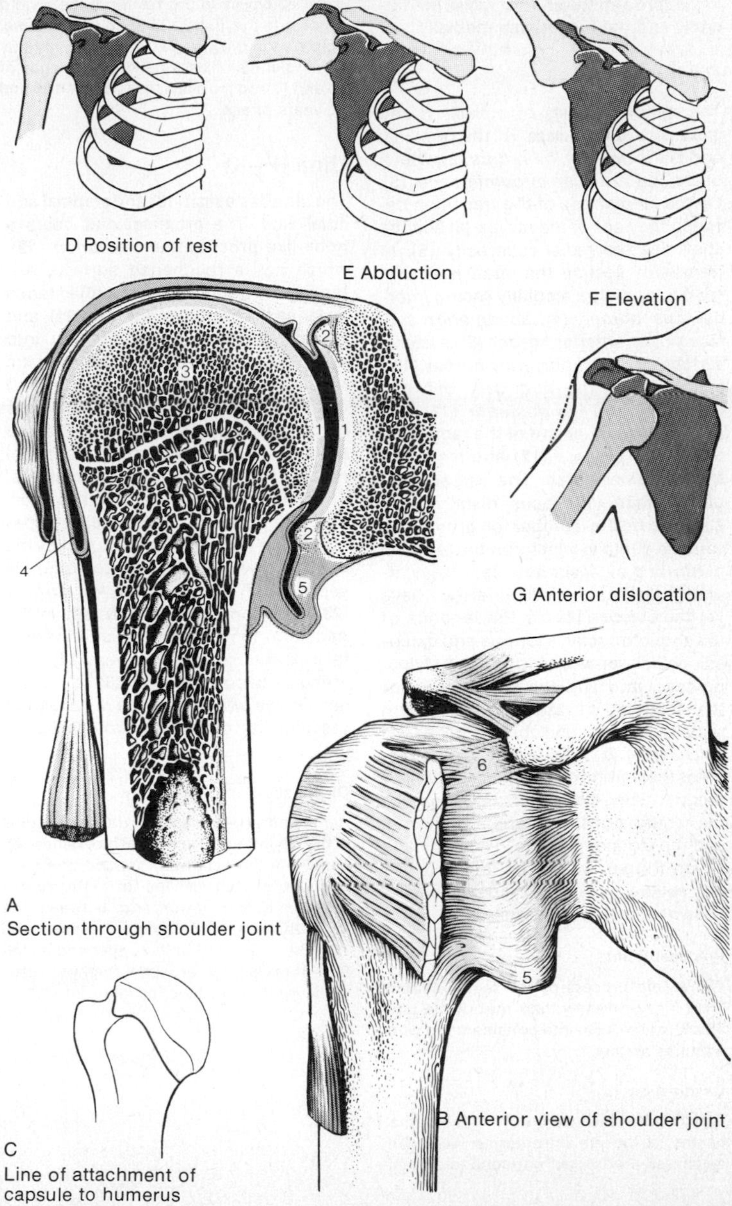

D Position of rest

E Abduction

F Elevation

G Anterior dislocation

A
Section through shoulder joint

B Anterior view of shoulder joint

C
Line of attachment of capsule to humerus

In the **forearm** the shorter **radius** lies laterally and the longer **ulna** medially.

Radius (A–E)

The **radius** consists of a **shaft** (**1**) and **proximal** and **distal ends**. At the proximal end is the *head of the radius* (**2**), which bears the *articular circumference* (**3**). On the medial side of the transition between the *neck of the radius* (**4**) and the shaft lies the *radial tuberosity* (**5**). In transverse section the shaft is almost triangular with a medially facing *interosseous border* (**6**), an *anterior surface* (**7**), an *anterior border* (**8**), a *lateral surface* (**9**) and a *posterior border* (**10**), which forms the boundary between the *lateral* and the *posterior* (**11**) *surfaces*. At the lower end of the radius lies the *styloid process* (**12**) and medial to it is the *ulnar notch*. The *carpal articular surface* (**13**) faces distally. Dorsally we find a number of grooves of variable depth in which run the tendons of the long extensor muscles. From lateral (radial) to medial (ulnar) we have *1st* the *sulcus* (**14**) for the tendons of the abductor pollicis longus and extensor pollicis brevis lying on the styloid process, and *2nd* the *sulcus* (**15**) for the tendons of the extensor carpi radialis longus and brevis. The *3rd sulcus* (**16**) is oblique and accommodates the tendon of the extensor pollicis longus. The *4th sulcus* (**17**) carries the tendons of the extensor digitorum and the extensor indicis. The bony elevation (ridge), which lies lateral to the 3rd sulcus, is usally palpable and is known as the **dorsal tubercle.**

Practical Points

The styloid process of the radius extends 1 cm further distally than that of the ulna. This must be taken into consideration when fractures are set.

Ossification

Perichondral ossification of the radial shaft begins in the 7th intrauterine week. The epiphyses are formed endochondrally, the distal epiphysis in the 1st–2nd, the styloid process in the 10th–12th, and the proximal epiphysis in the 4th–7th year. The proximal epiphysial disk closes between the ages of 14 and 17 and the distal disk between 20 and 25 years of age.

Ulna (F–K)

The **ulna** has a **shaft** (**18**) and **proximal** and **distal ends**. The proximal end bears a hook-like process, the *olecranon* (**19**), which has a roughened surface. Anteriorly the *trochlear notch* (**20**) extends as far as the *coronoid process* (**21**), and laterally is the *radial notch* (**22**) into which the articular circumference of the radius fits. At the junction with the shaft lies the *ulnar tuberosity* (**23**). The *crest of the supinator muscle* (**24**) is directed laterally in an extension of the radial notch. The shaft is triangular in shape. The *interosseous border* (**25**) lies laterally. The *anterior surface* (**26**) is separated from the *medial surface* (**29**) by the *anterior border* (**27**). The latter in turn is separated from the *posterior surface* (**28**) by the *posterior margin* (**30**). In the middle of the ulna, on its anterior surface, is the *nutrient foramen* (**31**). The *articular circumference* (**33**) is on the *head of the ulna* (**32**). At the distal end of the ulna is the small *styloid process* (**34**).

Ossification

Perichondral ossification of the shaft begins in the 7th intrauterine week. The ossification centers in the epiphyses are laid down endochondrally between the 4th–11th years of life (Y), at the lower end between the 4th–7th years, in the styloid process in the 7th–8th years and at the upper end by the 9th–11th year. The proximal epiphysis fuses earlier and the distal ones later.

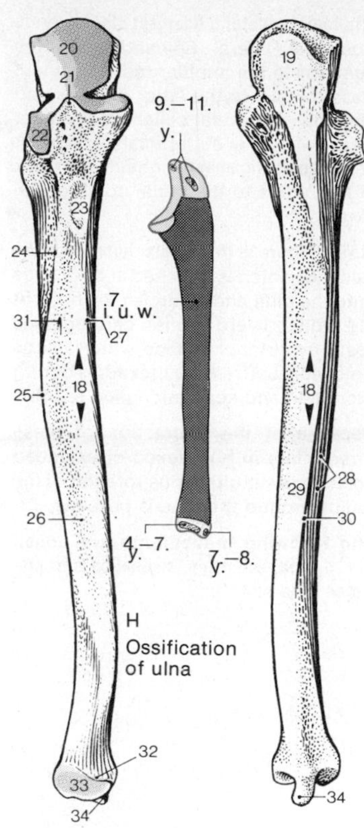

H
Ossification
of ulna

F Anterior view of right ulna

G Posterior view of right ulna

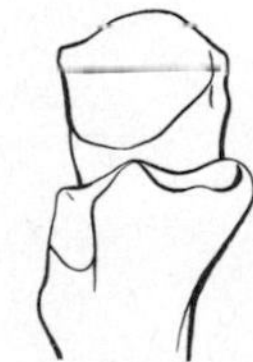

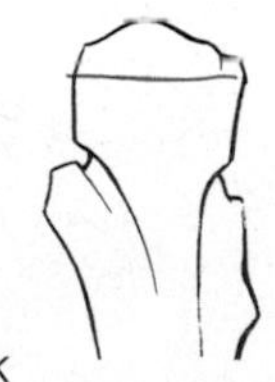

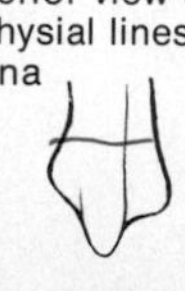

J
Anterior view of epiphysial lines of ulna

K
Posterior view of epiphysial lines of ulna

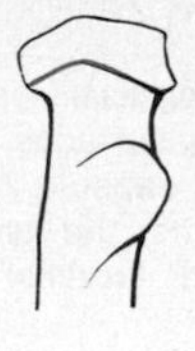

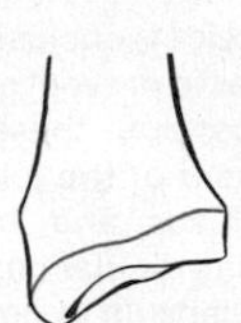

D
Anterior view of epiphysial lines of radius

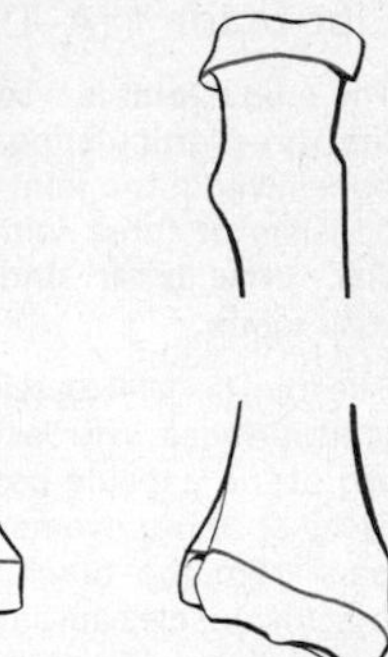

E
Posterior view of epiphysial lines of radius

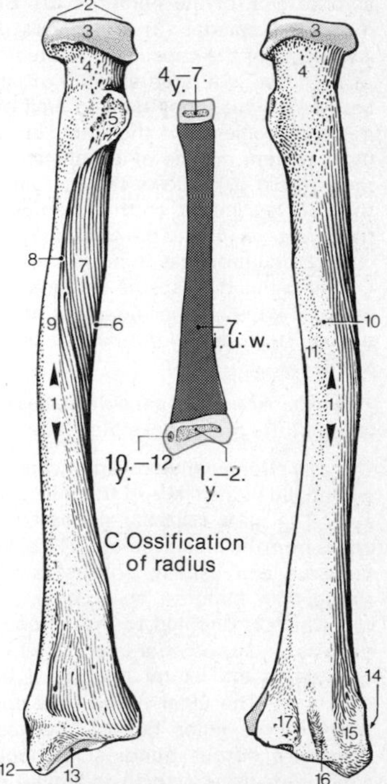

C Ossification of radius

A Anterior view of right radius

B Posterior view of right radius

Elbow Joint (A–D)

The **elbow joint** is a **compound joint** with the three articulating surfaces of the bones within the joint capsule. It really consists of three joints, the **humeroradial, humeroulnar** and **proximal radioulnar** joints.

The thin, lax **joint capsule** (**1**) encloses the joint surfaces. In order to prevent pinching of the capsule between these surfaces during movement of the joint, fibers from the brachialis and biceps brachii muscles act as articular muscles and radiate into the capsule in order to tense it. Both *humeral epicondyles* (**2**) are outside the capsule (**D**). The synovial membrane surrounds the olecranon fossa and both fossae on the anterior side of the humerus (**D**). Between the **synovial** (**3**) and **fibrous** (**4**) **membranes** of the capsule in the region of the fossa is a large amount of fatty tissue (**5**), which may help to limit extreme movements of the joint. In the ulnar region, the line of attachment of the capsule (**D**) follows the margin of the trochlear notch, so that the tips of the *olecranon* (**6**) and the *coronoid process* (**7**) still project within the capsule. On the radius the capsule extends as a sac below the *annular ligament of the radius* (**8**), the *superior recessus sacciformis* (**9**).

This extension of the capsule makes rotation of the radius possible.

The very strong collateral ligaments are embedded in the sides of the joint capsule. The **ulnar collateral ligament** (**10**) arises from the medial epicondyle of the humerus and usually possesses *two strong fiber bundles*, an *anterior one* (**11**) which is directed to the coronoid process, and a *posterior one* (**12**) which extends to the lateral margin of the olecranon. The ulnar nerve runs posterior to the latter bundle. Between these two fibrous bundles lies loose connective tissue, which is limited on the ulnar side by *oblique fibers* (**13**).

The **radial collateral ligament** (**14**) extends from the lateral epicondyle of the humerus to the annular radial ligament and proximal to the latter radiates into the ulna. The radial collateral ligament fuses with the superficial extensors. The **quadrate ligament** connects the neck of the radius to the radial notch of the ulna.

Finally, there is the **annular ligament of the radius** (**8**) which is attached at both ends onto the ulna and encircles the head of the radius. There is often cartilaginous tissue on its inner surface, which acts as a movable buttress for the radius during pronation and supination (see p. 118).

Because of the interaction of these three joints in any flexed or extended position, a simultaneous rotation of the radius around the ulna is possible.

The following movements are possible: flexion, extension, supination and **pronation** (see p. 118).

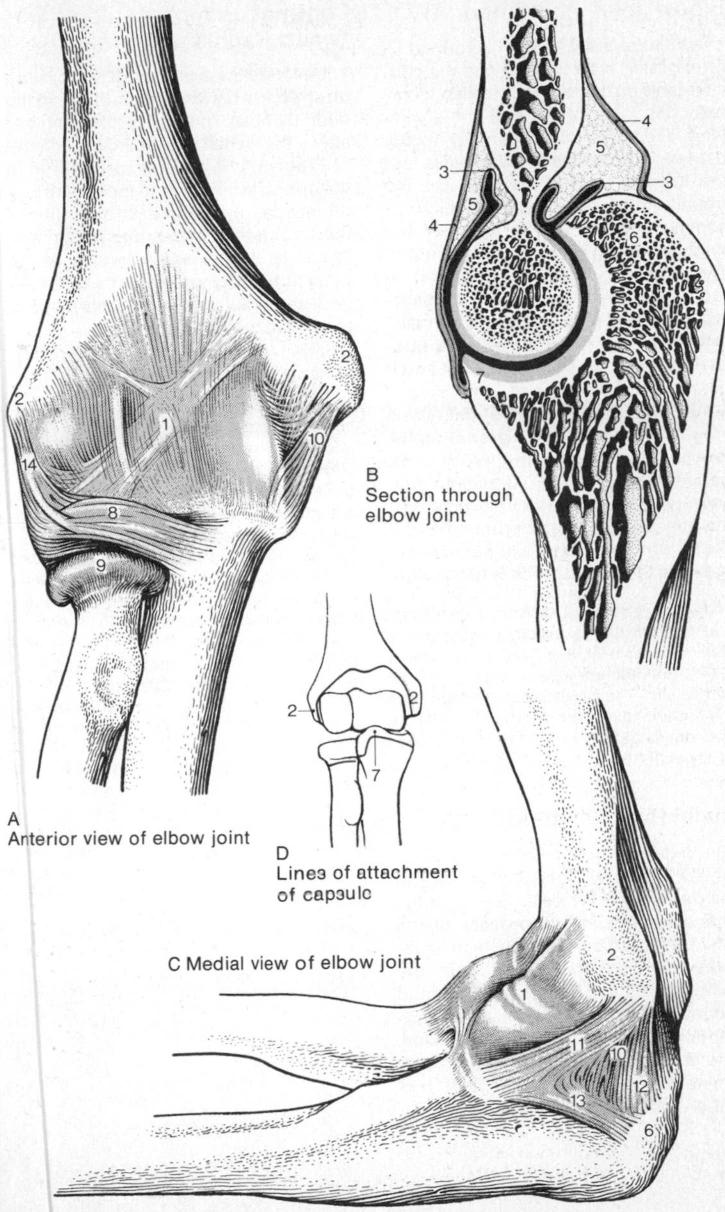

A
Anterior view of elbow joint

B
Section through elbow joint

C Medial view of elbow joint

D
Lines of attachment of capsule

Elbow Joint, continued (A)

The **humeroradial joint** (**1**) is formed by the **capitulum of the humerus** and the concave **fovea** on the **head of the radius**. It corresponds in form to a ball-and-socket joint. The **humeroulnar joint** (**2**) occurs between the **trochlea of the humerus** and the **trochlear notch of the ulna**. On the trochlea there is a *channel* (**3**) which accommodates the leading edge of the trochlear notch. This is a hinge joint. The **proximal radioulnar joint** (**4**) is formed between the **articular circumference of the head of the radius** and the **radial notch of the ulna,** together with the **annular ligament** (**5**). This is a pivot joint and it permits movements of the radius around the ulna. Rotation of the radius around the ulna is called **pronation** (**B**) (bones cross over each other) or **supination** (**C**) (bones lie parallel to one another). The axis of this movement of the bones of the forearm runs from the center of the fovea on the head of the radius to the styloid process of the ulna.

The **anteriorly measured angle** between the arm and forearm during maximal extension is slightly larger in females (180°) than in males (175°). Children are able to overextend the elbow joint. The **radially measured angle** with the forearm fully extended (the angle of abduction) ranges from 158 – 180°, with a mean of about 168,5°.

Distal Radioulnar Joint (D)

The **distal radioulnar joint** (**6**), a pivot joint is formed by the **head of the ulna** and the **ulnar notch of the radius.** Between the radius and the styloid process of the ulna lies an articular disk, which separates the distal radioulnar from the radiocarpal joint. The **capsule** is lax and extends from the *inferior recessus sacciformis* (**7**) up to the shaft of the ulna. The **proximal** and **distal radioulnar joints** are necessarily combined joints to permit pronation and supination.

Continuous Fibrous Joint Between Radius and Ulna (D)

The **interosseous membrane** of the forearm (**8**) stretches between the radius and the ulna. Its fibers run from proximal laterally to the medial side of the ulna distally. Fibers of the *oblique cord* (**9**) run in the opposite direction to those of the interosseous membrane. It strengthens the interosseus membrane proximally. The cord begins approximately at the ulnar tuberosity and extends to the interosseous border of the radius distal to the radial tuberosity.

Practical Points

The interosseous membrane not only prevents parallel displacement of the radius and ulna but also allows pulling and pressure stresses to be transmitted from one bone to the other. It is so strong that during overstrain of the forearm the bones tend to fracture before the fibers are torn.

The commonest of all fractures (described by Colles in 1814) is at a **classical site on the radius**, and is due to a fall on the palm of the hand with the arm extended. The weight of the body is transmitted through the humerus and the ulna and then passes through the interosseous membrane to the radius. The distal end of the radius resists the counterpressure, so that maximal stress develops and causes a fracture of the lower radius. The distal fragment is displaced radially and dorsally as the fibers of the interosseous membrane fix the shaft of the radius to the ulna (bayonet position).

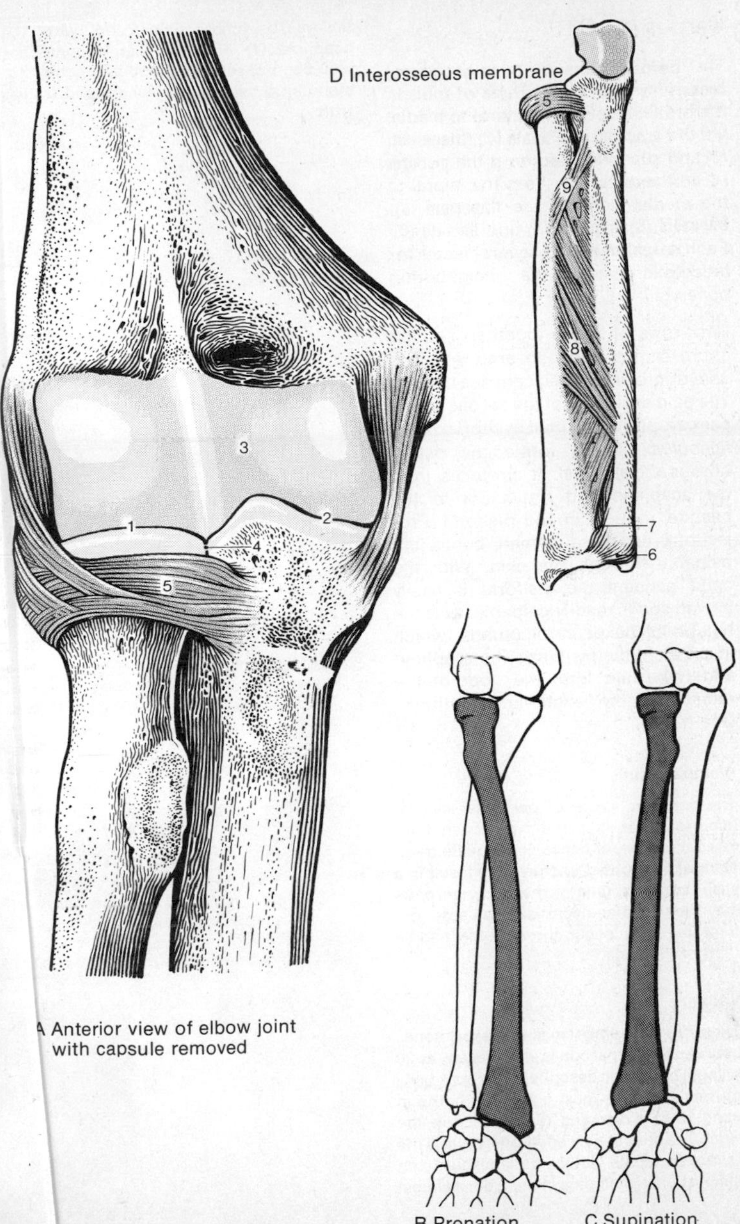

A Anterior view of elbow joint with capsule removed

B Pronation

C Supination

Carpus (A–C)

The **carpus** consists of eight **carpal bones** arranged in two rows of four. In the proximal row from lateral to medial are the **scaphoid** (**1**), **lunate** (**2**), **triquatrum** (**3**) and superimposed on it the **pisiform** (**4**). In the distal row from the lateral to the medial side are the **trapezium** (**5**), **trapezoid** (**6**), **capitate** (**7**) and **hamate** (**8**). Each carpal bone has several facets for articulation with the neighboring bones.

Both rows of bones together, i.e., the entire carpus, form an arch which is convex proximally and concave distally. The palmar surface of the carpus is also concave and is spanned by the *flexor retinaculum,* which forms the osteofibrous **carpal tunnel.** It stretches from the scaphoid and trapezium to the hamate, triquetrum and pisiform. Projections on these named bones are palpable through the skin. With the hand pendent the pisiform is easily moved and is readily palpable, as is the tendon of flexor carpi ulnaris, which inserts into the pisiform. The scaphoid and trapezium form the floor of the radial fossa, the "anatomical snuffbox" (see p. 376).

Practical Points

The scaphoid (**1**) is of particular clinical importance as it is the most often fractured of all carpal bones. Inadequate treatment of a scaphoid fracture may result in a pseudarthrosis. One of the fractured parts may even become necrotic. Of all scaphoid fractures 70% occur through the middle third of the bone.

Variants

There are sometimes small accessory bones between the carpal bones and as many as 20 of them have been described. The possibility of their presence must always be borne in mind when examining radiographs of the wrist. The commonest additional bone is the **os centrale** (**9**). Its cartilaginous anlage is an almost constant finding in man, but it almost always becomes synostosed with the scaphoid (**1**). Fusion of carpal bones has also been described, the most frequent fusion being between the lunate and triquetrum.

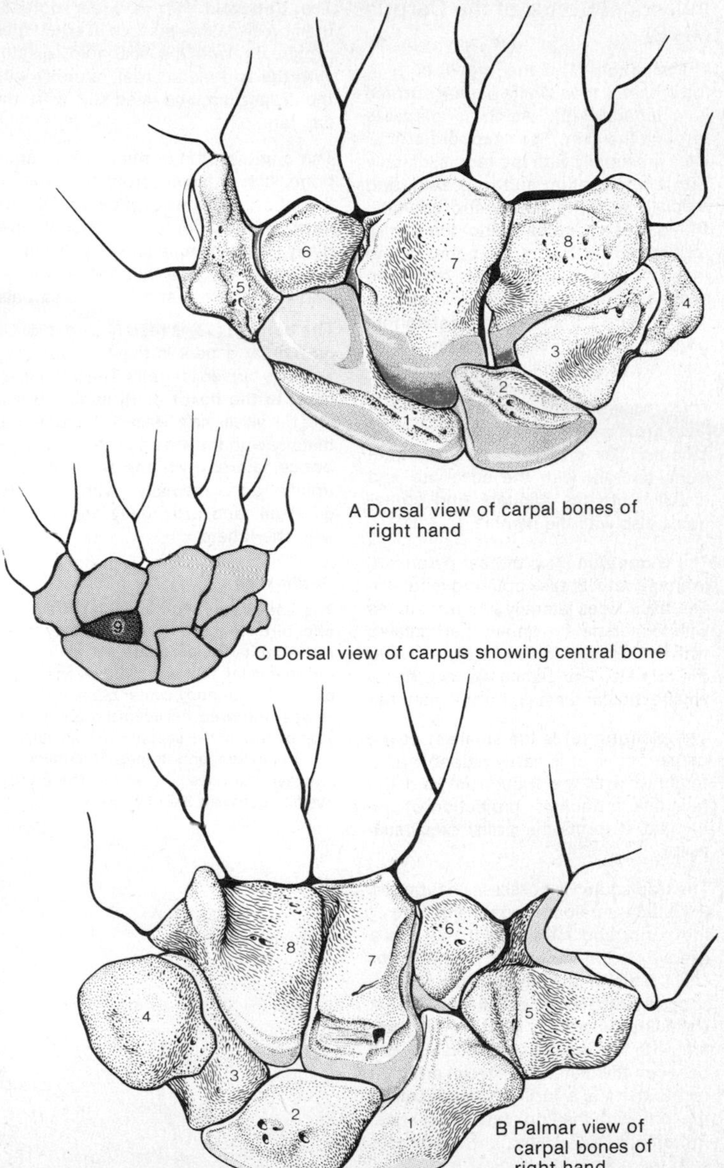

A Dorsal view of carpal bones of right hand

C Dorsal view of carpus showing central bone

B Palmar view of carpal bones of right hand

Individual Bones of the Carpus (A–B)

The **scaphoid** (**1**) is the largest bone in the proximal row. On its palmar surface is a *tubercle* (**2**), which is palpable through the skin. The scaphoid articulates proximally with the radius, distally with the trapezium and trapezoid, and medially with the lunate and capitate. Blood vessels enter along the entire roughened surface of the bone. In one third of cases, blood vessels reach the scaphoid bone only on its distal face and in them a fracture of the scaphoid bone (see p. 120) may be followed by necrosis of the proximal fragment.

The crescent-shaped **lunate** (**3**) articulates proximally with the radius and the articular disk, medially with the triquetrum, laterally with the scaphoid and distally with the capitate and sometimes also with the hamate.

The **triquetrum** (**4**) is almost pyramidal in shape with its apex pointing medially. The base faces laterally and articulates with the lunate. Proximally it articulates with the articular disk and distally with the hamate. The palmar surface has a small articular facet (**5**) for the pisiform.

The **pisiform** (**6**) is the smallest of the carpal bones. It is easily palpable and, together with the triquetrum and the hamulus, a hooklike projection of the hamate, it forms the **medial carpal eminence.**

The **trapezium** (**7**) possesses a *tubercle* (**8**), which is palpable on dorsiflexion of the hand, and medial to it there is a groove (**9**) for the tendon of the flexor carpi radialis. Distally it has a saddle-shaped articular facet (**10**) for the 1st metacarpal bone. A facet for articulation with the trapezoid lies medially, and between the distal and medial articular facets there is a further small facet for the joint with the 2nd metacarpal bone. Proximally the trapezium articulates with the scaphoid.

The **trapezoid** (**11**) is wider dorsally than on its palmar surface. It articulates proximally with the scaphoid, distally with the 2nd metacarpal, laterally with the trapezium and medially with the capitate.

The **capitate** (**12**) is the largest carpal bone. It has facets proximally for articulation with the scaphoid and the lunate, laterally for the trapezoid, medially for the hamate and distally mainly for the 3rd metacarpal bone, as well as partly for the 2nd and 4th metacarpals.

The **hamate** (**13**) is readily palpable. On its palmar aspect is the *hamulus* (**14**), which is curved laterally. The latter is related to the flexor digiti minimi brevis and the **pisohamate ligament**. It articulates distally with the 4th and 5th metacarpal bones, laterally with the capitate, proximally and medially with the triquetrum, and proximally and laterally with the lunate.

Ossification

The centers develop endochondrally only after birth. In the 1st year of life they appear in the capitate and hamate, and in the 2nd to 3rd year in the triquetrum. Between the ages of 2 and 6 the bony center of the lunate develops, followed between the 3rd and 6th year by that in the scaphoid. Ossification in the trapezium and trapezoid commences between the ages of 4 and 6. The pisiform ossifies between 8 and 12 years of age.

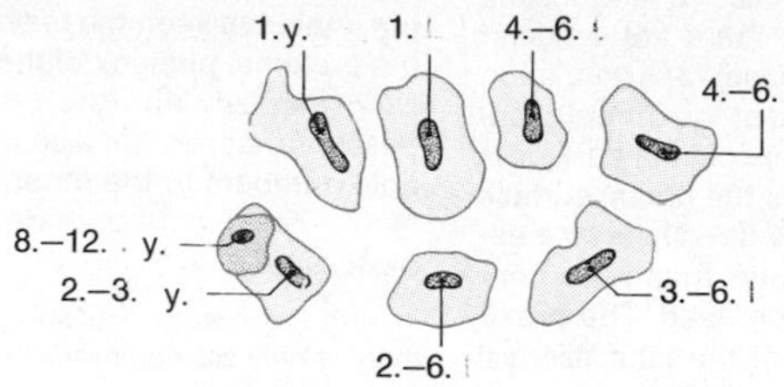

B Development of carpal bones

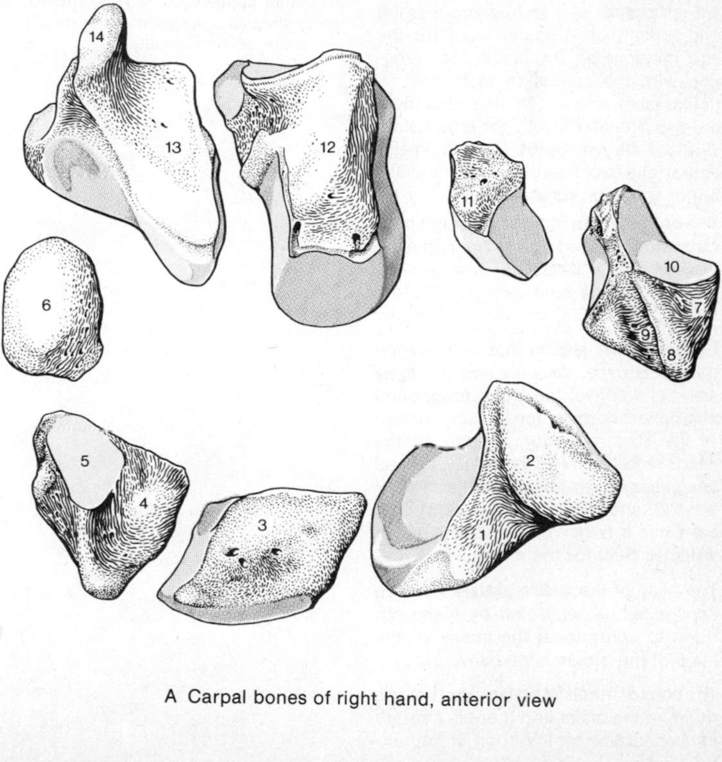

A Carpal bones of right hand, anterior view

Bones of the Metacarpus and Digits (A–C)

The five **metacarpals** of the hand each have a *head* (**1**), a *shaft* (**2**) and a *base* (**3**). On all of them there are articular facets at one end (base) for articulation with the carpals and at the other (head) for the phalanges. The palmar surface is slightly concave and the dorsal surface slightly convex. The dorsal surface exhibits a characteristic triangular configuration toward the head. The proximal articular facet of the **1st metacarpal** is saddle-shaped; the **2nd metacarpal** has a notched base proximally for articulation with the carpus and on the medial side with the 3rd metacarpal. On the dorsoradial side of the base of the **3rd metacarpal** is a *styloid process* (**4**) and radially an articular facet for the 2nd metacarpal. Proximally, for junction with the carpus there is one articular facet, and on the ulnar side there are two articular facets for articulation with the **4th metacarpal.** The 4th metacarpal has two articular facets radially but only one on its ulnar side.

The **bones of the digits**: Each digit consists of more than one bone, namely a **proximal** (**5**), a **medial** (**6**) and a **distal phalanx** (**7**). The sole exception is the thumb, which has only two phalanges.

Each **proximal phalanx** has a flattened palmar surface, dorsally and transversally it is convex and has roughened sharpened borders for the attachment of the fibrous tendon sheaths of the flexor muscles. It has a *shaft* (**8**), a distal *phalangeal head* (also called a "trochlea") (**9**) and a proximal *base* (**10**). The base has a transverse oval socket, an articular facet for the metacarpals.

The base of the **middle phalanx** has two convex facets separated by a smooth ridge to conform to the shape of the head of the proximal phalanx.

The base of the **distal phalanx** also bears a ridge. At the distal end there is a rough palmar surface for insertion of the tendon of the flexor digitorum profundus as well as a palmar-facing roughened, spade-shaped *plate* (**11**) at its terminus.

Sesamoid bones are regularly found in the joints between the metacarpals and the proximal phalanx of the thumb, one lying medially and the other laterally. Sesamoid bones are also found in variable numbers in the other fingers.

Ossification

In both the metacarpals and the phalanges there is only **one** epiphysial center of ossification in addition to the perichondral diaphysis (3rd intrauterine month). In the metacarpals the distal epiphysial centers develop in the 2nd year of life, except for the 1st metacarpal, in whose proximal end the center appears in the 2nd–3rd year. In the phalanges epiphysial ossification centers occur only proximally.

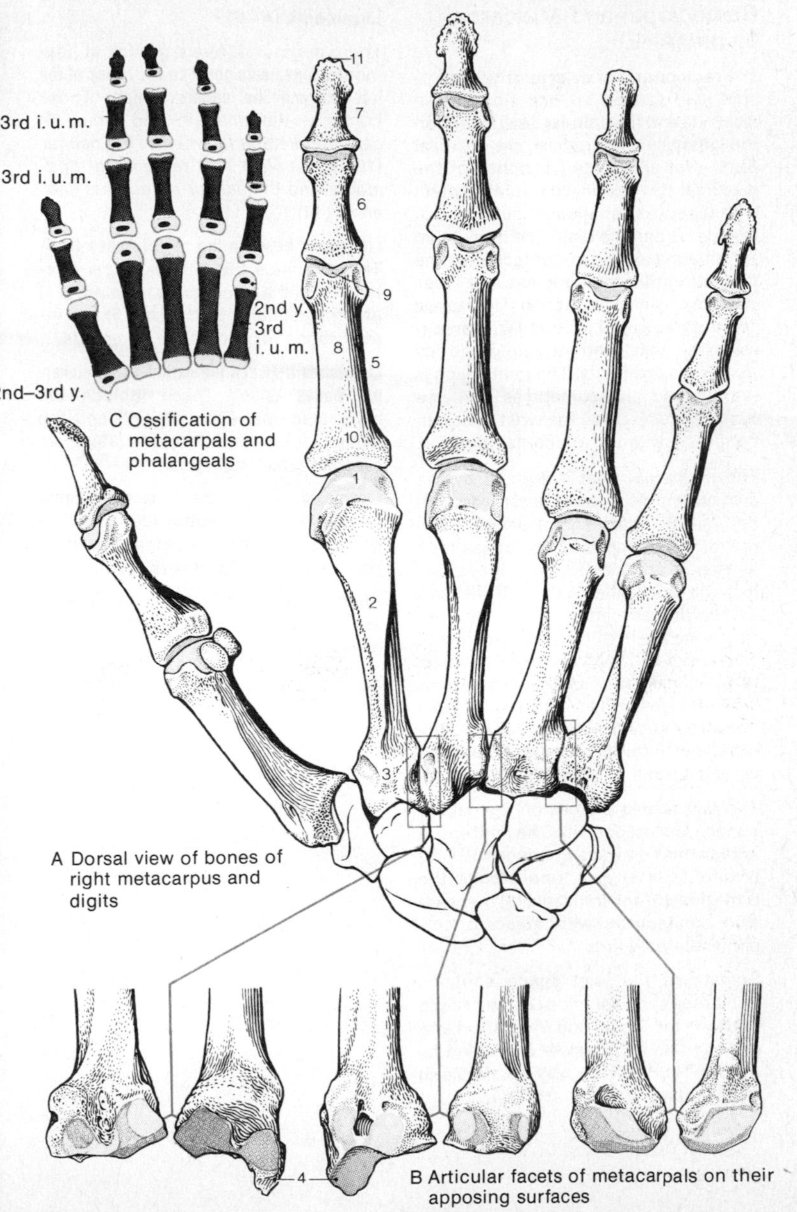

C Ossification of metacarpals and phalangeals

A Dorsal view of bones of right metacarpus and digits

B Articular facets of metacarpals on their apposing surfaces

Radiocarpal and Midcarpal Joints (A–E)

The **radiocarpal** or **wrist joint** is an ellipsoid joint formed on one side by the **radius** (**1**) and the **articular disk** (**2**) and on the other by the **proximal row of carpal bones**. Not all the carpal bones of the proximal row are in continual contact with the socket-shaped articular face of the radius and the disk. The triquetrum (**3**) only makes close contact with the disk during ulnar abduction and loses contact on radial abduction. The **capsule** of the radiocarpal joint is lax, dorsally relatively thin, and is reinforced by numerous ligaments, The joint space is unbranched and sometimes contains *synovial folds.* Often the wrist joint is in continuity with the midcarpal joint.

The **midcarpal joint** is formed by the **proximal** and **distal row** of **carpal bones** and has an "S"-shaped joint space. Each row of carpal bones can be considered as a single articular body and they interlock with each other. Although there is a certain limited degree of mobility between members of the proximal row of carpal bones, this is not true of the distal row because they are joined one to another (**4**) as well as to the metacarpal bones by strong ligaments. Thus, the distal row of carpal bones and the metacarpals form a functional entity.

The **joint capsule** is tense on the palmar surface and lax dorsally. The joint space is branched and has connections with the radiocarpal joint, and around the trapezium (**5**) and trapezoid (**6**) there are also connections with adjacent carpometacarpal joints.

Sometimes the joint space contains numerous *synovial folds* (**7**). The space between the lunate and triquetrum and the capitate and hamate is padded by synovial folds which may be visible in radiographs.

Ligaments (A–E)

There are four different groups of ligaments. **Ligaments between the bones of the forearm and the carpus (violet).** These comprise the *ulnar* (**8**) and *radial* (**9**) *carpal collateral ligaments*, the *palmar* (**10**) and *dorsal* (**11**) *radiocarpal ligaments* and the *palmar ulnocarpal ligament* (**12**).

Ligaments between the carpal bones (red). These include the *radiate carpal ligament* (**13**), the *pisohamate ligament* (**14**) and the *palmar* (**15**), *dorsal* (**16**) and *interosseous* (**4**) *intercarpal ligaments.*

Ligaments between the carpal and metacarpal bones (blue). These include the *pisometacarpal ligament* (**17**) and the *palmar* (**18**) and *dorsal* (**19**) *carpometacarpal ligaments.*

Ligaments between the metacarpal bones (yellow). These are subdivided into *dorsal* (**20**), *interosseous* (**21**) and *palmar* (**22**) *metacarpal ligaments.*

Almost all of these ligaments strengthen the joint capsules and partly direct the movements of the wrist.

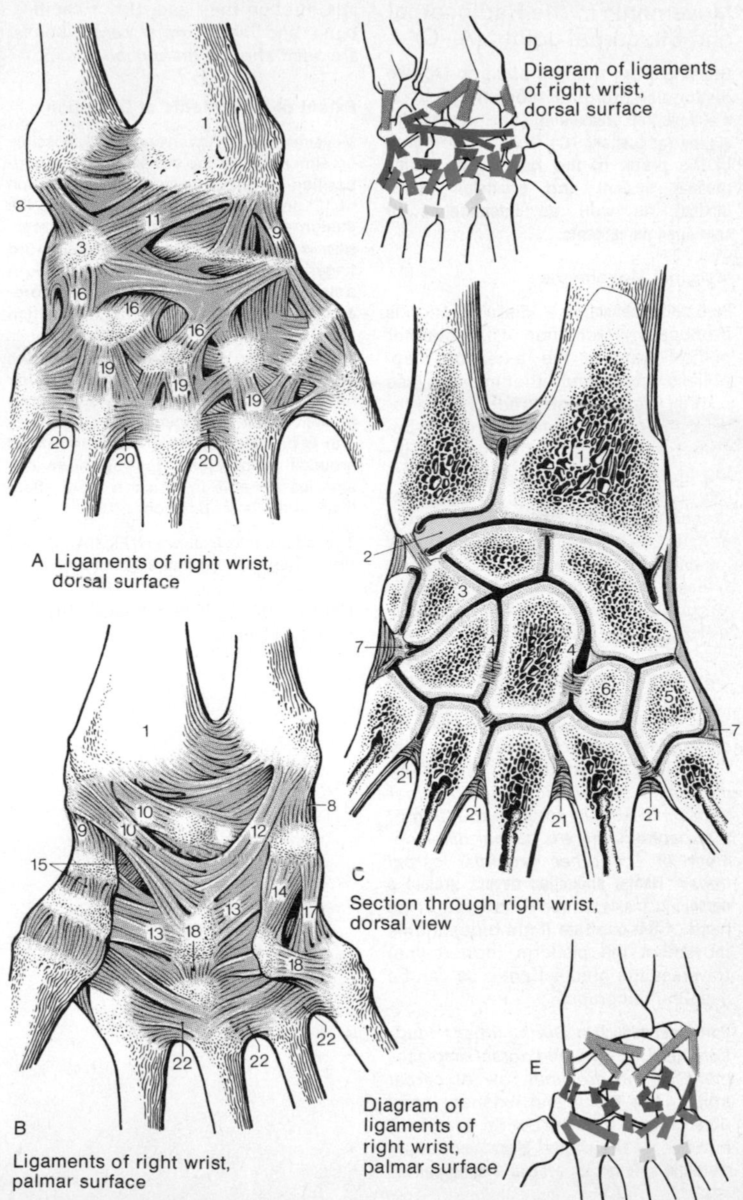

A Ligaments of right wrist, dorsal surface

B Ligaments of right wrist, palmar surface

C Section through right wrist, dorsal view

D Diagram of ligaments of right wrist, dorsal surface

Diagram of ligaments of right wrist, palmar surface

Movements in the Radiocarpal and Midcarpal Joints (A–C)

Starting from the mid-position (**A**), we distinguish **marginal movements** of **radial deviation (abduction)** (**B**) and **ulnar deviation (adduction)** (**C**) from **movements in the plane of the hand,** i. e., **flexion (palmar flexion)** and **extension (dorsiflexion)** as well as **intermediate or combined movements.**

Marginal Movements

Pure radial abduction: Radial abduction is produced by interaction of the abductor pollicis longus, the extensor carpi radialis longus and other muscles (see p. 168). The scaphoid (red) is tilted toward the palmar surface, where it becomes palpable through the skin. Tilting of this bone allows the trapezium (blue) and trapezoid (green) to approach the radius. Since the trapezoid and the 2nd metacarpal bone are rigidly joined together and the flexor carpi radialis and extensor carpi radialis longus are inserted into the 2nd metacarpal bone, radial abduction represents a pulling action on this functional unit. The trapezoid glides along the scaphoid and, as the latter bone is not fixed, it can be moved, and since it cannot free itself from its other articulations, it is forced to tilt. *This tilting movement occurs along a radioulnar transverse axis. In addition to tilting of the scaphoid, there is palmar displacement of the other proximal carpal bones.* **Radial abduction occurs around a dorsopalmar axis**, which runs through the head of the capitate (light blue). In this movement the pisiform (dotted line) traverses the greatest path, as can be seen in radiographs.

Pure ulnar adduction: *During ulnar adduction there is tilting and dorsal displacement, of the proximal row of carpal bones.* The flexor and extensor carpi ulnaris act together with the long muscles of the digits. **Movement toward the ulnar side occurs around a dorsopalmar axis** through the head of the capitate bone, and the *proximal carpal bones are tilted about a radioulnar axis.*

Extent of Movements of Deviation

Movements of deviation are equally possible on either side of the **mid-position**. The mid-position corresponds to an ulnar deviation of 12° and must not be confused with the straight position of the hand. The **straight position** is one in which the long axis of the 3rd finger runs over the capitate bone and is in a straight line with the long axis of the forearm. Starting from the straight position radial deviation is smaller, namely 15°, while ulnar deviation is about 40°. These values are only true when the arm is in strict supination; in strict pronation they are slightly greater. The angle is much larger if the forearm is pronated and the humerus rotated around the elbow joint. Possibly the various muscles are able to function more effectively in the latter position.

The radiographs from which Figs. A–C were drawn were taken with the arm in pronation.

Hamate (pink), lunate (black), triquetrum (yellow).

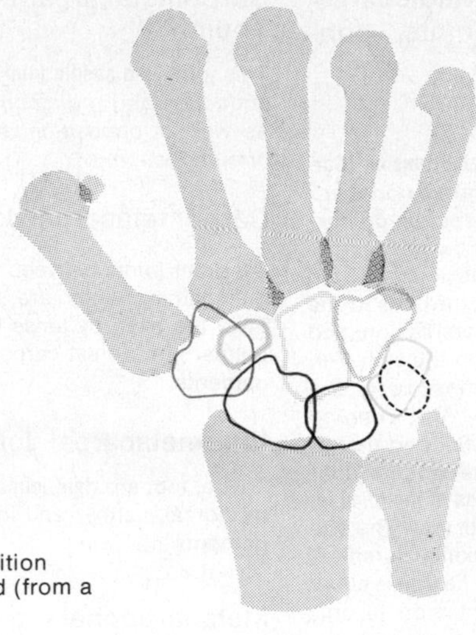

A Straight position of right hand (from a radiograph)

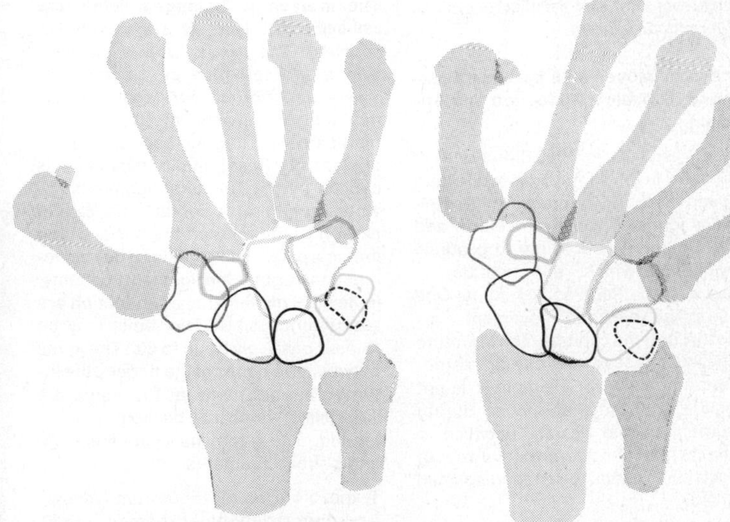

B Radial abduction of right hand (from a radiograph)

C Ulnar adduction of right hand (from a radiograph)

Movements in the Radiocarpal and Midcarpal Joints, continued (A–C)

Flexion and Extension

Flexion (Palmarflexion) and Extension (Dorsiflexion): *The proximal carpal bones are displaced in a palmar direction on dorsiflexion and dorsally on palmar flexion.* This is particularly obvious in the scaphoid (red), which protrudes in the palmar direction on dorsiflexion and may be palpated through the skin. *The axes of movement run transversely; the line of the proximal row running through the lunate (black), and that of the distal row through the capitate (light blue).* **Flexion and extension of the hand include movements about both axes.** The size of the angle between maximal dorsiflexion and maximal palmar flexion is about 170°. The angle of excursion is only limited by ligaments and muscles. **Palmar flexion** takes place *mostly in the radiocarpal joint* and **dorsiflexion** *mainly in the midcarpal joint.*

Accessory Movements between Flexion and Extension, Abduction and Adduction

These result from the directions in which the involved muscles work, and through them and the movements of the various joints, including the elbow and the shoulder, it is possible to produce movements which approximate to those of a ball-and-socket joint. One focus of all joint and movement axes runs through the capitate. The structure of the wrist necessitates certain restrictions of mobility; for example, it is not possible to produce abduction during maximum palmar flexion, because in the latter position the proximal row of carpal bones cannot be either displaced or tilted.

Carpometacarpal Joint of the Thumb

This joint is a **saddle joint**, which allows *abduction* and *adduction* of the thumb, as well as *opposition, reposition* and *circumduction.*

Carpometacarpal Joints

All other joints between the carpal and metacarpal bones are **amphiarthroses.** They are fixed by tense ligaments, the palmar and dorsal carpometacarpal ligaments.

Intermetacarpal Joints

These, too, are **rigid joints** and are fixed by dorsal, palmar and interosseous ligaments.

Metacarpophalangeal and Digital Joints (D–E)

The **metacarpophalangeal joints** are **ball-and-socket joints in shape** with *lax capsules. The palmar side of the capsule is strengthened by palmar ligaments and fibrous cartilage.* The articulation is between the head of the metacarpal (**1**) and the base of the 1st phalanx (**2**). Restriction of movement is caused by the collateral ligaments (**3**), whose origin (**4**) is dorsal to the axis of motion of the joint on the heads of the metacarpals. The greater the movement, the tighter the ligaments become. In flexion, movements of abduction are almost impossible. The joints may be rotated passively by up to 50°. The joints between the bones of the fingers, the **interphalangeal joints of the hand**, are **hinge joints**, which may be flexed and extended. They, too, have collateral (**5**) and palmar ligaments.

Trapezoid (green), triquetrum (yellow), trapezium (dark-blue), hamate (pink), pisiform (black interrupted line).

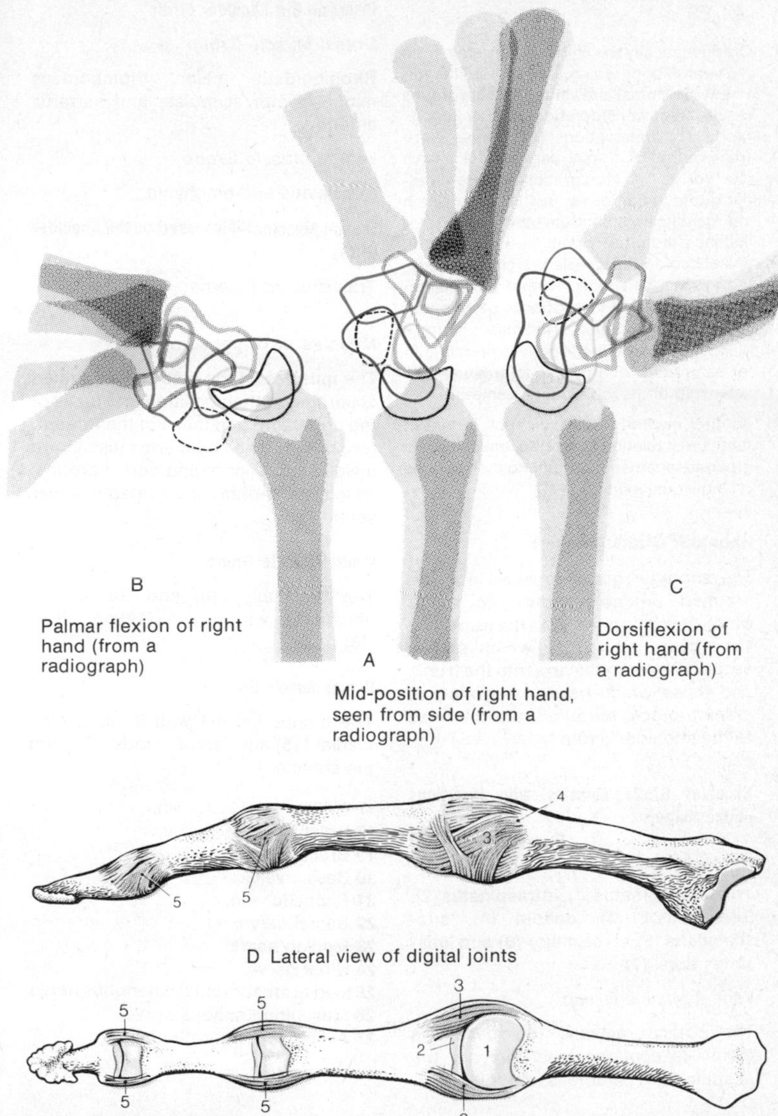

B

Palmar flexion of right hand (from a radiograph)

A

Mid-position of right hand, seen from side (from a radiograph)

C

Dorsiflexion of right hand (from a radiograph)

D Lateral view of digital joints

E Palmar view of metacarpophalangeal and digital joints with capsule removed

Classification of the Muscles (A–C)

Ontogenetically the limb muscles stem from the ventral body wall musculature. Their division into dorsal and ventral muscle groups results from consideration of their topography and innervation. The nerves arise from ventral or dorsal parts of the plexus (see Vol. 3). The immigration into the shoulder girdle region of various muscles which ontogenetically stem from other regions, for instance, from the branchial musculature, has obscured the simple principle underlying this classification. Further information should be sought in textbooks of embryology. In any description of the musculature, it is important to retain the genetic principle as far as possible and by this to prove the relationship of the individual muscles.

Another method of classification is that of functional relationship. Here muscles are grouped together according to their actions on individual joints.

Shoulder Girdle Muscles

The shoulder girdle muscles may be grouped ontogenetically into those which have migrated from the trunk into the upper limb, those which extend secondarily from the arm into the trunk, and those which have immigrated as craniothoracic muscles from the head to the shoulder girdle.

Shoulder Girdle Muscles with Insertions on the Humerus

Dorsal Muscle Group

The supraspinatus (**1**), infraspinatus (**2**), teres minor (**3**), deltoid (**4**), subscapularis (**5**), teres major (**6**) and latissimus dorsi (**7**).

Ventral Muscle Group

The coracobrachialis (**8**), pectoralis minor (exception: insertion on the scapula) and pectoralis major (**9**).

Migrated Trunk Muscles Which Insert on the Shoulder Girdle

Dorsal Muscle Group

Rhomboideus major, rhomboideus minor, levator scapulae and serratus anterior.

Ventral Muscle Group

Subclavius and omohyoid.

Cranial Muscles Which Insert on the Shoulder Girdle

Trapezius and sternocleidomastoid.

Muscles of Upper Arm

The muscles of the limb are separated according to their position into those of the upper arm and those of the forearm (see p. 154). The upper arm muscles are divided into ventral and dorsal groups, which are separated by intermuscular septa.

Ventral Muscle Group

The brachialis (**10**) and the biceps brachii (**11**) with its long (**12**) and short (**13**) heads.

Dorsal Muscle Group

The triceps brachii with its long (**14**), medial (**15**) and lateral heads (**16**), and the anconeus.

17 Axillary artery and vein,
18 Brachial artery,
19 Brachial veins,
20 Basilic vein,
21 Cephalic vein,
22 Radial nerve,
23 Median nerve,
24 Ulnar nerve,
25 Medial antebrachial cutaneous nerve,
26 Musculocutaneous nerve,
27 Axillary or circumflex nerve.

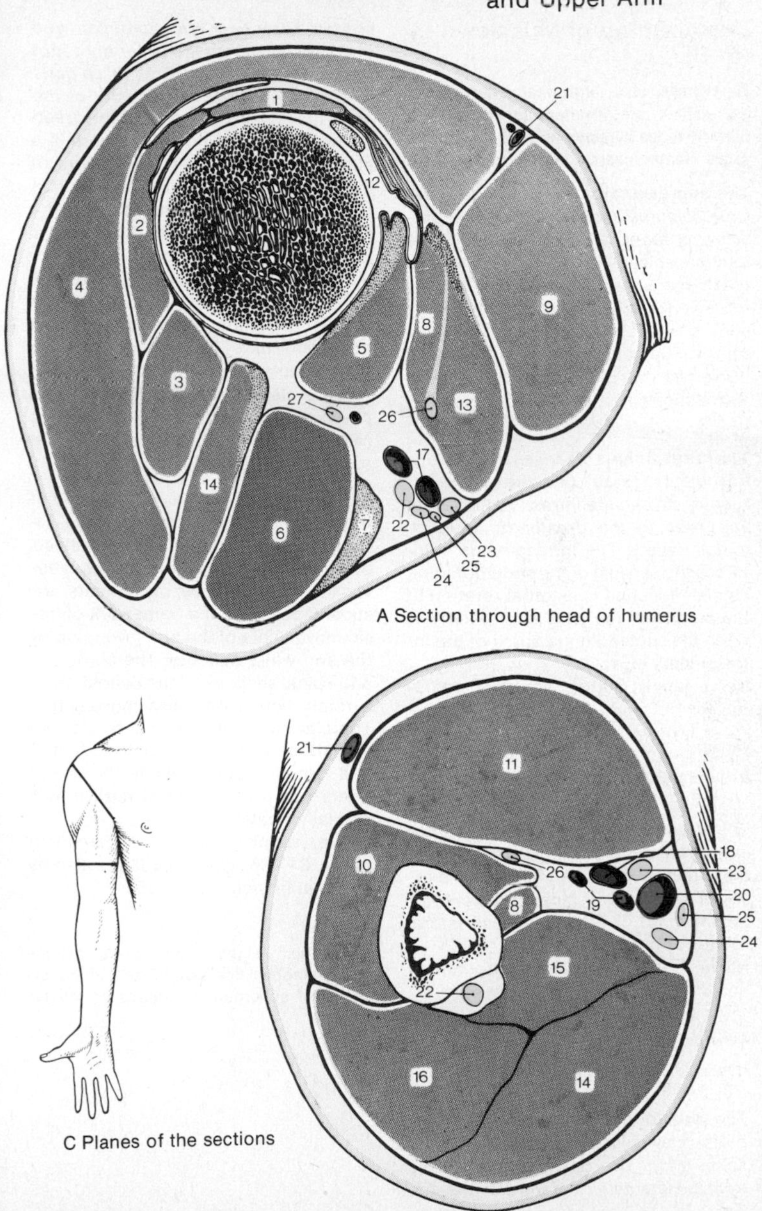

A Section through head of humerus

C Planes of the sections

B Section through middle of arm

Dorsal Group of Muscles (A–B)

The supraspinatus, infraspinatus, teres minor and deltoid are inserted on the greater tubercle of the humerus as well as the crest of the greater tubercle and its continuation.

The supraspinatus (**1**) *arises from the supraspinatus fascia and the supraspinatus fossa* (**2**). It passes over the joint capsule, with which it is fused, to reach the upper facet of the greater tubercle (**3**). It holds the humerus in its socket, tenses the capsule and abducts the arm. Sometimes there is a synovial bursa near the glenoid cavity.
Nerve supply: Suprascapular nerve (C4 to C6).

The infraspinatus (**4**) *arises from the infraspinatus fossa* (**5**), *the spine of scapula* (**6**) *and the infraspinatus fascia and runs to the greater tubercle* (**7**; middle facet). The infraspinatus reinforces the capsule of the shoulder joint. Its main function is external rotation of the arm. Near the joint socket there is often the subtendinous bursa of the infraspinatus muscle.
Nerve supply: Suprascapular nerve (C4 to C6).

Variants

It is frequently fused with the teres minor.

The **teres minor** (**8**) *arises from the lateral border of the scapula* (**9**) superior to the origin of the teres major, and *is inserted on the lower facet of the greater tubercle* (**10**). It acts as a weak lateral rotator of the arm.
Nerve supply: Axillary (circumflex) nerve (C5 and C6).

Variants

It may be fused with the infraspinatus.

The **deltoid** (**11**) is divided into three parts – clavicular (**12**), acromial (**13**) and spinal (**14**). The **clavicular fibers** *arise from the lateral third of the clavicle,* the **acromial fibers** *from the acromion* and the **spinal fibers** *from the lower border of the spine of the scapula. All three parts insert on the deltoid tuberosity of the humerus* (**15**). In the region of the greater tubercle of the humerus, there is a subdeltoid bursa. The three sections of the muscle act partly as synergists and partly as *antagonists.* The deltoid is the most important **abductor** of the shoulder joint. Abduction up to about 90° is mostly performed by the deltoid, at first only by the acromial fibers. Only after the first two thirds of the movement of abduction have been completed, do the clavicular and spinal fibers become responsible for the movement. The clavicular and spinal fibers are able to **adduct** the arm after it has been lowered to a third of its range of movement.

The clavicular fibers, aided by some of the acromial fibers, can produce **anteversion**, and the spinal fibers, helped by other acromial fibers, produce **retroversion**. These angular movements are superimposed on the framework of basic movements of the arm (swinging of the arm while walking). The clavicular and spinal sections of the deltoid exert a rotary action on these movements. The clavicular fibers can produce **medial rotation** in an arm which is adducted and laterally rotated, while the spinal fibers can produce **lateral rotation** in a medially rotated arm.
Nerve supply: Axillary (circumflex) nerve (C4–C6); clavicular fibers also by pectoral branches (C4–C5).

Variants

Fusion with neighboring muscles; absence of the acromial fibers of the deltoid; occurrence of supernumary groups of muscle fibers.

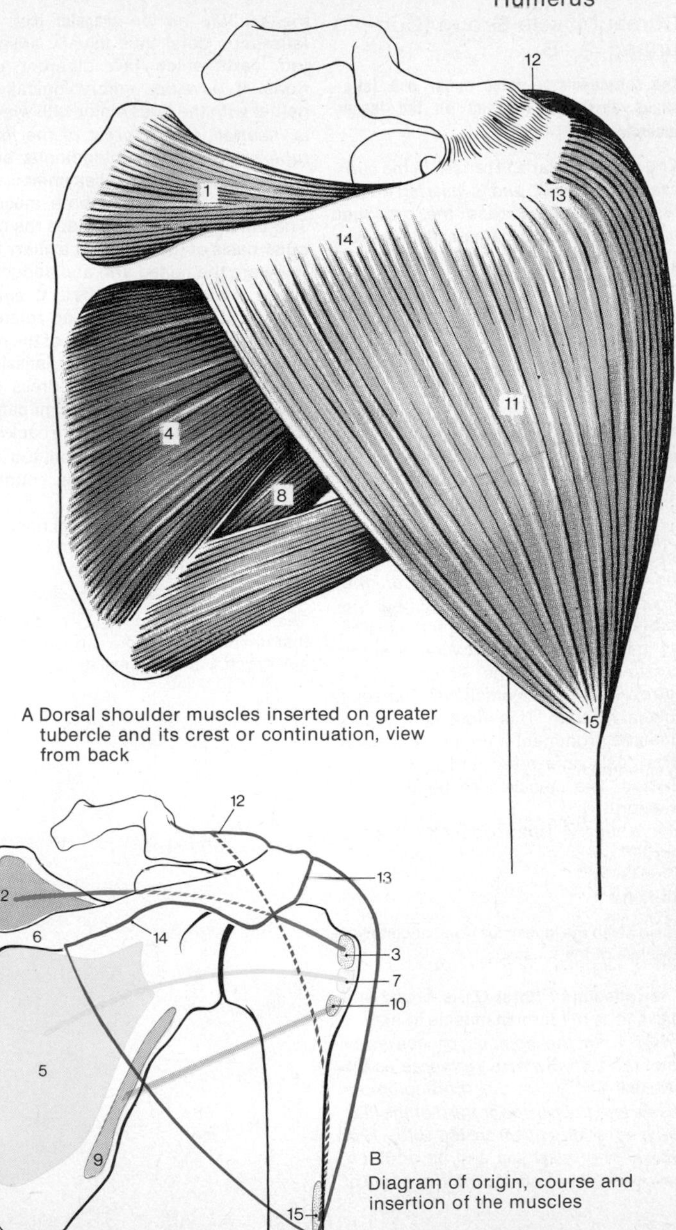

A Dorsal shoulder muscles inserted on greater tubercle and its crest or continuation, view from back

B
Diagram of origin, course and insertion of the muscles

Dorsal Muscle Group (Continued, A–B)

The subscapularis, teres major and latissimus dorsi are inserted on the lesser tubercle and its crest.

The **subscapularis** (**1**) *arises in the subscapular fossa* (**2**) *and is inserted on the lesser tubercle* (**3**) *and the proximal part of its crest.* It causes medial rotation of the arm.
Nerve supply: Subscapular nerve (C5–C8).

Variants

The occurence of accessory bundles.

Practical Points

Paralysis of the subscapularis produces maximal lateral (external) rotation of the upper limb, which indicates that it is a particularly strong medial rotator of the arm.

The **teres major** (**4**), which *arises from the lateral border (***5***) of the scapula near the inferior angle, is inserted on the crest of the lesser tubercle* (**6**) near the subtendinous bursa of the teres major. Its main function is retroversion of the arm toward the midline, which requires retroversion and a small simultaneous medial rotation. This movement is particularly prominent if the arm has been previously anteverted and slightly abducted. The muscle also helps in adduction.
Nerve supply: Thoracodorsal nerve (C6 and C7).

Variants

Fusion with the latissimus dorsi or complete absence of the muscle.

The **latissimus dorsi** (**7**) is broad and flat and is the largest muscle in man. *It arises from the spinous processes of the 7th–12th thoracic vertebrae* as the **vertebral part,** *from the thoracolumbar fascia and the posterior third of the iliac crest* as the **iliac part,** *from the 10th–12th ribs* as the **costal part** and, in addition, very often also *from the inferior angle of the scapula* as the **scapular part.** The latissimus dorsi thus usually arises in four parts which have different functions. It develops embryologically together with the teres major with which it *is inserted on the crest of the lesser tubercle* (**8**). The subtendinous bursa of the latissimus dorsi lies immediately before the junction of both muscles. The latissimus dorsi provides the muscular basis of the posterior axillary fold. It lowers the raised arm and adducts it. When the arm is adducted, it pulls it backward and medially, and rotates it so far medially that the back of the hand can cover the buttock. The latissimus dorsi is often called the "dress coat pocket" muscle. Both latissimi can act together to pull the shoulders backward and downward. They function, too, during forced expiration and in coughing (coughing muscle).
Nerve supply: Thoracodorsal nerve (C6 to C8).

Variants

The occurrence of aberrant muscle fibers that run into the pectoralis major as a muscular arch across the axilla.

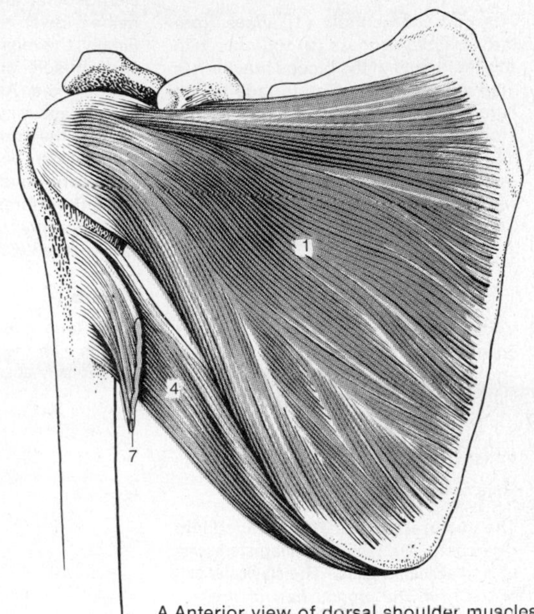

A Anterior view of dorsal shoulder muscles inserted on lesser tubercle and its crest

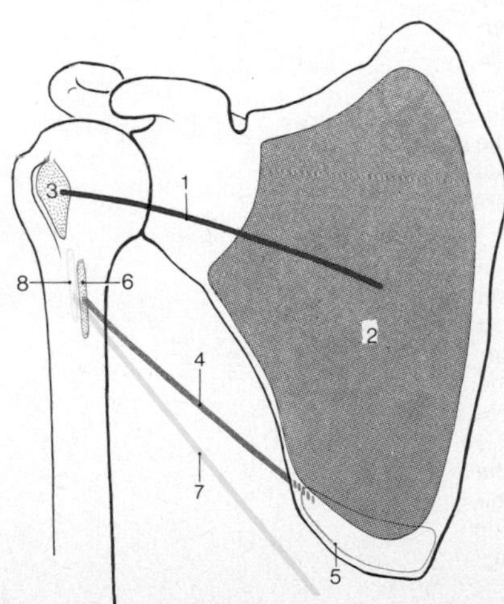

B Diagram of origin, course and insertion of the muscles

Ventral Muscle Group (A–B)

The **coracobrachialis** (**1**) *arises from the coracoid process (***2**) together with the short head of the biceps brachii. *It is inserted on the medial surface of the humerus on the continuation of the crest of the lesser tubercle* (**3**). It anteverts the arm and also holds the head of the humerus in its joint socket.
Nerve supply: Musculocutaneous nerve C6 and C7).

The **pectoralis minor** (**4**) is the only shoulder girdle muscle which is not inserted on bone in the free limb. *It arises from the 3rd–5th ribs* (**5**) *and is inserted on the coracoid process (***6**). It lowers and rotates the scapula.
Nerve supply: Medial pectoral nerves (C6 to C8).

Variants

More or fewer slips of origin.

The **pectoralis major** (**7**) is divided into three parts, i. e., the **clavicular, sternocostal** and **abdominal parts**. The **clavicular part** *arises from the medial half of the anterior surface of the clavicle* (**8**), while the **sternocostal part** *comes from the sternal membrane and the cartilages of the 2nd–6th ribs* (**9**). The weaker **abdominal part** *stems from the anterior layer of the uppermost part* (**10**) *of the rectus sheath. The pectoralis major is inserted on the crest of the greater tubercle* (**11**) in such a manner that the fibers are twisted, so that the abdominal part is attached most proximally and forms a pocket which is open above.

It is a strong muscle, four-sided when the arm hangs down, and when the arm is raised, its borders form a triangle. It forms the muscular basis of the anterior axillary fold. With the arm abducted the clavicular and sternal parts can produce anteversion, a movement which is familiar from swimming. All parts of the pectoralis major acting together, forcibly and rapidly lower the raised arm. In addition, the whole muscle can adduct the arm and rotate it medially. The sternocostal and abdominal parts together lower the shoulder anteriorly. Finally, the muscle can act as an accessory muscle during inspiration if the arm is fixed. An exhausted sportsman after a race may be seen to prop up his arms on his trunk, so that the pectorales majores can be brought into action as accessory muscles of respiration to move the thorax.
Nerve supply: Lateral and medial pectoral nerves (C5 to Th1).

Variants

It may form a muscular axillary arch connecting with the latissimus dorsi. It is very occasionally absent.

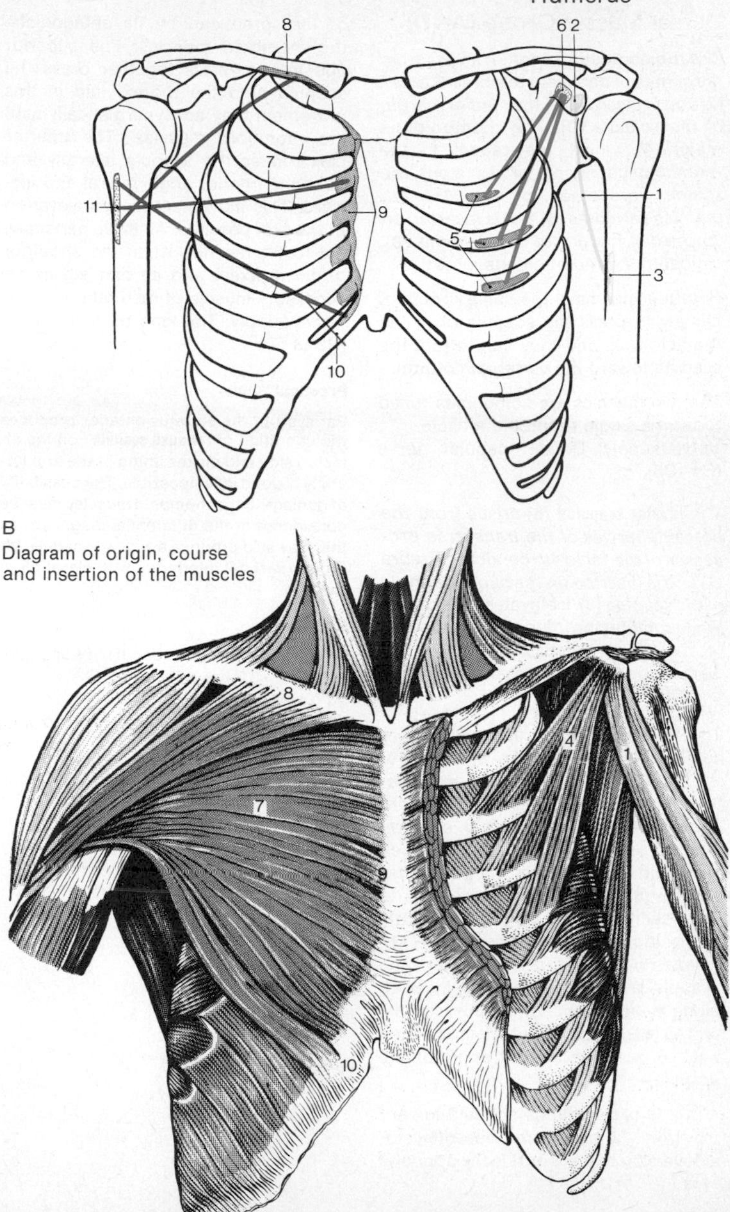

B
Diagram of origin, course and insertion of the muscles

A Ventral shoulder muscles, anterior view

Immigrant Trunk Muscles Inserting on the Shoulder Girdle

Dorsal Muscle Group (A–D)

The **rhomboideus minor** (**1**) *arises from the spines of cervical vertebrae 6 and 7 (***2***) and is inserted on the medial margin of the scapula (***3***)*. The **rhomboideus major** (**4**), which lies caudal to the rhomboideus minor, *arises from the spinous processes of the 1st–4th thoracic vertebrae* (**5**) and *is inserted on the medial margin of the scapula (***3***)*, caudal to the rhomboideus minor.

Both muscles have the same function, namely to press the scapula onto the thoracic wall, and they can retract the scapula toward the vertebral column.

The two muscles are sometimes fused to form a single rhomboid muscle.
Nerve supply: Dorsal scapular nerve (C4–C5).

The **levator scapulae** (**6**) *arises from the dorsal tubercles of the transverse processes of the 1st to 4th cervical vertebra (***7***)* and *is inserted on the superior angle of the scapula* (**8**). It elevates the scapula while rotating the inferior angle medially.
Nerve supply: Dorsal scapular nerve (C4 and C5).

The **serratus anterior** (**9**) *usually arises by nine slips from the 1st–9th ribs* (**10**) but sometimes from ribs 1–8. In the later case two slips arise from the 2nd rib. The *insertion of the muscle extends from the superior to the inferior angles along the entire medial margin of the scapula (***3***)*. The muscle is divided into three sections according to the points of insertion, namely a **superior part** (**11**), inserted near the superior angle of the scapula, an **intermediate part** (**12**), inserted along the medial margin of the scapula, and an **inferior part** (**13**) which is attached near to or at the inferior angle of the scapula.

All three parts pull the scapula toward the front, a movement essential for anteversion of the arm. It is the opposite of that produced by its antagonists, the rhomboid muscles. The superior and inferior parts together press the scapula onto the thorax, and in this movement they act synergistically with the rhomboid muscles. The inferior part rotates the scapula laterally and pulls the inferior angle lateral and forward. This movement makes elevation of the arm possible. All three parts may act to lift the ribs when the shoulder girdle is fixed, and so can act as an accessory muscle of respiration.
Nerve supply: The long thoracic nerve (C5 to C7).

Practical Points

Paralysis of the serratus anterior produces the condition of "**winged scapula**" on the affected side and makes lifting of the arm laterally beyond 90° impossible. The possibility of damage to the rhomboid muscles must be considered in the differential diagnosis, as this may also produce a winged scapula, although without interfering with elevation of the arm.

Variants

A larger or smaller number of slips of origin.

14 Teres major,
15 Clavicle.

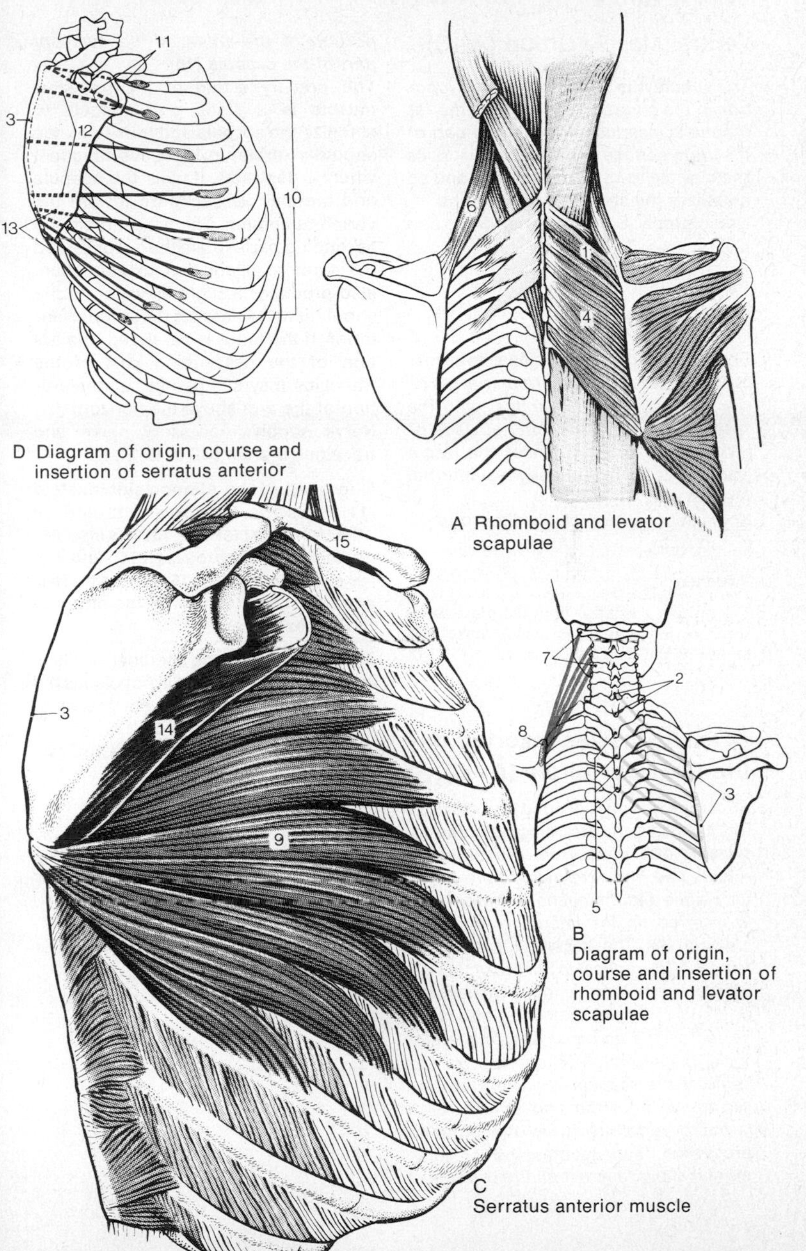

D Diagram of origin, course and insertion of serratus anterior

A Rhomboid and levator scapulae

B
Diagram of origin, course and insertion of rhomboid and levator scapulae

C
Serratus anterior muscle

Ventral Muscle Group (A–C)

The **subclavius** (**1**) *arises from the junction of the bone and cartillage of the 1st rib and is inserted on the lateral part of the undersurface of the clavicle*. It pulls the clavicle toward the sternum and so stabilizes the sternoclavicular joint.
Nerve supply: Subclavian nerve (C5 and C6).

Variants

This muscle may be absent.

The **omohyoid** has two bellies. Its **inferior belly** (**2**) *arises from the upper margin of the scapula* (**3**) *and reaches* with the **superior belly** (**4**) *to the inner surface of the hyoid bone* (**5**). It tenses the fascia and dilatates the underlying internal jugular vein.
Nerve supply: Ansa cervicalis profunda (C1 to C3).

Variants

The muscle may arise from the clavicle instead of the scapula, in which case it is known as the **cleidohyoid muscle.**

Cranial Muscles Inserted on the Shoulder Girdle (A–C)

The **trapezius** (**6**) is divided into **descending, transverse** and **ascending parts. The descending part** *arises from the superior nuchal line, the external occipital protuberance and the nuchal ligament and is inserted on the lateral third of the clavicle* (**7**). The **transverse part** *arises from the 7th cervical to 3rd thoracic vertebrae* (from their spinous processes and supraspinous ligaments) and *is inserted on the acromial end of the clavicle, the acromion* (**8**) *and part of the spine of the scapula* (**9**). The **ascending part** *arises from the 2nd or 3rd–12th thoracic vertebrae* (from the spinous processes and supraspinous ligaments) and *is inserted on the triangular portion of the spine or the adjacent part of the scapula* (**10**).
The primary action of the trapezius muscle is a static one, namely to stabilize the scapula and thus to fix the shoulder girdle. In its active function, when it contracts, it pulls the scapula and the clavicle backward toward the vertebral column. The descending and ascending parts rotate the scapula, and the former, in addition to adduction, also produces a slight elevation of the shoulder and so assists the serratus anterior. If the latter is paralyzed, the action of the descending part of the trapezius may still permit some elevation of the arm above the horizontal.
Nerve supply: Accessory nerve and trapezius branch (C2 to C4).

One head of the **sternocleidomastoid** (**11**) *arises from the sternum* (**12**) and the other *from the clavicle* (**13**). *It is inserted on the mastoid process* (**14**) and *the superior nuchal line* (**15**), where there is a tendinous junction with the origin of the trapezius.

As its action one the shoulder girdle is of minor importance, it is not discussed here, but subsequently with the muscles of the head (see p. 314).
Nerve supply: Accessory nerve and cervical plexus (C1 and C2).

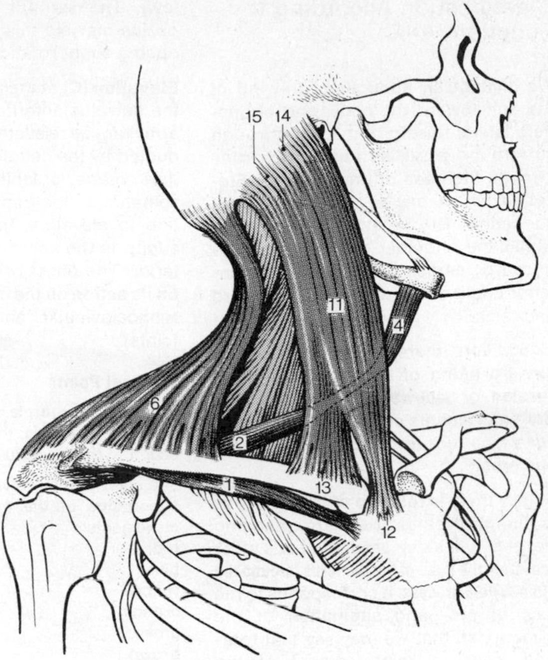

A
Immigrant trunk muscles inserted on shoulder girdle; lateral view of ventral group

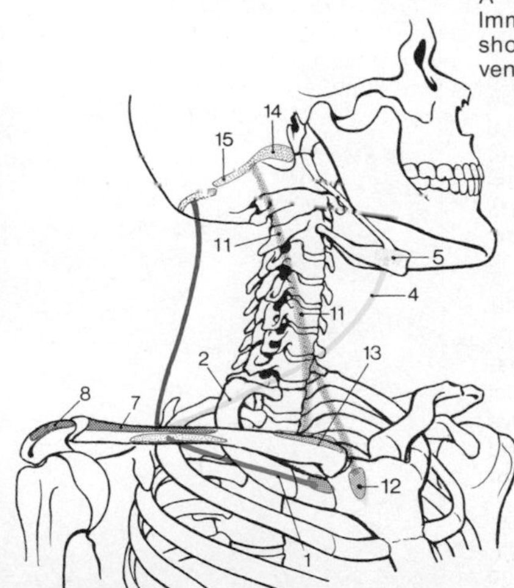

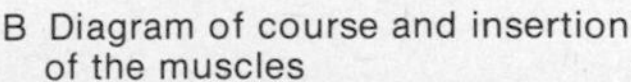
B Diagram of course and insertion of the muscles

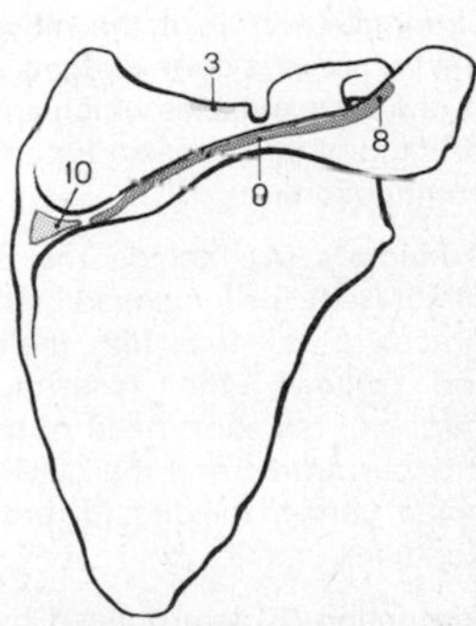

C Diagram of attachment of muscles to scapula

Classification According to Function (A–C)

We distinguish **adduction**, drawing of the arm toward the body, and **abduction**, lateral raising of the arm through 90° around a **sagittal axis**, which runs through the head of the humerus. **Elevation**, which may be a continuation of abduction, is due not to movement within the shoulder joint, but is produced by **rotation of the scapula**, the inferior angle of which is moved forward and laterally.

In addition, there is **anteversion** or forward lifting of the arm, and **retroversion** or backward lifting of the arm. Both movements occur around a **frontal axis** which runs through the head of the humerus.

Finally there is **rotation** of the arm. This is due to pivoting of the arm (hanging down by the side) around an **axis which runs from the head of the humerus through the ulnar styloid process**. It corresponds to the axis of pro- and supination of the forearm, so that we may say that rotation leads to reinforcement of the movements of pronation and supination. We distinguish between **lateral** (external) and **medial** (internal) **rotation.** The compound movement of **circumduction** may also be either a lateral or medial circumduction. In it the movement of the humerus is cone-shaped. Obviously, the same muscles which are active in rotation of the arm also function in circumduction.

Adductors (**A**) include the pectoralis major (red), the long head of the triceps brachii (blue, see p. 152), the teres major (yellow), the latissimus dorsi (orange), the short head of the biceps brachii (green) and the clavicular and spinal parts of the deltoid (brown, broken line).

Abduction (**B**) is produced by the deltoid (red), the supraspinatus (blue) and the long head of the biceps brachii (yellow). The serratus anterior and trapezius may aid this movement by producing slight rotation of the scapula.

Elevation (**C**) of the arm is produced by the serratus anterior (red). Before the arm can be elevated, it must be abducted by the deltoid, the long head of the biceps brachii and the supraspinatus. In the transition from abduction to elevation, the trapezius (blue) supports the action of the serratus anterior. The effect of the latter depends on its action on the clavicular joints (acromioclavicular and sternoclavicular joints).

Practical Points

If the serratus muscle is paralyzed, elevation of the arm is limited to the 15° produced by action of the trapezius.

The color of the arrows shows the order of importance of the muscles in individual movements:
red,
blue,
yellow,
orange,
green,
brown.

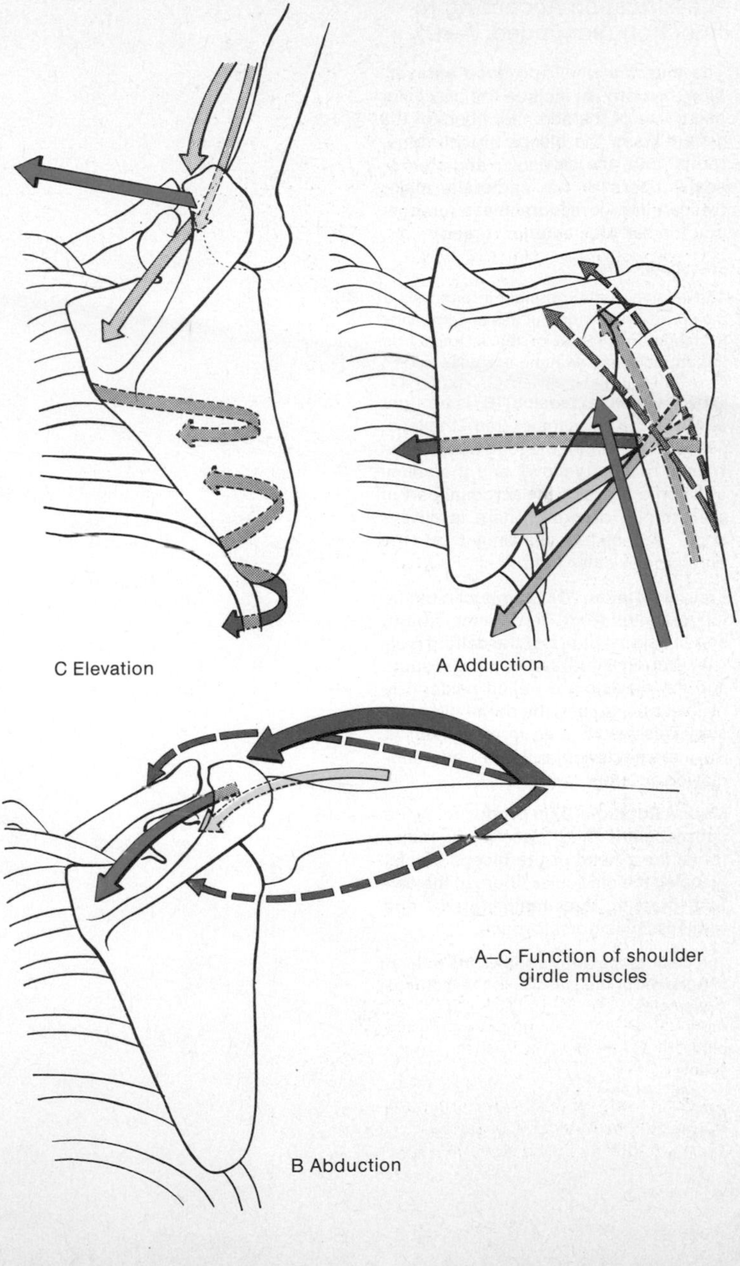

C Elevation

A Adduction

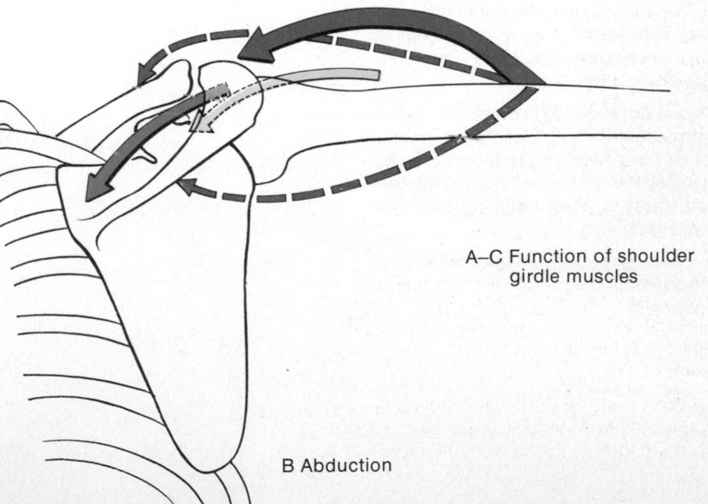

B Abduction

A–C Function of shoulder girdle muscles

Classification According to Function (continued, A–D)

The muscles which produce **anteversion** (flexion) (**A**) include the clavicular and some of the acromial fibers of the deltoid (red), the biceps brachii (blue, see p. 150), the clavicular and sternocostal fibers of the pectoralis major (yellow), the coracobrachialis (orange) and the serratus anterior (green).

Practical Points

Anteversion is still possible in paralysis of the serratus anterior, but it is accompanied by marked elevation of the scapula from the thoracic wall (winged scapula).

Retroversion (extension) (**B**) is brought about by the teres major (red), the latissimus dorsi (blue), the long head of the triceps brachii (yellow), and the spinal and some fibers of the acromial part of the deltoid (orange). There is always some associated movement at the acromioclavicular joint.

Lateral Rotation (**C**) is produced by the infraspinatus (red), teres minor (blue) and the spinal fibers of the deltoid (yellow). During lateral rotation the scapula and the clavicle are pulled posteriorly by the trapezius and the rhomboid muscles. This results also in movement at the sternoclavicular and acromioclavicular joints.

Medial Rotation (**D**) is produced by the subscapularis (red), pectoralis major (blue), long head of the biceps brachii (yellow), the clavicular fibers of the deltoid (orange), teres major (green) and the latissimus dorsi (brown).

The color of the arrows shows the order of importance of the muscles in the individual movements:
red
blue
yellow
orange
green
brown.

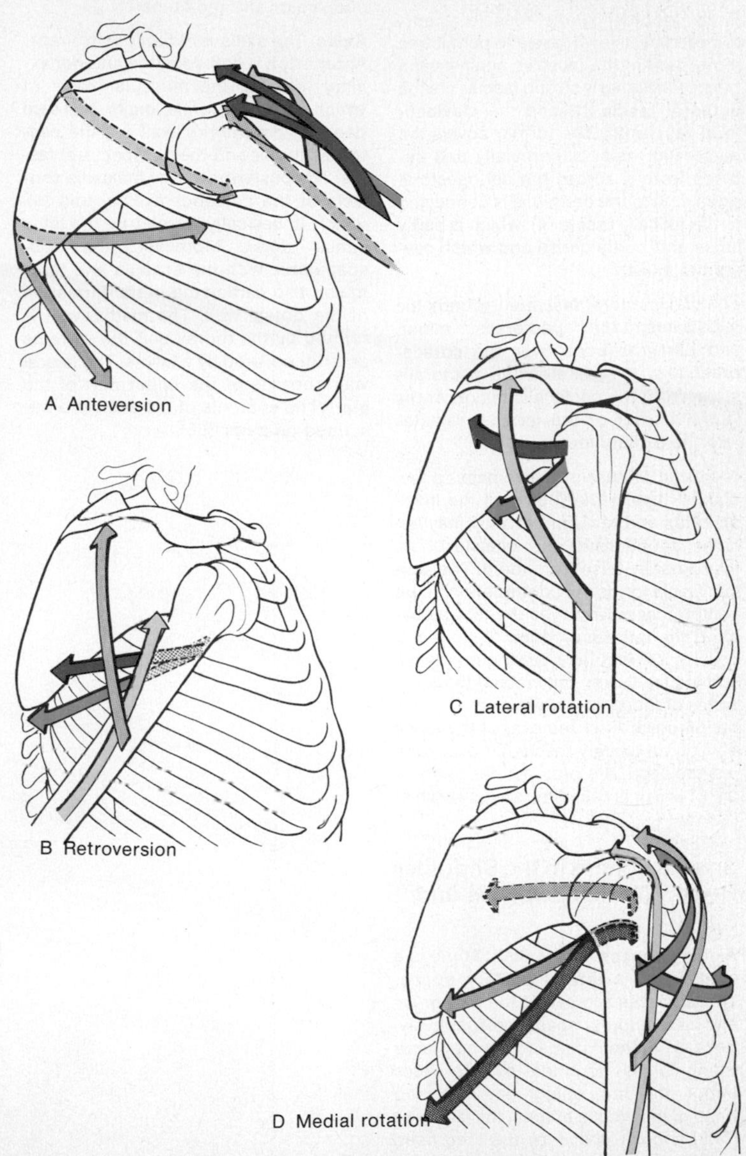
A Anteversion

B Retroversion

C Lateral rotation

D Medial rotation

Fascias (A–B)

Each shoulder girdle muscle is surrounded by its own fascia to permit free movement of the muscles against each other. Particularly strong fascias are the **pectoral fascia** (**1**) and the **clavipectoral fascia** (**2**). The former covers the pectoralis major superficially and extends from it across the deltopectoral groove (**3**) to the deltoid. It is connected to the **axillary fascia** (**4**), which is partly loose and partly dense and which covers the axilla.

The *clavipectoral fascia* surrounds the subclavius, the pectoralis minor, and partly extends over the coracobrachialis. It separates the pectoralis major from the pectoralis minor. At the lateral border of the latter it radiates into the axillary fascia.

A special feature of the remaining fascias is, that in the region of the infraspinatus and teres minor they may become aponeurotic and muscle fibers may actually arise from them. The axillary fascia forms the continuation of the pectoral fascia as far as the fascia covering the latissimus dorsi. It does not consist of regularly arranged, dense connective tissue, but instead there are zones of loose tissue, which may easily be removed. After removal of the loose part of the axillary fascia, an oval zone may be seen, the proximal fascial border of which is called the axillary arch of *Langer*.

Special Spaces in the Shoulder Region (Axillary Spaces and Axilla)

Axillary Spaces (see p. 360): There is a **medial** and a **lateral axillary space**. These spaces are called the *triangular* and *quadrangular* spaces, respectively, because of their shapes. The medial or triangular is bounded by the teres minor, the teres major and the long head of the triceps brachii, the lateral or quadrangular space by the long head of the triceps brachii, the teres minor and major and the humerus.

Axilla. The axilla is *pyramidal* in shape. Anteriorly it is limited by the anterior axillary fold (**5**), the muscular basis of which is the pectoralis major, and also deep in the anterior wall are the pectoralis minor and the clavipectoral fascia. The posterior wall of the axilla consists of the posterior axillary fold (**6**), which is basically formed by the latissimus dorsi. Moreover, the subscapularis, with the scapula and teres major also participate in the formation of the dorsal wall. The medial wall is formed by the thorax and the serratus anterior covered by a fascia. The lateral wall consists of the upper part of the arm. (The contents of the axilla are described on page 358).

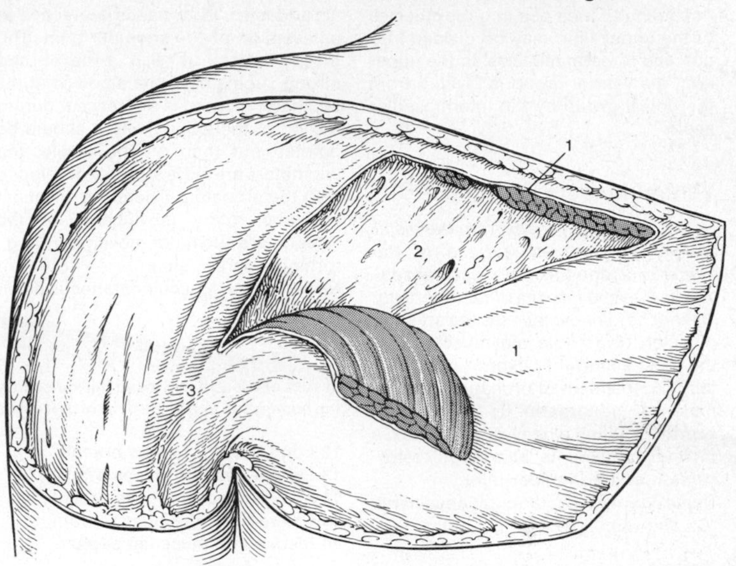

A Fascias in region of deltopectoral triangle

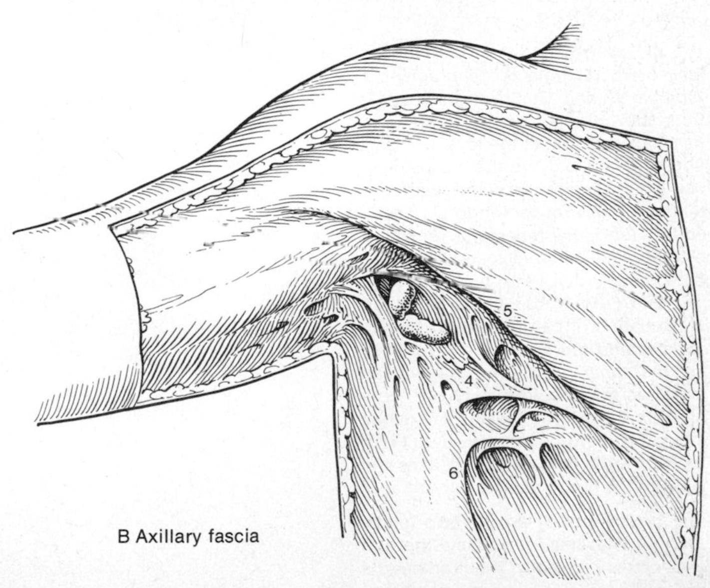

B Axillary fascia

According to their position the muscles of the upper limb may be divided into arm and forearm muscles. In the upper arm, the ventral group is divided from the dorsal group by the intermuscular septa.

Ventral Muscle Group (A–C)

The **brachialis** (**1**) *arises from the distal half of the anterior surface of the humerus* (**2**) *and the intermuscular septa. It is inserted into the ulnar tuberosity* (**3**) *and the joint capsule* (as the articular muscle). It is a single joint muscle and is the most important flexor of the elbow joint independent of pronation or supination of the forearm. Its full power is exerted in lifting a heavy load. In such a movement there is also slight retroversion at the shoulder joint.
Nerve supply: Musculocutaneous nerve (C5 and C6).

Variants

Insertion into the oblique cord or into the radius.

The **biceps brachii** (**4**) arises with its **long head** (**5**) from the *supraglenoid tubercle* (**6**) and with its **short head** (**7**) from the *coracoid process* (**8**). Both heads usually join at the level of insertion of the deltoid into the biceps muscle, which again terminates with two tendons. The stronger tendon is *inserted into the radial tuberosity* (**9**) with a bicipitoradial bursa enclosed. The other flattened tendon, *the bicipital aponeurosis* (**10**), whose fibers form the continuation of part of the short head, *radiates into the fascia of the forearm on the ulnar side*. The long head traverses the shoulder joint and, covered by a synovial sheath, it extends along the intertubercular groove (**11**) of the humerus. In its action it uses the head of the humerus as a fulcrum.

The biceps brachii acts on two joints. With its long head it abducts the arm and rotates it medially. The short head is an adductor. Both heads are active in anteversion of the shoulder joint. The biceps brachii is also a flexor and strong supinator of the elbow joint. Its supinator action is increased during flexion of the elbow joint. It should be pointed out that, on the whole, the supinators are more strongly developed than the pronators. Therefore, the most essential rotary movements of the forearm are supinator movements (e.g., turning a screw, etc.).
Nerve supply: Musculocutaneous nerve (C5 and C6).

Variants

In 10% of cases a 3rd head may arise from the humerus to join to the belly of the biceps.

12 Long head of triceps brachii,
13 Lateral head of triceps brachii,
14 Medial head of triceps brachii,
15 Lateral intermuscular septum,
16 Medial intermuscular septum.

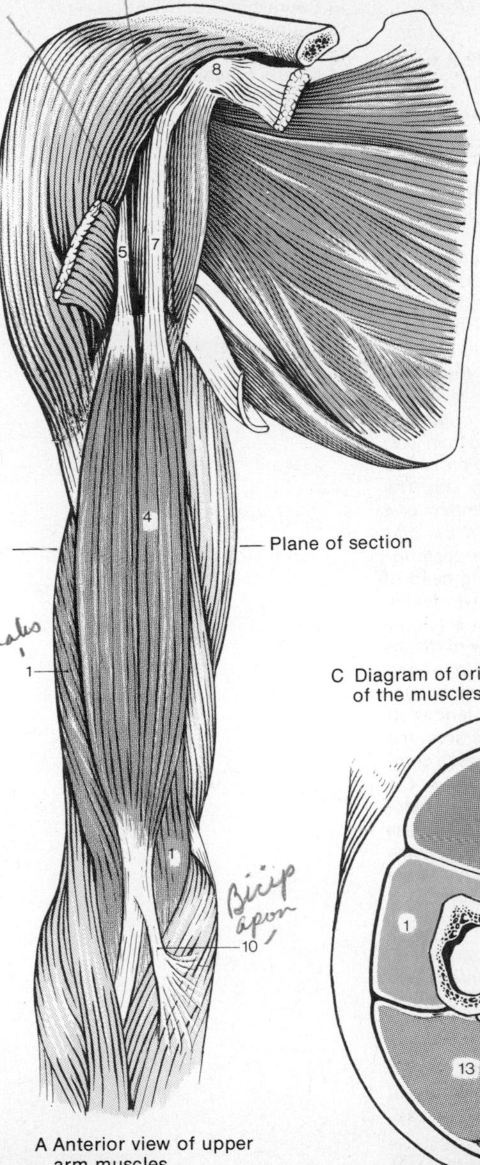

Plane of section

A Anterior view of upper arm muscles

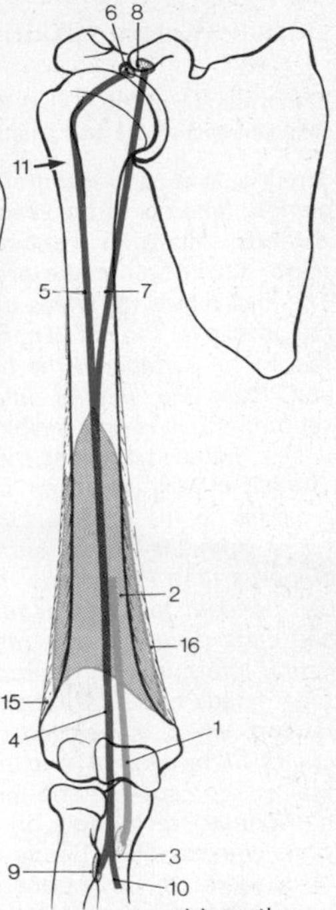

C Diagram of origin, course and insertion of the muscles

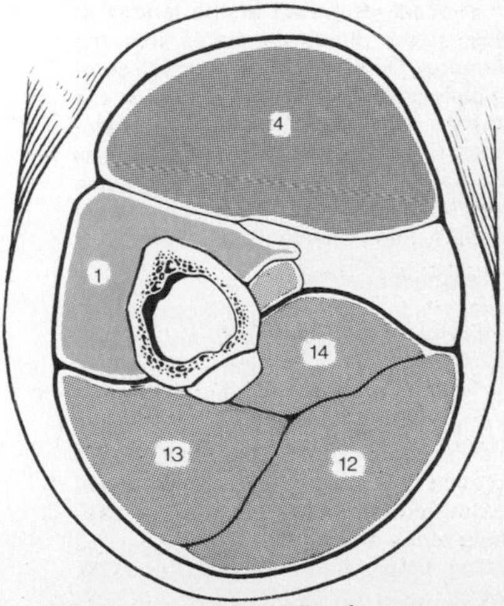

B Section through middle of upper arm

Dorsal Muscle Group (A–C)

The **triceps brachii** (**1**) has three heads, **long** (**2**), **medial** (**3**) and **lateral** (**4**).

The **long head** (**2**) *arises from the infraglenoid tubercle of the scapula* (**5**) and extends distally in front of the teres minor (**6**) and behind the teres major (**7**). The **medial head** (**3**) *arises distally from the groove for the radial nerve* (**8**), *from the dorsal surface of the humerus* (**9**) *and from the medial intermuscular septum* (**10**). It is only visible distally as it lies flattened against the humerus. The **lateral head** (**4**) *arises laterally and proximal to the groove for the radial nerve from the dorsal surface of the humerus (*(**11**). *Proximally it originates just beneath the greater tubercle* (**12**) *and ends distally in the region of the lateral intermuscular septum* (**13**). The three heads fuse in a flat common end tendon, which is *inserted on the olecranon of the ulna* (**14**) *and the posterior wall of the capsule.* The long head of the triceps brachii acts on two joints, while with the other heads it acts only on one joint. It is an extensor of the elbow joint. At the shoulder the long head is involved in retroversion and adduction of the arm. Part of the tendon of the triceps brachii radiates into the forearm fascia and may almost completely cover the anconeus (**15**). In the region of its attachment to the olecranon there are often bursae: the bursa subcutanea olecrani and bursa subtendinea m. tricipitis brachii. Nerve supply: Radial nerve (C6 to C 8).

The **anconeus** (**15**) *arises from the dorsal surface of the lateral epicondyle* (**16**) *and the lateral collateral ligament and is inserted into the proximal one-fourth of the dorsal side of the ulna* (**17**), close to the medial head of the triceps brachii. Its function is to assist the triceps brachii in producing the movement of extension, and it also tenses the capsule of the elbow joint.
Nerve supply: Radial nerve (C7 and C8).

18 Supraspinatus,
19 Deltoid,
20 Infraspinatus,
21 Biceps brachii,
22 Brachialis,
23 Coracobrachialis,
24 Humerus.

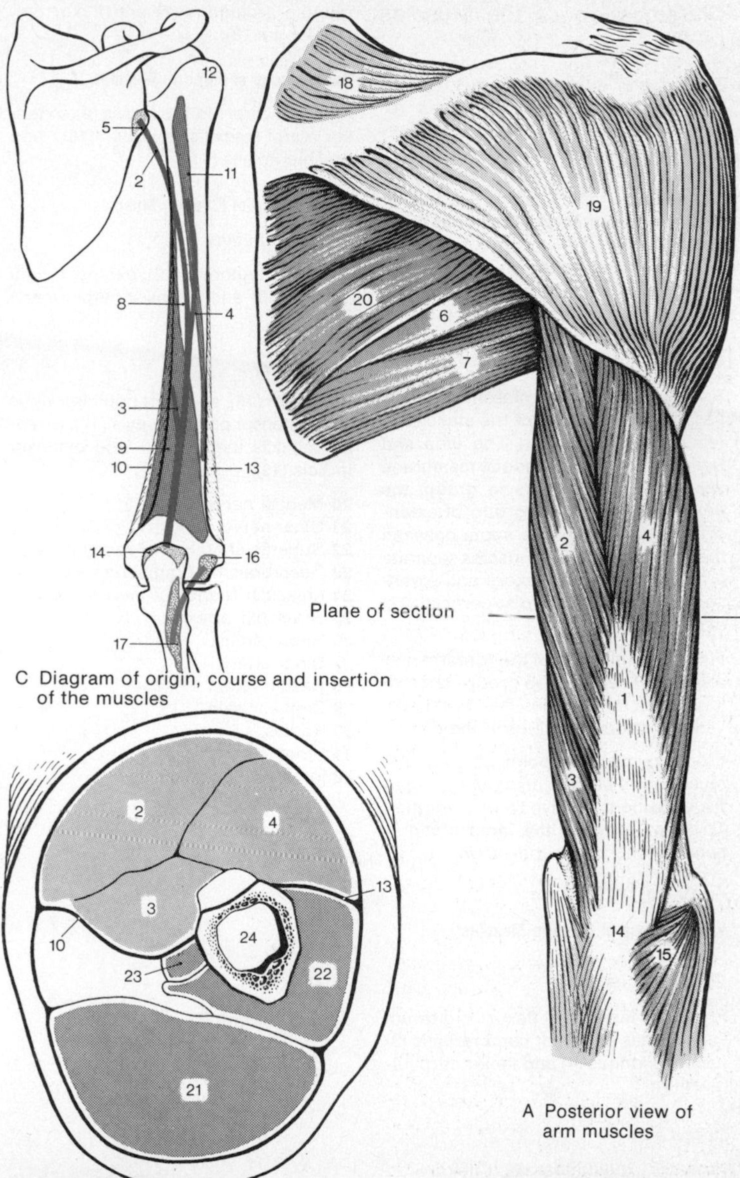

C Diagram of origin, course and insertion of the muscles

A Posterior view of arm muscles

B Section through middle of arm

Classification of the Muscles (A–D)

The forearm muscles are divided into three groups, according to their relationship to the various joints, their attachments and their mode of action. One group comprises muscles attached to the radius, which are only involved in movements of the bones of the forearm. The 2nd group of forearm muscles extends to the metacarpus and produces movement at the wrist. The 3rd group comprises those muscles that extend to the phalanges and are responsible for finger movements.

Another system of classification is based on the position of the muscles in relation to each other. The ulna and radius with the interosseous membrane separate a ventral muscle group, the flexors, from a dorsal group of extensors. Connective tissue septa between the ventral and dorsal muscles separate a radial group. The flexors and extensors can be divided into superficial and deep muscles.

Finally, the muscles of the forearm may also be divided into two groups according to their innervation – from either the ventral or dorsal portions of the plexus.

From the practical point of view, the muscles will be classified according to their positions relative to one another. This also provides the most comprehensive functional subdivision.

Ventral Group of Forearm Muscles

Superficial Layer

Pronator teres (**1**), flexor digitorum superficialis (**2**), flexor carpi radialis (**3**) palmaris longus (**4**) and flexor carpi ulnaris (**5**).

Deep Layer

Pronator quadratus (**6**), flexor digitorum profundus (**7**) and flexor pollicis longus (**8**).

Radial Group of Forearm Muscles

Extensor carpi radialis brevis (**9**), extensor carpi radialis longus (**10**) and brachioradialis (**11**).

Dorsal Group of Forearm Muscles

Superficial Layer

Extensor digitorum (**12**), extensor digiti minimi (**13**) and extensor carpi ulnaris (**14**).

Deep Layer

Supinator (**15**), abductor pollicis longus (**16**), extensor pollicis brevis (**17**), extensor pollicis longus (**18**) and extensor indicis (**19**).

20 Median nerve,
21 Ulnar nerve,
22 Superficial branch of radial nerve,
23 Deep branch of radial nerve,
24 Muscular branch of median nerve,
25 Brachialis artery,
26 Radial artery,
27 Ulnar artery,
28 Basilic vein,
29 Cephalic vein,
30 Radius,
31 Ulna,
32 Interosseous membrane.

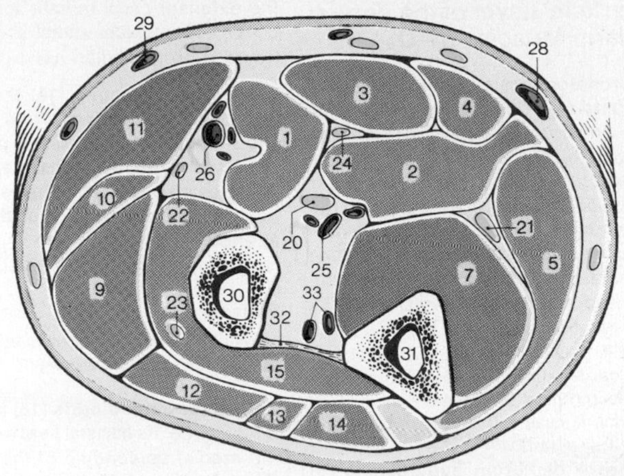

A Section through proximal third of forearm

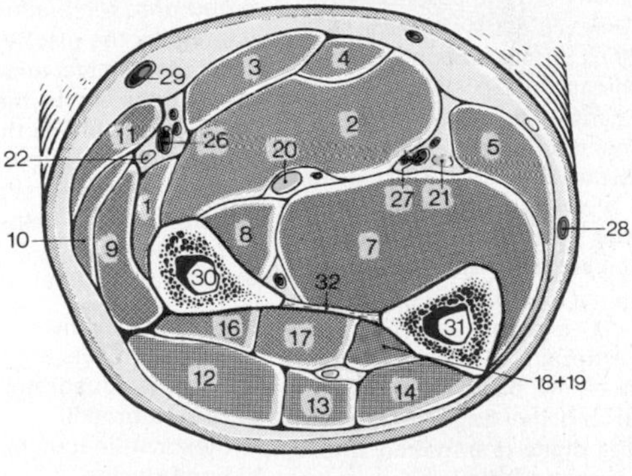

B Section through middle third of forearm

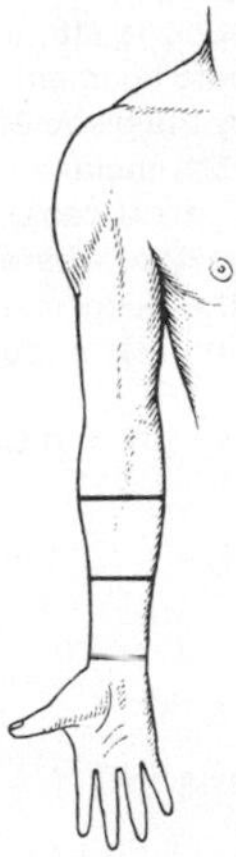

D Planes of the sections

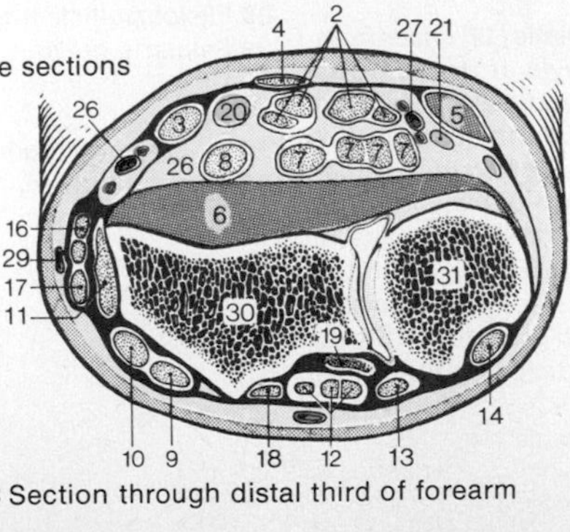

C Section through distal third of forearm

Superficial Layer of the Ventral Forearm Muscles (A–D)

The **pronator teres** (**1**) *arises by its* **humeral head** *from the medial epicondyle of the humerus* (**2**), *as well as from the medial intermuscular septum,* and its **ulnar head** *takes origin from the coronoid process of the ulna* (**3**). *It is inserted* into the rough area in the middle of the *lateral surface of the radius* (**4**). It pronates the forearm and flexes the elbow joint.
Nerve supply: Median nerve (C6 and C7).

Variants

The ulnar head may be absent. If a supracondylar process is present (see p. 110), the humeral head will also arise from it.

The **flexor digitorum superficialis** (**5**) *arises by its* **humeral head** *from the medial epicondyle of the humerus* (**6**), by its **ulnar head** *from the coronoid process of the ulna* (**7**), and by its **radial head** *from the radius* (**8**). Its tendons run in a common sheath (see p. 176) through the carpal canal. The muscle ends in four tendons, each inserted onto the lateral bony crests (**9**) *in the center of the middle phalanges of the 2nd–5th fingers.* At this point the tendons divide two slips, the **perforatus muscle** (**10**) and the tendons of the flexor digitorum profundus (**11**) slip through them, as if through a trough. It is a very weak flexor of the elbow, but a strong flexor of the wrist and the finger joints. Its action on the digits is impaired when the wrist is maximally flexed.
Nerve supply: Median nerve (C7 to Th1).

The **flexor carpi radialis** (**12**) *arises from the medial epicondyle of the humerus* (**6**) *and from* the superficial *fascia of the forearm. It inserts into the palmar surface of the base of the 2nd metacarpal* (**13**) and also in some cases on the 3rd metacarpal. It runs in the carpal canal in a groove in the trapezium, which is closed to form an osteofibrous canal. It is a weak flexor and pronator of the elbow joint and participates in palmar flexion of the wrist, and, together with the extensor carpi radialis longus (see p. 160), it produces radial abduction.
Nerve supply: Median nerve (C6 to C8).

The **palmaris longus** (**14**) *arises from the medial epicondyle of the humerus and radiates into the palmar surface of the hand* with the **palmar aponeurosis** (**15**); (see also p. 174). It flexes the hand toward the palm and tenses the palmar aponeurosis.
Nerve supply: Median nerve (C8 to Th1).

Variants

It may be absent, but even then the palmar aponeurosis is always present.

The **flexor carpi ulnaris** (**16**) lies on the medial side. Its **humeral head** *arises from the medial epicondyle of the humerus* (**6**) and its **ulnar head** *from the olecranon and the upper two thirds of the posterior margin of the ulna* (**17**). *It is inserted onto the pisiform bone* (**18**) and extends by the pisohamate ligament as far as the hamate, and by the pisometacarpal ligament to the 5th metacarpal (**20**). It runs outside the carpal canal. It participates in palmar flexion, where it is more effective than the flexor carpi radialis and also helps in ulnar adduction of the hand.
Nerve supply: Ulnar nerve (C7 and C8).

21 Brachioradialis,
22 Flexor pollicis longus,
23 Pronator quadratus,
24 Biceps brachii,
25 Flexor retinaculum,
26 Lumbricales,
27 Abductor pollicis brevis
28 Flexor pollicis brevis
29 Palmaris brevis,
30 Ulna,
31 Radius,
32 Vinculum longum,
33 Vinculum breve.

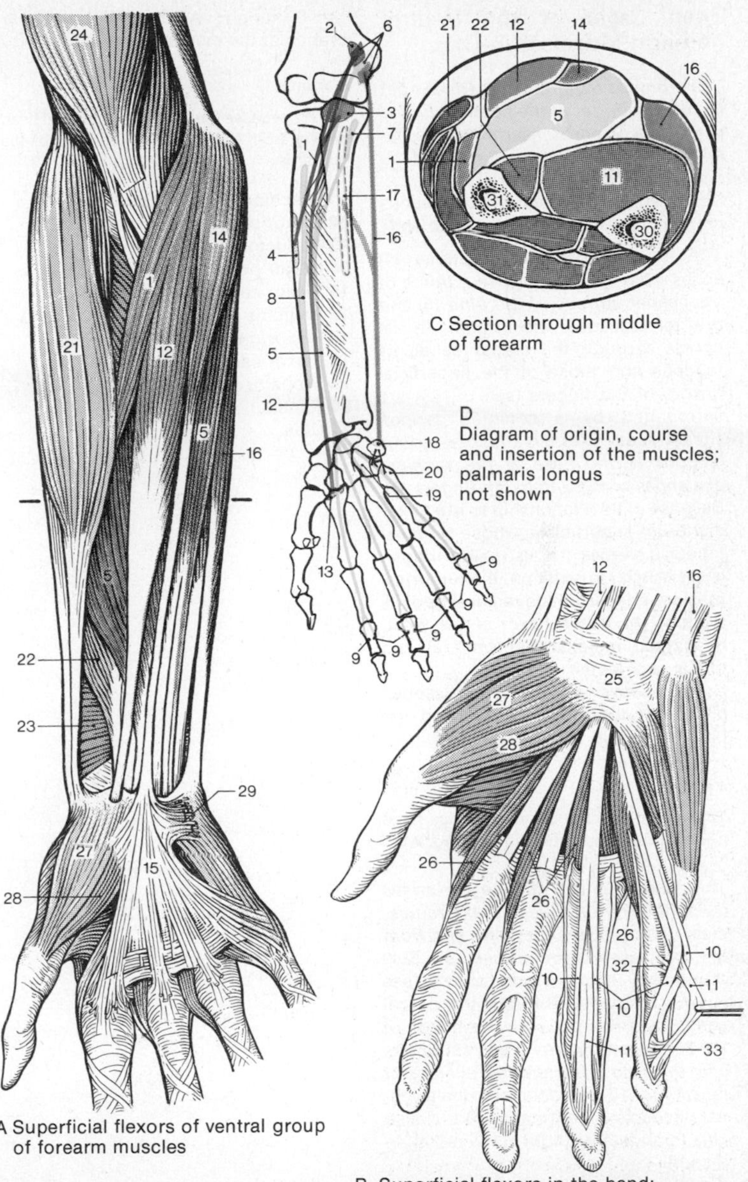

C Section through middle of forearm

D Diagram of origin, course and insertion of the muscles; palmaris longus not shown

A Superficial flexors of ventral group of forearm muscles

B Superficial flexors in the hand; palmar aponeurosis removed

Deep Layer of the Ventral Forearm Muscles (A–C)

The **pronator quadratus** (**1**) *arises from the distal quarter of the palmar surface of the ulna* (**2**) and *is inserted on the distal quarter of the palmar surface of the radius* (**3**). It takes part in pronation.
Nerve supply: Anterior interosseous branch of the median nerve (C 6 to Th 1).

The **flexor digitorum profundus** (**4**) *arises from the proximal two thirds of the palmar surface of the ulna* (**5**) *and the interosseous membrane.* In its course through the carpal canal, its tendons and those of the superficial flexors of the fingers (see p. 156) are surrounded by a common tendon sheath (see p. 176). *It is attached by four tendons to the base of the terminal phalanges of the 2nd to 5th fingers* (**6**). Because of its relationship to the flexor digitorum superficialis whose terminal tendon it pierces, it is also called the **perforans muscle**. In addition, the lumbrical muscles arise from the radial side of its tendons (**7**). It is a flexor of the wrist, midcarpal, metacarpophalangeal and phalangeal joints.
Nerve supply: Anterior interosseous branch of the median nerve and the ulnar nerve (C6 to Th1).

Variants

The tendon which reaches the index finger often has a belly of its own (see Fig. **A**).

The **flexor pollicis longus** (**8**) *arises from the anterior surface of the radius*, distal to the radial tuberosity, *and from the interosseous membrane* (**9**). Surrounded by its own tendon sheath (see p. 176) it extends through the carpal canal, then lies between the heads of the flexor pollicis brevis and *continues onto the base of the terminal phalanx of the thumb* (**10**). It is a flexor of the terminal phalanx of the thumb and it is also able to abduct it a little in the radial direction.

Nerve supply: Anterior interosseous branch of the median nerve (C6 to C8).

Variants

In 40% of cases there is also a humeral head arising from the medial epicondyle of the humerus.

11 Brachioradialis,
12 Flexor retinaculum,
13 Abductor pollicis brevis,
14 Flexor pollicis brevis,
15 Flexor carpi radialis,
16 Palmaris longus,
17 Flexor digitorum superficialis,
18 Flexor carpi ulnaris,
19 Pronator teres,
20 Radius,
21 Ulna.

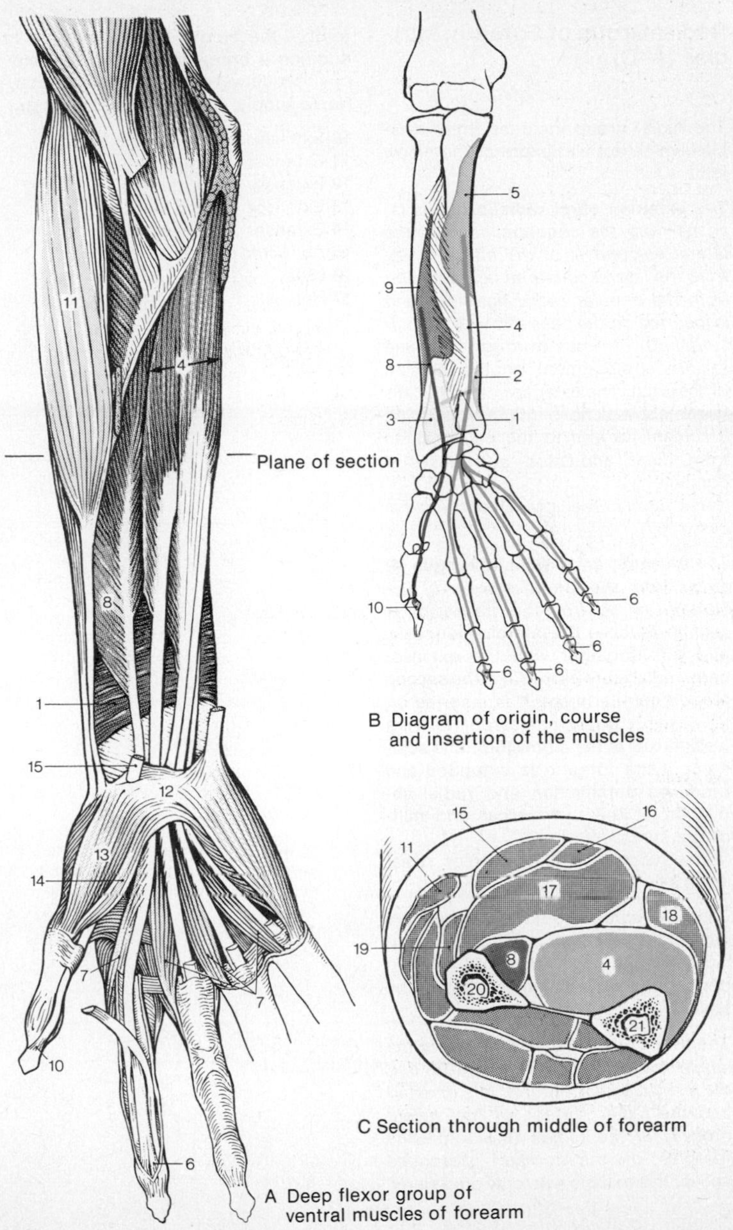

A Deep flexor group of ventral muscles of forearm

B Diagram of origin, course and insertion of the muscles

C Section through middle of forearm

Radial Group of Forearm Muscles (A–D)

The radial group includes three muscles which act as flexors at the elbow joint.

The **extensor carpi radialis brevis** (**1**) *arises from the common head of the lateral epicondyle of the humerus* (**2**), *from the lateral collateral ligament and from the annular radial ligament, and is inserted on the base of the 3rd metacarpal* (**3**). It runs through the 2nd tendon compartment on the dorsum of the wrist. The extensor carpi radialis brevis is a weak flexor of the elbow joint. It brings the arm to the mid-position from ulnar adduction and flexes it dorsally.
Nerve supply: Deep branch of the radial nerve (C7).

The **extensor carpi radialis longus** (**4**) *arises from the lateral margin of the humerus* (**5**) *and from the intermuscular septum* as far as the lateral epicondyle, and runs together with the extensor carpi radialis brevis through the second tendon compartment. *It is inserted on the base of the 2nd metacarpal* (**6**). It is a weak flexor at the elbow joint and supinator if the forearm is extended and produces dorsiflexion and radial abduction at the radiocarpal and midcarpal joints.
Nerve supply: Deep branch of radial nerve (C5 to C7).

The two muscles just described are called **"fist clenchers"**, as during clenching the hand must be slightly flexed dorsally to permit maximal action by the flexors.

The **brachioradialis** (**7**) *arises from the lateral margin of the humerus* (**8**) *and the intermuscular septum. It is inserted into the radial surface of the styloid process of the radius* (**9**). Unlike the muscles of the forearm described above, this muscle acts only on a single joint – the elbow – and flexes it. In addition it brings the arm to the mid-position between pro- and supination.
Nerve supply: Radial nerve (C5 and C6).

10 Extensor digitorum,
11 Extensor digiti minimi,
12 Extensor carpi ulnaris,
13 Extensor pollicis longus,
14 Extensor pollicis brevis,
15 Abductor pollicis longus,
16 Ulna,
17 Radius.

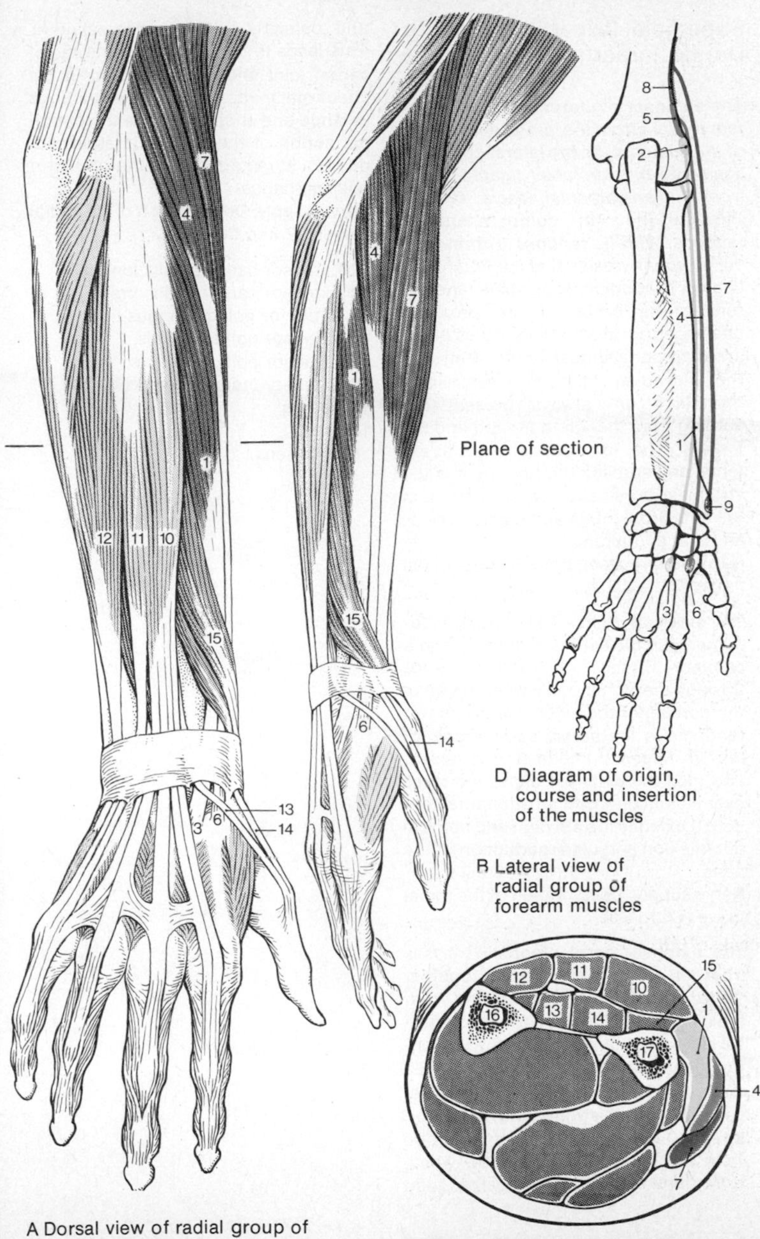

D Diagram of origin, course and insertion of the muscles

B Lateral view of radial group of forearm muscles

A Dorsal view of radial group of forearm muscles

C Section through middle of forearm

Superficial (Ulnar) Layer of the Dorsal Forearm Muscles (A–C)

The **extensor digitorum** (**1**) *has* a flattened *origin from the lateral epicondyle of the humerus* (**2**), *the lateral collateral ligament, annular radial ligament and from the antebrachial fascia.* It runs through the 4th compartment of tendons. *With its tendons it forms the dorsal aponeurosis* (**3**) *of the 2nd to 5th fingers.* In addition, slips of the tendons run to the bases of the proximal phalanges (**4**) and to the capsules of the metacarpophalangeal joints. Between the individual tendons **intertendinous connections** are always present (**5**), starting from the 4th to the 3rd and 5th fingers. The extensor digitorum extends and spreads the fingers. It is the strongest dorsiflexor of the wrist and the midcarpal joints and it acts, too, as an ulnar adductor.
Nerve supply: Deep branch of the radial nerve (C6 to C8).

The **extensor digiti minimi** (**6**) *arises together with the extensor digitorum in a common head* (**2**) and extends through the 5th tendon compartment of the dorsum of the wrist, usually as two tendons, *to the dorsal aponeurosis of the 5th finger.* Sometimes it is absent and then the extensor digitorum takes over its function with an additional tendon. It extends the 5th digit and helps in dorsiflexion and ulnar adduction of the hand.
Nerve supply: Deep branch of the radial nerve (C6 to C8).

The **extensor carpi ulnaris** (**7**) *arises from the common* head (**2**) together with the extensor digitorum, *and from the ulna* (**8**), and runs on the mediodorsal side of the ulna through the 6th tendon compartment to *the base of the 5th metacarpal* (**9**). It is really misnamed because it acts as a strong ulnar adductor, an action that is most easily understood from the course of its tendon, which runs dorsally to the radiocarpal joint and palmarly to the midcarpal joint. This leads to dorsiflexion of the radiocarpal joint and palmar flexion in the midcarpal joint, i. e., the two functions balance one another. Hence the principal action of the muscle is as an adductor. Its antagonist is the abductor pollicis longus.
Nerve supply: Deep branch of the radial nerve (C7 and C8).

10 Extensor carpi radialis longus,
11 Extensor carpi radialis brevis,
12 Abductor pollicis longus,
13 Extensor pollicis brevis,
14 Extensor pollicis longus,
15 Extensor indicis,
16 Radius,
17 Ulna,
18 Anconeus.

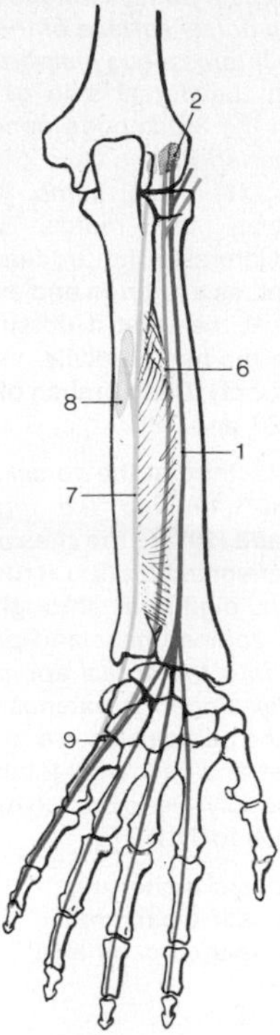

Plane of section

C Diagram of origin, course and insertion of the muscles

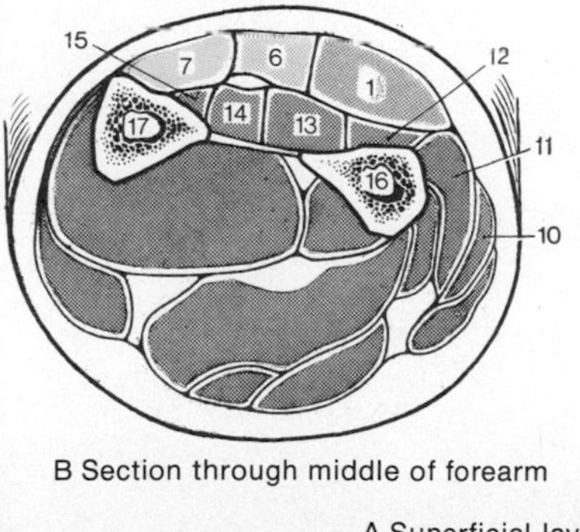

B Section through middle of forearm

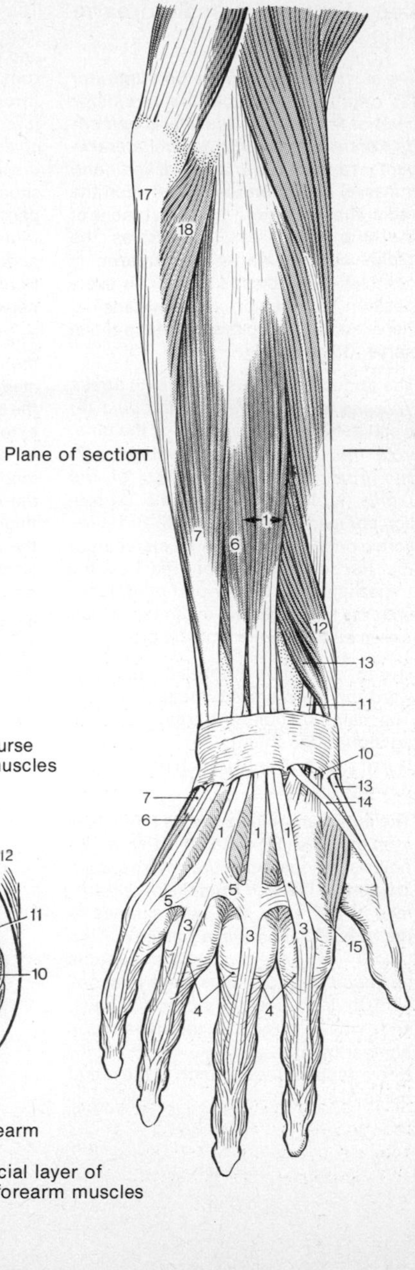

A Superficial layer of dorsal forearm muscles

Deep Layer of Dorsal Forearm Muscles (A–C)

The *surfaces from which the* **supinator** (**3**) *originates* include the *supinator crest of the ulna* (**1**), *the lateral epicondyle of the humerus* (**2**), *the collateral ligament and the annular radial ligament. It inserts on the radius* (**4**) between the radial tuberosity and the attachment of the pronator teres. It encircles the radius and supinates the forearm, in contrast to the biceps brachii, in every position of flexion and extension.
Nerve supply: Deep branch of the radial nerve (C5 and C6).

The **abductor pollicis longus** (**5**) *arises from the dorsal surface of the ulna* (**6**) distal to the supinator crest of the ulna, *from the interosseous membrane* (**7**) *and from the dorsal surface of the radius* (**8**). It runs through the 1st tendon compartment (see p. 176) and is *inserted on the base of the 1st metacarpal* (**9**). Part of the tendon reaches the trapezium and another part often fuses with the tendon of the extensor pollicis brevis and abductor pollicis brevis.

Due to its position it flexes the hand toward the palm and abducts it radially. The main function of this muscle is abduction of the thumb.
Nerve supply: Deep branch of the radial nerve (C7 and C8).

The **extensor pollicis brevis** (**10**) *arises from the ulna* (**11**) distal to the abductor pollicis longus *from the interosseous membrane* (**12**) *and from the dorsal surface of the radius* (**13**), and *extends to the base of the proximal phalanx of the thumb* (**14**). It extends and abducts the thumb because of its close relationship to the abductor pollicis longus, with which it runs in the 1st tendon compartment.
Nerve supply: Deep branch of the radial nerve (C8–Th1).

The **extensor pollicis longus** (**15**) *arises from the dorsal surface of the ulna* (**16**) *and the interosseous membrane* (**17**). It runs on the dorsal side of the wrist through the 3rd tendon compartment. *It is inserted on the base of the distal phalanx* (**18**) *of the thumb.* It uses the crest on the radius, which is situated lateral to the 3rd tendon compartment, as a fulcrum and extends the thumb. At the wrist it dorsiflexes and abducts the hand radially.
Nerve supply: Deep branch of the radial nerve (C7 and C8).

The distal third of the *dorsal surface of the ulna* (**19**) *and the interosseous membrane* (**20**) *are the sites of origin* of the **extensor indicis** (**21**). It runs with the extensor digitorum through the 4th tendon compartment and *projects its tendon into the dorsal aponeurosis of the index finger.* It extends the index finger and participates in dorsiflexion at the wrist and midcarpal joints.
Nerve supply: Deep branch of the radial nerve (C8 to Th1).

22 Extensor digitorum,
23 Extensor digiti minimi,
24 Extensor carpi ulnaris,
25 Ulna,
26 Radius.

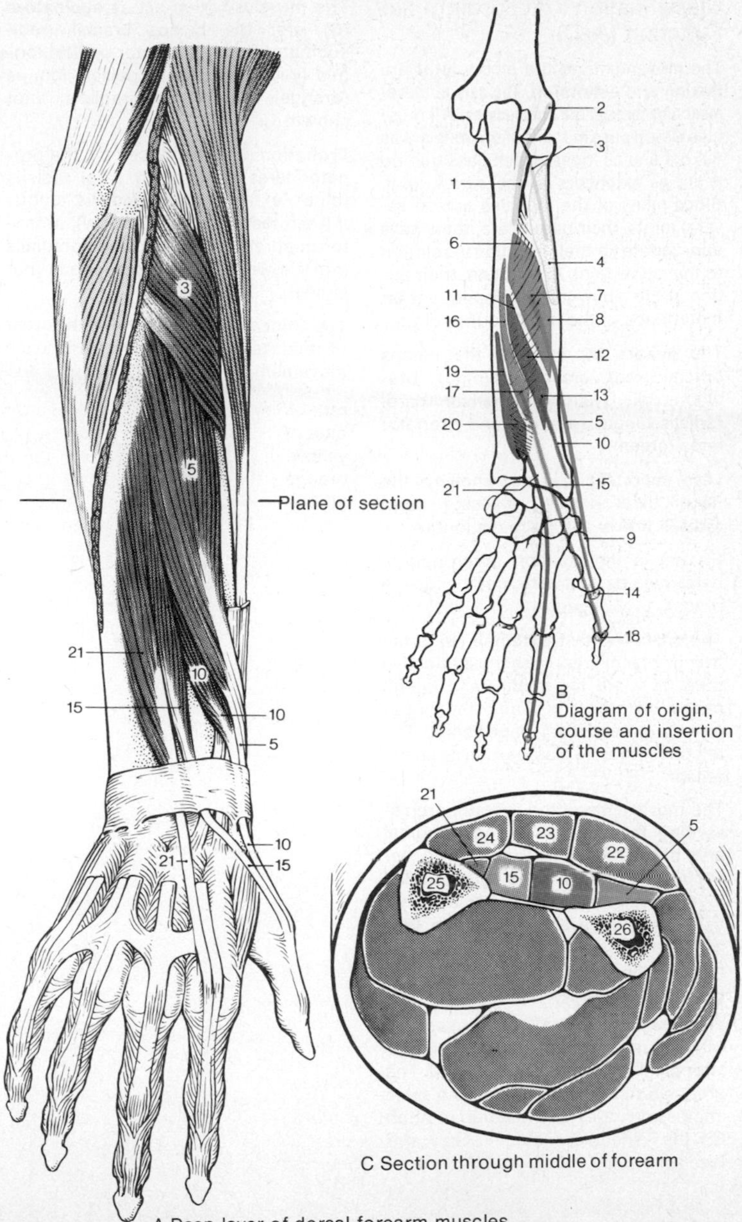

B
Diagram of origin, course and insertion of the muscles

C Section through middle of forearm

A Deep layer of dorsal forearm muscles

Classification According to Function (A–D)

The movements at the elbow joint are **flexion** and **extension. The axis of movement runs through the epicondyles.** All muscles which pass in front of the axis act as flexors and all those which pass behind it act as extensors at the elbow joint. Since many of the muscles act on several joints, their names are not always appropriate for their function in relation to the elbow joint. In addition, their action at the elbow joint is dependent on the attitude of the neighboring joints.

The **flexors** (**A**) include: the biceps brachii (red), brachialis (blue), brachioradialis (yellow), extensor carpi radialis longus (orange) and pronator teres (green).

Less important are (not shown): the flexor carpi radialis, extensor carpi radialis brevis and palmaris longus.

Flexion in the position of pronation, performed by contraction of the biceps brachii, is strongest.

The only important **extensor** (**B**) is the triceps brachii (red). The most effective parts of it are the medial and lateral heads, while the long head of the triceps is only of secondary importance. The anconeus may be disregarded as an extensor.

The movements of the forearm are **reversing movements** at the proximal and distal radioulnar joints, with associated movement at the humeroradial joint. These reversing movements are called **pronation** and **supination** (see p. 118) and they **occur around an axis which runs from the fovea on the head of the radius to the styloid process of the ulna.**

Pronation and supination are executed with almost equal force but with greater strength if the elbow joint is flexed. The preponderance of pronation is a false impression due to a medial rotation in the shoulder joint (*Lanz and Wachsmuth*).

The muscles which act as **supinators** (**C**) are: the biceps brachii (red), supinator (blue), abductor pollicis longus (yellow), extensor pollicis longus (orange) and brachioradialis (not shown).

Pronation (**D**) is produced by: the pronator teres (red), flexor carpi radialis (blue), extensor carpi radialis longus if the forearm is flexed (yellow), pronator quadratus (orange), brachioradialis (not shown) and palmaris longus (not shown).

The color of the arrows shows the order of importance of the muscles in each movement:

red
blue
yellow
orange
green

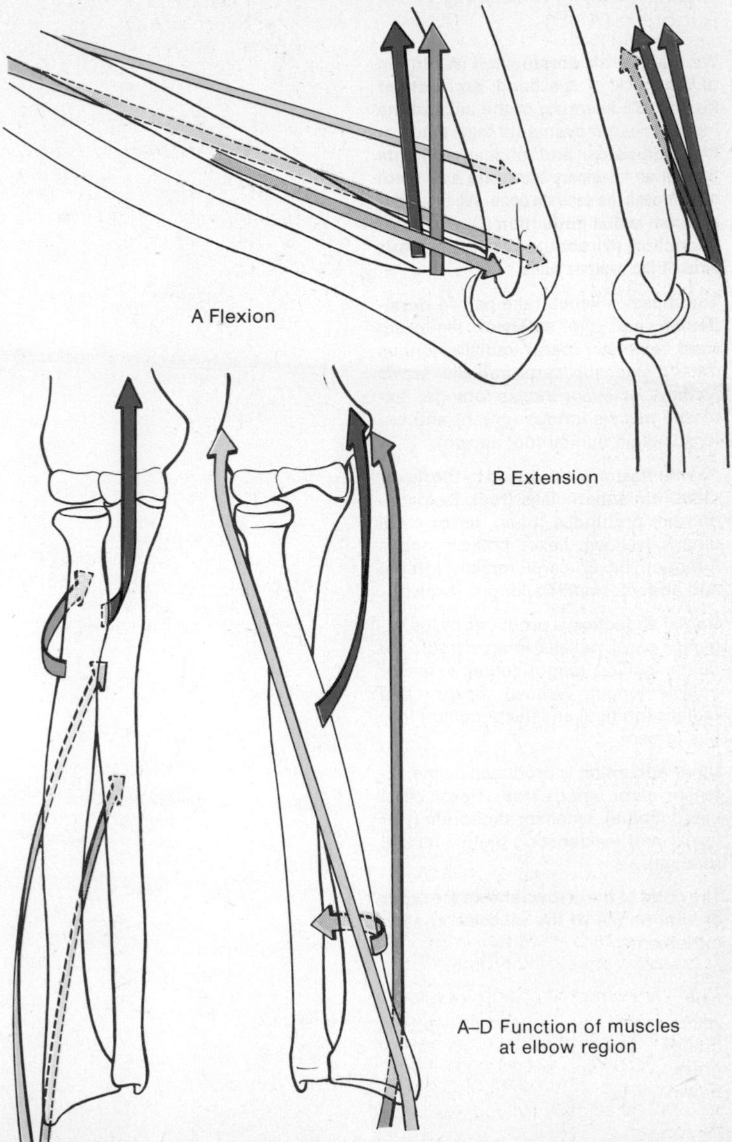

A Flexion

B Extension

C Supination

D Pronation

A–D Function of muscles at elbow region

Classification According to Function (A–D)

We distinguish **dorsiflexion** (**A**), lifting of the back of the hand, and **palmar flexion** (**B**), lowering of the back of the hand. These movements take place at the radiocarpal and midcarpal joints **through an imaginary transverse axis which runs through the capitate bone**. We also distinguish **radial abduction** (**C**) and **ulnar adduction** (**D**) about a **dorsopalmar axis through the capitate bone.**

The muscles which take part in **dorsiflexion** are: the extensor digitorum (red), extensor carpi radialis longus (blue), extensor carpi radialis brevis (yellow), extensor indicis (orange), extensor pollicis longus (green) and extensor digiti minimi (not shown).

Palmar flexion is produced by the flexor digitorum superficialis (red), flexor digitorum profundus (blue), flexor carpi ulnaris (yellow), flexor pollicis longus (orange), flexor carpi radialis (green) and abductor pollicis longus (brown).

Radial abduction is produced by the extensor carpi radialis longus (red), abductor pollicis longus (blue), extensor pollicis longus (yellow), flexor carpi radialis (orange) and flexor pollicis longus (green).

Ulnar adduction is produced by the extensor carpi ulnaris (red), flexor carpi ulnaris (blue), extensor digitorum (yellow) and extensor digiti minimi (orange).

The color of the arrows shows the order of importance of the muscles in each movement:

red
blue
yellow
orange
green
brown

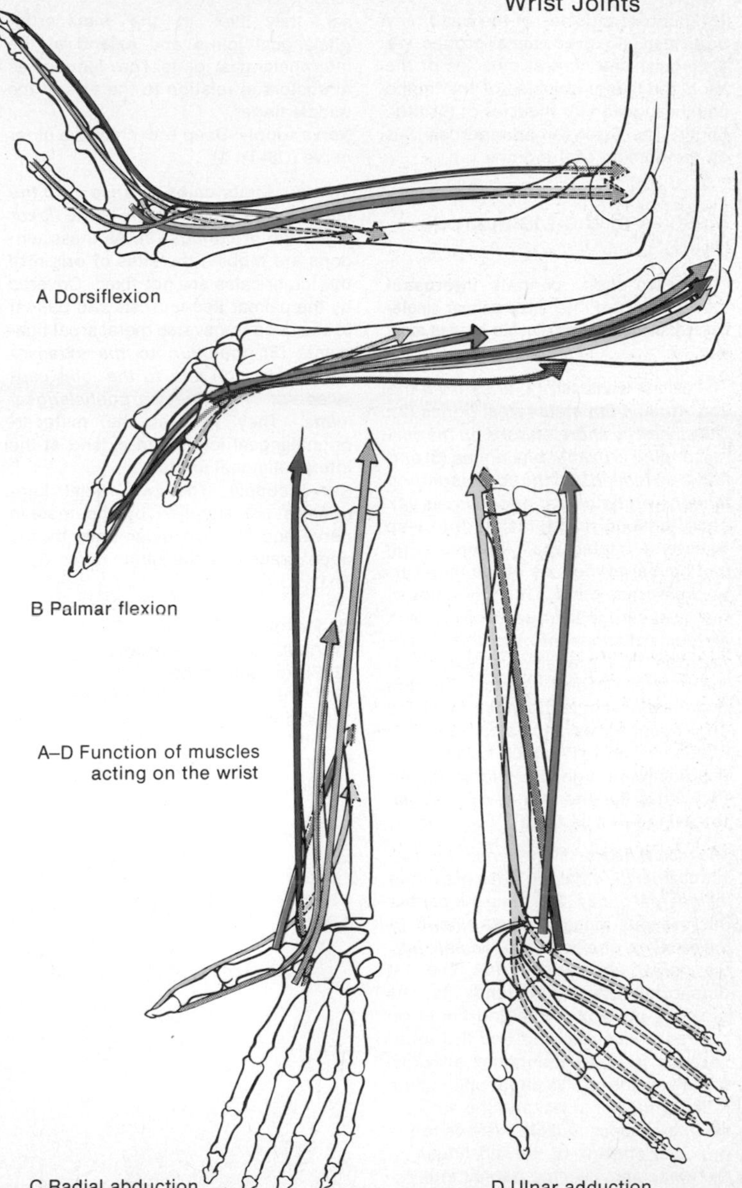

A–D Function of muscles acting on the wrist

The intrinsic muscles of the hand may be divided into three palmar groups. We distinguish the central muscles of the hand, the thenar muscles of the thumb and the hypothenar muscles of the little finger. The extensor aponeurosis lies on the dorsum of the digits.

Muscles of the Metacarpus (A–D)

The seven short, pennate **interossei** may be divided into **three palmar single-headed and four dorsal double-headed muscles**.

The **palmar interossei**; (**1**) *arise from the 2nd, 4th and 5th metacarpal bones* (**2**). *They insert by short tendons on the corresponding proximal phalanges* (**3**) *and they also radiate into the corresponding tendons of the dorsal aponeurosis* (**4**). Their tendons run dorsal to the deep transverse metacarpal ligaments (**5**) and palmar to the axis of the metacarpophalangeal joints. Thus, they flex at the metacarpophalangeal joints, and by their radiations into the dorsal aponeurosis they are able to extend at the interphalangeal joints. Through their relationship to the metacarpal and phalangeal bones, they also adduct in relation to an axis which passes longitudinally through the middle finger; they move the 2nd, 4th and 5th finger toward the middle finger.

The **dorsal interossei** (**6**) *arise by two heads from the adjacent sides of the five metacarpal bones* (**2,7**). Like the palmar interosseous muscles, *they extend to the proximal phalanges and radiate into the dorsal aponeurosis* (**4**). The 1st dorsal interosseous extends to the proximal phalanx of the 2nd finger on the radial side, the 2nd and 3rd interosseous muscles reach the proximal phalanx of the middle finger on both the radial and ulnar sides, and the 4th dorsal interosseous muscle extends to the proximal phalanx of the 4th finger on the ulnar side. Like the palmar interossei, they flex at the metacarpophalangeal joints and extend at the interphalangeal joints. They function as abductors in relation to the axis of the middle finger.
Nerve supply: Deep branch of the ulnar nerve (C8–Th 1).

The four **lumbricales** (**8**) *arise from the radial sides of the tendons of the flexor digitorum profundus* (**9**). As these tendons are mobile, the sites of origin of the lumbricales are not fixed. Covered by the palmar aponeurosis and palmar to the deep transverse metacarpal ligaments (**5**), *they run to the extensor aponeurosis* (**4**) *and to the joint capsules of the metacarpophalangeal joints.* They flex at the metacarpophalangeal joints and extend at the interphalangeal joints.
Nerve supply: The two radial lumbricales are supplied by the median nerve and the two ulnar ones by the deep branch of the ulnar nerve (C8–Th1).

10 Flexor retinaculum,
11 Abductor pollicis brevis,
12 Flexor pollicis brevis,
13 Transverse head of the adductor pollicis,
14 Abductor digiti minimi,
15 Flexor carpi ulnaris,
16 Flexor carpi radialis.

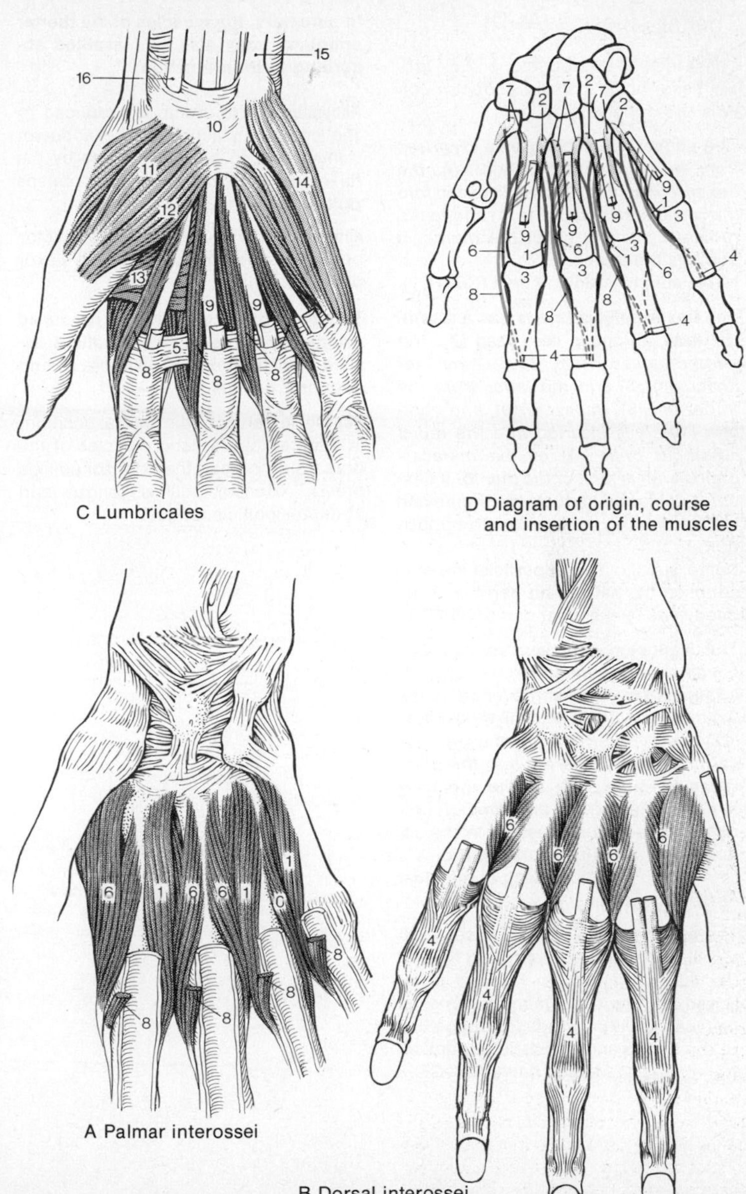

C Lumbricales

D Diagram of origin, course and insertion of the muscles

A Palmar interossei

B Dorsal interossei

Thenar Muscles (A–D)

These include the abductor pollicis brevis, flexor pollicis brevis, adductor pollicis and opponens pollicis.

The **abductor pollicis brevis** (**1**) *arises from the scaphoid tubercle* (**2**) *and the flexor retinaculum* (**3**). *It is inserted into the radial sesamoid bone* (**4**) *and to the proximal phalanx* (**5**) *of the thumb.* It abducts the thumb.
Nerve supply: Median nerve (C8–Th 1).

The **flexor pollicis brevis** has a **superficial head** (**6**) and a **deep head** (**7**). *The former arises from the flexor retinaculum* (**3**) *and the latter from the trapezium* (**8**), *trapezoid* (**9**), *and capitate* (**10**). *It is inserted into the radial sesamoid bone* (**4**) *of the metacarpophalangeal joint of the thumb.* It flexes, adducts and abducts the thumb and is able to bring the thumb into opposition.
Nerve supply: The superficial head is supplied by the median nerve and the deep head by the ulnar nerve (C8–Th1).

The **adductor pollicis** *also has two heads of origin,* the **transverse head** (**11**) *originating from the entire length of the 3rd metacarpal* (**12**), and the **oblique head** (**13**) *originating from the adjacent carpal bones. It is inserted into the ulnar sesamoid bone* (**14**) *of the metacarpophalangeal joint of the thumb.* It produces adduction and assists in the opposition and flexion of the thumb.
Nerve supply: Deep branch of the ulnar nerve (C8 –Th 1).

The **opponens pollicis** (**15**) *arises from the tubercle of the trapezium* (**16**) *and the flexor retinaculum* (**3**), *and is inserted into the radial margin of the 1st metacarpal* (**17**). It produces opposition of the thumb and assists in adduction.
Nerve supply: Median nerve (C6–C7).

In summary, the muscles of the thenar eminence may also be classified according to their function:

Adduction of the thumb is produced by the combined action of the adductor pollicis and to a lesser degree by the flexor pollicis brevis and opponens pollicis.

Abduction is produced by the abductor pollicis brevis and partly by the flexor pollicis brevis.

The position of **opposition** is produced principally by the opponens pollicis, assisted by the flexor pollicis brevis and adductor pollicis.

Reposition (return to the neutral position) is effected by the long muscles of the dorsal side, namely the extensor pollicis brevis, extensor pollicis longus and abductor pollicis longus.

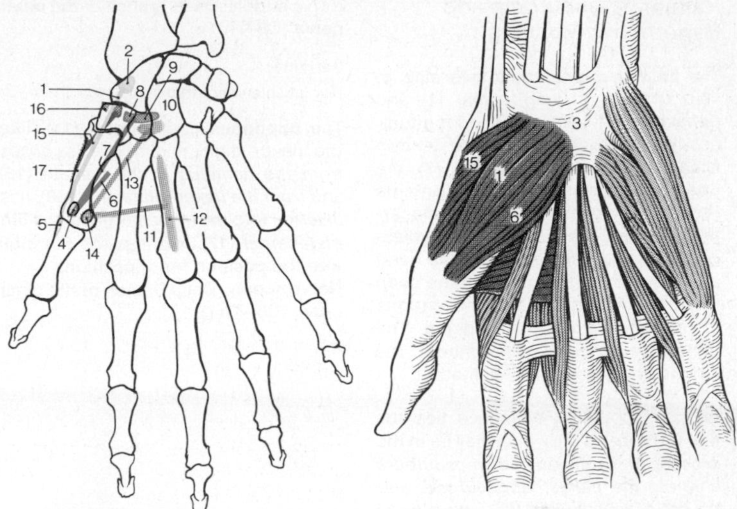

D Diagram of origin, course and insertion of the muscles

A Thenar muscles, 1st layer

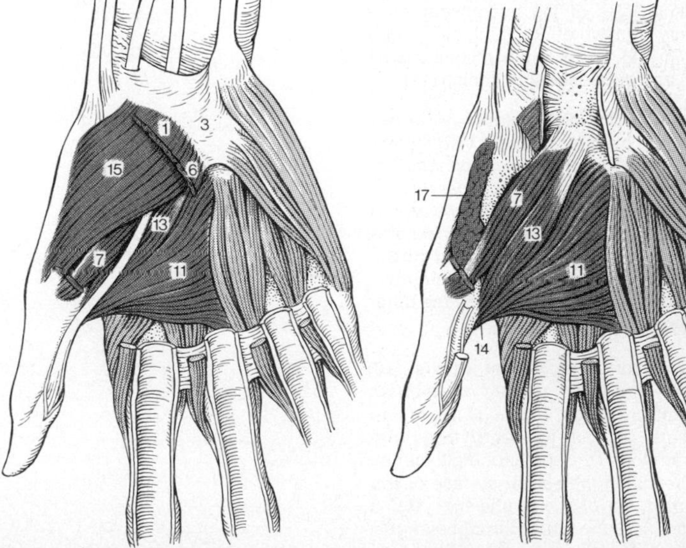

B Thenar muscles, 2nd layer

C Thenar muscles, 3rd layer

Palmar Aponeurosis and Hypothenar Muscles

The **palmar aponeurosis** (see also p. 156) consists of *longitudinal* (**1**) and *transverse* (**2**) *fascicles*. The longitudinal fibers are attached to the tendon sheaths of the flexor tendons (**3**), the deep transverse metacarpal ligaments (**4**) and the ligaments of the metacarpophalangeal joints. They also radiate into the corium of the palm of the hand (**5**) and send eight septa (**6**) to the deep fascia to compartmentalize the tendons of the long flexors of the digits. The transverse fasciculi (**2**) connect the longitudinal fibers with each other.

In the hypothenar eminence lies the **palmaris brevis** (**7**), which may be in the process of involution *and whose fibers connect the palmar aponeurosis and the flexor retinaculum* (**8**) *to the skin of the ulnar border of the hand.*
Nerve supply: Superficial branch of the ulnar nerve (C8–Th 1).

The muscles of the hypothenar eminence consist of the abductor digiti minimi (**9**), flexor digiti minimi brevis (**10**) and opponens digit minimi (**11**).

The **abductor digiti minimi** (**9**) *arises from the pisiform* (**12**), *the pisohamate ligament* (**13**) *and the flexor retinaculum* (**8**) *and is inserted into the ulnar margin of the base of the proximal phalanx of the 5th digit* (**14**). In part it also radiates into the extensor aponeurosis of the 5th digit. It functions as a pure abductor.
Nerve supply: Deep branch of the ulnar nerve (C8–Th 1).

The **flexor digiti minimi brevis** (**10**) *arises from the flexor retinaculum* (**8**) *and also from the hamulus of the hamate* (**15**). At its insertion it fuses with the tendon of the abductor digiti minimi and *ends on the palmar surface of the base of the proximal phalanx* (**16**). It flexes at the metacarpophalangeal joint.
Nerve supply: Deep branch of the ulnar nerve (C8–Th 1).

Variants

The muscle very often is absent.

The **opponens digiti minimi** (**11**), like the flexor digiti minimi brevis, *arises from the hamulus of the hamate* (**15**) *and from the flexor retinaculum* (**8**). *It is inserted into the ulnar margin of the 5th metacarpal* (**17**). It brings the 5th digit into the position for opposition.
Nerve supply: Deep branch of the ulnar nerve (C8–Th1).

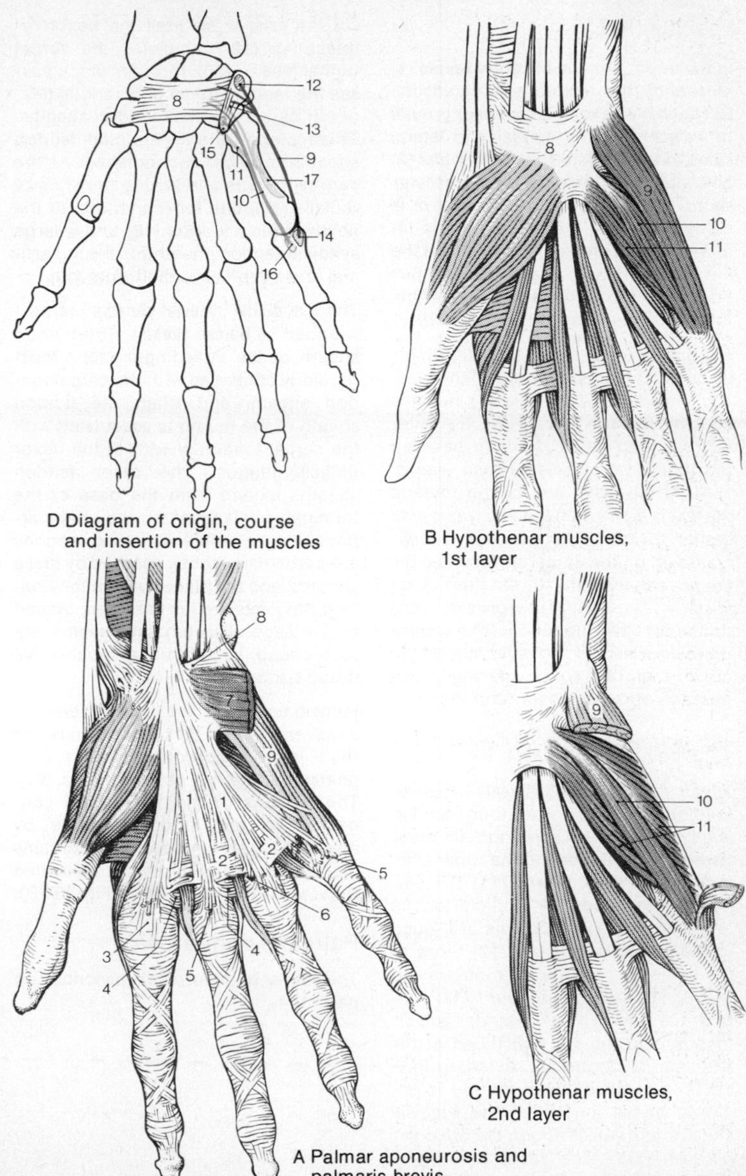

D Diagram of origin, course and insertion of the muscles

B Hypothenar muscles, 1st layer

C Hypothenar muscles, 2nd layer

A Palmar aponeurosis and palmaris brevis

Fascias (A–C)

In the upper arm the **brachial fascia** (**1**) surrounds the flexors and extensors. Between the flexor and extensor groups of muscles on the medial and lateral sides of the humerus are the *medial* (**2**) and *lateral* (**3**) *brachial intermuscular septa*. The fascia of the upper arm is continuous with the axillary fascia (**4**) and with the forearm fascia (**5**). On the anterior surface of the upper arm just above the elbow there is an aperture, the *hiatus basilicus* (**6**) (see p. 362).

The **antebrachial fascia** (**5**) is tightly attached to the dorsal surface of the ulna. The *bicipital aponeurosis* (**7**) radiates into the forearm fascia, and the latter sends strong septa (**8**) deep between the individual muscle groups (see p. 154). At the distal end of the forearm the fascia is strengthened by transverse bands to form the *extensor retinaculum* (**9**) on the dorsal surface and the *flexor retinaculum* (**10**) on the palmar surface. The retinacula provide conduits for the tendons of various muscles. Deep to the extensor retinaculum there are six compartments for passage of the extensor tendons.

Tendon Sheaths (D–E)

These six **dorsal compartments** (**vaginae tendinum**) contain the long tendon sheaths for nine muscles and are numbered from the radial to the ulnar side. In the *1st compartment* (**11**) the tendons of the abductor pollicis longus and extensor pollicis brevis are found in the *2nd compartment* (**12**) those of the extensor carpi radialis longus and brevis. The *3rd compartment* (**13**) contains the tendon of the extensor pollicis longus, and the *4th* (**14**) those of the extensor digitorum and extensor indicis. The extensor digiti minimi is enclosed in the longest of the synovial sheaths and runs through the *5th compartment* (**15**). The *6th compartment* (**16**) contains the extensor carpi ulnaris.

On the **palm of the hand** the flexor retinaculum (**10**) completes the carpal tunnel (see p. 120), through which passes the median nerve and various flexors in carpal synovial tendon sheaths. Three carpal and five digital tendon sheaths may be distinguished. At the carpus there is one for the flexor carpi radialis (**17**), one for the tendon of the flexor pollicis longus (**18**) and a large synovial tendon sheath for the superficial and deep flexor digitorum (**19**).

The **five digital synovial sheaths** are surrounded by **fibrous sheaths**. The tendon sheath of the little finger (**20**) almost regularly continues with the carpal tendon sheath, and often the tendon sheath of the thumb is associated with the carpal tendon sheath of the flexor pollicis longus. The other tendon sheaths extend from the base of the terminal phalanges to the metacarpophalangeal joints. The long tendons are particularly tightly secured by these sheaths, and the places where they run over the joints are further strengthened by cartilage. The tendon sheaths are surrounded by additional connective tissue bands.

Immediately over the joints there are *transverse fibers* (**21**), and in between them, in the region of the corpus of a phalanx, there are *oblique fibers* (**22**). The tendons of the flexors are connected to the tendon sheaths by mesotendons. A mesotendon contains blood vessels and nerves and is called the *vinculum* tendinum (see Fig. 157 B).

Palmar Aponeurosis

The palmar aponeurosis is described on page 174.

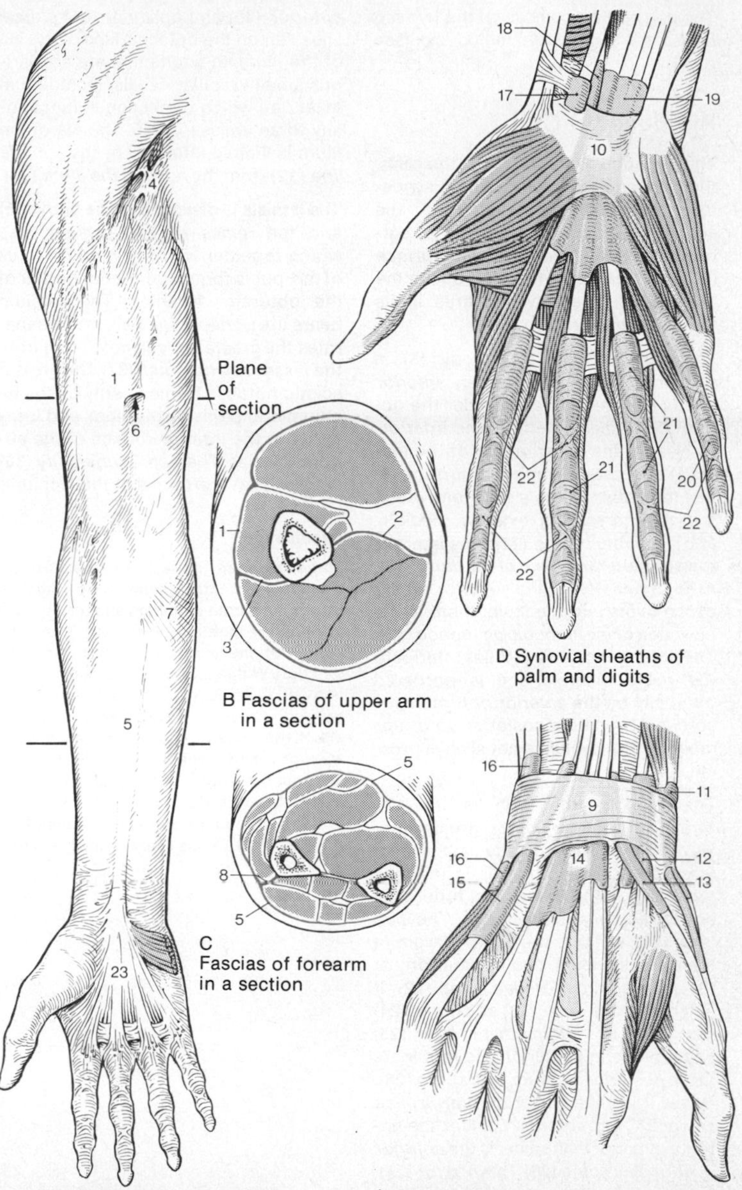

A Fascias of the upper limb

B Fascias of upper arm in a section

C Fascias of forearm in a section

D Synovial sheaths of palm and digits

E Synovial sheaths of dorsum of hand

The bony **pelvis** consists of the two hip bones, the sacrum and the coccyx (see p. 48).

Hip Bone (A–C)

The **hip bone** has three parts, the **pubis**, the **ilium** and the **ischium**, which synostose within the acetabulum in the *acetabular fossa* (**1**), which is surrounded by the *lunate articular surface* (**2**). The *acetabular notch* (**3**) opens the acetabulum inferiorly and thus limits the *obturator foramen* (**4**).

The **pubis** consists of a *body* (**5**), a *superior ramus* (**6**) and an *inferior ramus* (**7**). The two rami border the obturator foramen anteriorly and inferiorly. Near to the superior end of the medially orientated *symphysial surface* (**8**) lies the *pubic tubercle* (**9**), from which the *pubic crest* (**10**) extends medially and the *pubic pecten* (**11**) runs laterally toward the *arcuate line of the ilium* (**12**). At the transition of the superior ramus of the pubis into the ilium, there is the elevation of the *iliopubic eminence* (**13**). The *obturator groove* (**14**) lies inferior to the pubic tubercle and is bordered internally by the *anterior obturator tubercle* (**15**) and the *posterior obturator tubercle* (**16**), which is not always present.

The **ilium**, together with its *ala* (**17**), forms the boundary of the greater pelvis. On the inner surface is the *iliac fossa* (**18**), posterior to this is the *iliac tuberosity* (**19**). Below the tuberosity lies the *auricular surface* (**20**). The *iliac crest* (**21**), which is the upper margin of the ala of the ilium, begins anteriorly at the *anterior superior iliac spine* (**22**). It extends as the *outer* (**23**) and *inner* (**24**) *lips*, with an *intermediate line* (**25**) superiorly and posteriorly, to terminate at the *posterior superior iliac spine* (**26**). Below it lies the *posterior inferior iliac spine* (**27**), and anteriorly, under the anterior superior iliac spine, is the *anterior inferior iliac spine* (**28**). The *inferior* (**29**), *anterior* (**30**) and *posterior* (**31**) *gluteal lines* run on the outer surface of the ala of the ilium. In addition, there are various small vascular canals, including at least one which corresponds functionally to an emissary vein. The ala of the ilium is limited inferiorly by the *arcuate line* (**12**) from the *body of the ilium* (**32**).

The **ischium** is divided into the *body* (**33**) and the *ramus of the ischium* (**34**), which together with the inferior ramus of the pubis forms the inferior border of the obturator foramen. The ischium bears the *ischial spine* (**35**), which separates the *greater sciatic notch* (**36**) from the *lesser sciatic notch* (**37**). The greater sciatic notch is formed partly by the ischium and partly by the ilium, and it extends to the inferior surface of the auricular facies. The *ischial tuberosity* (**38**) develops on the ramus of the ischium.

Ossification

Three anlagen appear: in the 3rd intrauterine month (ilium), 4th–5th intrauterine month (ischium) and the 5th–6th intrauterine month (pubis). They fuse in the center of the acetabulum in a Y-shaped junction. Within the acetabulum one or more individual ossification centers develop between the ages of 10 and 12 years. Synostosis of the three bones occurs between the ages of 5 and 7 years, but within the acetabulum itself not until between the ages of 15 and 16 years. Epiphysial centers of ossification occur in the spines at the age of 16, in the ischial tuberosity and in the iliac crest between the ages of 13 and 15.

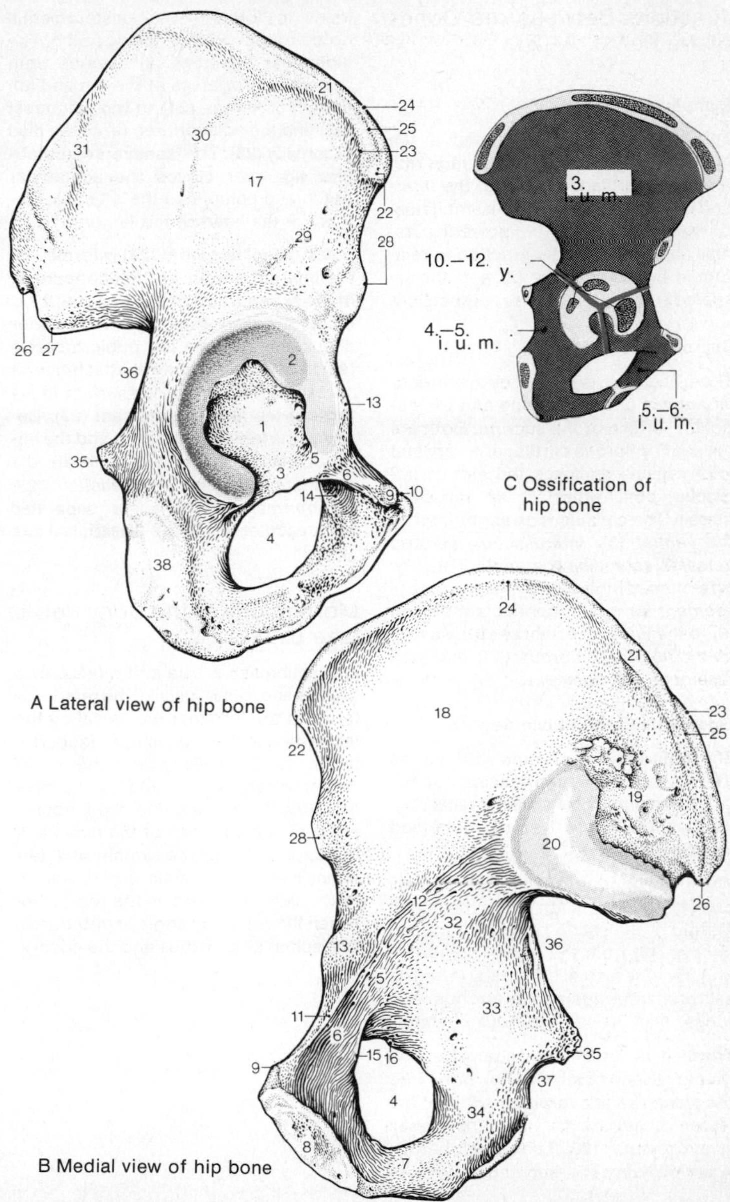

A Lateral view of hip bone

B Medial view of hip bone

C Ossification of hip bone

Junctions Between the Bones of the Pelvis (A–B)

Symphysis

The two hip bones are joined at the symphysis (**1**) by a fibrous cartilage with a hyaline cartilage covering, the *interpubic disk.* Within the disk a small nonsynovial cavity may be present. Cranially and caudally the junction is reinforced by the *superior* (**2**) and the *arcuate* (**3**) *pubic ligaments*, respectively.

Sacroiliac Joint (4)

The articulation is formed by the auricular surface of the hip bone and the auricular surface of the sacrum. Both are covered by fibrous cartilage. A very taut joint capsule encloses the almost immobile joint, which is an amphiarthrosis. The capsule is strengthened by the *ventral* (**5**), *interosseous* (**6**) and *dorsal* (**7**) *sacroiliac ligaments*. The joint is reinforced indirectly by the *iliolumbar ligament* (**8**), which connects the ilium (**9**) to the lumbar vertebrae (**10**), as well as by the *sacrotuberous* (**11**) and *sacrospinous* (**12**) *ligaments*.

Ligaments in the Pelvic Region

The **obturator membrane** (**13**) closes the obturator foramen, except for the small opening of the **obturator canal** (**14**), through which pass the obturator blood vessels and nerve.

The **sacrospinous** (**12**) and **sacrotuberous (11) ligaments** fan out to the lateral margin of the sacral bone (**15**) and the coccyx (**16**) from the ischial spine (**17**) and from the ischial tuberosity (**18**). The sacrotuberous ligament is stronger and longer than the sacrospinous ligament.

These two ligaments complete the greater sciatic notch and convert it into the *greater sciatic foramen* (**19**) and the lesser sciatic notch into the *lesser sciatic foramen* (**20**). The sacrotuberous ligament joins the sacrospinous ligament in forming the posteromedial border of the greater sciatic notch. The **iliolumbar ligament** (**8**) extends from the costal processes of the 4th and 5th lumbar vertebrae (**21**) to the iliac crest (**22**) and the adjacent region of the iliac tuberosity (**23**). The **transverse acetabular ligament** closes the acetabular notch and completes the articular surface for the head of the femur.

The **inguinal ligament** (**24**) is formed by the inferior margin of the aponeurosis of the external abdominal oblique. It extends between the anterior superior iliac spine (**25**) and the pubic tubercle (**26**). At the latter point of attachment it spreads out along a broad surface in the form of the lacunar ligament (**27**). Between the inguinal ligament and the anterior margin of the hip bone are the *muscular* (**29**) and the *vascular* (**29**) *compartments,* which are separated from each other by the **iliopectineal arch** (**21**).

Morphology of the Bony Pelvis (see p. 182)

We distinguish a true and a false, or a greater and lesser, pelvis. The region inferior to the terminal line is called the lesser pelvis. The *pelvic inlet* (superior pelvic aperture) leads into the lesser pelvis, which is bordered by the promontory, the arcuate line, the iliopubic eminence, the pecten of the pubis and the upper edge of the symphysis ("terminal line"). The *pelvic outlet*, the inferior pelvic aperture, is the region between the subpubic angle or pubic arch, the ischial tuberosities and the coccyx.

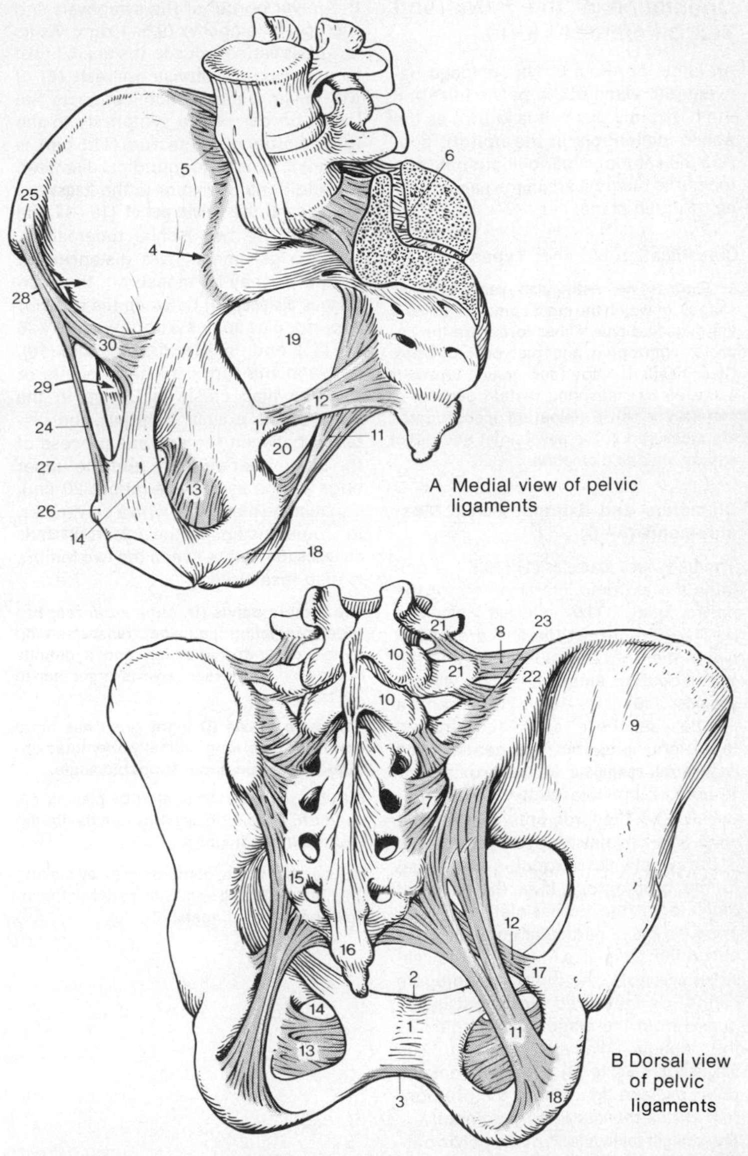

A Medial view of pelvic ligaments

B Dorsal view of pelvic ligaments

Orientation of the Pelvis and Sex Differences (A–F)

An angle of about 60° is enclosed between the plane of the pelvic inlet and the horizontal plane. It is known as the **pelvic inclination**. In the upright posture the anterior superior iliac spine and the pubic tubercle are in the same vertical (frontal) plane.

Classification of Pelvic Types

In females we distinguish various pelvic shapes, of which the most common (50%) is the gynecoid type. Other forms are the android, anthropoid and platypelloid types. Classification into four main types is achieved by measuring certain pelvic diameters. The pelvic **diameters** or **conjugates** are measured at the pelvic inlet and outlet and as oblique diameters.

Diameters and External Pelvic Measurements (A–C)

The **transverse diameter** (**1**) (13.5–14 cm) joins the extreme lateral points of the pelvic inlet. The **oblique diameter** (**2**) (12–12.5 cm) ist the line drawn between the right sacroiliac joint and the left iliopubic eminence. The **oblique diameter II** (**3**) (11.5–12 cm) represents a line between the left sacroiliac joint and the right iliopubic eminence. The **anatomical conjugate** (**4**) (approximately 12 cm) is the line between the symphysis and the promontory. The *true conjugate* (**5**) joins the posterior surface of the symphysis (retropubic eminence) to the promontory. It is the shortest diameter of the pelvic inlet (11.5 cm); because it is of particular importance in parturition, it is also known as the "**obstetric conjugate**". As the true conjugate cannot be measured directly, it is deduced from the diagonal conjugate as the "oblique diameter" (13 cm). The **diagonal conjugate** (**6**) extends from the pubic arcuate ligament to the promontory and is measured per vaginam.

The **straight conjugate** (**7**) at the pelvic outlet represents the connection between the lower border of the symphysis and the tip of the coccyx (9.5–10 cm). As its length is variable due to the flexibility of the coccyx, the **median conjugate** (**8**) of the pelvic outlet, which connects the lower border of the symphysis to the lower border of the sacrum (11.5 cm), is a more important longitudinal diameter. An additional measure is the **transverse diameter of the pelvic outlet** (10–11 cm) between the two ischial tuberosities. Using a pelvimeter, two distances on the pelvis may be measured; the **interspinous distance** (**9**) between the anterior superior iliac spines is approximately 26 cm (♀), and the **intercristal distance** (**10**), between the furthest lateral points of the two iliac crests is 29 cm in the female. The **external conjugate**, the distance between the spinous process of the 5th lumbar vertebra and the upper edge of the symphysis (about 20 cm), can also be measured with a pelvimeter. In some instances the **intertrochanteric distance** (31 cm) between the two femurs is also measured.

The **female pelvis** (**D**, outlined in red) has wider projecting iliac alae, transversely directed obturator foramina and a definite pubic arch. The lesser pelvis is larger than in the male.

The **male pelvis** (**D**, light gray) has more erect iliac alae, longitudinally orientated obturator foramen and a subpubic angle.

E Pubic arch, demonstrated by placing the hand on it; the arch lies between the thumb and the index finger.

F Subpubic angle, demonstrated by placing the hand on it; the angle lies between the index and middle fingers.

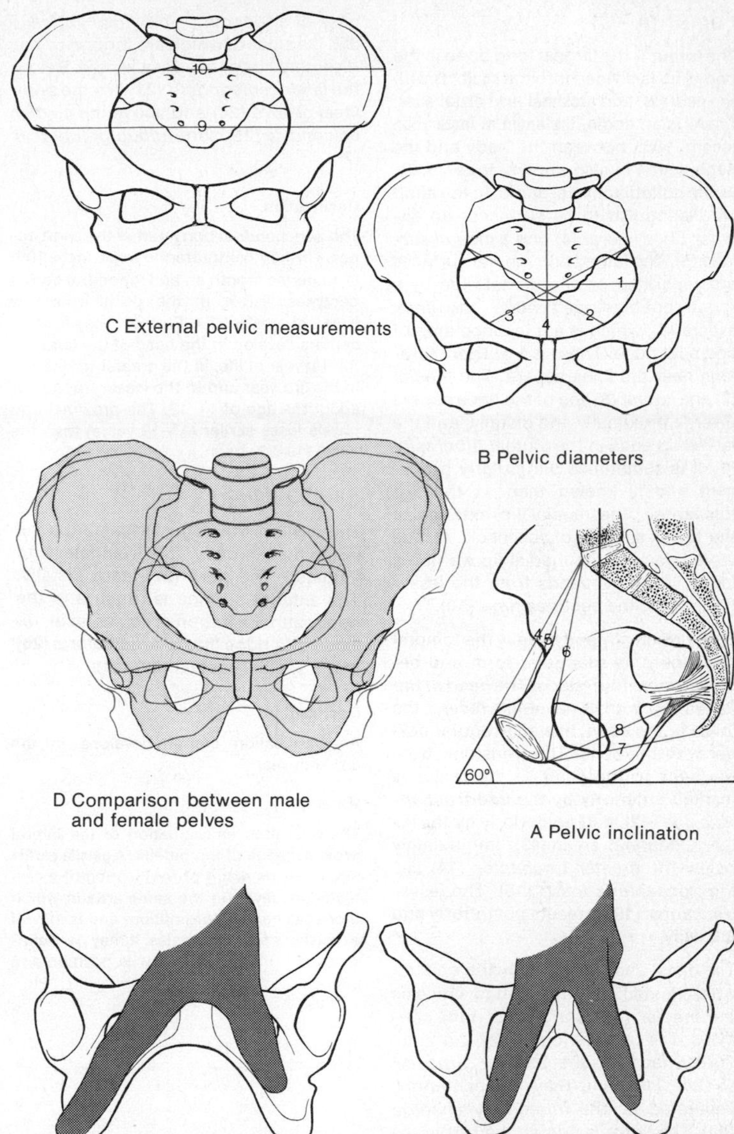

C External pelvic measurements

B Pelvic diameters

D Comparison between male and female pelves

A Pelvic inclination

E Pubic arch

F Subpubic angle

Femur (A–C)

The **femur** is the largest long bone in the body and is divided into the **shaft** (**1**) with the **neck** (**2**), and **proximal** and **distal ends**. There is an angle, **the angle of inclination** (see p. 186), between the body and the neck which is also known, incorrectly, as the collodiaphysial angle. In the shaft we distinguish three surfaces: an *anterior* (**3**), a *lateral* (**4**) and a *medial surface* (**5**). The lateral and medial surfaces are separated on the dorsal side by a rough double-lipped ridge, the *linea aspera* (**6**), which is a thickened area of compact bone. There is a nutrient foramen near the linea aspera. The *medial* (**7**) and *lateral* (**8**) *lips* of the linea aspera diverge proximally and distally, and the lateral lip ends in the *gluteal tuberosity* (**9**). It is sometimes particularly prominent and is known then as the *3rd trochanter*. The medial lip extends to the lower surface of the neck. A little more lateral to the medial lip we find a ledge which descends from the lesser trochanter, the *pectineal line* (**10**).

Both proximally and distally the femoral shaft loses its triangular form and becomes more four-sided. The *head of the femur* (**11**) with its navel-like recess, the *fovea of the head*, has an irregular border with the neck. The transition from the neck to the shaft of the femur is marked anteriorly by the *intertrochanteric line* (**12**), and posteriorly by the *intertrochanteric crest* (**13**). Immediately below the *greater trochanter* (**14**) lies the *trochanteric fossa* (**15**). The *lesser trochanter* (**16**) projects posteriorly and medially.

The distal end is formed by the epicondyles, immediately adjacent to which lie the *medial* (**17**) and *lateral* (**18**) *condyles.* The two are joined on the anterior surface by the *patellar articular surface* (**19**), and they are posteriorly separated by the *intercondylar fossa* (**20**). The latter is demarcated from the posterior surface of the shaft by the *intercondylar line* (**21**), which forms the base of a triangle (= *popliteal surface*; **22**), the sides of which are formed by the divergent lips of the linea aspera. Below the *lateral epicondyle* (**23**) lies the *popliteal groove* (**24**) and above the *medial epicondyle* (**25**) is the *adductor tubercle* (**26**).

Ossification

The perichondrial bony cuff of the shaft appears in the 7th intrauterine week. In the 10th intrauterine month an endochondral center becomes visible in the distal epiphysis (**sign of maturity**). Further ossification centers develop in the head of the femur in the 1st year of life, in the greater trochanter in the 3rd year and in the lesser trochanter about the age of 11–12. The proximal epiphysis fuses earlier (17–19 years) than the distal (19–20 years).

Patella (D–F)

The **patella** is the largest sesamoid bone in the human body. It is triangular and flattened. The *apex* (**27**) faces distally. The anterior surface is rough and the dorsal surface has an articular facet, divided by a ridge into a larger lateral (**28**) and a smaller medial (**29**) face.

Ossification

An ossification center develops in the 3rd–4th year.

Variants

There is often emargination of the lateral proximal edge of the patella. A **patella partita** usually is the result of ossification of a cartilaginous layer, in the same area in which there has been emargination, and is almost exclusively found in males. It may be distinguished from a fracture by its position and shape.

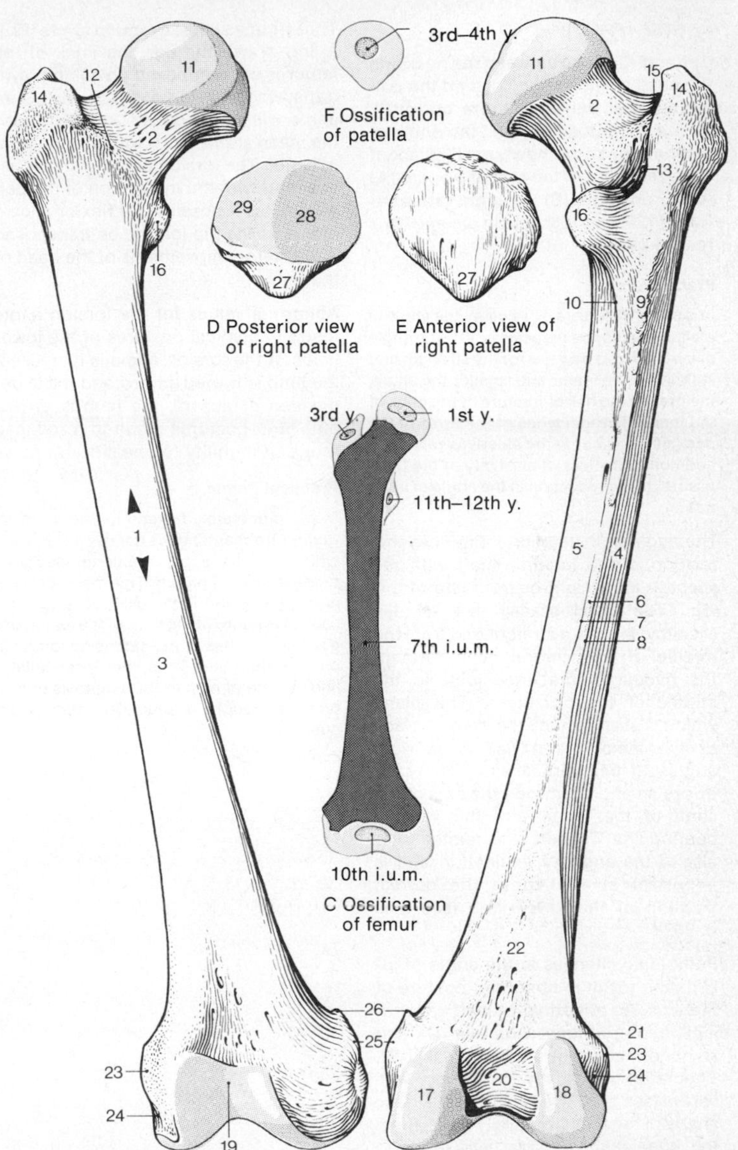

F Ossification of patella

D Posterior view of right patella

E Anterior view of right patella

C Ossification of femur

A Anterior view of right femur

B Posterior view of right femur

Femur (A–G)

The angle formed between the neck and the shaft of the femur is called the collodiaphysial angle or, more correctly, the **neck-shaft angle,** i. e., the **angle of inclination**. In the newborn it is about 150°, reducing at the age of 3 years (**A**) to 145°. In adults (**B**) the angle varies between 126° and 128°, and in old age (**C**) it reaches 120°.

Practical Points

In disease of bone (e.g., rickets), the angle of inclination may be reduced to 90°. The angle of inclination is decisive for the strength and stability of the femur, the smaller the angle, the greater the risk of fracture of the neck of the femur. The incidence of fractures of the neck of the femur in the elderly is related in addition to the loss of elasticity of the bony tissues, to the reduction in the angle of inclination.

The angle of inclination influences the relation of the femoral shaft with respect to the weight-bearing line of the leg. The **weight-bearing line of the** (healthy) **leg** lies a straight line from the middle of the femoral head through the middle of the knee joint to the middle of the calcaneus. The plane which passes through the lower surface of the femoral condyles is at right angles to this vertical line. This produces an angle between the axis of the shaft of the femur and the weight-bearing line. This angle is related inter alia to the angle of inclination and is important in relation to the correct position of the lower limb (see also p. 202).

Pathologic changes in the angle of inclination result in abnormal posture of the legs. An abnormally small angle of inclination produces **coxa vara** (**D**), and an abnormally large angle **coxa valga** (**E**). The latter is usually combined with varum (see p. 202), as any change in the shape of the femur naturally must affect the knee joint. A coxa vara leads to genu valgum (see p. 202).

The femur also has a **torsion angle** (**F**). If a line drawn through the neck of the femur is superimposed on a line drawn transversely through the condyles, an angle will be produced. In a European the mean angle is 12°, with a range from 4° to 20°. The torsion angle, which is associated with the inclination of the pelvis, makes it possible for flexion movements of the hip joint to be transposed into rotatory movements of the head of the femur.

Abnormal values for the torsion angle result in atypical postures of the lower limbs. If the torsion angle is increased, the limb is turned inward, and if it is decreased or absent, the limb is turned out; both postures result in a reduced range of mobility to one side.

Practical Points

In the moderately flexed hip, the tip of the greater trochanter does not rise above a line which joins the superior anterior iliac spine to the ischial tuberosity. This theoretical line is known as the **Roser-Nélaton line** (**G**). In a case of fracture of the neck of the femur, or a dislocation, these three points no longer lie on a straight line. Thus, the Roser-Nélaton line may be of help in the diagnosis of fractures, although its practical value is disputed.

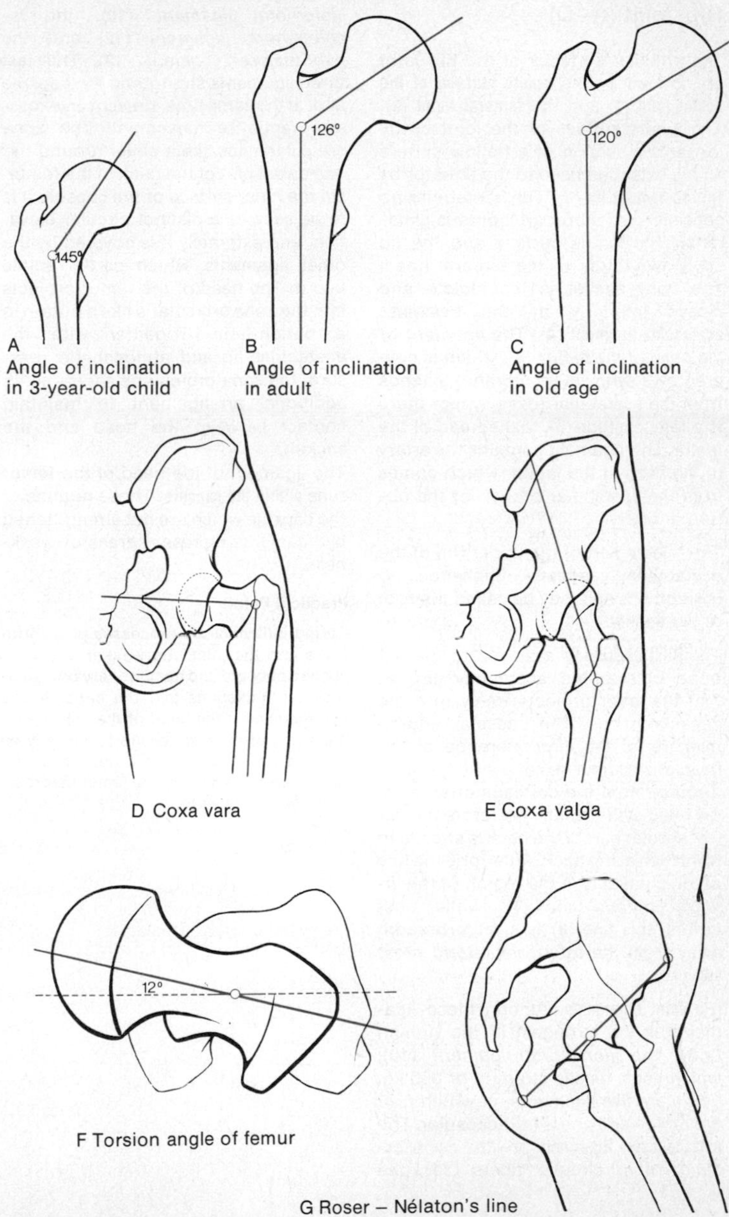

A
Angle of inclination in 3-year-old child

B
Angle of inclination in adult

C
Angle of inclination in old age

D Coxa vara

E Coxa valga

F Torsion angle of femur

G Roser – Nélaton's line

Hip Joint (A–D)

The articular surfaces of the **hip joint** are formed by the **lunate surface of the acetabulum** (**1**) and the **femoral head** (**2**). The lunate surface of the joint cavity presents a section of a hollow sphere and is extended beyond the equator by the **acetabular lip** (**3**). The acetabular lip consists of fibrocartilaginous material. The lunate surface and the lip cover two-thirds of the femoral head. The bony socket is incomplete and closed inferiorly by the **transverse acetabular ligament** (**4**). The *ligament of the head of the femur* (**6**), which is covered by a synovial membrane, extends from the acetabular fossa, where there is a fatty cushion (**5**), to the head of the femur. This ligament contains the artery to the head of the femur, which comes from the acetabular branch of the obturator artery.

The middle part of the upper rim of the acetabulum appears thickened in radiographs and may be called the roof of the socket.

The **joint capsule** is attached to the hip bone outside the acetabular lip, so that the latter projects freely into the capsular space. The capsular attachment (**8**) at the circumference of the head of the femur lies at about the same distance from the cartilaginous rim of the head of the femur. Therefore the extracapsular part of the neck is shorter in front than at the back. Anteriorly the line of attachment is in the region of the *intertrochanteric line* (**7**), while posteriorly this line (**8**) is a fingerbreadth away from the *intertrochanteric crest* (**9**).

Hip Joint Ligaments. Among these ligaments is the strongest in the human body, the *iliofemoral ligament* (**10**), which has a tensile strength of 350 kg. There are five ligaments, of which four are extra – and one is intracapsular. The **extracapsular ligaments** are the *zona orbicularis* or circular fibers (**11**), the *iliofemoral ligament* (**10**), the *ischiofemoral ligament* (**12**) and the *pubofemoral ligament* (**13**). The last three ligaments strengthen the capsule and, at the same time, prevent an excessive range of movement. The zona orbicularis lies like a collar around the narrowest part of the neck of the femur. On the inner surface of the capsule it is to be seen as a distinct circular elevation, and externally it is covered by the other ligaments, which partly radiate into it. The head of the femur projects into the zona orbicularis like a button in a button-hole. Together with the acetabular lip and atmospheric pressure, the zona orbicularis serves as an additional arrangement to maintain contact between the head and the socket.

The ligament of the head of the femur runs **within the capsule**. Those regions of the capsule which are not strengthened by ligaments represent areas of weakness.

Practical Points

During inflammatory processes, e. g., effusions into the joint, the weaker areas are pushed outward and become very pressure-sensitive. Luxations tear the capsule and the ligament of the head of the femur with the artery of the head of the femur may be severed. This may produce nutritional deficiencies in the head of the femur (necrosis of the femoral head).

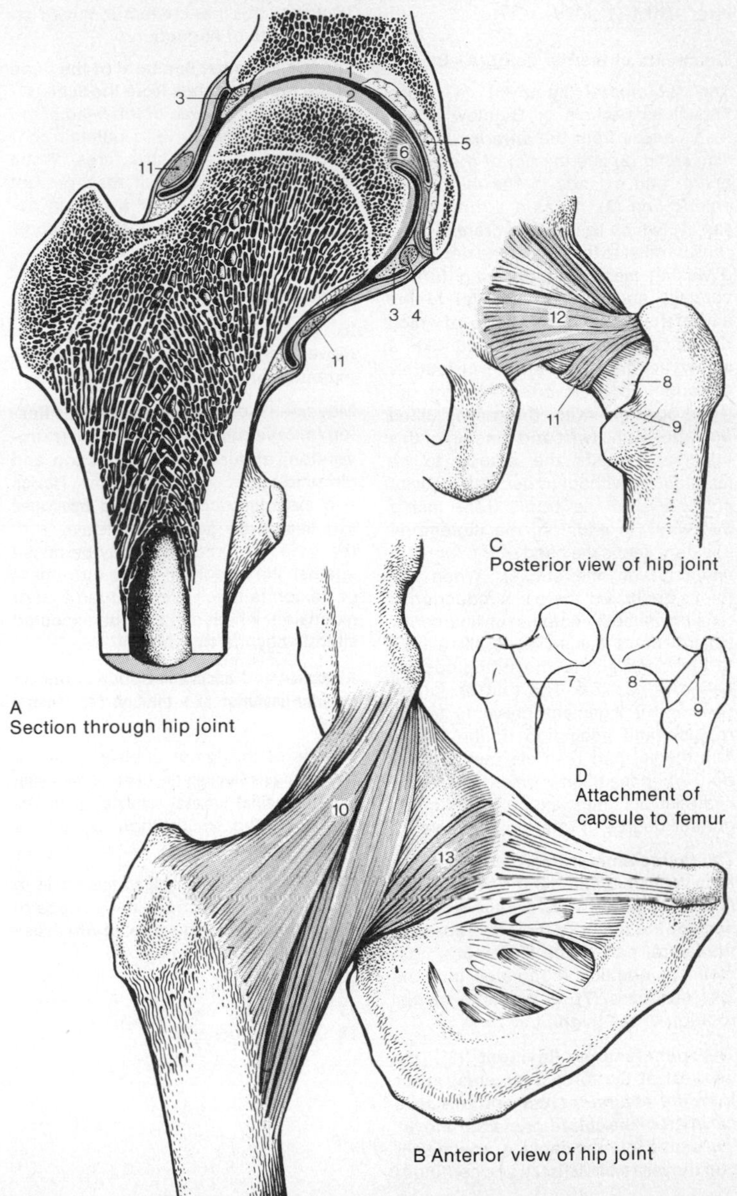

A
Section through hip joint

B Anterior view of hip joint

C
Posterior view of hip joint

D
Attachment of capsule to femur

Hip Joint (continued)

Ligaments of the Hip Joint (A–B)

The **iliofemoral ligament** (**1**), also known as Bertin's or Bigelow's ligament, arises from the *anterior inferior iliac spine* (**2**) and the *rim of the acetabulum* and extends to the *intertrochanteric line* (**3**). It has a strong **lateral part** (**4**), which lies further cranially and runs parallel to the axis of the neck, and a weaker **medial part** (**5**) lying further caudally and running parallel to the axis of the shaft. The two parts, of which the lateral portion is twisted like a screw, act differently and form roughly the outline of an inverted Y. In the upright position, with the pelvis tilted posteriorly, the twist and tension of this ligament permits the stance to be maintained without muscular activity and prevents the trunk from falling backward. In addition, the iliofemoral ligament keeps the head of the femur in contact with the socket. When the thighs are flexed, there is a reduction in tension in both iliofemoral ligaments, which allows the pelvis to tilt a little further back, so that the sitting posture becomes possible. The thicker, lateral part of the ligament prevents lateral rotation and adduction of the femur. The medial part restricts medial rotation. When the thigh is flexed, the entire ligament becomes lax, so that a much greater degree of rotation is possible.

The **ischiofemoral ligament** (**6**) arises from the *ischium* below the acetabulum and runs almost horizontally over the neck of the femur to the attachment of the lateral part of the iliofemoral ligament. In addition it radiates into the **zona orbicularis** (**7**). It prevents medial rotation of the thigh.

The **pubofemoral ligament** (**8**), the weakest of the three ligaments, arises from the *obturator crest* and the adjacent part of the *obturator membrane* (**9**). It radiates into the capsule, specifically into the **zona orbicularis** (**7**), and continues by way of this into the femur. It restricts movements of abduction.

The intracapsular **ligament of the head of the femur** extends from the *acetabular notch* to the *fovea of the head of the femur*. It does not serve to maintain contact between these structures. When the hip is dislocated, it may prevent further displacement to a certain degree, since only then does it become stretched.

Movements of the Hip Joint

In life, muscle tone restricts joint movement, most noticeably when the extended limb is anteriorly elevated.

Movements of the hip joint include **flexion (anteversion)** and **extension (retroversion), abduction** and **adduction**, and **circumduction** and **rotation**. **Flexion** and **extension** occur about a **transverse axis through the head of the femur.** With the knee bent, the thigh may be raised against the abdomen. This movement of flexion is much greater than that of extension, which can only be executed slightly beyond the vertical.

Abduction and **adduction** occur about an **anterior-posterior axis through the femoral head.**

Rotation of the femur occurs around a **(vertical) axis through the head of the femur and the medial femoral condyle.** With the leg extended, a rotation of 60° is possible.

Circumduction is a compound movement in which the leg describes the surface of an irregular cone, the apex of which lies in the head of the femur.

10 Acetabular lip,
11 Ischial tuberosity,
12 Greater trochanter.

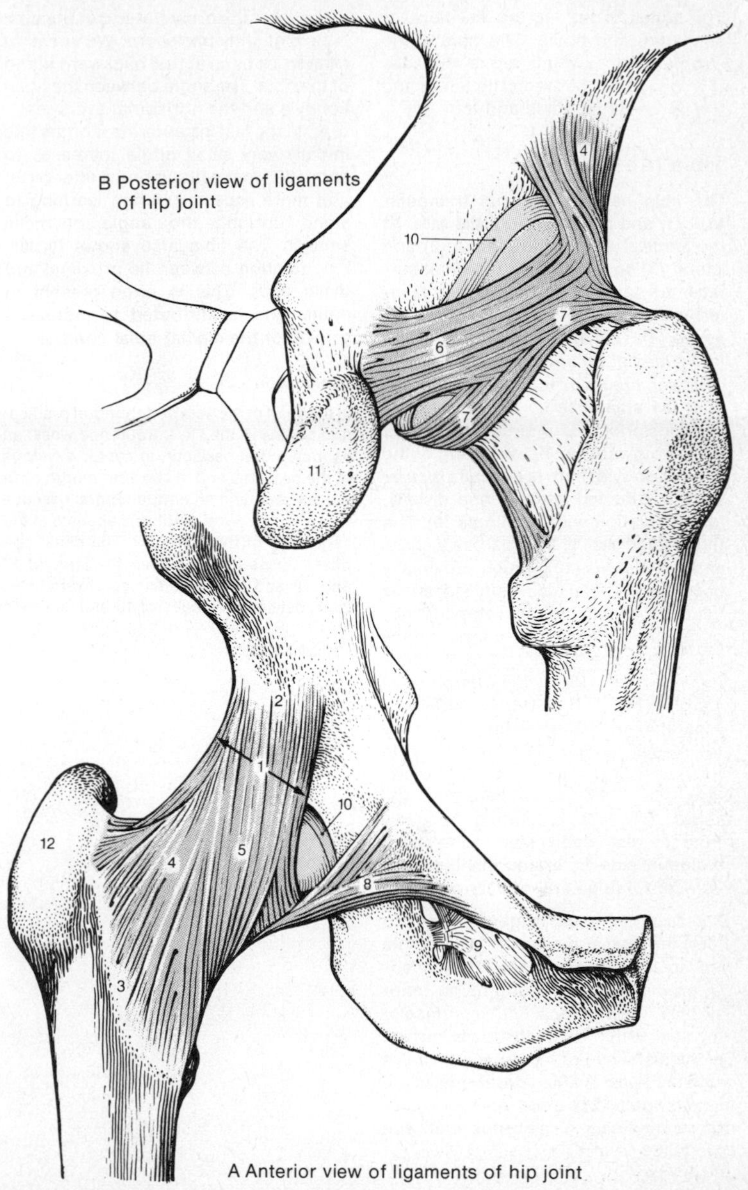

B Posterior view of ligaments of hip joint

A Anterior view of ligaments of hip joint

The bones of the leg are the tibia, or shinbone, and fibula. The tibia is the stronger bone which alone provides the connection between the femur and the bones of the ankle and foot.

Tibia (A–D)

The **tibia** has a somewhat triangular **shaft** (**1**) and **proximal** and **distal ends**. At the **proximal end** lie the *medial* (**2**) and *lateral* (**3**) *condyles*. The proximal surface, the *superior articular facet,* is interrupted by the *intercondylar eminence* (**4**). This elevation is subdivided into a *medial* (**5**) and a *lateral* (**6**) *intercondylar tubercle*. In front of and behind the eminence lie the *anterior* (**7**) and *posterior* (**8**) *intercondylar area* On the outward-facing overhang of the lateral condyle there is a small *articular surface,* directed laterally and distally, for articulation with the fibula (**9**). The three-sided **shaft of the tibia** has a sharp *anterior margin* (**10**), which proximally becomes the *tibial tuberosity* (**11**) and is flattened distally. It separates the *medial surface* (**12**) from the *lateral surface* (**13**). The lateral surface joins the *posterior surface* (**15**) at the *interosseous margin* (**14**). The posterior surface is separated from the medial surface by the *medial margin* (**16**). Proximally on the posterior surface of the shaft of the tibia is a slightly roughened area, the *soleal line* (**17**), extending obliquely from the distomedial side to the proximolateral side. Lateral to this there is a *nutrient foramen* (**18**) of varying size.

The **distal end** is prolonged medially to form the *medial malleolus* (**19**) with its *malleolar articular surface.* The *malleolar groove* (**20**) runs along its posterior surface. The *inferior articular surface* of the tibia, which lies on the lower surface of the distal end of the tibia, articulates with the talus. On the lateral side, in the *fibular notch* (**21**), there is a syndesmotic connection, i. e., a fibrous joint, with the fibula.

In the adult the proximal end of the tibia is bent slightly backward. We speak of **retroversion** or an actual backward tilting of the tibia. The angle between the tibial condyle and the horizontal averages 4° to 6°. In the last intrauterine months this initially very small angle increases to about 30°. In the first months after birth, and more especially when learning to stand upright, the angle becomes smaller. The tibia also shows **torsion**, i. e., rotation between its proximal and distal ends. This is often present in adults and is attributed to increased growth of the medial tibial condyle.

Ossification

In the shaft of the tibia perichondral ossification begins in the 7th intrauterine week, an endochondral ossification center develops at the proximal end in the 10th month or in the 1st year, and an endochondral osseous center in the distal epiphysis appears at the beginning of the 2nd year. The distal epiphysis fuses first, between the ages of 17 and 19 and the proximal epiphysis fuses later, between the ages of 19 and 20 years.

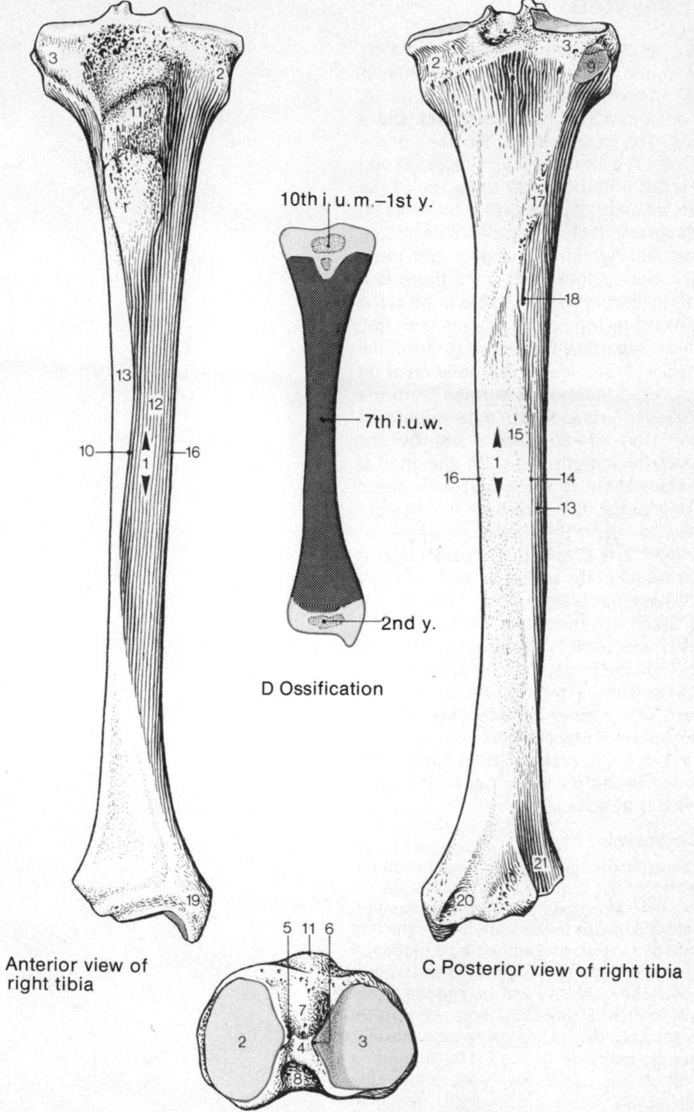

A Anterior view of right tibia

D Ossification

C Posterior view of right tibia

B Superior view of right tibia

Fibula (A–D)

The **fibula** corresponds approximately in length to the tibia, but is a slimmer and therefore more flexible bone. It, too, consists of **two extremities and a shaft.** The **proximal end** is the *head of the fibula* (**1**) with its *articular facet* (**2**) and a small protuberance, the *apex of the fibular head* (**3**). The **shaft of the fibula** (**4**) is approximately triangular in its middle part and has three margins and three surfaces. In the distal third there is a fourth margin. The sharpest edge is the forward-facing *anterior margin* (**5**), which separates the *lateral* (**6**) from the *medial* (**7**) *surface.* The *medial crest* **(8)** separates the medial surface from the *posterior surface* (**9**). It is separated from the *lateral surface* (**6**) by the *posterior margin* (**10**). On the medial surface there is a low but very sharp bony ridge, the *interosseous margin* (**11**), to which the *interosseous membrane* (**12**) is attached. Approximately in the center of the posterior surface or on the posterior margin, there is a nutrient foramen. On the lateral surface of the **distal end,** which expands distalward, there is the large, flat *lateral malleolus* (**13**) with *a facet for articulation with the talus on its inner surface* (**14**). On the posterior surface there is a deep groove, the *lateral malleolar fossa* (**15**), to which the posterior talofibular ligament is attached.

Ossification

The perichondral bony cuff develops in the region of the shaft in the 2nd intrauterine month. An endochondral ossification center develops in the malleolus in the 2nd year and in the head of the fibula in the 4th year. The distal epiphysis fuses earlier, between the ages of 16 and 19, and the proximal somewhat later, between 17 and 20 years. The junction line of the proximal epiphysis runs below the head of the fibula, and that of the distal epiphysis above the malleolus. Clinically, care must be taken not to confuse these epiphysial disks, particularly that of the distal epiphysis, with fracture lines.

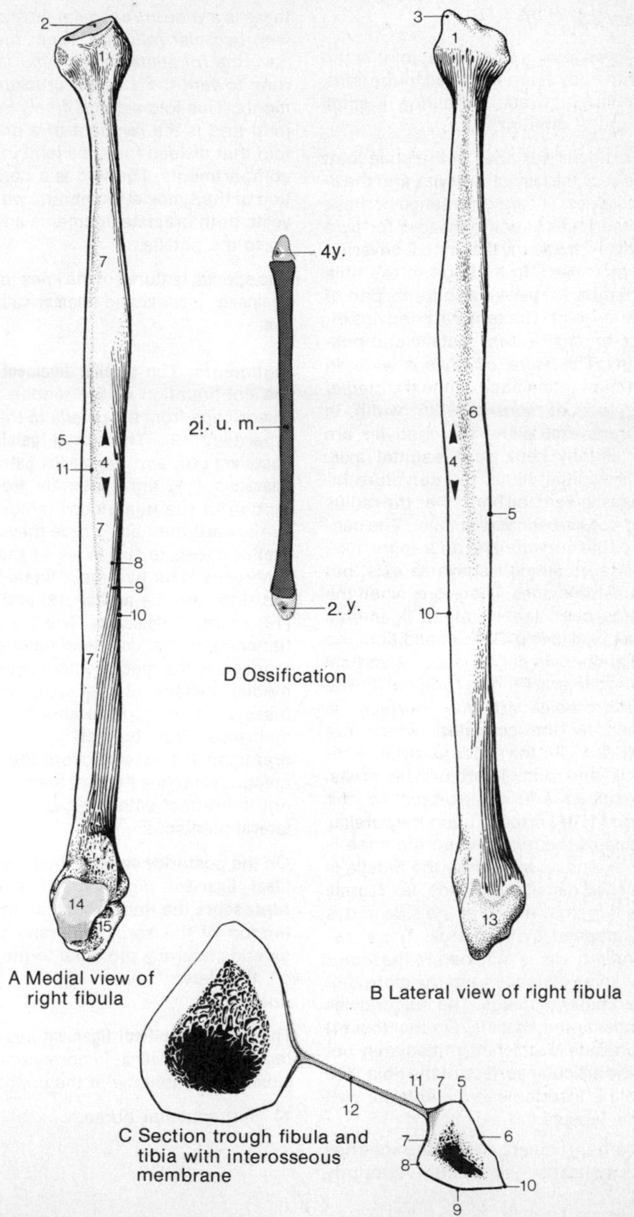

A Medial view of right fibula

B Lateral view of right fibula

D Ossification

C Section trough fibula and tibia with interosseous membrane

Knee Joint (A–C)

The **knee joint** is the largest joint in the human body. It is a modified hinge joint, a trochoginglymus permitting a small amount of rotation.

The articular surfaces of the knee joint consist of the **femoral condyles** and the **tibial condyles**. The incongruence of these joint surfaces is compensated for by a relatively thick cartilaginous covering and by **menisci**. In addition to the tibia and femur, the **patella** also forms part of the knee joint. The femoral condyles diverge to some extent distally and posteriorly. The *lateral condyle* is wider in front than at the back, while the *medial condyle* is of more constant width. In the transverse plane the condyles are only slightly bent on a sagittal axis. In the sagittal plane, the curvature increases toward the back, i. e., the radius of curvature becomes smaller. The centers of the curvature lie on a spiral, i. e., there is no single transverse axis, but innumerable ones. Therefore, when the knee is bent, the collateral ligaments are relaxed (see p. 200). In addition, the medial condyle curves about a vertical axis (curvature of rotation). The *superior tibial articular surface* is formed by the condyles, which are separated by the intercondylar eminence, and both intercondylar areas. The ridged *articular surface of the patella* (**1**) lies directly upon the *patellar surface of the femur* when the knee is fully extended. In flexion, the patella is displaced distally. The wide, lax **capsule** (**2**) is thin in front and at the side and is strengthened by ligaments. The *synovial membrane* is attached to the *femur* (**3**) at some distance from the margin of the articular cartilage. The epicondyles lie outside the capsule. On the *tibia* (**4**) the capsule is attached immediately below the articular surface of the tibia. The patella is inserted into the anterior wall of the capsule.

The large articular cavity of the knee has a complicated structure. Anteriorly there is a wide *infrapatellar fatty pad* (**5**) with *two alar folds* (**6**). From the fatty pad, the *infrapatellar synovial fold* (**7**) runs toward the anterior cruciate ligaments. This fold extends freely into the joint and is the remnant of a primitive fold that divided the knee joint into two compartments. The fold is a continuation of the synovial membrane which invests both cruciate ligaments and runs up to the patella.

The special features of the knee joint are **ligaments, menisci** and **communicating bursae.**

Ligaments. The **patellar ligament** (**8**) is the continuation of the tendon of the quadriceps from the *patella to the tibial tuberosity* (**9**). The **lateral patellar retinaculum** (**10**) and the **medial patellar retinaculum** (**11**) arise laterally from the tendon of the quadriceps femoris and run toward the tibia, where they are attached close to the sides of the tibial tuberosity. The two main ligaments at the sides are the **medial** (**12**) and **lateral** (**13**) **collateral ligaments**. The triangular, flattened medial collateral ligament extends from the medial epicondyle to the medial surface of the tibia, where it fuses with the capsule and the medial meniscus. The rounded lateral collateral ligament extends from the lateral epicondyle to the head of the fibula. It is not in contact with the capsule or the lateral meniscus.

On the posterior surface the **oblique popliteal ligament** *(ligament of Winslow)* represents the lateral emanation of the tendon of the semimembranosus and extends laterally proximal to the origin of the lateral head of the gastrocnemius.

The **arcuate popliteal ligament** lies in the region of the lateral femoral condyle in close relationship with the popliteus.

14 Suprapatellar bursa.

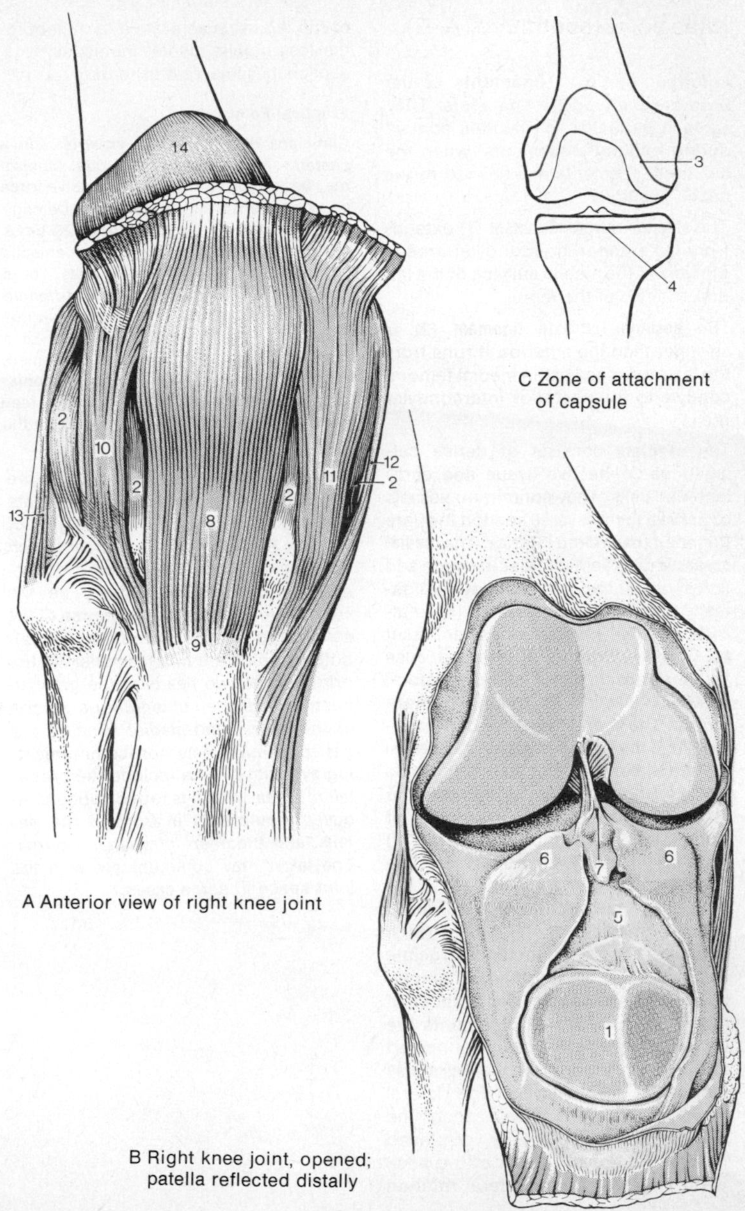

C Zone of attachment of capsule

A Anterior view of right knee joint

B Right knee joint, opened; patella reflected distally

Knee Joint (continued, A–B)

A further group of **ligaments** of the knee are the *cruciate ligaments.* They serve in particular to maintain contact during rotatory movements, when the collateral ligaments are relaxed in the flexed position.

The **anterior cruciate ligament** (**1**) extends from the anterior intercondylar area of the tibia to the medial surface of the lateral condyle of the femur.

The **posterior cruciate ligament** (**2**) is stronger than the anterior. It runs from the lateral surface of the medial femoral condyle to the posterior intercondylar area.

The **menisci** consists of dense collagenous connective tissue and cartilage-like cells. They contain no vessels or nerves. In transverse section they are flattened toward the interior. The **medial meniscus** (**3**) is semicircular in shape and is fused with the medial collateral ligament (**4**). The **lateral meniscus** (**5**) is almost circular, its points of attachment being close together. It does not fuse with the capsula or the lateral collateral ligament (**6**) and is therefore more mobile. The lateral meniscus may be attached to the inner surface of the medial femoral condyle by ligaments. From its posterior horn (see below) the **posterior meniscofemoral ligament** (ligament of Robert or ligament of Weisberg) (**7**) frequently extends dorsal to the posterior cruciate ligament (**2**). Less frequently an **anterior meniscofemoral ligament** (ligament of Humphrey) (**8**) is noted ventral to the posterior cruciate and extending to the medial femoral condyle. In an even smaller number of cases (see Fig. **C**) both ligaments are present. The two menisci are connected and fixed anteriorly by the **transverse ligament of the knee** (**9**). The lateral meniscus is more mobile than the medial one and can be displaced further during movements of the knee joint. However, during lateral rotation of the leg because of its attachment to the less mobile medial meniscus, it is especially vulnerable to tearing.

Practical Points

Clinicians differentiate an *anterior* and a *posterior horn* in each meniscus. Menisci may be torn by continuous excessive force or by uncoordinated movements. Damage to the medial meniscus is about 20 times more frequent than to the lateral meniscus because of its more limited mobility. There may be a *longitudinal tear (bucket-handle tear)* or *fracture of the anterior or posterior horn.* After partial surgical removal of a meniscus, meniscoid tissue may be formed, which takes over the function of the meniscus. The meniscofemoral ligaments may cause difficulties during operations on the posterior horn.

There are numerous **bursae** around the knee joint, some of which communicate with the articular cavity. The largest of these is the *suprapatellar bursa*, which lies anteriorly and increases the joint space proximally. Posteriorly lie the *subpopliteal recess* and the bursa of the semimembranosus *(Brodie's bursa),* both of which are much smaller. At the origin of the two heads of the grastrocnemius are the *subtendinous bursae of the lateral* and *medial head of the gastrocnemius.* The non-communicating synovial bursae include the *prepatellar bursa,* which is found subcutaneously immediately in front of the patella, and the *deep infrapatellar bursa*. The latter may communicate with the joint space in some cases.

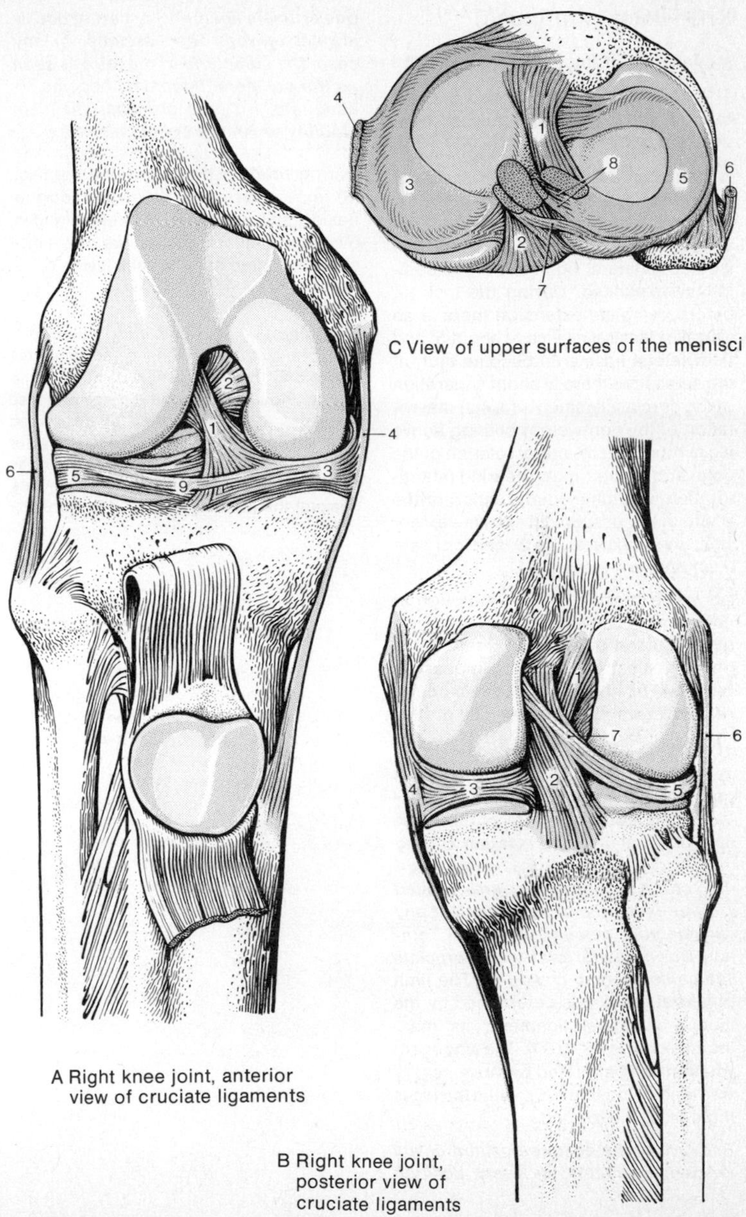

C View of upper surfaces of the menisci

A Right knee joint, anterior view of cruciate ligaments

B Right knee joint, posterior view of cruciate ligaments

Knee Joint (continued)

Movements of the Knee Joint (A–E)

The knee joint may be **flexed** and **extended**, and in the flexed position **rotation** is possible.

In the **extended knee** (**A**) *both collateral ligaments* (**1,2**) *are taut.* During the extension femoral condyles glide into the almost extreme position in which the medial collateral ligament (**1**) is completely expanded. During the last 10° before complete extension there is an **obligatory terminal rotation** of about 5° and both lateral ligaments become taut; at the same time there is slight separation of the cruciate ligaments (**3, 4**). Final rotation of the non-weight bearing active leg is produced by lateral rotation of the tibia, and in the weight-bearing (standing) leg through medial rotation of the thigh. In the position of extreme extension, the collateral (**1, 2**) and cruciate ligaments are tensed (**A**).

Normal extension is 180°, although in children and adolescents the leg may be overextended by about 5°. In the newborn maximal extension is impossible because of the physiological occurrence of tibial retroversion (see p. 192).

In the **flexed knee** (**B**), *the collateral ligaments* (**1, 2**) *are relaxed.* Rotation is possible in the flexed position. The extent of **medial rotation** (**C**) **of the leg** is less than that of **lateral rotation**. *During medial rotation of the tibia on the femur, the cruciate ligaments are twisted around each other and so prevent any considerable amount of medial rotation. During lateral rotation, the cruciate ligaments become unwound.* The limit of lateral rotation is determined by the medial collateral ligament; its maximum extent is 45° to 60°. The amount of rotation can be verified by movement of the head of the fibula (**5**), when the leg is lifted from the ground.

Because of the oblique position of the cruciate ligaments, in every position one cruciate ligament, or part of one, is always tensed. They assume, in any case, the command in the joint as soon as the collateral ligaments become inadequate, i.e., the cruciates maintain stability when the collaterals relax.

During rotation the femur and menisci (**6**) move over the tibia, and during flexion and extension the femur glides over the menisci, so that we may consider the knee as a "**mobile joint**".

Practical Points

The relatively large and incongruent joint surfaces are subjected to considerable stress and they often show damage to the cartilaginous covering in old age and also bony changes. In the case of a ruptured cruciate ligament (**D**), the so called **"drawer phenomenon"** (**E**) is observed, i. e., in the flexed position (with the collateral ligaments relaxed) the leg can be pushed forward (arrow).

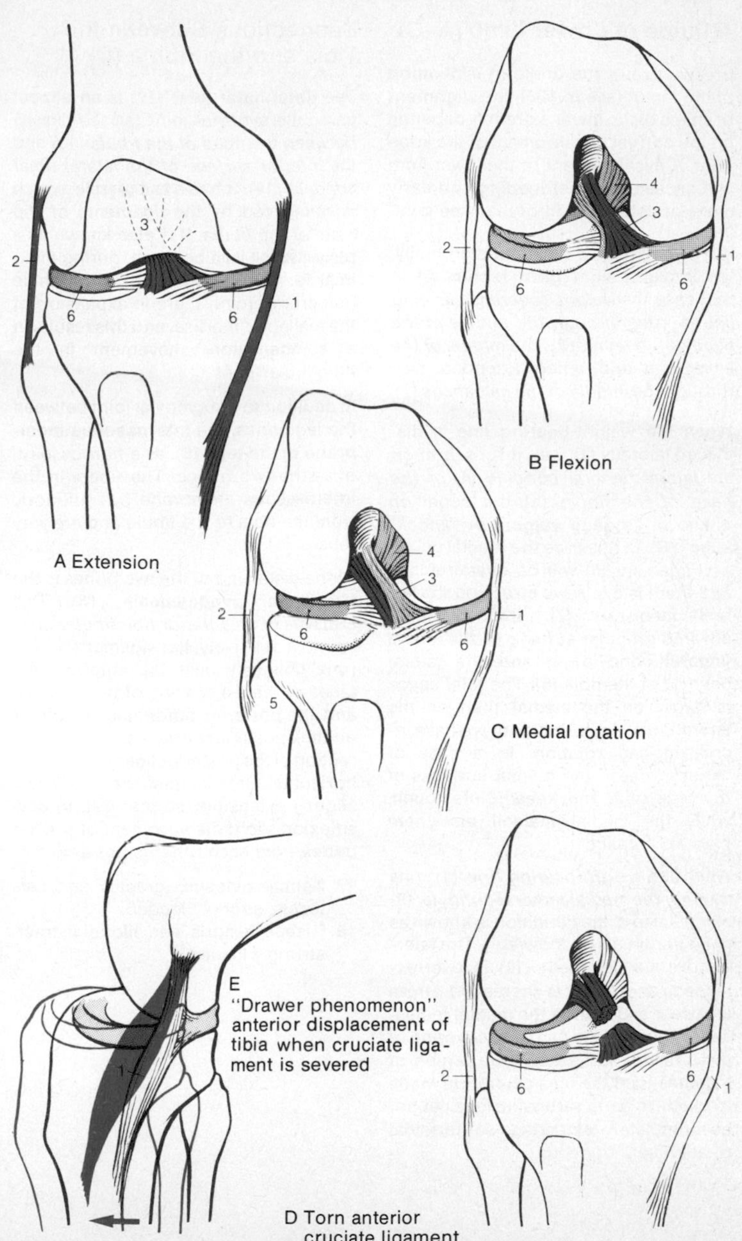

A Extension

B Flexion

C Medial rotation

D Torn anterior cruciate ligament

Attitude of Lower Limb (A–C)

Irrespective of the angle of inclination of the femur (see p. 186), the alignment or shape of the lower extremity depends on the correct development of the knee joint. A misalignment of the lower limb will cause abnormal loading and early signs of deterioration of the knee joint.

If the knee joint is developed normally, the limb is straight (**genu rectum, A**). In that case the *weight-(bearing) carrying line* (**1**) runs *through the middle of the head of the femur* (**2**), the *middle of the knee joint* and, when extended, also through the *middle of the calcaneus* (**3**).

When the weight-bearing line is displaced laterally (**1**), i.e., it runs *through the lateral femoral condyle* (**4**) *or the head of the fibula* (**5**) the condition is known as **genu valgum** or *"knock-knee"* (**B**). In this case the medial collateral ligament (**6**) will be overstretched and there is excissive stress on the lateral meniscus (**7**), the cartilage-covered articular surface of the lateral femoral condyle (**4**) and the lateral condyle of the tibia (**8**). The joint space is larger on the medial than on the lateral side. In genu valgum we have increased end rotation. In a case of "knock-knees" the medial surfaces of the legs near the knee joints touch, while the medial maleoli elsewhere have no contact.

When the *weight-bearing line* (**1**) runs *through the medial femoral condyle* (**9**) or medial to it, the condition is known as **genu varum** (**C**) or *"bowleg"*. The lateral collateral ligament (**10**) is over-extended, and there is increased stress and wear and tear on the medial meniscus (**11**) and on the cartilage covering of the articular surfaces. In the region of the knee joint the legs cannot be made to touch. In genu varum the legs cannot be completely extended, so terminal rotation cannot occur.

Connections Between the Tibia and the Fibula (D)

The **tibiofibular joint** (**12**) is an almost immobile synovial joint **(amphiarthrosis)** between the *head of the fibula* (**13**) and the *inferior surface of the lateral tibial condyle* (**14**). It has a **taut capsule**, which is reinforced by the *ligaments of the head of the fibula*. It is also known as a **compensation joint** because, during maximal forward dorsiflexion in the ankle (talocrural) joint, there is expansion of the malleolar mortise, and this results in a compensatory movement in the tibiofibular joint.

In addition to the synovial joint between the leg bones, the **interosseous membrane of the leg** (**15**), as a fibrous joint, fixes the two bones. The fibers in the interosseous membrane run inferiorly from the tibia to the fibula and are very tense.

At the distal end of the two bones is the **tibiofibular syndesmosis** (**16**). This consists of an *anterior tibiofibular ligament*, a relatively flat ligament which runs obliquely over the anterior surfaces of the distal ends of both bones, and the *posterior tibiofibular ligament* on their posterior surfaces. The fiber direction of the posterior ligament is more horizontal. Both ligaments are only very slightly extensible, so that during dorsiflexion slight displacement of the leg bones from each other is possible.

17 Semitendinosus, gracilis and sartorius, strongly loaded,
18 Biceps femoris and iliotibial tract, strongly loaded.

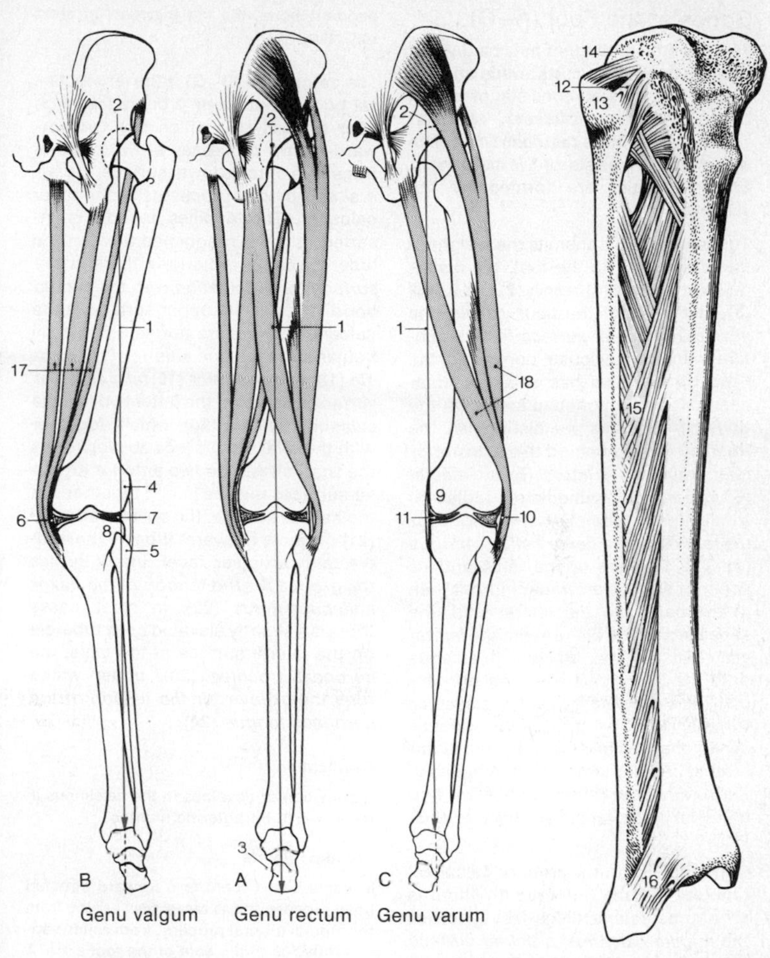

D Connections between tibia and fibula

A–C Posture of the lower limb and knee joint (after Lanz-Wachsmuth)

Bones of the Foot (A–G)

The skeleton of the foot may be divided into the **tarsus**, the **metatarsus** and the **digits**. The **tarsus** consists of seven bones, the **talus, calcaneus, navicular, cuboid** and the three **cuneiform bones**. The **metatarsus** consists of **five metatarsals**, and the **digits** are formed by the **phalanges.**

The **talus** (**A–C**) transmits the weight of the entire body to the foot. We distinguish in it a **head** (**1**), a **body** (**2**) and a **neck** (**3**). The head of the talus carries the *navicular articular surface* for articulation with the navicular bone, and the neck of the talus has small vascular channels and roughened areas. On the body of the talus we distinguish the *trochlea* (**4**) and behind this a *posterior talar process* with *lateral* (**5**) and *medial* (**6**) *tubercles.* Immediately adjacent to the medial tubercle is the *groove for the tendon of the flexor hallucis longus* (**7**). The trochlea of the talus and its superior surface are wider in front than at the back. On the lateral side, the superior surface blends with the *lateral malleolar surface* (**8**), which extends onto the *lateral talar process* (**9**). Medially lies the smaller *medial malleolar surface* (**10**). The three joint surfaces serve for articulation with the malleolar mortise. As an inferior continuation of the navicular articular surface we find the *anterior calcaneal articular surface* (**11**).

Continuous with the anterior calcaneal articular surface (infrequently there is an intermediate cartilage-free zone) lies the *middle calcaneal articular surface* (**12**). Posterior to the latter the *talar sulcus* (**13**) and the large *posterior calcaneal articular surface* (**14**) are found.

Ossification

An ossification center appears in the talus in the 7th–8th intrauterine month.

Variants

In exceptional cases, the lateral tubercle of the posterior talar process forms an independent bone, the **"os trigonum" or accessory talus.**

The **calcaneus (D–G)** is the largest tarsal bone. Posteriorly it bears the large **tuber calcanei** (**15**) which has two forward-facing processes at the point of transition onto its lower surface, the *lateral and medial processes* of the tuber calcanei. The Achilles tendon is inserted into the roughened area on the tuber calcanei. Anteriorly there is the *surface for articulation with the cuboid bone* (**16**). On the upper surface of the calcaneus, there are normally three articular surfaces, the *anterior* (**17**), *middle* (**18**) and *posterior* (**19**) *talar articular surfaces.* Between the latter two lies the *calcaneal sulcus* (**20**), which, together with the talar sulcus (see above), forms the **tarsal sinus**. The two anterior articular surfaces may be joined together. On the medial surface, the **sustentaculum tali** (**21**) projects outward. It bears the middle talar articular facet. Inferiorly lies the *groove for the tendon of the flexor hallucis longus* (**22**). In most cases there is a slightly elevated bony tubercle on the lateral surface of the talus, the *peroneal trochlea* (**23**), under which runs the *groove for the tendon of the peroneus longus* (**24**).

Ossification

A bony center develops in the calcaneus in the 4th–7th intrauterine months.

Practical Points

In some cases there is a forward directed bony process, the **calcaneal spur**, arising from the medial tuberal process, from which various muscles of the sole of the foot arise. A calcaneal spur may be very painful.

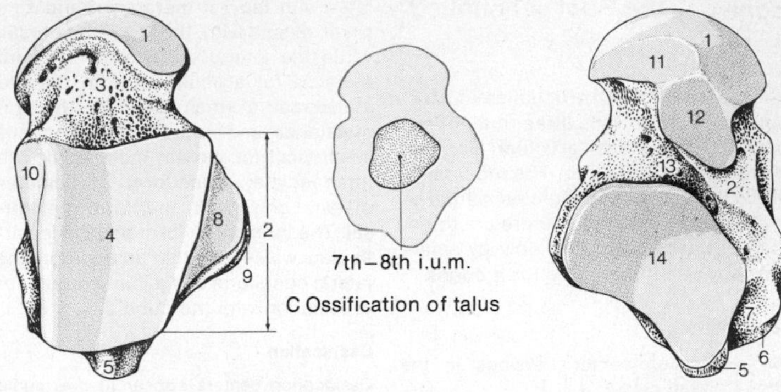

A Superior view of right talus

C Ossification of talus

B Inferior view of right talus

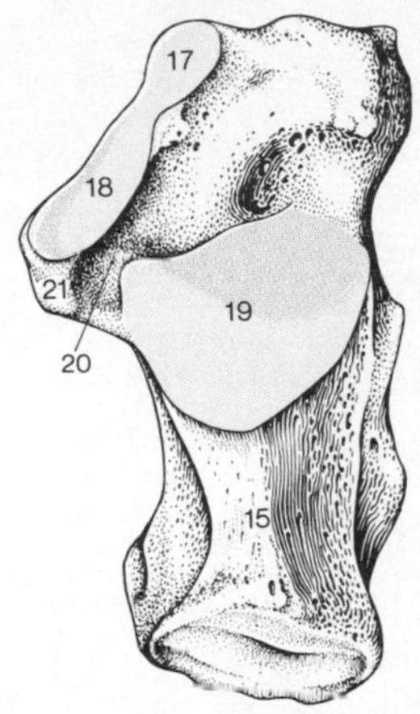

D Superior view of right calcaneus

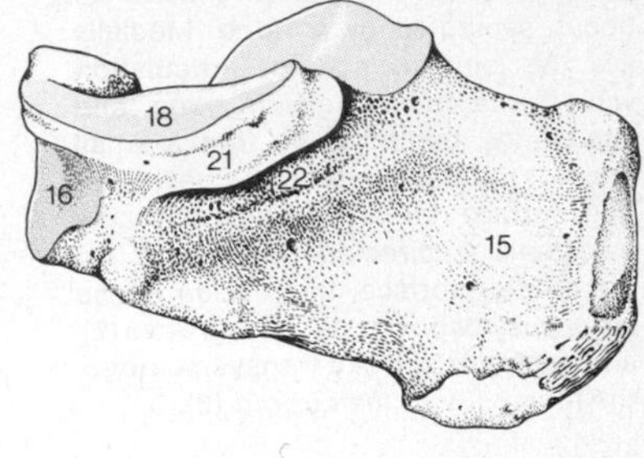

E Medial view of right calcaneus

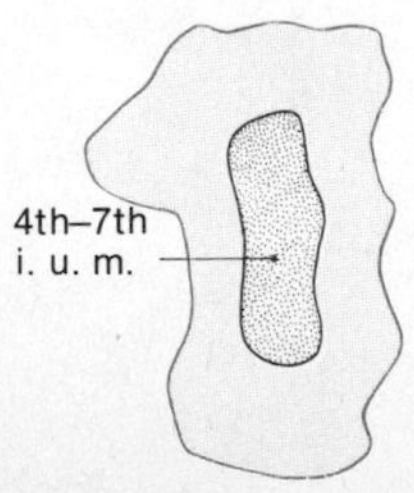

G Ossification of calcaneus

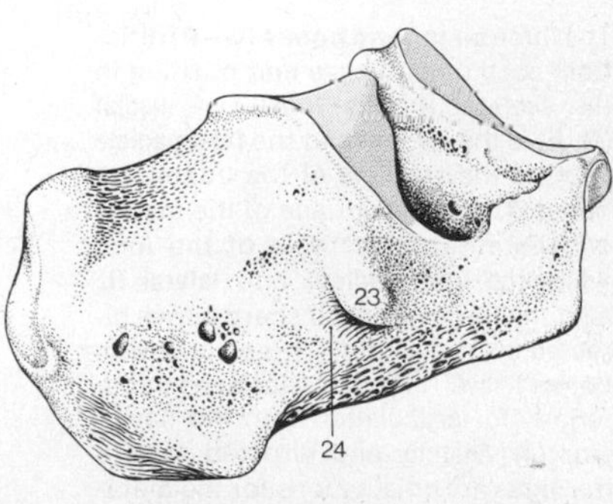

F Lateral view of right calcaneus

Bones of the Foot (continued A–P)

The **navicular (A–C)** articulates with the talus and with the three cuneiform bones. A concave articular surface faces the head of talus. The *tuberosity of the navicular* (**1**) is directed *plantarly* and medially. Anteriorly there are three joint surfaces separated only by small crests for the three cuneiform bones.

Ossification

An ossification center develops in the 3rd–4th year.

The **cuboid (D–F)** is shorter laterally than medially. Distally there are joint surfaces for the 4th and 5th metatarsal bones separated by a ridge. Medially lies the joint surface for articulation with the lateral cuneiform bone, and sometimes, behind it, we find a small area for articulation with the navicular. The surface for articulation with the calcaneus is directed posteriorly. On the inferior surface, the *tendon of the peroneus longus* runs in a groove (**2**), and posterior to it is a transverse ridge, the *tuberosity of the cuboid* (**3**).

Ossification

The ossification center in the cuboid develops in the 10th intrauterine month (**sign of maturity**).

The three **cuneiform bones (G–P)** differ from each other in size and position in the skeleton of the foot. The **medial** (**G, H**) is the largest and the **intermediate** (**J, K**) is the smallest of the cuneiform bones. The broad surface of the medial cuneiform faces the sole of the foot, while the intermediate and **lateral** (**L, M**) cuneiform have their sharp edges directed plantarward. All three cuneiform bones have articular surfaces posteriorly for articulation with the navicular (**4**). Distally and directed toward the digits are articulations for the metatarsals. The medial cuneiform articulates with the 1st metatarsal and, to a small extent, with the 2nd metatarsal, while the lateral cuneiform has joint surfaces for articulation with the 3rd metatarsal, a small facet for the 2nd metatarsal and sometimes an equally small facet for the 4th metatarsal. The intermediate cuneiform articulates distally only with the 2nd metatarsal. The three cuneiform bones also articulate with each other. In addition, the lateral cuneiform has a joint surface for articulation with the cuboid.

Ossification

Ossification centers appear in the medial cuneiform in the 2nd–3rd year, in the intermediate cuneiform in the 3rd year, and in the lateral cuneiform in the 1st–2nd year.

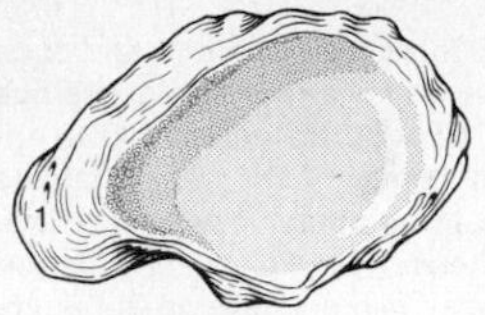

A Posterior view of right navicular

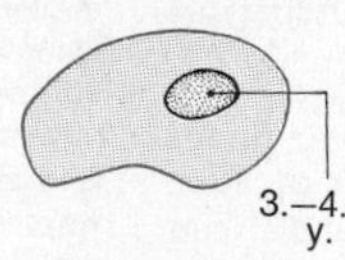

C Ossification of navicular

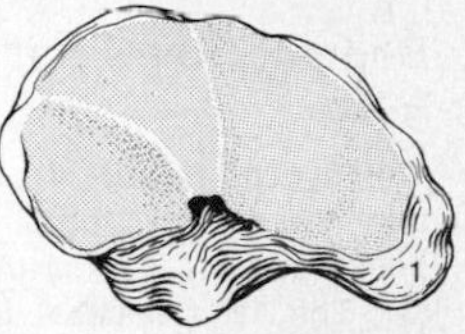

B Anterior view of right navicular

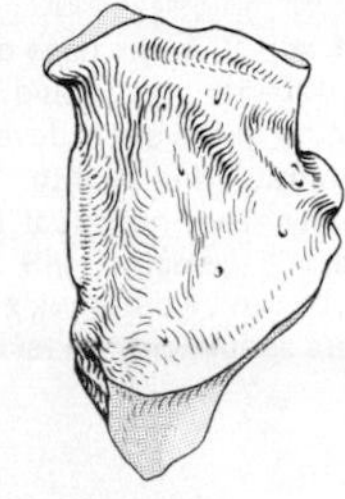

D Dorsal view of right cuboid

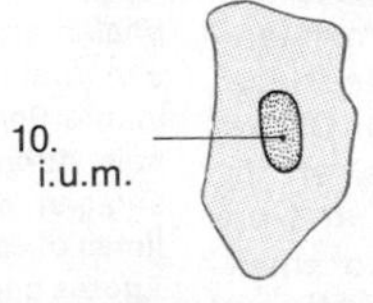

F Ossification of cuboid

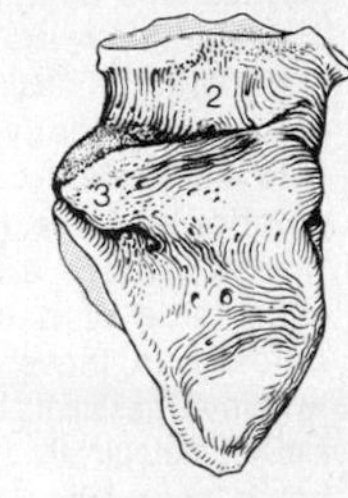

E Plantar view of right cuboid

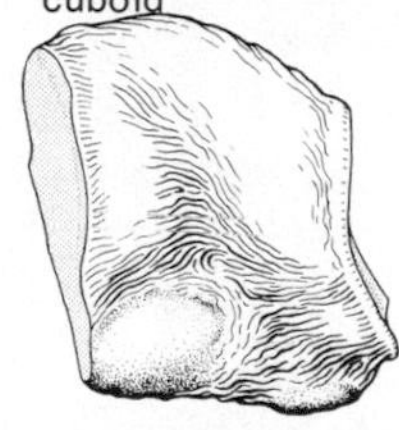

G Medial view of right medial cuneiform

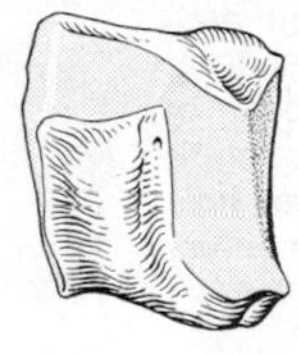

J
Medial view of right intermediate cuneiform

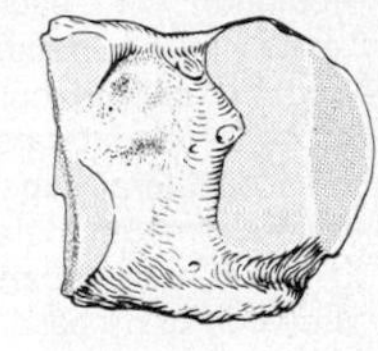

L Medial view of right lateral cuneiform

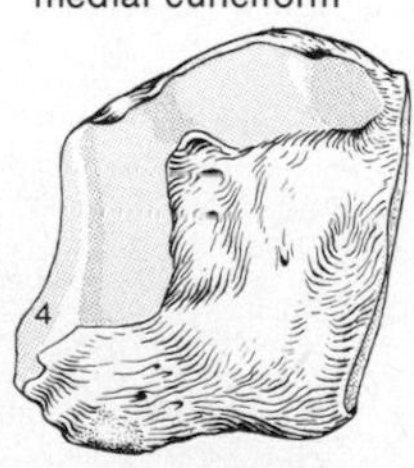

H Lateral view of right medial cuneiform

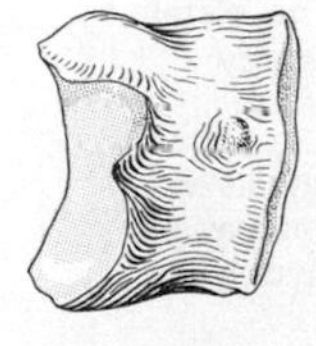

K
Lateral view of right intermediate cuneiform

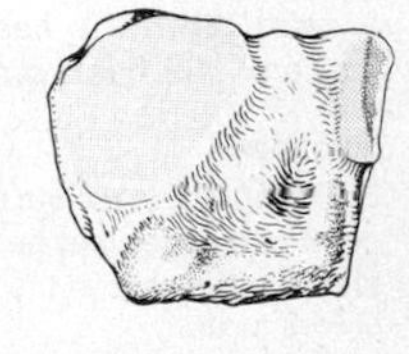

M Lateral view of right lateral cuneiform

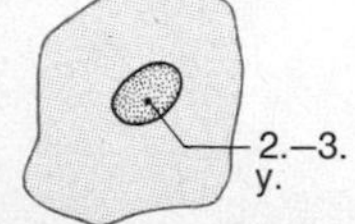

N Ossification of medial cuneiform

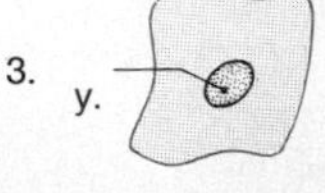

O Ossification of intermediate cuneiform

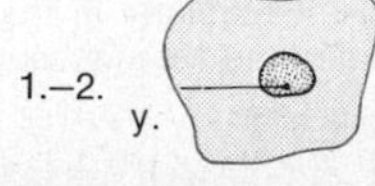

P Ossification of lateral cuneiform

Bones of the Foot (continued A–B)

The five **metatarsals** are long bones and are convex dorsally. All of them possess a *base* (**1**), a *shaft* (**2**) and a *head* (**3**). The **1st metatarsal** is the shortest and thickest. There is a *tuberosity* at the base of the 1st metatarsal on its plantar surface. In the region of this tuberosity and lateral to it, the bone articulates laterally with the base of the 2nd metatarsal, and posteriorly via a curved surface with the medial cuneiform (**4**). On its anterior end the head carries, on its plantar surface a small ridge, and on either side of it there are two small grooves. In these are regularly found two small **sesamoid bones** (**5**). The **2nd, 3rd and 4th metatarsals** are slimmer and their bases are wider dorsally than on their plantar sides. On their sides facing one another there are joint surfaces for articulation with each other, and posteriorly joint surfaces for the cuneiform und the cuboid bones. The heads of these three metatarsal bones are compressed laterally so that they ressemble rollers. The 5th metatarsal bone differs in that it has a *tuberosity* (**6**) on the lateral side of its base.

Bones of the Digits. The 2nd–5th digits each have a **proximal, middle** and **distal phalanx**, while the 1st digit has only two phalanges. Each phalanx has a *base* (**7**), a *shaft* (**8**) and a *head* (**9**). The distal phalanx (**10**) has a *distal tuberosity*.

Variants

Occasionally, in the 5th digit the middle and distal phalanges may be joined. This may already be the case in the cartilaginous stage before birth.

Sesamoid Bones. Near the metatarsophalangeal joints there may be many sesamoid bones, although they are only present regularly in the region of the head of the 1st metatarsal.

Ossification

The cartilaginous metatarsal anlagen develop a perichondral bony cuff in the shaft in the 2nd–3rd intrauterine month, and occasionally there is also an epiphysial ossification center. Like the metacarpals, the epiphysial bony center of the 1st metatarsal is in its base, in the other metatarsals it is always in the head. The epiphysial endochondral ossification centers develop in the 2nd–4th years. In some instances there may be additionally a 2nd epiphysial anlage in the 1st and 5th metatarsal bones.

Epiphysial centers appear in the base of the phalanges in the 1st–5th year, while perichondral ossification in the shaft develops in the 2nd–8th intrauterine month. They fuse during puberty. The individual bony anlagen are relatively variable and their times of appearance can be different, so the figures quoted here should only be taken as a general guide.

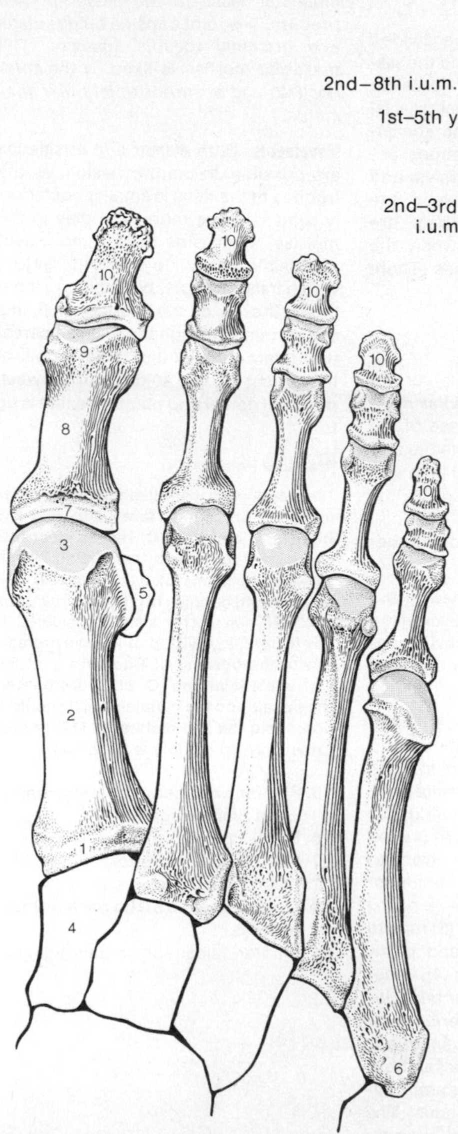

A Dorsal view of metatarsals and phalanges of right foot

2nd–8th i.u.m.

1st–5th y.

2nd–3rd i.u.m.

2nd–4th y.

B Ossification

Joints of the Foot (A–C)

The **joints of the foot** may be divided into the **ankle (talocrural) joint** and the **subtalar** and **talocalcaneonavicular joints**. In addition, there is the **calcaneocuboidal joint** and the **cuneonavicular joint**. The **tarsometatarsal joints** are articulations between the tarsals and metatarsals, and the **intermetatarsal joints** between the bases of the metatarsals. There are **metatarsophalangeal joints** between the metatarsals and the phalanges. There are also **interphalangeal joints.**

Ankle Joint

The **articular surfaces** of the talocrural joint are formed by the *malleolar mortise* (**1**) and the superior surface of the *talar trochlea* along with its medial and lateral malleolar surfaces. The tibia and fibula form a mortise or "clasp" for the roll of the talus (see p. 204). The joint surface of the fibula extends further distally than the tibia.

The **joint capsule** (**2**) is attached to the margins of the cartilaginous layer of the articular surfaces. The joint cavity contains anterior and posterior synovial folds.

Ligaments of the Ankle Joint. The largest ligament on the medial side is the *deltoid (or medial) ligament* (**3**), which consists of tibionavicular (**4**), tibiocalcaneal (**5**) and anterior and posterior (**6**) tibiotalar parts. The tibionavicular part (**4**) extends from the tibia (**7**) to the navicular (**8**) and covers the anterior tibiotalar part, which reaches to the neck of the talus. The tibiocalcaneal part (5) runs to the sustentaculum tali (**9**) and partly covers the tibionavicular part (**4**). Other ligaments include the *anterior talofibular ligaments* (**10**), the *posterior talofibular ligament* and the *calcaneofibular ligament* (**11**). The anterior talofibular ligament connects the lateral malleolus to the neck of the talus. The posterior talofibular ligament runs almost horizontally from the lateral malleolar fossa to the posterior talar process. The joint capsule bulges distal and proximal to this ligament. The malleolar mortise is fixed by the *anterior* (**12**) and *posterior tibiofibular ligaments.*

Movements. Both **plantar** and **dorsiflexion** are possible. In plantar flexion, as the trochea of the talus is smaller posteriorly which leaves more free play in the mortise, slight side-to-side movement is possible. The ankle joint is a **hinge joint** with a **transverse axis**, beginning just beneath the tip of the medial malleolus and running through the thickest part of the lateral malleolus. The range of movement of the ankle joint between maximal dorsal and plantar flexion is up to 70°.

Practical Points

Two joint lines permit amputation of the fore-foot or of the fore- and mid-foot. **Chopart's joint line** (**C**, red) is incorrectly called the "transverse tarsal joint." It runs between the talus (**13**), calcaneus (**14**), navicular (**8**) and cuboid (**15**). The *bifurcate ligament* (**16**; see p. 214) is also considered the key feature, as division of it is the prerequisite to the opening of Chopart's joint line. **Lisfranc's joint line** (**C**, blue) lies between the tarsals and the metatarsals. It should be noted that the 2nd metatarsal (**17**) projects proximally, so the line is not straight.

18 Plantar calcaneocuboid ligament,
19 Long plantar ligament,
20 Medial cuneiform,
21 Intermediate cuneiform,
22 Lateral cuneiform,
23 Medial tubercle of the posterior talar process,
24 Plantar calcaneonavicular ligament.

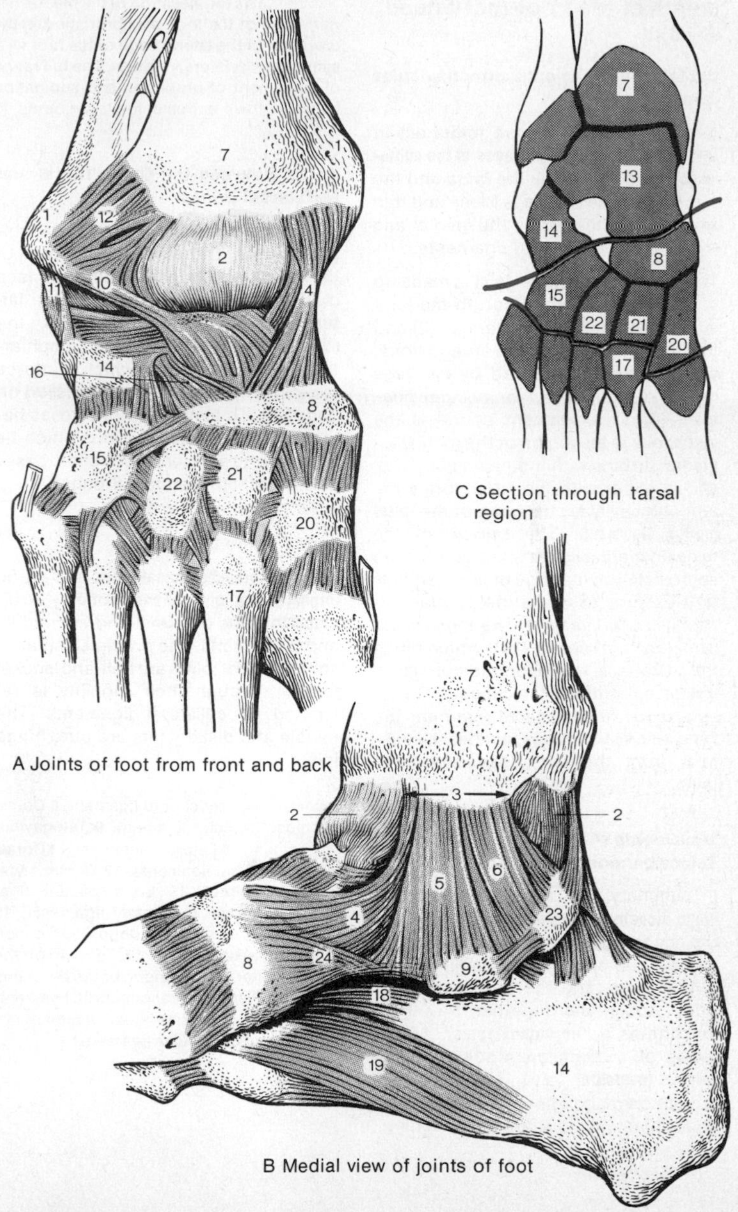

A Joints of foot from front and back

C Section through tarsal region

B Medial view of joints of foot

Joints of the Foot (continued A–B)

Subtalar and Talocalcaneonavicular Joints

Although separate, these joints act in unison. The **articular surfaces of the subtalar joint** are formed by the *talus* and the *clacaneus*. The **capsule** is loose and thin and is strengthened by the *medial* and *lateral* (**1**) *talocalcaneal ligaments*.

The **talocalcaneonavicular joint** is made up of three bones. In addition to the joint surfaces of the *talus, calcaneus* (**2**) and the *navicular* (**3**), there is an additional articular surface covered by cartilage on the *plantar calcaneonavicular ligament* (**4**). This ligament connects the calcaneus in the region of the medial articular surface with the navicular bone, and together with the latter forms the articular cavity for the head of the talus **(spring ligament)**. The **capsule** of the talocalcaneonavicular joint is attached immediately at the edge of the cartilage or it extends as far as the plantar calceonavicular ligament. The tense *bifurcate ligament* (see p. 214), which binds the calcaneus, navicular and cuboid together, strengthens the capsule. The *interosseous talocalcaneal ligament* (**5**), lying in the tarsal sinus, divides the subtalar from the talocalcaneonavicular joint.

Movements of the Ankle, Subtalar and Talocalcaneonavicular Joints

In summary, the ankle joint permits **hinge movements** while the subtalar and the talocalcaneonavicular joints permit **rotation**. The ankle joint is a **hinge joint**, a ginglymus, arid the others are **pivot joints**, trochi and together the three function as a **"trochoginglymus"**. Movements of rotation are known as **pronation (eversion)** and **supination (inversion)** corresponding to the pronating and supinating movements of the hand. Supination is the elevation of the medial (inner) edge of the foot, and pronation is the elevation of the lateral edge of the foot with simultaneous lateral rotation. The full range of movement of pronation and supination between their extreme limits amounts to 130°.

Joints Between the Other Tarsal and Metatarsal Bones

The **calcaneocuboid joint** (**6**) ist an amphiarthrosis. The joint cavity is a part of the so-called Chopart's joint line (see p. 210). The **cuneonavicular** and the **tarsometatarsal joints** as well as the **cuneocuboid joint** are also amphiarthroses. The ligaments which reinforce the joint capsules will be discussed on page 214. To these amphiarthroses belong the **intermetatarsal joints**, which lie between the adjacent sides of the bases of the 2nd–5th metatarsal bones.

Joints of the Digits

The **metatarsophalangeal joints** and the **interphalangeal joints** of the foot may be divided into the proximal and the middle and distal joints. The proximal metatarsophalangeal joints are ball-and-socket joints, although their mobility is restricted by collateral ligaments. The middle and distal joints are pure hinge joints.

7 Dorsal calcaneocuboid ligament, **8** Dorsal cuboideonavicular ligament, **9** Talonavicular ligament, **10** Lateral cuneiform, **11** Dorsal tarsometatarsal ligaments, **12** Dorsal metatarsal ligaments, **13** Long plantar ligament, **14** Plantar metatarsal ligaments, **15** Tendon of the peroneus longus, **16** Tendon of the tibialis anterior, **17** Tendon of the tibialis posterior, **18** Tendon of the peroneus brevis, **19** Plantar calcaneocuboid ligament; **20** Plantar cuboideonavicular ligament, **21** Plantar cuneonavicular ligaments.

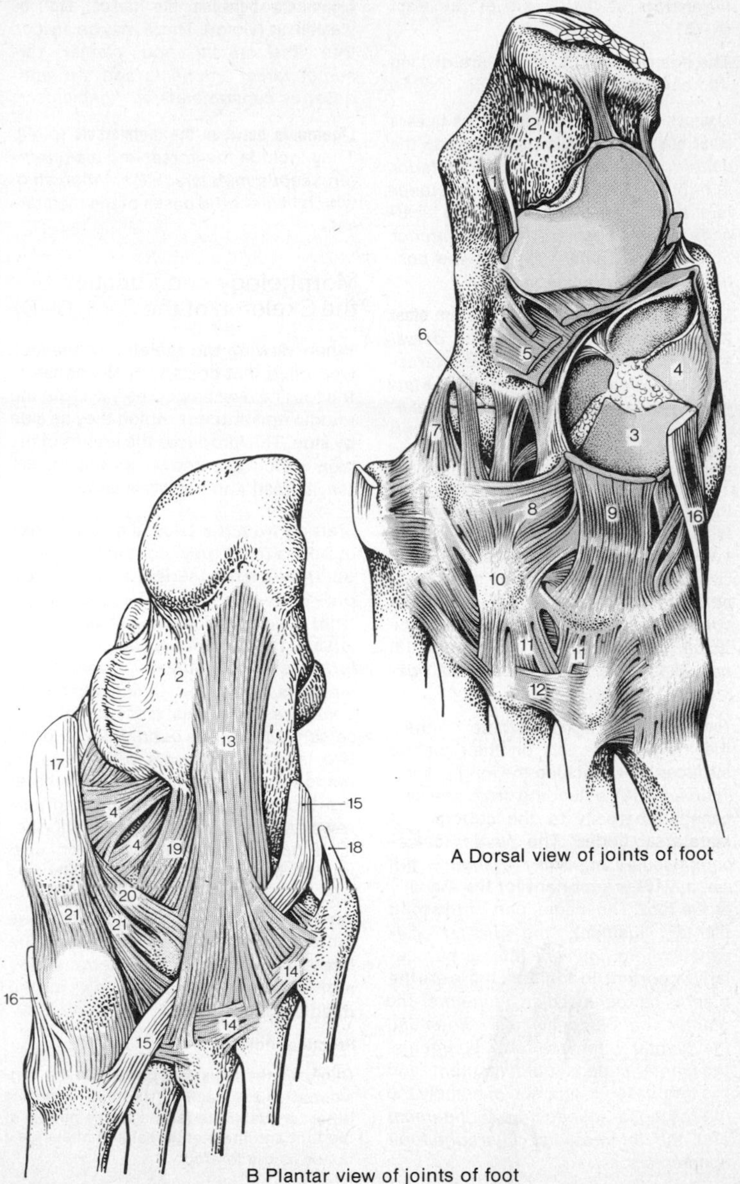

A Dorsal view of joints of foot

B Plantar view of joints of foot

Ligaments of the Joints of the Foot (A–B)

The ligaments of the tarsus are divided into several groups.

Ligaments which join the leg bones to each other and to the tarsals (red) include the *deltoid ligament* (**1**), the *anterior talofibular ligament* (**2**), the *posterior talofibular ligament* (**3**), the *calcaneofibular ligament* (**4**), the *anterior tibiofibular ligament* (**5**) and the *posterior tibiofibular ligament* (**6**).

Ligaments which join the talus to the other tarsals (green) include the *dorsal talonavicular ligament* (**7**), the *interosseus talocalcaneal ligament* (**8**), the *lateral* (**9**) and *medial* (**10**) *talocalcaneal ligaments* and the *posterior talocalcaneal ligament* (**11**).

The remaining dorsal tarsal ligaments (yellow) include the *bifurcate ligament* (**12**) with its calcaneonavicular and calcaneocuboid fibers, the *dorsal intercuneiform ligaments* (**13**), the *dorsal cuneocuboid ligament* (**14**), the *dorsal cuboideonavicular ligament* (**15**), the *dorsal cuneonavicular ligaments* (**16**) and the *dorsal calcaneocuboid ligaments* (**17**).

The plantar tarsal ligaments (blue) connect the individual tarsals on their plantar surfaces. They include the *long plantar ligament* (**18**) extending from the calcaneal tuberosity to the cuboid and metatarsal bones. The *plantar calcaneonavicular* or *spring ligament* (**19**); see p. 216) is important for the stability of the foot. The medial part of the long plantar ligament, the *plantar calcaneocuboid ligament* (**20**), is particularly important. In addition, there are the *plantar cuneonavicular ligaments,* the *plantar cuboideonavicular ligament,* the *plantar intercuneiform ligaments*, the *plantar cuneocuboid ligament* and the interosseous ligaments, namely the *interosseous cuneocuboid ligament* and the *interosseous intercuneiform ligaments.*

Ligaments between the tarsus and the metatarsus (violet). These may be divided into the *dorsal* and *plantar tarsometatarsal ligaments* and the *interosseous cuneometatarsal ligaments.*

Ligaments between the metatarsals (pink). They include the *dorsal* and *plantar interosseous metatarsal ligaments,* all of which lie near the bases of the metatarsals.

Morphology and Function of the Skeleton of the Foot (C–D)

When viewing the skeleton of the foot, we notice that posteriorly the bones of the foot lie over each other, while in the middle and anterior region they lie side by side. This produces the arches of the foot, which are known as the **sagittal (longitudinal)** and **transverse arches.**

Starting from the talus, a medial series of bones (light gray) continues straight on, while a lateral series (dark gray) fans out from the calcaneus toward the front. The **medial series** consists of the *talus* (**21**), the *navicular* (**22**), the *cuneiform bones* (**23**) and the *three medial metatarsals* with their associated *phalanges.* The **lateral series** contains the *calcaneus* (**24**), the *cuboid* (**25**) and the two lateral *metatarsals* with their corresponding phalanges. This results in the foot being wide in front and narrower at the back; it is also higher behind than in front. Finally, the foot also has an arch which faces medially and is curved both longitudinally and transversely. The longitudinal curvature is more marked on the medial than the lateral edge of the foot. The transverse arch is well developed only in the middle and forefoot.

Practical Point

Clinically the talus and calcaneus are considered as the back of the foot, while the other tarsals are regarded as the middle of the foot and the metatarsal and phalangeal bones as the forefoot.

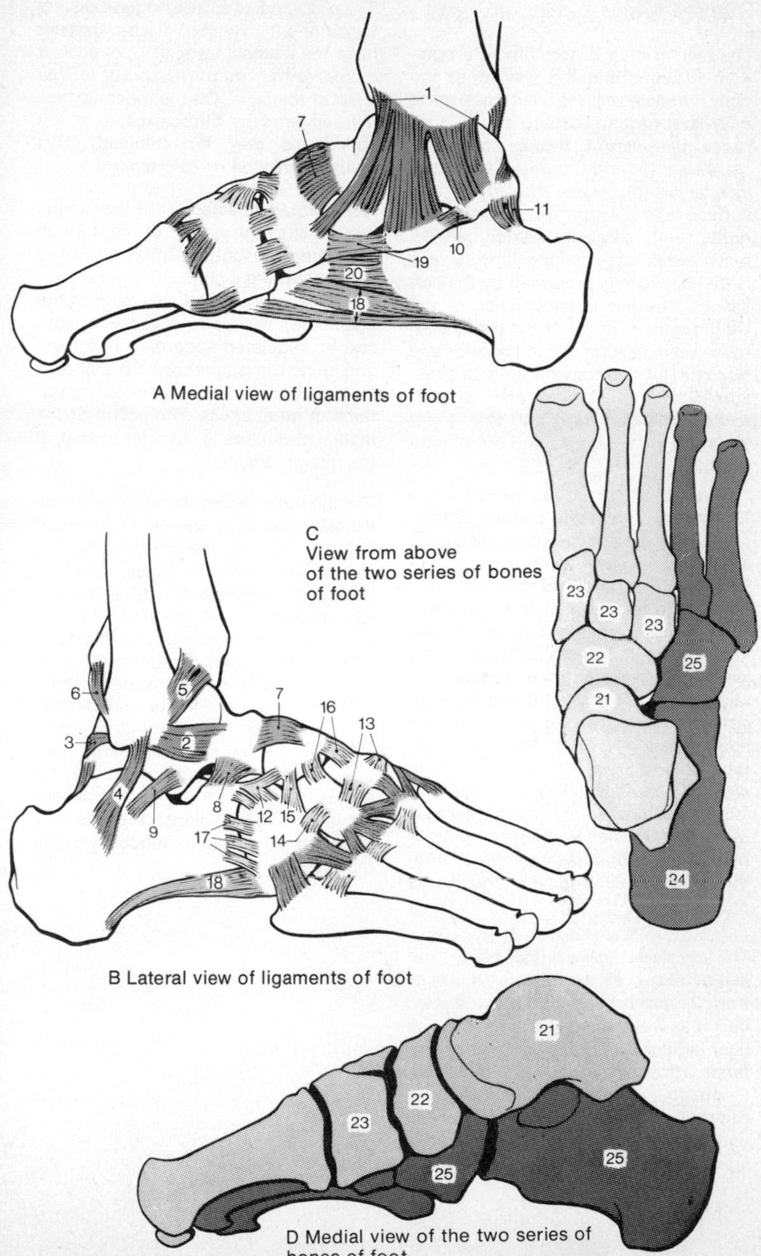

A Medial view of ligaments of foot

B Lateral view of ligaments of foot

C
View from above
of the two series of bones
of foot

D Medial view of the two series of
bones of foot

Plantar Arch (A–C)

The plantar arch is normally in a position of supporting the weight of the body. The **bony points of support of the arch** on a level ground surface are the *calcaneal tuberosity* (**1**), the *head of the 1st metatarsal* (**2**) and the *head of the 5th metatarsal* (**3**). Thus, the supporting surface is in the form of a triangle (**A**, dotted red). If a **footprint** is examined (**B**), a somewhat larger supporting surface is found, which is produced by the soft tissues. The **line of transmission** of the weight of the body runs from the *tibia* (**4**) to the *calcaneus* (**5**) and to the *mid-* and *forefoot* (**6**). The transmission of pressure to the arch in both directions tends to flatten its curvature, and this is opposed by the ligaments and the plantar muscles.

Ligaments. *Ligaments cannot fatigue and have a greater resistance to stress than muscles.* Their resistance does not vary but if they are overstretched they are unable to return to their previous shape. The ligaments may be divided into the **plantar aponeurosis** (**7**), the **long plantar ligament** (**8**), the **plantar calcaneonavicular ligament** (**10**) and the **short plantar ligaments**. The superficial plantar aponeurosis (**7**) joins the calcaneal tuberosity to the plantar surface of the digits. It acts especially in the standing (static) position. In the metatarsal part of the foot, tension in the transverse fibers of the aponeurosis supports both the longitudinal and the transverse arches.

The **long plantar ligament** (**8,9**) braces the lateral series of the tarsals. It arises from the plantar side of the calcaneus, becomes wider distally and extends as a *long, superficial fibrous layer* (**8**) inferior to the tendon of the peroneus longus to the bases of the metatarsals. Short fibers reach the tuberosity of the cuboid as the *plantar calcaneocuboid ligament* (**9**).

The **plantar calcaneonavicular ligament** (**10**) together with the **short plantar ligaments** form the deepest layer of ligaments. *It increases the size of the socket for the head of the talus.* On the inner surface it is covered by fibrocartilage, which sometimes may be calcified. This ligament may be up to 5 mm thick.

The **plantar muscles.** They also resist the effect of the weight of the body in spreading the foot, and they surround the arches like a clamp. They are subject to fatigue and are weaker than the ligaments. However, muscle tension can be regulated according to stress, and recent investigations have shown that it is brought into play under conditions of great stress. The action of the medial abductors is superior to that of the lateral abductors.

The plantar muscles are divided into the **intrinsic muscles of the foot** (**11**), which stretch between the tarsals and the metatarsals and phalanges, and the **tendons of the extrinsic muscles of the foot,** which descend from the leg and are inserted on the various tarsals, metatarsals and phalanges. The intrinsic muscles of the foot permit movements of the digits with respect to the metatarsals and tarsals. In the standing or static position, the digits and metatarsals are pressed onto the ground, and the intrinsic muscles of the foot function as tensor muscles of the plantar arch, as they counteract the sagging tendency of the metatarsals.

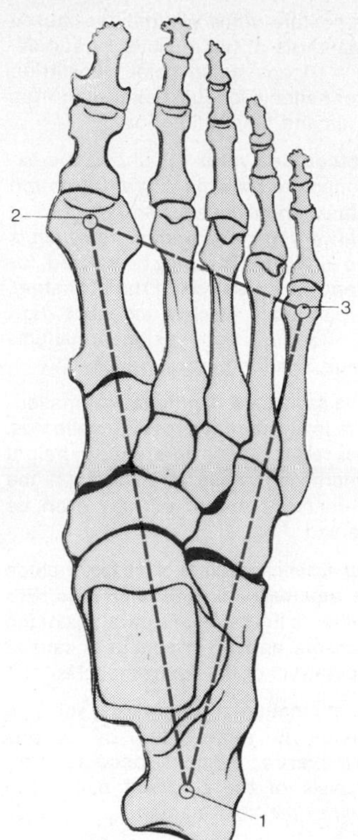

A Skeleton of foot, showing weight-bearing points; view from above

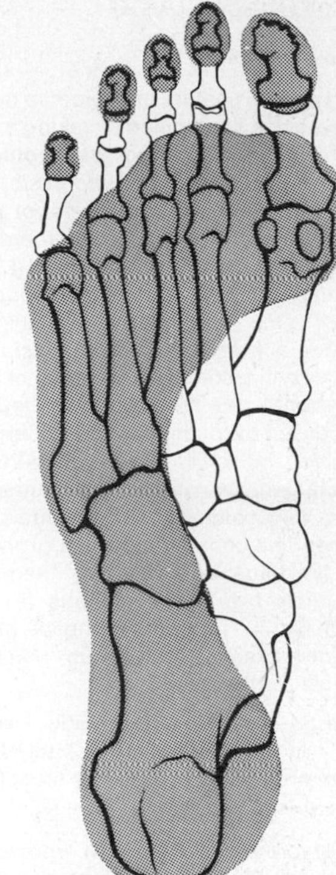

B
Footprint of right foot with outline of its bony skeleton; view from below

C Medial view of plantar arch of foot

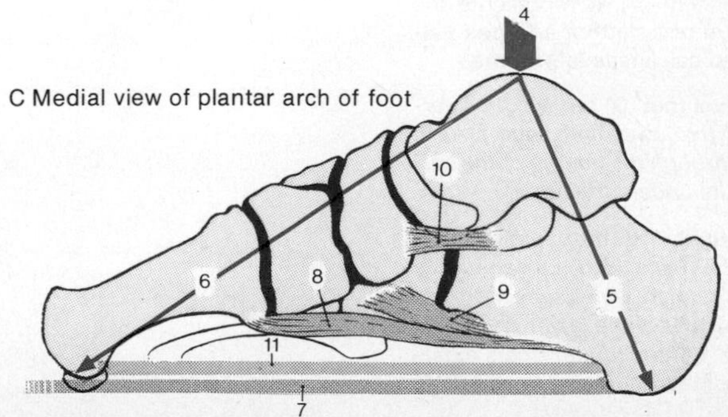

Foot Shapes (A–J)

Practical Points

The normal posture of the foot in the living may be determined by taking a footprint. In the **healthy foot, pes rectus** (**A**), the *print should show impressions of five digits anterior and posterior parts of the sole and a strip joining them.* The *main load* on the healthy foot (**E**) *lies medially on the calcaneus* (**1**) *and the head of the 1st metatarsal* (**2**). If the print shows a *wide, flattened impression* (**B**) of the entire sole, then the subject has a **"flatfoot", pes planus**. Flattfootedness is caused by inadequacy of the intrinsic plantar muscles, which leads to an overextension of the ligaments and thus to a collapse of the plantar arch. When this occurs, there is a pronation of the talus, and this may then slide medially over the calcaneus (**F**). The end result is a remodeling of all the involved tarsals (calcaneus, talus, navicular and cuboid).

During development of flatfoot severe pain in the foot and leg occurs, due to overstretching of the long muscles of the sole.

A *footprint in two parts* (**C**) represents **a high longitudinal arch, pes cavus (C).** Here the calcaneus is supinated while the other skeletal parts of the foot are pronated.

A **pes planovalgus** has a *footprint that bulges medially* (**D**). It represents the combination of a flatfoot and **pes valgus (H)**; the calcaneus is pronated.

In the **normal foot** (**G**) *the weight-bearing line of the lower limb* (see also p. 202) *runs through the middle of the calcaneus to its undersurface.*

In **pes valgus (H)** *the vertical axis through the talus and calcaneus is sharply angulated with respect to the longitudinal axis of the lower limb, thus forming an obtuse angle, open externally.* The foot is everted (pronated). This posture of the foot may be caused by paralysis of the muscles of supination – triceps surae, tibialis posterior, flexor hallucis longus, flexor digitorum longus and tibialis anterior.

Clubfoot, pes varus (**J**), shows the exact opposite. *Here the long axis through the talus and calcaneus and the axis of the lower limb form and angle which is open medially.* This may be caused, for instance, by paralysis of the pronators, the peroneal muscles, extensor digitorum longus and the extensor hallucis longus, resulting in supination.

In the **normal foot** (**G**) the lateral malleolus is lower than the medial malleolus. In **pes valgus** (**H**) this difference in height is increased, while in **clubfoot** (**J**) the difference is absent or may even be reversed.

Other abnormal postures of the foot include **pes equinus** and **pes calcaneus.** Pes equinus is the result of a paralysis of the extensors, and pes calcaneus is caused by paralysis of the flexor muscles.

A combination of pes varus and pes equinus is represented by a **pes equinovarus**, which occurs after paralysis of the peroneal nerve and injury to the tibialis anterior.

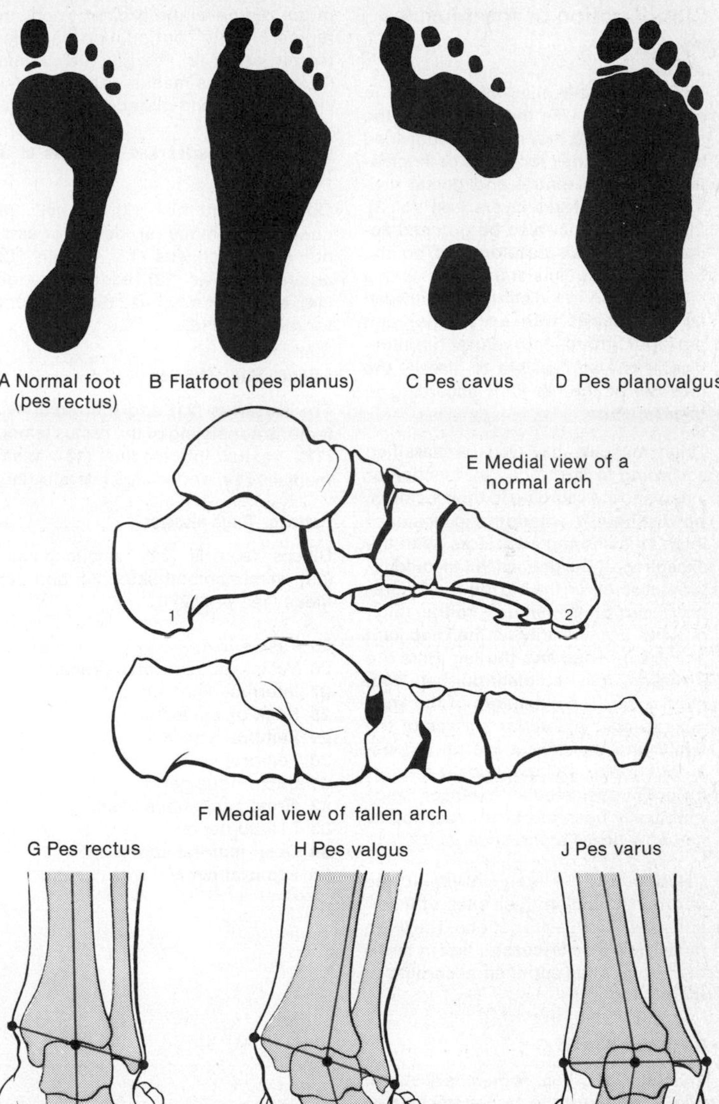
A Normal foot (pes rectus)
B Flatfoot (pes planus)
C Pes cavus
D Pes planovalgus
E Medial view of a normal arch
1
2
F Medial view of fallen arch
G Pes rectus
H Pes valgus
J Pes varus

Classification of the Muscles (A–C)

The hip muscles may be classified in several ways. Like the muscles of the shoulder girdle, they may be subdivided according to their locations or innervation from the ventral and dorsal divisions of the plexus layers (see Vol. 3). Further, they may also be grouped according to their development on the basis of their points of insertion. In this classification we distinguish between dorsal muscles with an anterior and posterior group, and ventral hip muscles. It is also possible to classify the muscles of the hip joint according to their function.

Thigh muscles may also be classified according to their location, function or innervation. According to their location, we distinguish anterior and posterior thigh muscles and adductors. With the exception of the gracilis, all the adductors act solely on the hip joint and therefore insert on the femur. The true thigh muscles act primarily on the knee joint and are inserted into the leg. Here the extensors must be distinguished from the flexors. The extensors of the knee joint lie on the anterior surface of the femur and the flexors are on its posterior surface. Ontogenetically the sartorius is considered an extensor, since it has only been displaced secondarily and now flexes at the knee joint.

Discussion of the hip muscles will take into consideration their sites of insertion as well as their functions. The thigh muscles will be discussed first in terms of their location and then according to their function.

Dorsal Hip Muscles

The anterior group, which is inserted in the region of the lesser trochanter, includes: the psoas major and iliacus = iliopsoas (**1**), psoas minor.
The posterior group, which is inserted in the region of the greater trochanter region and its continuation, includes: the piriformis (**2**), the gluteus minimus (**3**), the gluteus medius (**4**), tensor fasciae latae (**5**) and gluteus maximus (**6**).

Ventral Hip Muscles and Adductors of the Thigh

Obturator internus (**7**), gemelli (**8**), quadratus femoris (**9**), obturator externus (**10**), pectineus (**11**), gracilis (**12**), adductor brevis (**13**), adductor longus (**14**), adductor magnus (**15**) and adductor minimus (**16**).

Anterior Thigh Muscles

The sartorius (**21**) and the quadriceps femoris consisting of the rectus femoris (**17**), vastus intermedius (**18**), vastus medialis (**19**) and vastus lateralis (**20**).

Posterior Thigh Muscles

Biceps femoris (**22**), semitendinosus (**23**), semimembranosus (**24**) and popliteus (see p. 252).

25 Fascia lata,
26 Vasto-adductor membrane,
27 Intermuscular septum,
28 Neck of the femur,
29 Femoral artery,
30 Femoral vein,
31 Saphenous nerve,
32 Great saphenous vein,
33 Sciatic nerve,
34 Deep femoral artery,
35 Femoral nerve.

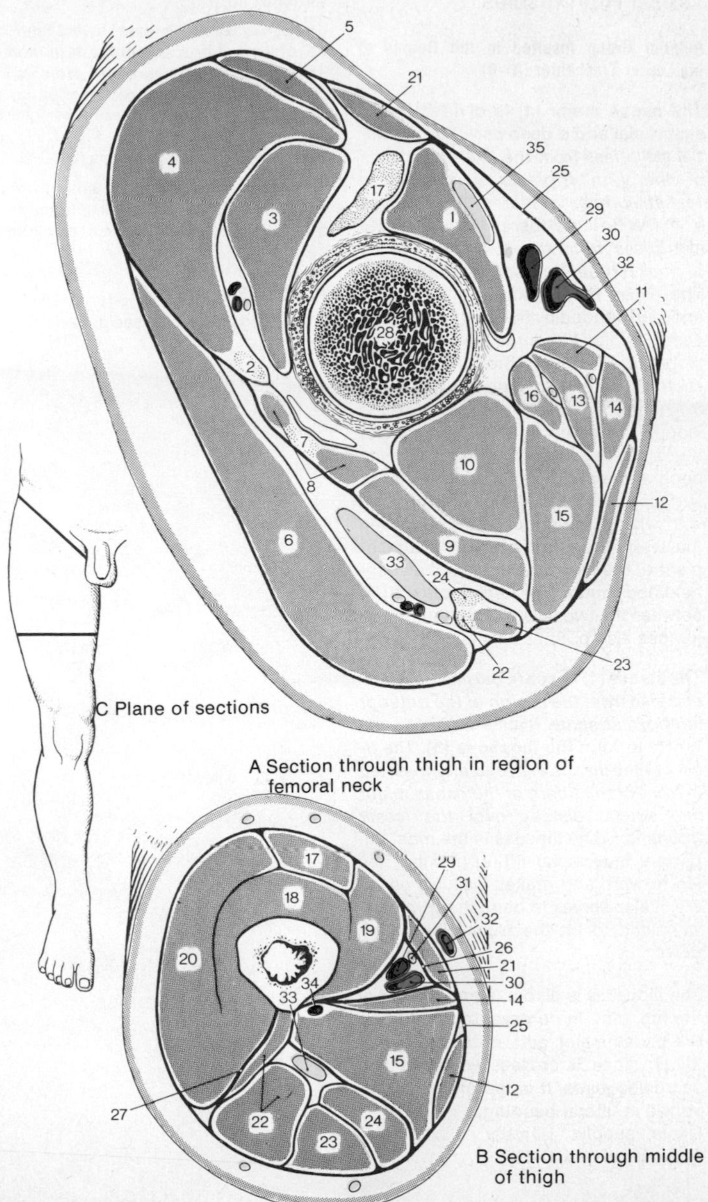

C Plane of sections

A Section through thigh in region of femoral neck

B Section through middle of thigh

Dorsal Hip Muscles

Anterior Group Inserted in the Region of the Lesser Trochanter (A–B)

The **psoas major** (**1**) is divided into a superficial and a deep part. The **superficial part** *arises from the lateral surfaces of the 12th thoracic vertebra and 1st–4th lumbar vertebrae* (**2**) *as well as from their intervertebral disks.* The **deep part** *arises from the costal processes of the 1st–5th lumbar vertebrae* (**3**). The psoas major joins the iliacus (**4**) and, surrounded by the iliac fascia, proceeds as the **iliopsoas** (**5**) across the iliopubic eminence through the muscular lacuna to be inserted on *the lesser trochanter* (**6**). In the region of the iliopubic eminence, the iliopectineal bursa lies between the muscle and the bone and extends as far as the anterior surface of the capsule of the hip joint with which it communicates. Between the lesser trochanter and the attachment of the iliopsoas lies the iliac subtendinous bursa. The lumbar plexus lies between the two layers of the psoas major (see also p. 92).

The **iliacus** (**4**) *arises in the iliac fossa* (**7**) *and also from the region of the anterior inferior iliac spine.* It joins the psoas major (**1**) to form the **iliopsoas** (**5**). *The fibers of the iliacus are regularly inserted in front of the fibers of the psoas major and extend distally over the lesser trochanter.* The ilipsoas is the most important muscle for lifting (flexing) the leg forward and makes walking possible. It also serves to bend the trunk forward and to lift the trunk when lying down.

The iliopsoas is also a lateral rotator of the hip joint. In contrast to the iliacus, the psoas major acts on a number of joints, since it crosses vertebral and sacroiliac joints. It is therefore also involved in lateral bending.
Nerve supply: Lumbar plexus and femoral nerve (L1–L4).

Variants

The **psoas minor** is present in less than 50% of subjects. *It arises from the 12th thoracic and 1st lumbar vertebra and projects into the iliac fascia.* It is either inserted on the ilio pubic eminence or radiates into the iliopectineal arch.
Nerve supply: Lumbar plexus (L1–L2).

The psoas major may also arise from the head of the 12th rib and the iliacus may arise from the capsule of the hip joint and from the sacrum.

Practical Points

Wandering abscesses, see p. 92.

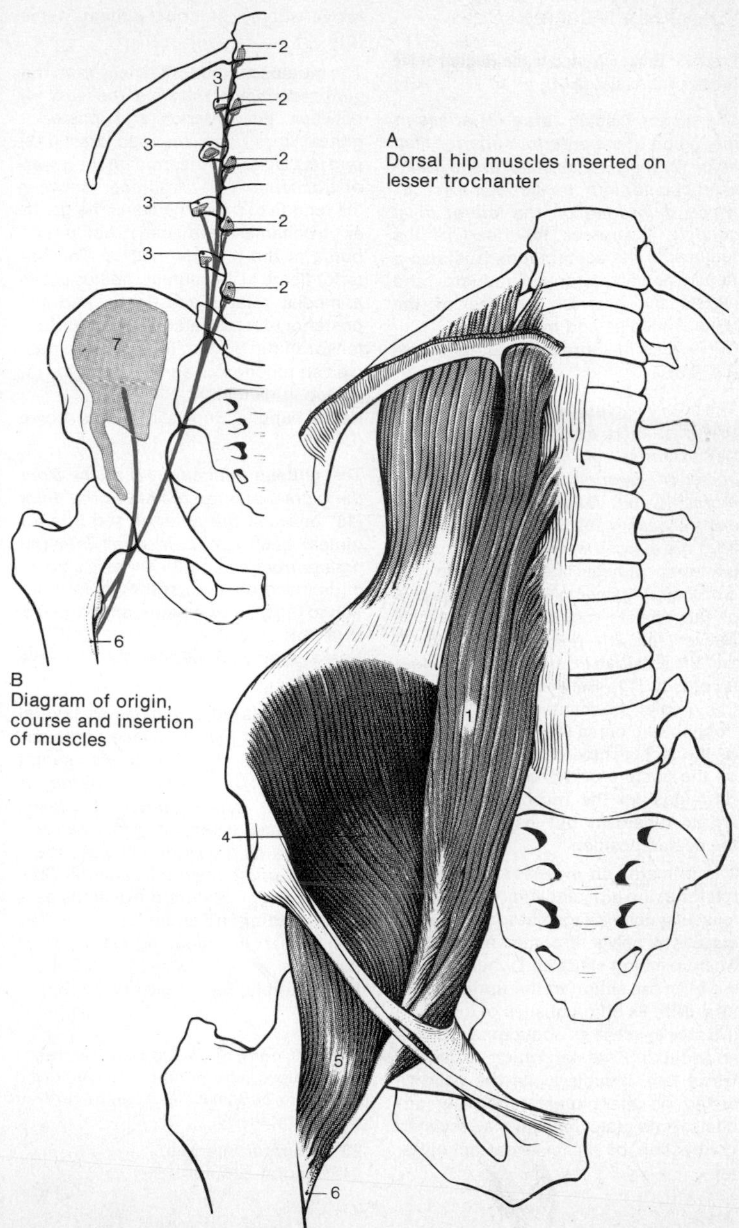

A
Dorsal hip muscles inserted on lesser trochanter

B
Diagram of origin, course and insertion of muscles

Dorsal Hip Muscles

Posterior Group Inserted in the Region of the Greater Trochanter (A–D)

The **tensor fasciae latae** (**1**) *arises in the region of the anterior superior iliac spine* (**2**) *and extends distal to the greater trochanter into the iliotibial tract* (**3**), *which is inserted on the lateral tibial condyle.* It presses the head of the femur into the acetabulum. It is also a flexor, medial rotator and abductor, and assists the anterior bundles of the gluteus medius and minimus.
Nerve supply: Superior gluteal nerve (L4–L5).

The powerful **gluteus maximus** (**4**) has a **superficial** and a **deep origin**. The **superficial fibers** *arise from the iliac crest* (**5**), *the posterior superior iliac spine* (**6**), *the thoracolumbar fascia, the sacrum* (**7**) *and the coccyx* (**8**). The **deep fibers** *arise from the ala of the ilium* (**9**) behind the posterior gluteal line, *from the sacrotuberal ligament* (**10**) *and the fascia of the gluteus medicus. The* **proximal part** *radiates into the iliotibial tract* (**3**) and the **distal part** *inserts* into *the gluteal tuberosity* (**11**). Between the latter and the greater trochanter lies the large trochanteric bursa (**12**). Its relationship to the ischial tuberosity is dependent on the posture of the body. In the upright posture the muscle covers the ischial tuberosity but leaves it free in the seated position.

It is primarily an extensor and lateral rotator at the hip joint and represents a muscular defense against excessive tilting of the pelvis. It comes into action when climbing stairs and when changing from the sitting to the upright posture. With its different sites of insertion it is able to act as an abductor as well as an adductor. That part which tenses the fascia lata abducts, while the part inserted on the gluteal tuberosity adducts. Both glutei maximi may assist in contraction of the external sphincter ani.

Nerve supply: Inferior gluteal nerve (L5–S2).

The **gluteus medius** (13) *arises from the gluteal surface of the ala of the ilium* (4) between the anterior and posterior gluteal lines, *from the iliac crest* (**15**) *and its fascia. It is inserted on the greater trochanter* (**16**) *like a cap.* Between the tendon of attachment and the greater trochanter lies the trochanteric bursa of the gluteus medius. The anterior fibers of the gluteus medius act as a medial rotator and flexor, and the posterior part as a lateral rotator and extensor of the hip, while the entire muscle can function as an abductor (for instance in dancing).
Nerve supply: Superior gluteal nerve (L4–L5).

The **gluteus minimus** (**17**) *arises from the gluteal area on the ala of the ilium* (**18**) between the anterior and inferior gluteal lines *and is inserted into the greater trochanter* (**19**). There is a bursa at its insertion. It corresponds in function to the gluteus medius, although it is a weaker abductor.
Nerve supply: Superior gluteal nerve (L4–S1).

The **piriformis** (**20**) *originates* as *several slips from the pelvic surface of the sacrum,* lateral to the pelvic sacral foramina (**21**), *and from the margin of the greater sciatic notch.* It passes through the greater sciatic foramen *and is inserted on the anteriomedial aspect of the tip of the greater trochanter* (**22**). In the upright posture it functions as a lateral rotator and abductor, and it also plays a part in producing extension of the thigh.
Nerve supply: Sacral plexus (L5–S2).

Variants

The muscle may be divided into several parts by the sciatic nerve or other branches of the sacral plexus. Sometimes it may be partly or completely absent.

23 Obturator internus,
24 Quadratus femoris.

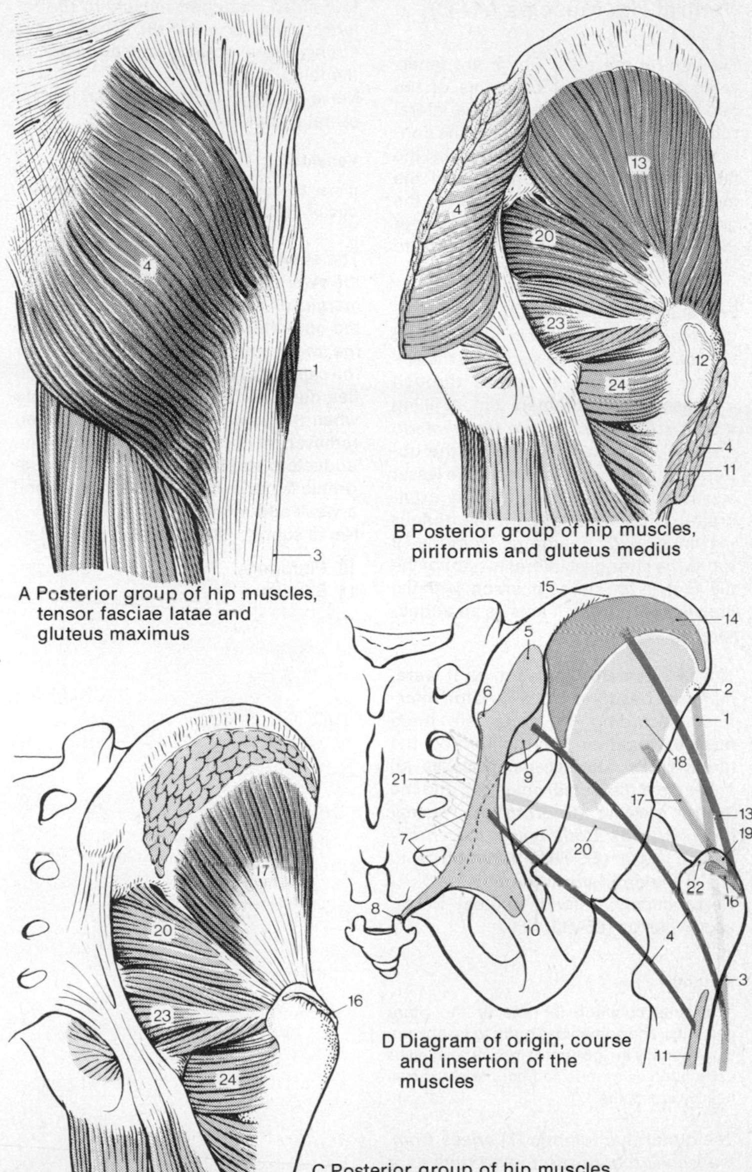

A Posterior group of hip muscles, tensor fasciae latae and gluteus maximus

B Posterior group of hip muscles, piriformis and gluteus medius

C Posterior group of hip muscles, piriformis and gluteus minimus

D Diagram of origin, course and insertion of the muscles

Ventral Hip Muscles (A–C)

The ventral muscles, which are innervated by the ventral branches of the nerve plexus layer, function as lateral rotators. They are important in the control of the body's balance. Basically, the lateral rotators are stronger than the medial rotators, and therefore, in the normal position of the limb, the apex of the foot points slightly outward to achieve better support for the body.

The **obturator internus** (**1**) *arises from the inner surface of the hip bone around the obturator foramen and from the obturator membrane.* It passes through the lesser sciatic foramen, almost filling it, *and is inserted into the trochanteric fossa (***2**). The ischial bursa of the obturator internus is found near the lesser sciatic notch. The bone acts as a fulcrum for this muscle. With the gluteus maximus and quadratus femoris it forms the strongest lateral rotator of the hip joint. In the sitting position, with the limb flexed in front, it acts as an abductor.

The two **gemelli** represent, as it were, marginal heads of the obturator internus. According to *Lanz* all three muscles together may be termed the **triceps coxae**. The **superior gemellus** (**3**) *arises from the ischial spine* (**4**), and the **inferior gemellus** (**5**) *from the ischial tuberosity* (**6**). *Both reach the trochanteric fossa* (**2**). Their function is to assist the obturator internus.
Nerve supply: Inferior gluteal nerve, sacral plexus (L5–S2).

Variants

It is quite common for one or the other gemellus, and sometimes both, to be absent. Occasionally the obturator internus receives extra bundles of muscle fibers arising from nearby ligaments.

The **quadratus femoris** (**7**) *arises from the ischial tuberosity* (**6**) and runs as a four-sided, flattened muscle *to the intertrochanteric crest* (**8**). It acts as a strong lateral rotator and adductor of the thigh.
Nerve supply: Inferior gluteal nerve, sacral plexus (L5–S2).

Variants

It may be absent or it may fuse with the adductor magnus.

The **obturator externus** (**9**) *arises from the external surface of the medial bony margin of the obturator foramen and the obturator membrane. It extends to the trochanteric fossa* (**2**) *and* (rarely) *to the capsule of the hip joint.* This muscle lies deep and it only becomes visible when the adjacent muscles have been removed. At its origin it is covered by the adductors and in the thigh by the quadratus femoris. It is a lateral rotator and a weak adductor.
Nerve supply: Obturator nerve (L1–L4).

10 Piriformis,
11 Sacrum.

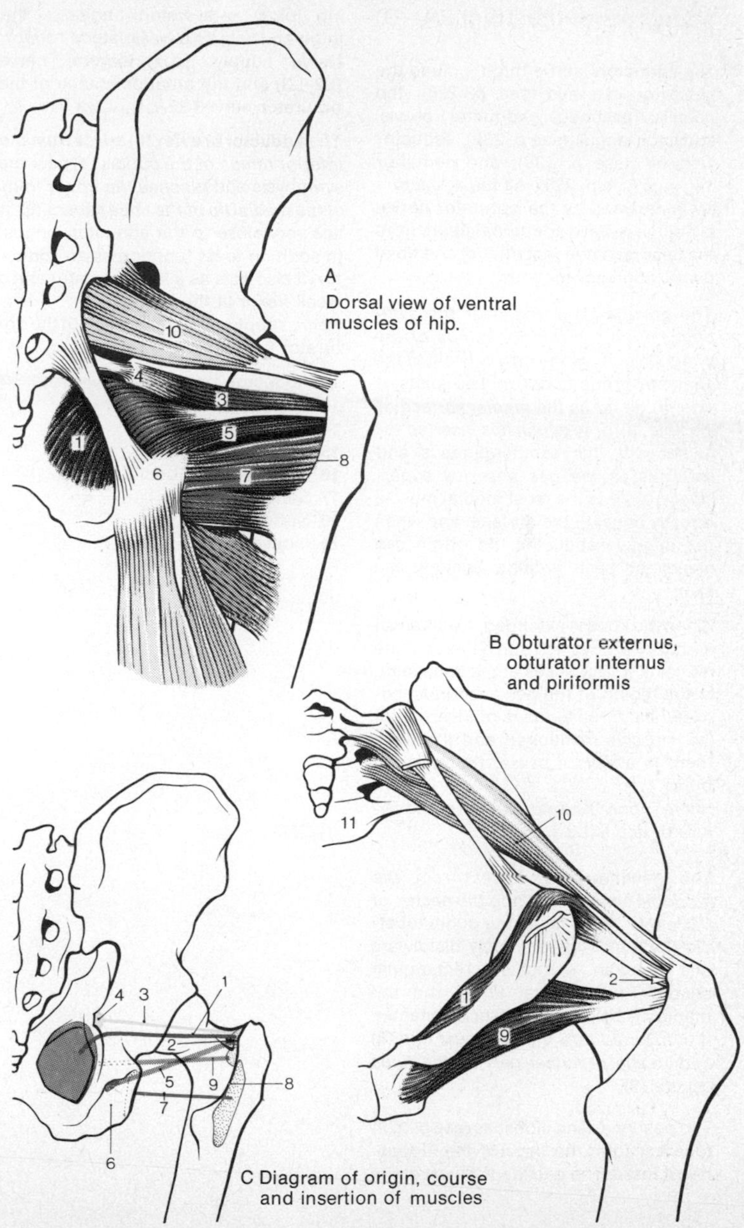

A
Dorsal view of ventral muscles of hip.

B Obturator externus, obturator internus and piriformis

C Diagram of origin, course and insertion of muscles

Adductors of the Thigh (A–D)

The adductors of the thigh include the obturator externus (see p. 226), the gracilis, pectineus, adductor brevis, adductor longus (see p. 230), adductor magnus (see p. 230), and adductor minimus (see p. 230). All the adductors are innervated by the obturator nerve, but some receive additional fibers from the femoral nerve (pectineus) and tibial nerve (adductor magnus).

The **gracilis** (**1**) *arises near the symphysis from the inferior ramus of the pubis* (**2**) and, as the only muscle of the adductor group to act on two joints, it *extends as far as the medial surface of the tibia* (**3**), *onto which it is inserted* together with the semitendinosus and sartorius *as the pes anserius superficialis* (**4**). It is the most medial muscle directly beneath the surface, and when the thigh is abducted, its origin can clearly be seen arching beneath the skin.

When the knee is extended, it acts as an adductor of the thigh and a flexor of the hip joint. It also flexes at the knee joint. In the region of the pes anserinus, between the three tendons of insertion of the muscles mentioned and the tibia, there is always a bursa, the anserine bursa.
Nerve supply: Anterior branch of the obturator nerve (L2–L4).

The **pectineus** (**5**) *arises from the iliopubic eminence, along the pecten of the pubis,* (**6**) as far as the pubic tubercle (**7**). It extends obliquely distalward and has an elongated rectangular shape. The proximal fibers run immediately behind the lesser trochanter. *It is inserted into the pectineal line* (**8**) *and to the proximal part of the linea aspera* (**9**).

The pectineus and iliopsoas (see p. 222) together form the floor of the iliopectineal fossa. The pectineus flexes at the hip joint (anteversion), adducts the thigh and acts as a weak lateral rotator.
Nerve supply: The femoral nerve (L2–L3) and the anterior branch of the obturator nerve (L2–L4).

The **adductor brevis** (**10**) *arises from the inferior ramus of the pubis* (**11**) near the symphysis and *reaches the upper third of the medial lip of the linea aspera* (**9**). It lies very close to the adductor longus. In addition to its function as an adductor, it also acts as a lateral rotator and a weak flexor at the hip joint.
Nerve supply: Anterior branch of the obturator nerve (L2–L4).

12 Adductor longus,
13 Adductor magnus,
14 Adductor minimus,
15 Obturator externus,
16 Quadratus femoris,
17 Semitendinosus,
18 Sartorius,
19 Iliopsoas.

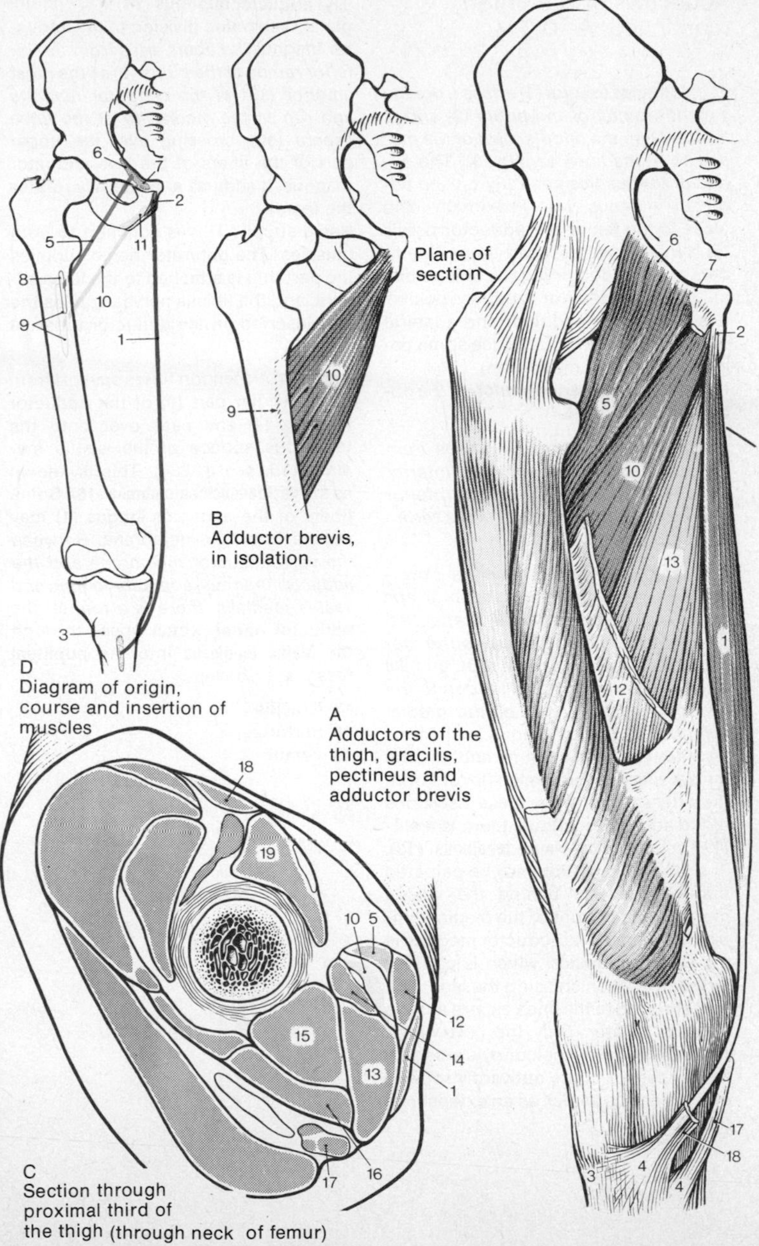

A
Adductors of the thigh, gracilis, pectineus and adductor brevis

B
Adductor brevis, in isolation.

C
Section through proximal third of the thigh (through neck of femur)

D
Diagram of origin, course and insertion of muscles

Adductors of the Thigh (continued, A–D)

The **adductor longus** (**1**) *arises from the superior ramus of the pubis* (**2**) *and is inserted into the middle third of the medial lip of the linea aspera* (**3**). The adductor longus lies ventrally on the adductor magnus (**4**). Proximally and close to the femur the adductor brevis (**5**) is interposed between them. The fibers of the adductor longus extend distally into the adductor canal (see below). It is primarily an adductor and a lateral rotator, but may also produce some degree of flexion (anteversion).
Nerve supply: Anterior branch of the obturator nerve (L2–L4).

The **adductor magnus** (**4**) *arises from the anterior surface of the interior ramus of the pubis* (**6**) *and the inferior ramus of the ischium* (**7**) *as far as the ischial tuberosity* (**8**).

The large muscle belly passes downward on the medial side of the thigh and divides into two. **One part** (**9**) *is attached directly by its muscle fibers to the medial lip of the linea aspera* (**10**), and **the other** (**11**) *is attached by a tendon to the adductor tubercle* (**12**) *of the medial epicondyle.* The tendinous part forms an intermuscular septum and on the medial side it separates the flexors from the extensors. Between these insertions of the adductor magnus, there is a slit-like opening, **the hiatus tendineus** (**13**). The tendinous portion may be palpated through the skin behind the vastus medialis and in front of the medial dimple of the knee. The adductor magnus is a powerful adductor, which is particularly active when crossing the legs. The part attached to the linea aspera acts as a lateral rotator. Only the part which reaches the medial epicondyle acts as a medial rotator of the outwardly rotated and flexed leg, as well as an extensor of the hip joint.

The **adductor minimus** (**14**) is an incompletely separated division of the adductor magnus. *Its fibers arise from the inferior ramus of the pubis* (**6**) *as the most anterior part of the adductor magnus and run to the medial lip of the linea aspera* (**10**), crossing over the upper part of the fibers of the true adductor magnus. It adducts and laterally rotates the femur.
Nerve supply: This is common to both muscles. The obturator nerve supplies the part that is attached to the linea aspera, and the tibialis nerve supplies the part inserted on the adductor tubercle (L3–L5).

Aponeurotic tendon fibers split off from the muscular part (**9**) of the adductor magnus (**4**) and pass over onto the tendinous surface of the vastus medialis (**15**; see p. 236). This is known as the **vastoadductor membrane** (**16**). Some fibers of the adductor longus (**1**) may radiate into this membrane. *Between the vastoadductor membrane and the adductor magnus, adductor longus and vastus medialis, there is a tunnel,* the **adductor canal**, which opens through the **hiatus tendineus** into the popliteal fossa (see above).

17 Gracilis,
18 Sartorius,
19 Femur.

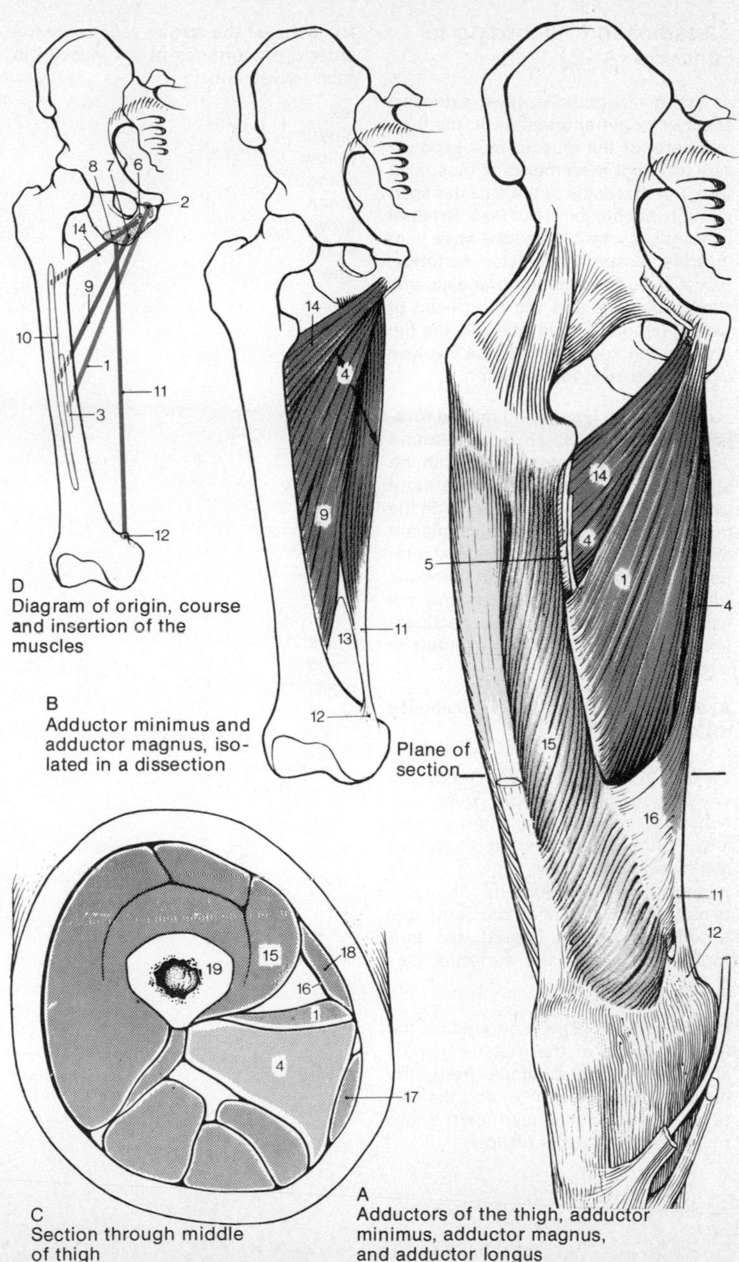

D
Diagram of origin, course and insertion of the muscles

B
Adductor minimus and adductor magnus, isolated in a dissection

C
Section through middle of thigh

A
Adductors of the thigh, adductor minimus, adductor magnus, and adductor longus

Classification According to Function (A–B)

As some hip muscles have extensive areas of origin and insertion, the various parts of the muscle may produce very different movements. It must also be noted that some of the muscles span not only the hip joint, but also vertebral joints (psoas major) and the knee joint (gracilis, tensor fasciae latae, sartorius, rectus femoris, semimembranosus and semitendinosus and the long head of biceps femoris). Thus not only the hip but also the thigh muscles are involved in movements at the hip joint.

We distinguish **lateral** and **medial rotation** movements which occur around the **longitudinal axis** of the limb. With the hip extended, medial rotation is more extensive than lateral rotation. With the hip flexed, the restrictive ligaments are tensed, so that the extent of lateral rotation is then greater than that of medial rotation. The movements around the **transverse axis** are **extension** (dorsiflexion, retroversion) and **flexion** (anteflexion, anteversion).

Abduction and **adduction** occur about a **sagittal axis**.

Lateral rotation (A) is produced by: the gluteus maximus (red), quadratus femoris (blue), obturator internus (yellow), gluteus medius and gluteus minimus with their dorsal fibers (orange), iliopsoas (green), obturator externus (brown) and all the adductors except the gracilis (violet), the piriformis (gray) and the sartorius (see p. 236; not shown).

Medial rotation (B) is produced by: the anterior fibers of the gluteus medius and the gluteus minimus (red), the tensor fasciae latae (blue) and the part of the adductor magnus inserted into the adductor tubercle (yellow).

The color of the arrows represents the order of importance of the muscles in each movement:

red
blue
yellow
orange
green
brown
violet
gray

(dorsal)
gluteus max, med, min
quad fem.
ob. int
iliopsoas
ob ex
all adductors
not gracilis
piriformis
Sart

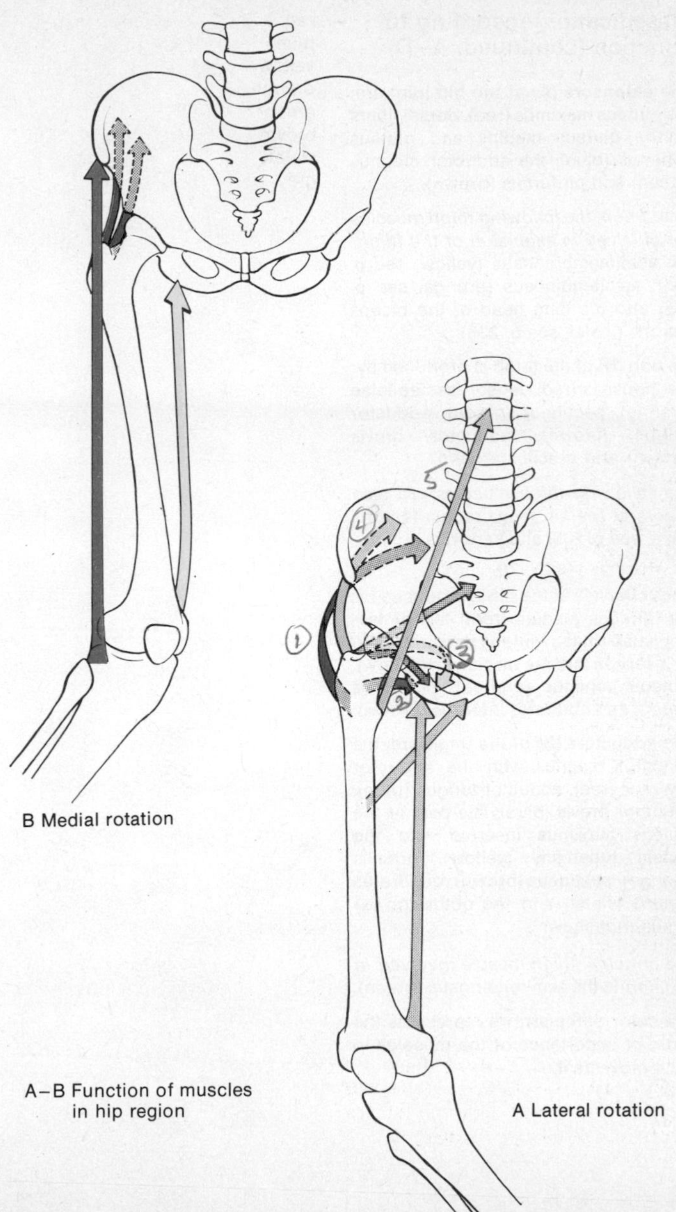

B Medial rotation

A Lateral rotation

A–B Function of muscles in hip region

Classification According to Function (continued, A–D)

red
blue
yellow
orange
green
brown
violet
gray

The **extensors** (**A**) at the hip joint are: the gluteus maximus (red), dorsal fibers of the gluteus medius and gluteus minimus (blue), the adductor magnus (green) and piriformis (brown).

In addition, the following thigh muscles are involved in extension of the thigh: the semimembranosus (yellow, see p. 238), semitendinosus (orange, see p. 238) and the long head of the biceps femoris (violet, see p. 238).

Flexion (**B**) of the thigh is produced by: the iliopsoas (red), tensor fasciae latae (orange), pectineus (green), adductor longus (brown), adductor brevis (brown) and gracilis (brown).

The following thigh muscles are also flexors at the hip joint: rectus femoris (blue, see p. 236) and sartorius (yellow, see p. 236).

Abduction (**C**) at the hip is produced by: the gluteus medius (red), tensor fasciae latae (blue), gluteus maximus with its insertion into the fascia lata (yellow), gluteus minimus (orange), piriformis (green) and obturator internus (brown).

The **adductors** (**D**) of the thigh are: the adductor magnus with the adductor minimus (red), adductor longus (blue), adductor brevis (blue), the part of the gluteus maximus inserted into the gluteal tuberosity (yellow), gracilis (orange), pectineus (brown), quadratus femoris (violet) and the obturator externus (not shown).

The principal thigh muscle involved in addition is the semitendinosus (green).

The color of the arrows represents the order of importance of the muscles in each movement.

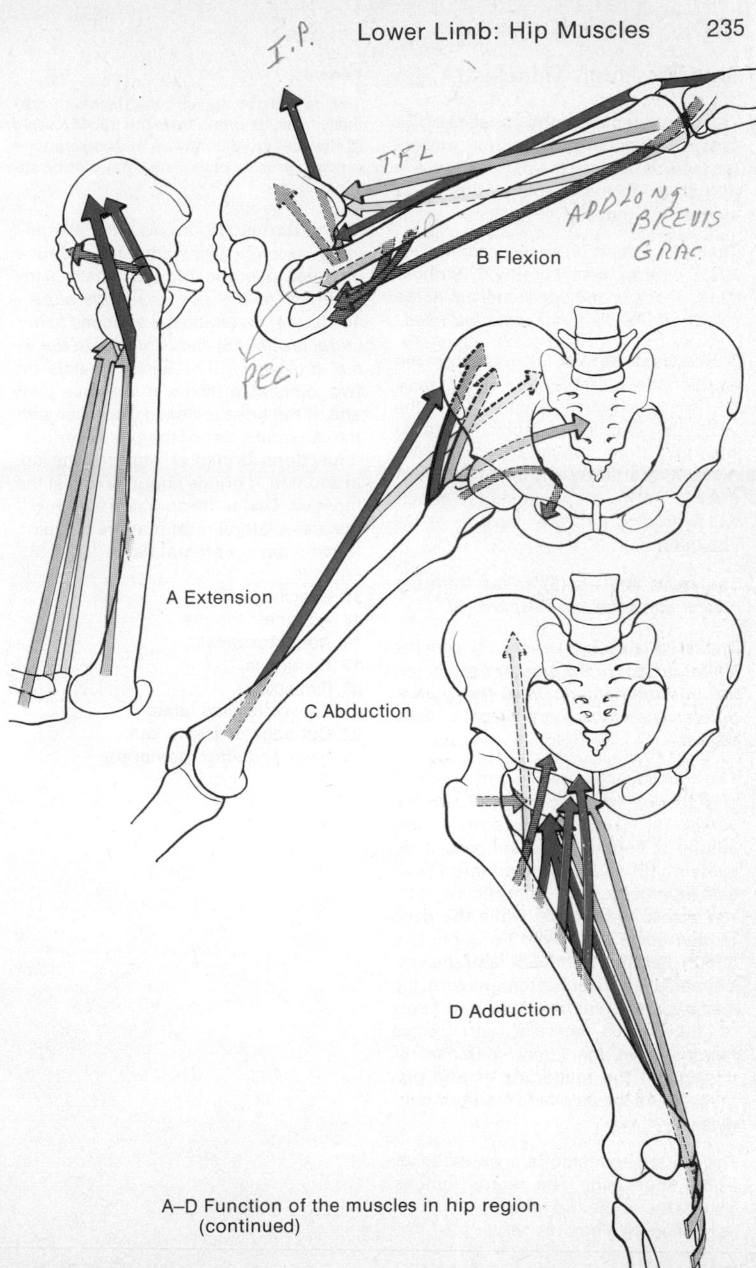

A–D Function of the muscles in hip region (continued)

Anterior Thigh Muscles (A–D)

The **quadriceps femoris** consists of **four parts**, of which the straight part, the rectus femoris, acting on two joints, runs in a channel formed by the other three single joint muscles.

The **rectus femoris** (**1**) *arises from the anterior inferior iliac spine* (**2**), *straight head, and from the upper margin of the socket of the hip joint, reflected head.*

The **vastus intermedius** (**3**) *arises from the anterior and lateral surface of the femur* (**4**). It is easily distinguished from the vastus lateralis but is more difficult to separate from the vastus medialis. Some of the fibers of the vastus intermedius form the articularis genus, which inserts into the capsule of the knee joint.

The **vastus medialis** (**5**) *arises from the medial lip of the linea aspera* (**6**).

The **vastus lateralis** (**7**) *arises* (**8**) *from the lateral surface of the greater trochanter, the intertrochanteric line, the gluteal tuberosity and the lateral lip of the linea aspera.*

The four muscles join to form a *common tendon which is inserted into the patella* (**9**). Distal to the patella, the tendon is continued as the *patellar ligament* (**10**) and is *inserted into the tibial tuberosity* (**11**). Superficial fibers run across the patella, while the deep tendon fibers insert into its upper and lateral margins. Some fibers of the vastus medialis and rectus femoris form the *medial patellar retinaculum*, and fibers of the vastus lateralis and rectus femoris form the *lateral patellar retinaculum*. The retinacula extend distally around the patella to the tibial condyles.

The quadriceps femoris is an extensor at the knee joint. The rectus femoris also flexes at the hip joint.
Nerve supply: Femoral nerve (L2–L4).

Variants

The part of the rectus femoris which normally takes its origin from the upper margin of the acetabulum may be missing, and the articular muscle of the knee may also be absent.

The **sartorius** (**12**) *arises from the anterior superior iliac spine* (**13**) and runs obliquely over the thigh in its fascial investment *to the pes anserinus superficialis* (**14**), by which it *is attached to the crural fascia* (**15**) *and is medial to the tibial tuberosity.* The sartorius acts on two joints as a flexor at the knee joint and, if the knee is flexed, together with the other muscles of the pes anserinus, it functions as medial rotator of the leg. In addition, it brings about flexion at the hip joint. Due to its course it also functions as a lateral rotator at the hip joint. Nerve supply: Femoral nerve (L1–L3).

16 Gracilis,
17 Adductor longus,
18 Adductor brevis,
19 Pectineus,
20 Iliopsoas,
21 Tensor fasciae latae,
22 Cut edge of fascia lata,
23 Vastoadductor membrane.

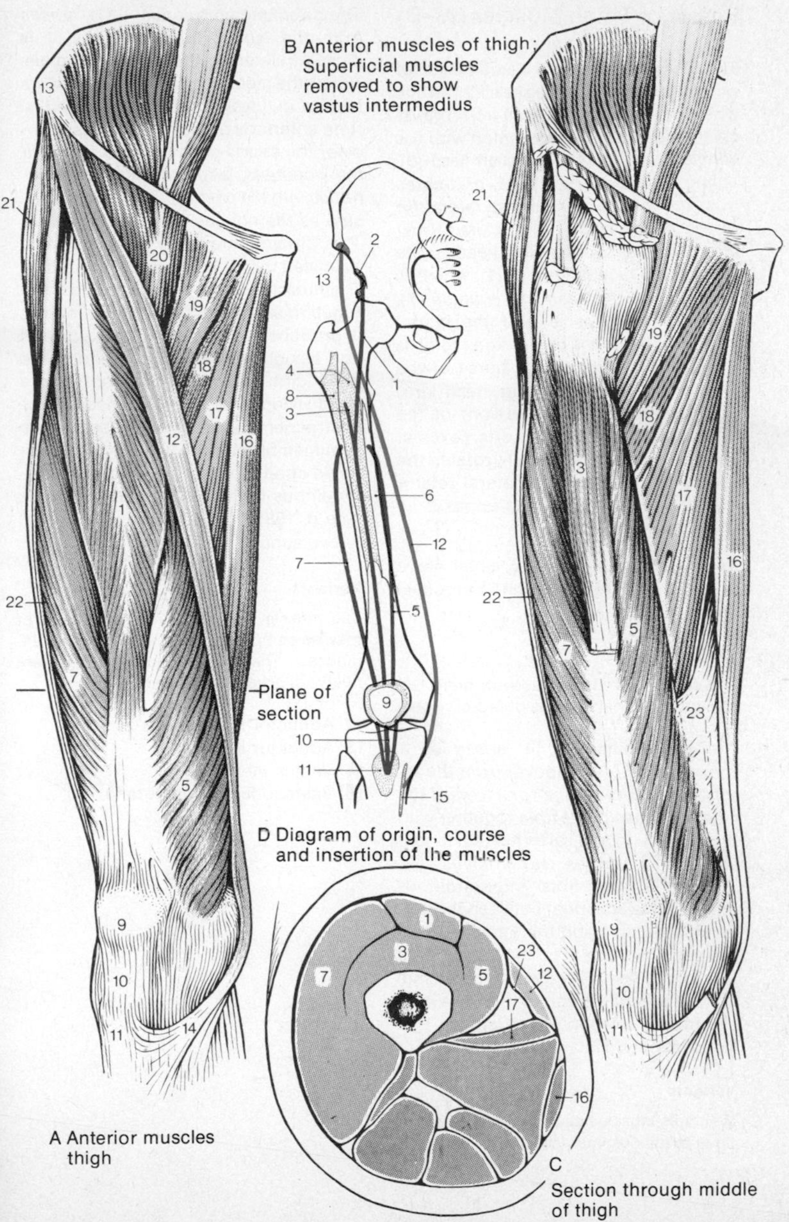

A Anterior muscles thigh

B Anterior muscles of thigh; Superficial muscles removed to show vastus intermedius

C Section through middle of thigh

D Diagram of origin, course and insertion of the muscles

Posterior Thigh Muscles (A–D)

The **biceps femoris** (**1**) has a **long head** and a **short head**. The **long head** (**2**), which acts over two joints, *arises from the ischial tuberosity* (**3**) in common with the semitendinosus (**4**). The **short head** (**5**), acting only over one joint, *originates from the middle third of the lateral lip of the linea aspera* (**6**) *and its lateral intermuscular septum.* The heads unite to form the biceps femors (**1**), which is *inserted into the head of the fibula* (**7**). Between the muscle and the lateral collateral ligament of the knee joint is the inferior subtendineal bursa of the biceps femoris. The long head produces extension (retroversion) of the hip joint. The biceps femoris flexes at the knee joint and laterally rotates the flexed leg. It is the only lateral rotator at the knee joint and thus opposes all the medial rotators.

Nerve supply: Long head, tibial nerve (L5–S2); short head, common peroneal nerve (S1–S2).

Variants

The short head may be absent; there may also be additional bundles of muscle fibers.

The **semitendinosus** (**4**) *arises by a common head* (see above) *from the ischial tuberosity (***3***) and runs toward the medial surface of the tibia* together with the gracilis (**9**) and sartorius (**10**) *to join the pes anserinus superficialis* (**8**). There is a large tibial intertendinous bursa (bursa anserina) between the surface of the tibia and the attachment to the pes anserinus. The muscle acts on two joints, being involved in extension at the hip joint, flexion at the knee joint and medial rotation of the leg.
Nerve supply: Tibial nerve (L5–S2).

Variants

Within its muscle belly there may be an oblique tendinous intersection.

The **semimembranosus** (**11**) *arises from the ischial tuberosity* (**3**). It is closely related to the semitendinosus. Below the medial collateral ligament, *its tendon divides into* **three parts**; the **first** *runs* anteriorly *to the medial tibial condyle,* the **second** *goes into the fascia of the popliteus,* and the **third** part *continues into the posterior wall of the capsule as the oblique popliteal ligament.* This division into three parts may also be called the *pres anserinus profundus.* The muscle acts on two joints and has a function similar to the semitendinosus. It produces extension at the hip joint and flexion with medial rotation at the knee joint. Between its tendon (before the division) and the medial head of the gastrocnemius lies the bursa of the semimembranosus, which is sometimes continuous with the medial subtendinous bursa of the gastrocnemius (see p. 198).
Nerve supply: Tibial nerve (L5–S2).

Variants

The muscle may sometimes be absent or may be completely fused with the semitendinosus. The oblique popliteal ligament need not always be present.

12 Adductor magnus,
13 Adductor longus,
14 Vastus medialis,
15 Vastoadductor membrane.

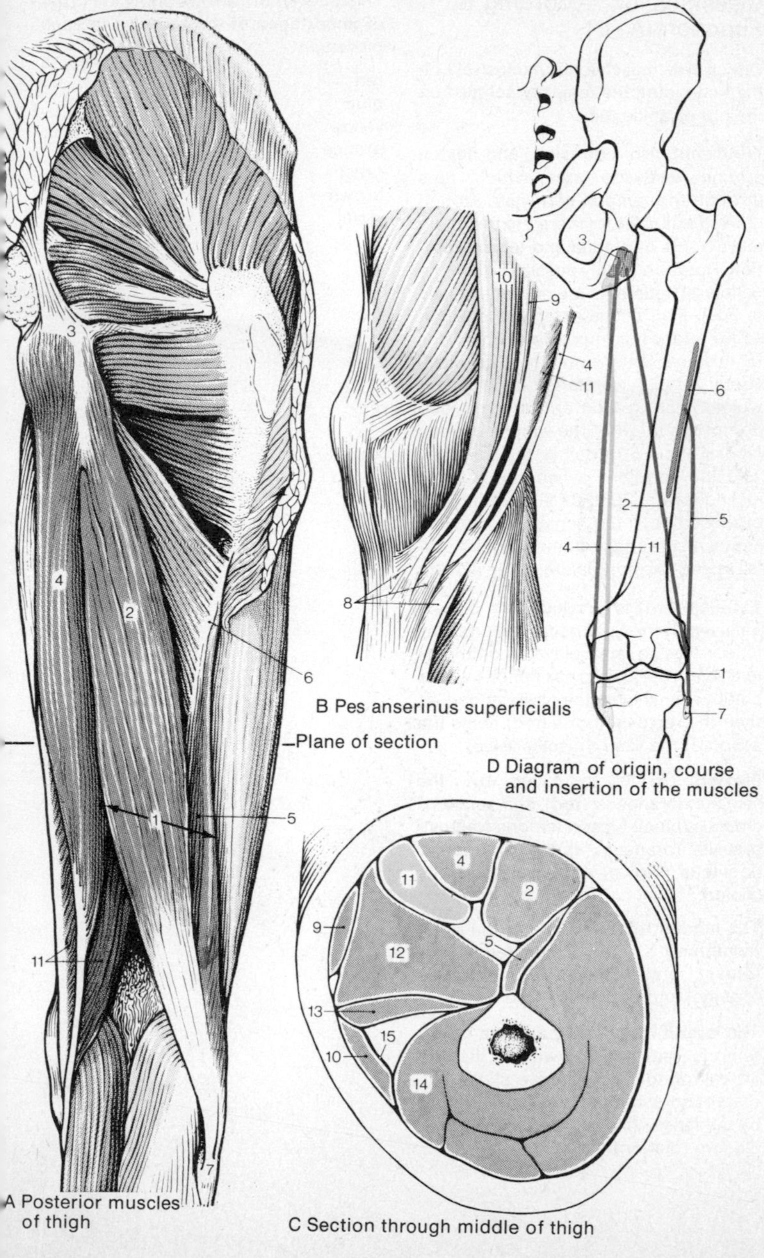

A Posterior muscles of thigh

B Pes anserinus superficialis

C Section through middle of thigh

D Diagram of origin, course and insertion of the muscles

Classification According to Function (A–D)

Only a few muscles act exclusively on the knee joint, the majority act also on the hip or ankle joint.

We distinguish **extension**, and **flexion** around **transverse axes** which runs through the femoral condyles. Around the **long axis of the leg** there are the rotary movements of **medial** and **lateral rotation**. Rotation is only possible when the collateral ligaments are not tensed (see p. 200), i. e., in the extended position active rotation is impossible. Passively, in maximal extension, there is some lateral rotation of the leg on the non-weight-bearing side and medial rotation of the thigh of the weight-bearing limb of about 5: possible, the so-called "closure rotation" when the joint is locked (see p. 200). Closure rotation is produced by the anterior cruciate ligament, the shape of the articular surfaces and the iliotibial tract (see p. 242).

Extension (**A**) is produced almost exclusively by the quadriceps femoris. The tensor fasciae latae plays an unimportant role. The quadriceps femoris works better when the hip joint is extended, as then the rectus femoris (red) helps the action of the vasti muscles (blue).

Flexion (**B**) is produced by: the semimembranosus (red), the semitendinosus (blue), biceps femoris (yellow), gracilis (orange), sartorius (green), popliteus (brown) and gastrocnemius (violet).

The **medial rotators (C)** are: the semimembranous (red), semitendinosus (blue), gracilis (yellow), sartorius (orange) and popliteus (green).

The **lateral rotators** (**D**) are: the biceps femoris (red), which is almost the only lateral rotator and opposes all the medial rotators. It may be assisted slightly by the tensor fasciae latae (not shown; closure rotation).

The color of the arrows show the order of importance of the muscles in each movement:

red
blue
yellow
orange
green
brown
violet

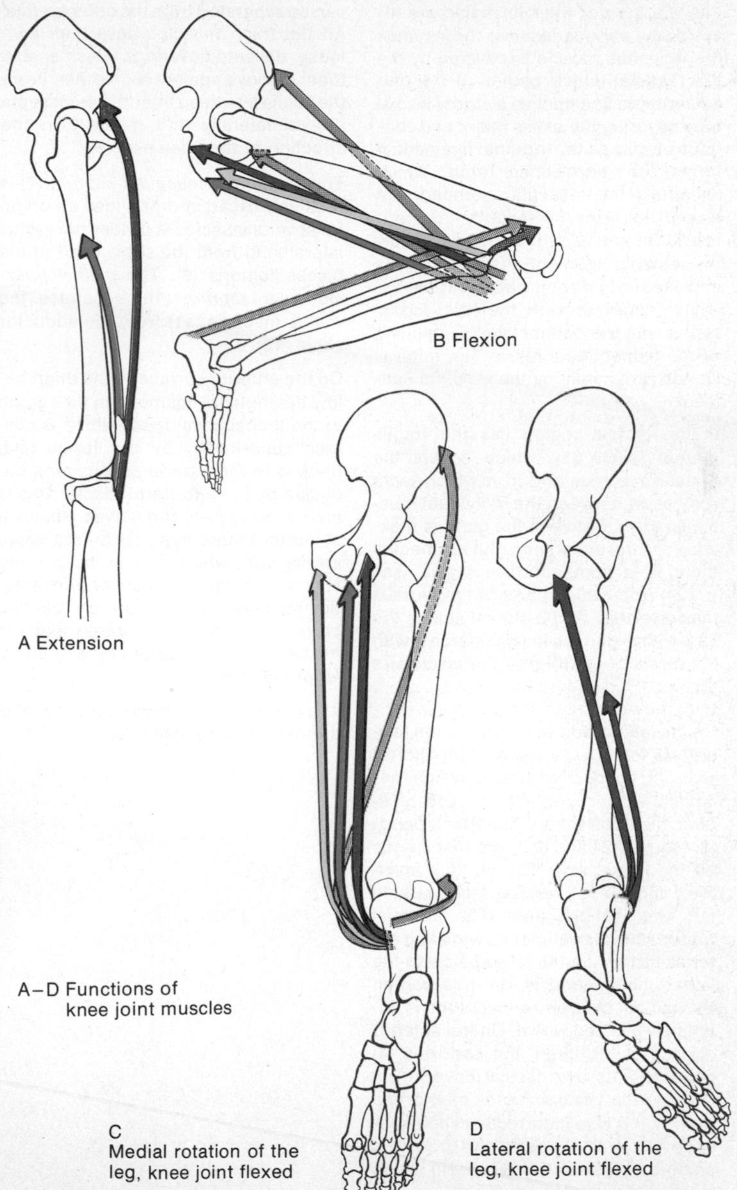

A–D Functions of knee joint muscles

The muscles of the hip region are invested by various fascias; for instance the iliopsoas muscle is covered by the **iliac fascia**, which begins at the medial arcuate ligament as a sturdy fascial tube covering the psoas major and continues as far as the inguinal ligament. It forms the iliopectineal arch, which separates the muscular compartment (see p. 98) from the vascular compartment. On the anterior surface, below the inguinal ligament, the pectineus is enclosed in a strong **pectineal fascia**, which, together with the iliac fascia, represents the connective tissue lining of the iliopectineal fossa. The latter is limited proximally by the inguinal ligament.

In the gluteal region lies the fragile **gluteal fascia** (**1**), which covers the gluteus maximus and from which septa run deeply between the individual muscle bundles. Between the gluteus maximus and the underlying gluteus medius there is a compact firm fascia (see p. 224) from which parts of the gluteus maximus arise. At the gluteal sulcus the superficial gluteal fascia merges with the fascia of the thigh – the fascia lata (**2**).

On the lateral side of the thigh, the **fascia lata** forms a dense, parallel fibered layer of connective tissue which becomes weaker medially. A band of fibers, the **iliotibial tract** (*Maissiat's band*) (**3**; see pp. 224 and 388) is conspicuous on the lateral side. The gluteus maximus and tensor fasciae latae radiate into this iliotibial tract. The iliotibial tract is several centimeters wide and extends distally on the lateral side to the lateral tibial condyle. In this region the lateral patellar retinaculum is intimately blended with it. On the anterior surface of the thigh, the sartorius (**4**) possesses its own fascial covering. It overlies the *vastoadductor membrane* (**5**) which is also incorrectly called subsartorial fascia. Similarly, the gracilis is enclosed in its own fascial sheath which can be separated from the other fascias. All the thigh muscles have their own loose, delicate coverings which enable them to move against each other. From the fascia lata deep intermuscular septa project laterally and medially in the direction of the linea aspera.

The *lateral intermuscular septum* (**7**) is relatively broad and provides an origin for several muscles. It divides the vastus lateralis (**8**) from the short head of the biceps femoris (**9**). The *medial intermuscular septum* (**10**) separates the vastus medialis (**11**) from the adductor canal (**12**).

On the anterior surface of the thigh below the inguinal ligament, in the region of the iliopectineal fossa which is covered superficially by the fascia lata, there is in the latter a porous area occupied by the **cribriform fascia**. This is pierced by vessels and nerves. Removal of this loose fascia reveals the **saphenous opening** (**13**), whose lateral margin, the *falciform margin,* or *Hey's* or *Burn's* ligament, (**14**) forms a sharply defined border. The falciform margin extends medially with a *superior* (**15**) and an *inferior* (**16**) *cornu*.

The femoral canal and femoral hernias are described on page 98.

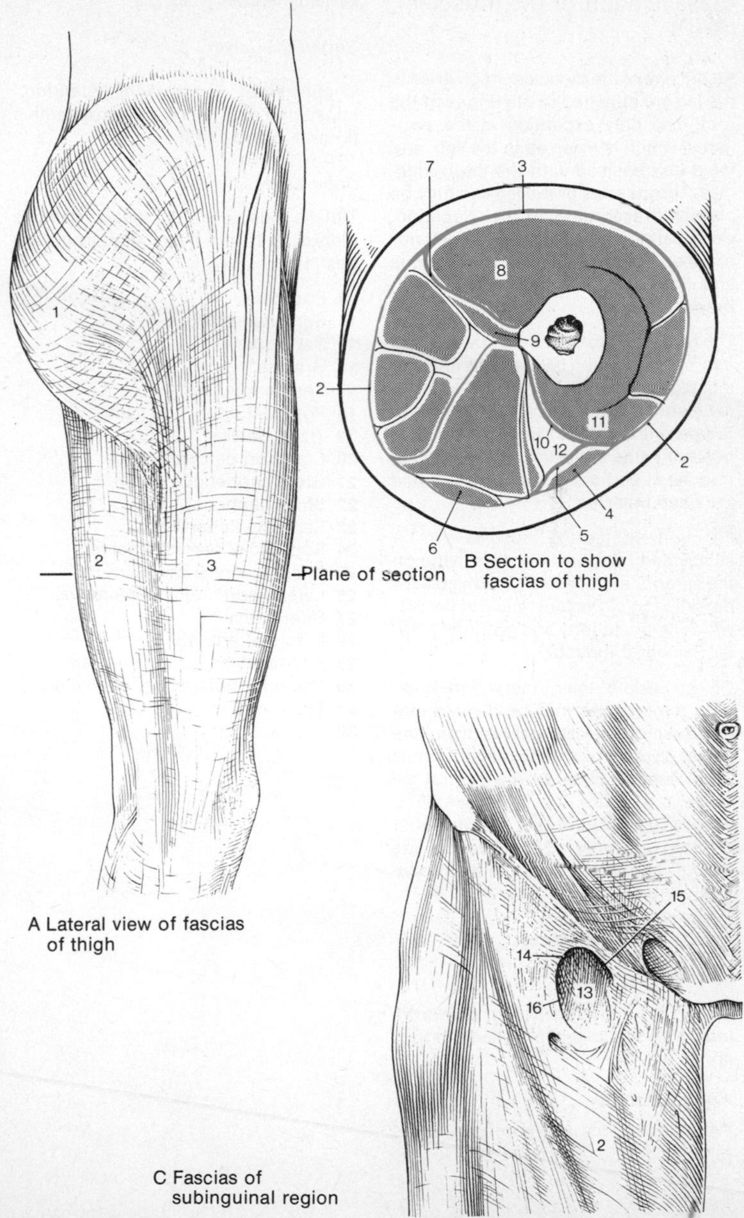

A Lateral view of fascias of thigh

B Section to show fascias of thigh

C Fascias of subinguinal region

Classification of the Muscles (A–D)

All but one of the muscles which arise in the leg are attached to the bones of the foot. The only exception is the popliteus, which is inserted in the leg and must be classified with the thigh muscles. The muscles of the leg can only be classified according to their location, principally into anterior and posterior groups. They are separated by the tibia and fibula and the interosseus membrane.

The two main groups are divided in turn into subgroups or layers. The anterior muscle group consists of the anterior extensors and the lateral subdivision of the peroneal group. The flexors on the posterior side of the leg are subdivided into the superficial or calf muscles and the deep muscles.

Functionally, the leg muscles can be subdivided into the extensors, lying on the anterior surface and responsible for dorsiflexion of the foot, and the flexors, which lie posteriorly and produce plantar flexion of the foot.

On the basis of their innervation, however, the muscles may be divided into those which receive nerves from the dorsal division of the plexus and those which are supplied by the ventral division.
For practical purposes the muscles of the leg, like those of the forearm, are best discussed according to their location.

Anterior Muscles of the Leg

Extensor Group

Tibialis anterior (**1**), extensor digitorum longus (**2**) and extensor hallucis longus (**3**).

Peroneal Group

Peroneus longus (**4**), peroneus brevis (**5**).

Posterior Muscles of the Leg

Superficial Layer

Triceps surae (**6**; with Achilles tendon), consisting of soleus (**7**), gastrocnemius (**8**) and plantaris (**9**).

Deep Layer

Tibialis posterior (**10**), flexor hallucis longus (**11**) and flexor digitorum longus (**12**).

13 Popliteus,
14 Semimembranosus,
15 Sartorius,
16 Gracilis,
17 Semitendinosus,
18 Popliteal artery and vein,
19 Tibial nerve,
20 Common peroneal nerve,
21 Great saphenous vein,
22 Small saphenous vein,
23 Saphenous nerve,
24 Superficial peroneal nerve,
25 Deep peroneal nerve,
26 Lateral sural cutaneous nerve,
27 Sural nerve,
28 Peroneal artery,
29 Anterior tibial artery and vein,
30 Posterior tibial artery and vein,
31 Tibia,
32 Fibula.

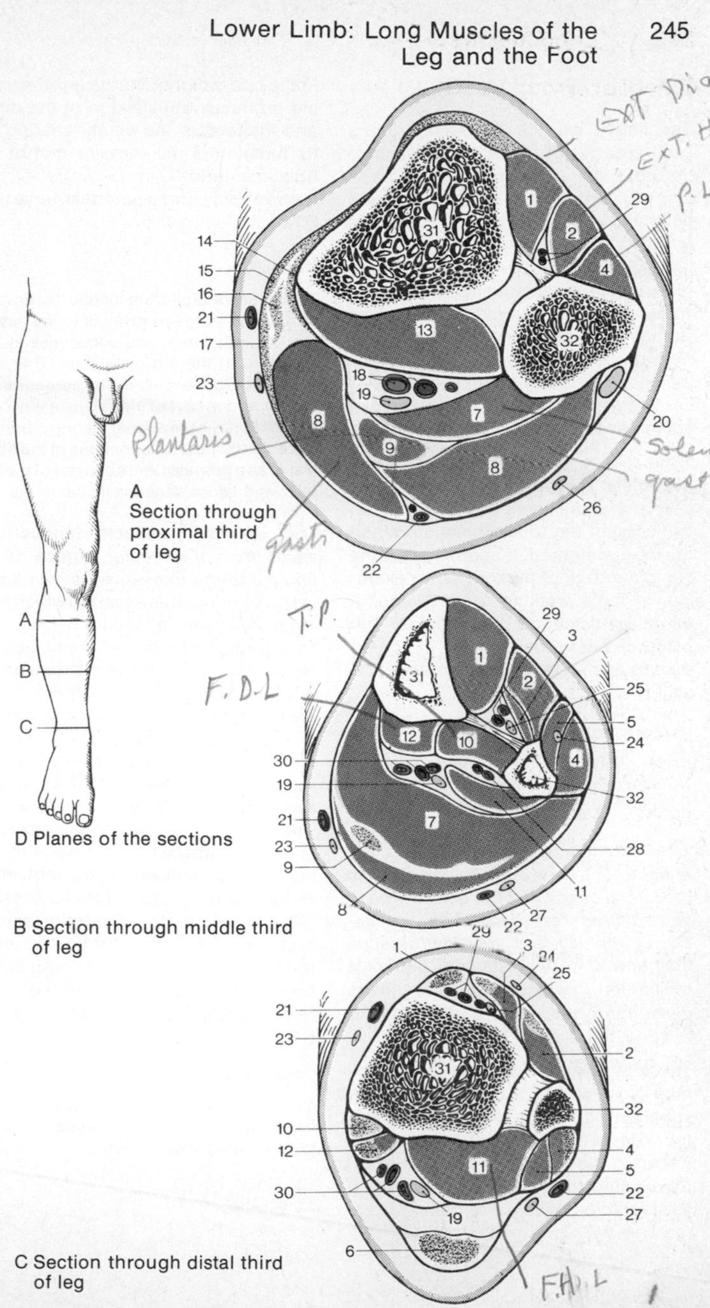

A
Section through proximal third of leg

D Planes of the sections

B Section through middle third of leg

C Section through distal third of leg

Extensor Group (A–C)

The **tibialis anterior** (**1**) *arises from* a wide area (**2**) of *the lateral surface of the tibia, the interosseous membrane and the crural fascia.* Its threesided belly ends in a tendon which extends beneath the superior extensor retinaculum (**3**) and the inferior extensor retinaculum (**4**) surrounded by a synovial sheath. *It is inserted in the plantar surface of the medial cuneiform bone* (**5**) *and the 1st metatarsal* (**6**). The subtendinous bursa of the tibialis anterior lies between its tendon and the medial cuneiform bone.

When the leg is not bearing any weight, the tibialis anterior flexes the foot dorsally and at the same time lifts the medial edge of the foot supination. When the leg is weighted, it approximates the leg to the back of the foot as, for example, in rapid walking, or in skiing. A slight participation in pronation has also been described.
Nerve supply: Deep peroneal nerve (L4–L5).

Practical Points

Under great stress the tibialis anterior may become fatigued resulting in pain along the muscle.

The **extensor digitorum longus** (**7**) *arises from* a large area (**8**), namely from *the lateral condyle of the tibia, the head and anterior crest of the fibula, the fascia of the leg and the interosseous membrane*. In the region of the ankle the tendon, in which the muscle ends, is divided into four parts and extends to the 2nd–5th digits.

These tendons are enclosed in a common synovial sheath and *run* under the superior extensor retinaculum (**3**) and the inferior extensor retinaculum (**4**), lateral to the tendon of the tibialis anterior; they extend over the dorsum of the foot *into the dorsal aponeuroses of the 2nd–5th digits.*

In the non-weight-bearing leg, the muscle produces dorsiflexion of the digits and the foot. In the weight-bearing leg its function is the same as that of the tibialis anterior.
Nerve supply: Deep peroneal nerve (L5–S1).

Variants

The extensor digitorum longus has an additional tendon which extends to the base of the 5th metatarsal and sometimes also to the base of the 4th metatarsal. This additional tendon is called the **peroneus tertius** (**9**), and as part of the extensor digitorum longus it may have a separate origin from the distal third of the anterior edge of the fibula. It acts as a pronator and abductor of the subtalar and talocalcaneonavicular joints.

The **extensor hallucis longus** (**10**) *arises from the medial surface of the fibula and the interosseous membrane* (**11**). It continues as a tendon which runs in its own synovial sheath between the sheath for the tendon of the tibialis anterior and that for the extensor digitorum longus beneath the superior extensor retinaculum (**3**) and inferior extensor retinaculum (**4**). It reaches across the 1st metatarsal to the dorsal aponeurosis of the great digit and is inserted into the *terminal phalanx* (**12**). The extensor hallucis longus flexes the great toe dorsally and in the unstressed leg it aids dorsiflexion of the foot. In the weight-bearing leg its function resembles that of the tibialis anterior, since it brings the leg nearer to the dorsum of the foot. To a small extent it also aids in pronation and supination of the foot.
Nerve supply: Deep peroneal nerve (L4–S1).

Variants

A separate muscle bundle may split off and be attached to the 1st metatarsal as the **extensor hallucis accessorius.**

13 Tibia,
14 Fibula.

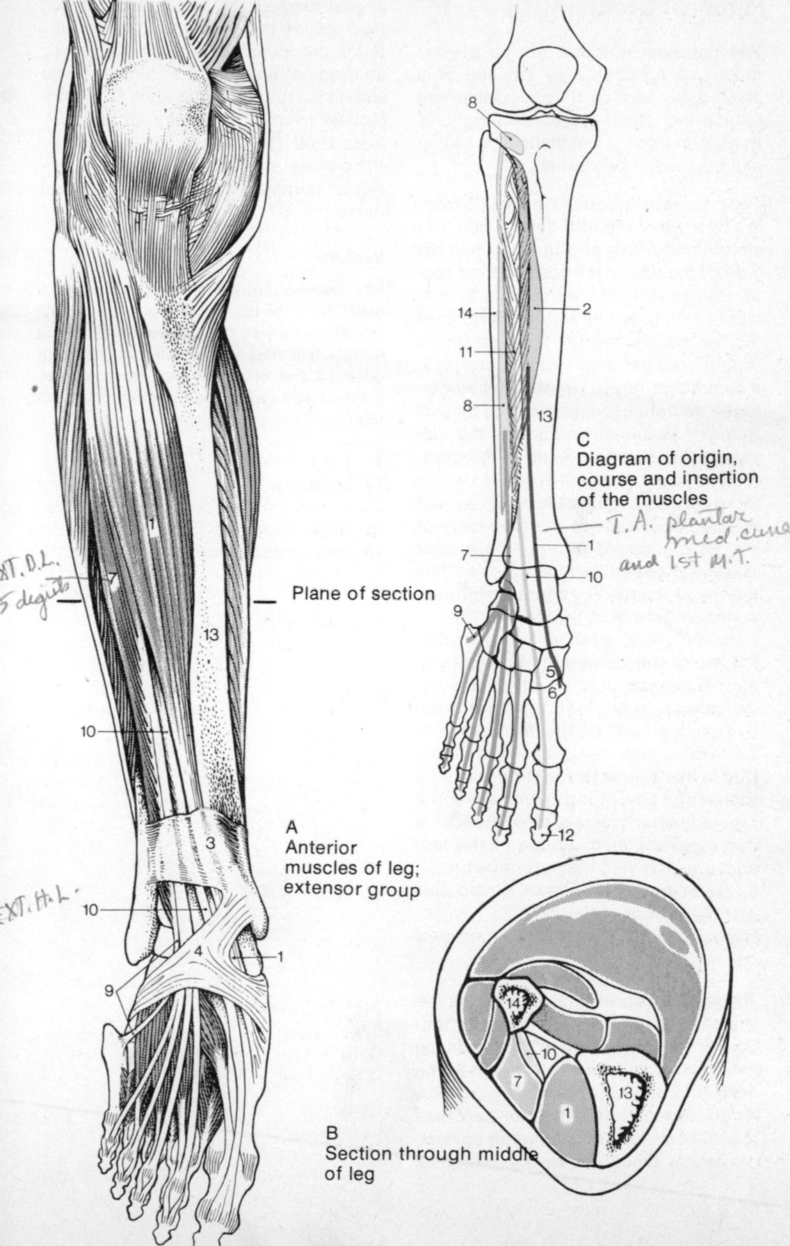

A
Anterior muscles of leg; extensor group

B
Section through middle of leg

C
Diagram of origin, course and insertion of the muscles

Peroneal Group (A–D)

The peroneal muscles act as plantar flexors, a function they attained only secondarily, due to their displacement behind the lateral malleolus. Originally they lay in front of the malleolus, as can still be seen in predators.

The **peroneus longus** (**1**) *arises* (**2**) *from the capsule of the tibiofibular joint, the head of the fibula and the proximal region of the fibula.* It ends in a long tendon which runs behind the lateral malleolus and, together with the tendon of the peroneus brevis (**3**), it passes under the superior peroneal retinaculum (**4**) in a common synovial sheath. The tendon of the peroneus longus *extends* distally from the peroneal trochlea of the calcaneus in an evagination of the common synovial sheath (fixed by the inferior peroneal retinaculum [**5**]), *across the plantar surface to the tuberosity of the 1st metatarsal* (**6**) *and the medial cuneiform bone* (**7**). Its tendon reaches the site of insertion by coursing through a tendon groove of the cuboid (**8**) in a special fibrous canal, which *runs* from the lateral side behind the tuberosity of the 5th metatarsal obliquely to the medial margin of the foot. Within this canal, on the sole of the foot, another synovial sheath encloses the tendon. Due to this course its function is similar to that of a bow string *(Kummer)* and it braces the transverse arch of the foot. It depresses the medial edge of the foot and, together with the peroneus brevis, it is the strongest pronator. It also aids plantar flexion.
Nerve supply: Superficial peroneal nerve (L5–S1).

The **peroneus brevis** (**3**) *arises from the lateral surface of the fibula* (**9**). Its tendon, together with that of the peroneus longus, runs in a synovial sheath in the groove for the tendon of the peroneus longus, beneath the superior peroneal retinaculum (**4**). On the lateral surface of the calcaneus, the tendon becomes fixed proximally, i.e., above the peroneal trochlea of the calcaneus, by the inferior peroneal retinaculum (**5**) where an evagination of the common synovial sheath surrounds the tendon. *This is attached to the tuberosity of the 5th metatarsal* (**10**). The muscle acts like the peroneus longus.
Nerve supply: Superficial peroneal nerve (L5–S1).

Variants

The **peroneus quartus** is seldom present. It arises from the fibula and is attached to the lateral surface of the calcaneus or to the cuboid. It is closely associated with the tendons of the extensor digitorum longus. It may also send a small tendon to the 5th digit.

11 Tibia,
12 Fibula,
13 Soleus,
14 Gastrocnemius,
15 Interosseus membrane.

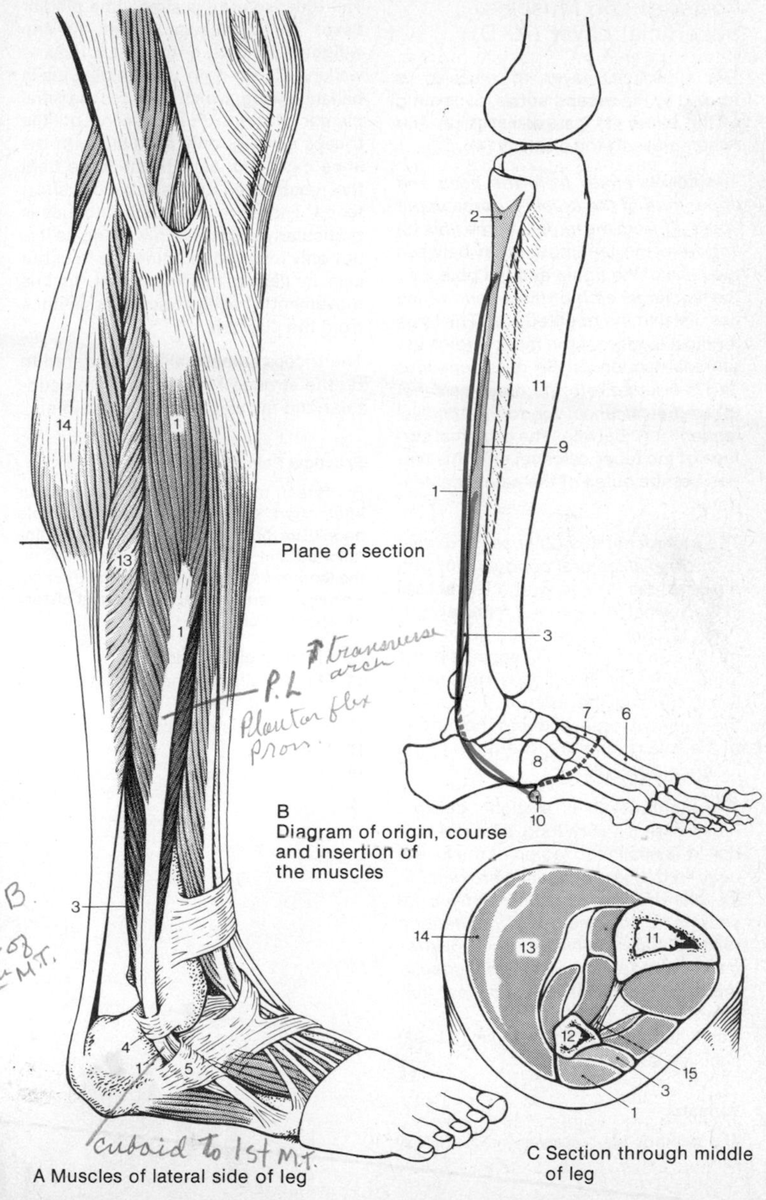

A Muscles of lateral side of leg

B
Diagram of origin, course and insertion of the muscles

C Section through middle of leg

Posterior Leg Muscles, Superficial Layer (A–D)

The superficial layer of muscles is formed by the **triceps surae**, consisting of the **soleus** (**1**), **gastrocnemius** (**2**) and (when present) the **plantaris** (**3**).

The **soleus** *arises from the head and upper third of the dorsal surface of the fibula* (**4**), *from the middle of the tibia* (**5**) *and from* the tendinous arch between the head of the fibula and the tibia, i. e., *the tendinous arch of the soleus* which lies distal to the popliteus (**6**). The large terminal tendon of the muscle joins the terminal tendon of the gastrocnemius and *is inserted into the tuber calcanei* (**8**) *as the calcaneal tendon ("Achilles' tendon"*; **7**). Between the proximal surface of the tuber calcanei and this tendon lies the bursa of the calcaneal tendon.

The **gastrocnemius** (**2**) *arises proximal to the medial femoral condyle* (**10**) with a **medial head** (**9**) and with a **lateral head** (**11**) *proximal to the lateral femoral condyle* (**12**). Some of the fibers from both heads also arise from the capsule of the knee joint. The two heads run distalward, forming the inferior borders of the popliteal fossa, and join the tendon of the soleus; they are *inserted into the tuber calcanei* (**8**).

The **plantaris** (**3**) is a slight, delicate muscle with a very long terminal tendon. *It arises* in the region of the lateral head of the gastrocnemius *proximal to the lateral femoral condyle and from the capsule of the knee joint. Its tendon* runs distally between the gastrocnemius and soleus and *is embedded in the medial edge of the calcaneal tendon*.
Nerve supply: The tibial nerve (S1–S2) supplies all the muscles.

Variants

The plantaris may be absent in 5–10% of cases.

The **triceps surae** is simply the plantar flexor par excellence. It can lift the weight of the body both in standing and walking. Its strength is most obvious in ballet dancing, which requires maximal plantar flexion. Full activity of the triceps surae is only possible with the knee extended, as with the knee bent the gastrocnemius is already shortened. Therefore, the gastrocnemius is particularly important in walking as it is not only involved in lifting the heel but also in flexing the knee joint. In this movement it receives some assistance from the plantaris.

The triceps surae is also considered to be the strongest supinator in the subtalar and talocalcaneonavicular joints.

Practical Points

Rupture of the Achilles' tendon may occur after short stress. The most vulnerable people are those who are athletically unconditioned and who suddenly put stress on the tendon without any preliminary training. However, there is usually also a past history of tendon injury.

13 Flexor digitorum longus,
14 Flexor hallucis longus,
15 Tibialis posterior,
16 Interosseous membrane,
17 Tibia,
18 Fibula.

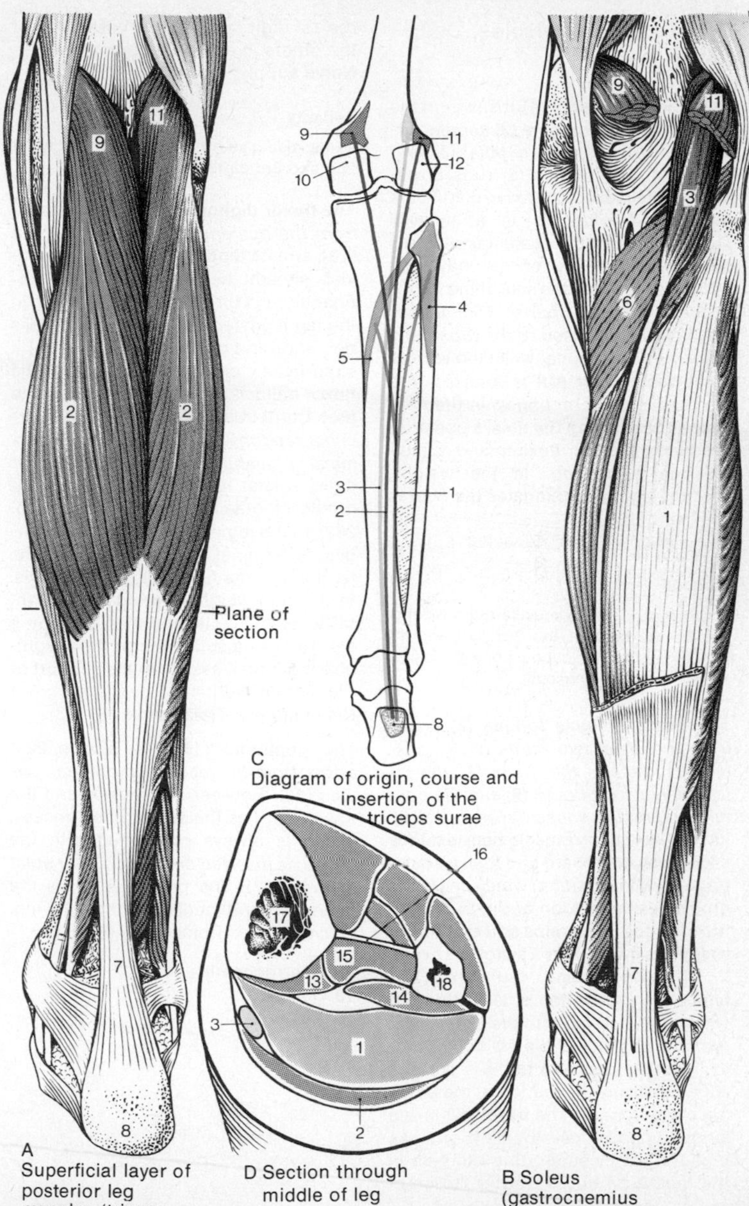

A
Superficial layer of posterior leg muscles (triceps surae)

B Soleus (gastrocnemius removed)

C
Diagram of origin, course and insertion of the triceps surae

D Section through middle of leg

Posterior Leg Muscles, Deep Layer (A–C)

The **tibialis posterior** (**1**) *arises from the interosseous membrane* (**2**) *and the adjoining surfaces of the tibia* (**3**) *and fibula* (**4**). The tendon (**5**) runs downward in the malleolar groove behind the medial malleolus (**6**) in a synovial sheath between the sustentaculum tali and the tuberosity of the navicular bone and reaches the sole of the foot. *It divides into two parts. The* **thicker, medial part** *is attached to the tuberosity of the navicular bone,* while the **lateral**, somewhat **weaker part** *is inserted into the three cuneiform bones.* In the non-weight-bearing leg the tibialis posterior produces plantar flexion and simultaneous supination. In the weight-bearing leg it approximates the heel to the calf of the leg.
Nerve supply: Tibial nerve (L4–L5).

Variants

The insertion of the muscle often extends also to the base of the 2nd, 3rd and 4th metatarsals and the cuboid bone. Occasionally the muscle is absent.

The **flexor hallucis longus** (**7**) *arises from the distal two-thirds of the posterior surface of the fibula* (**8**), *the interosseous membrane* (**9**) *and the posterior crural intermuscular septum* (**10**). Its relatively thick muscle belly extends a long way distalward and then is transformed into its tendon, which lies in the groove for the tendon of the flexor hallucis longus in the talus and calcaneus, where it is invested by a synovial sheath. It extends beneath the flexor retinaculum (**11**) to the sole of the foot where *it is inserted into the base of the terminal phalanx of the 1st digit.* Distal to the sustentaculum tali it is crossed superficially by the tendon of the flexor digitorum longus. The flexor digitorum longus opposes development of a pes planovalgus by supporting the arch of the foot. It produces plantar flexion of the 1st digit and in some cases also of the others. It assists in supination.
Nerve supply: Tibial nerve (S1–S3).

Variants

It may also give off terminal tendons to the 2nd and 3rd digits.

The **flexor digitorum longus** (**12**) *arises from the posterior surface of the tibia* (**13**), and its tendon (**14**) runs in a synovial sheath beneath the flexor retinaculum (**11**) to the sole of the foot. In the leg it posteriorly crosses the tibialis posterior and on the sole of the foot it superficially crosses the tendon of the flexor hallucis longus. In the sole of the foot the tendon divides into *four terminal tendons which extend to the terminal phalanges* of the lateral four digits. Distal to this division the quadratus plantae radiates into it (see p. 262). In the region of the middle phalanges its terminal tendons penetrate the tendons of the flexor digitorum brevis. In the non-weight-bearing leg it plantarflexes the digits and then the foot. It also acts as a supinator. In the weight-bearing limb it assists in the support of the plantar arch.
Nerve supply: Tibial nerve (S1–S3).

The **popliteus** (**15**; see also p. 220) *arises from the lateral femoral epicondyle* (**16**). Between the muscle and the knee joint lies the subpopliteal recess, which is always connected with the joint. *It is inserted on the posterior tibial surface* (**17**). The popliteus flexes the knee joint and medially rotates the leg.
Nerve supply: Tibial nerve (L4–S1).

18 Gastrocnemius,
19 Soleus,
20 Plantaris.

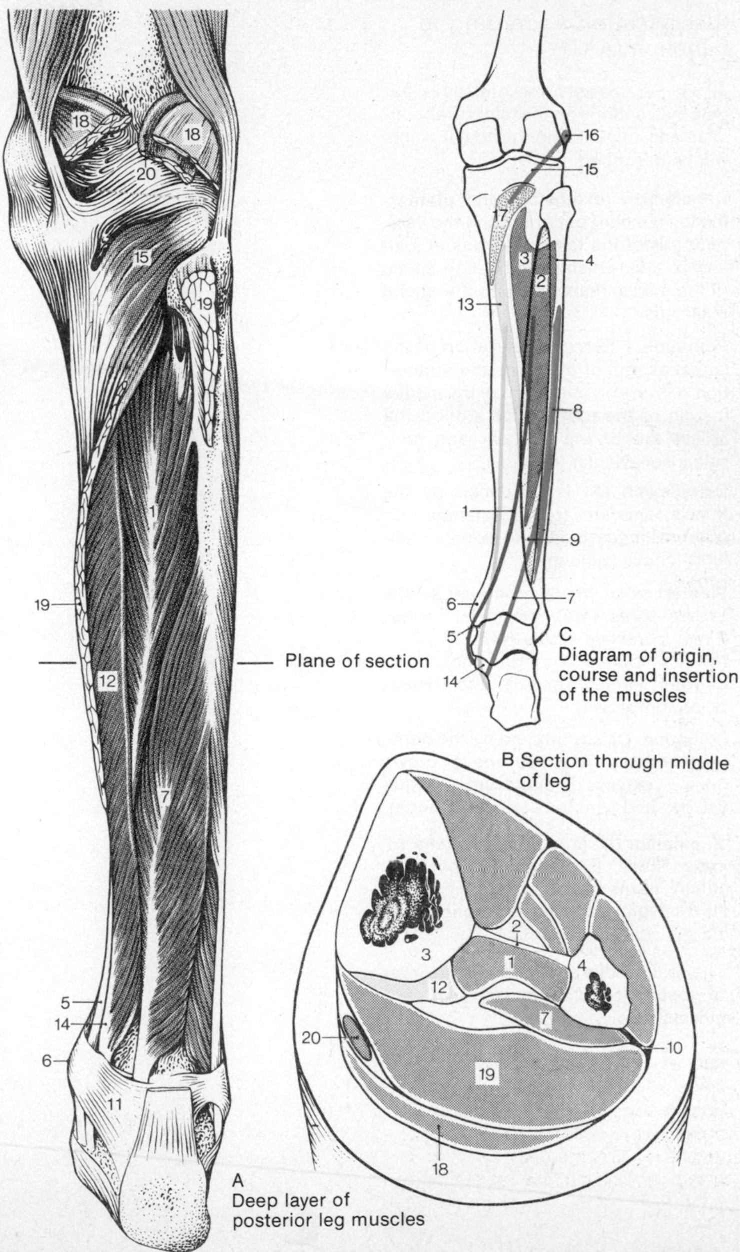

A
Deep layer of posterior leg muscles

B Section through middle of leg

C
Diagram of origin, course and insertion of the muscles

Classification According to Function (A–D)

All the muscles act on several joints, but only their actions on the talocrural, subtalar and talocalcaneonavicular joints will be described.

Dorsiflexion (extension) and **plantarflexion** (flexion) occur around the **transverse axis** of the talocrural (ankle) joint (see p. 210), which runs through the tip of the medial malleolus and the lateral malleolus.

Pronation = Eversion (elevation of the lateral margin of the foot) and **supination** = Inversion (elevation of the medial margin of the foot) occur around the **oblique axis** of the subtalar and talocalcaneonavicular joints.

Dorsiflexion (**A**) is produced by the tibialis anterior (red), extensor digitorum longus (blue) and extensor hallucis longus (yellow).

Plantarflexion (**B**) is produced by the triceps surae (red), peroneus longus (blue), peroneus brevis (yellow), flexor hallucis longus (orange), flexor digitorum longus (green) and tibialis posterior (brown).

Pronation (**C**) is produced by the peroneus longus (red), peroneus brevis (blue), extensor digitorum longus (yellow) and peroneus tertius (orange).

Supination (**D**) is produced by the triceps surae (red), tibialis posterior (blue), flexor hallucis longus (yellow), flexor digitorum longus (orange) and tibialis anterior (green).

The colors of the arrows show the order of importance of the muscles in each movement:

red
blue
yellow
orange
green
brown.

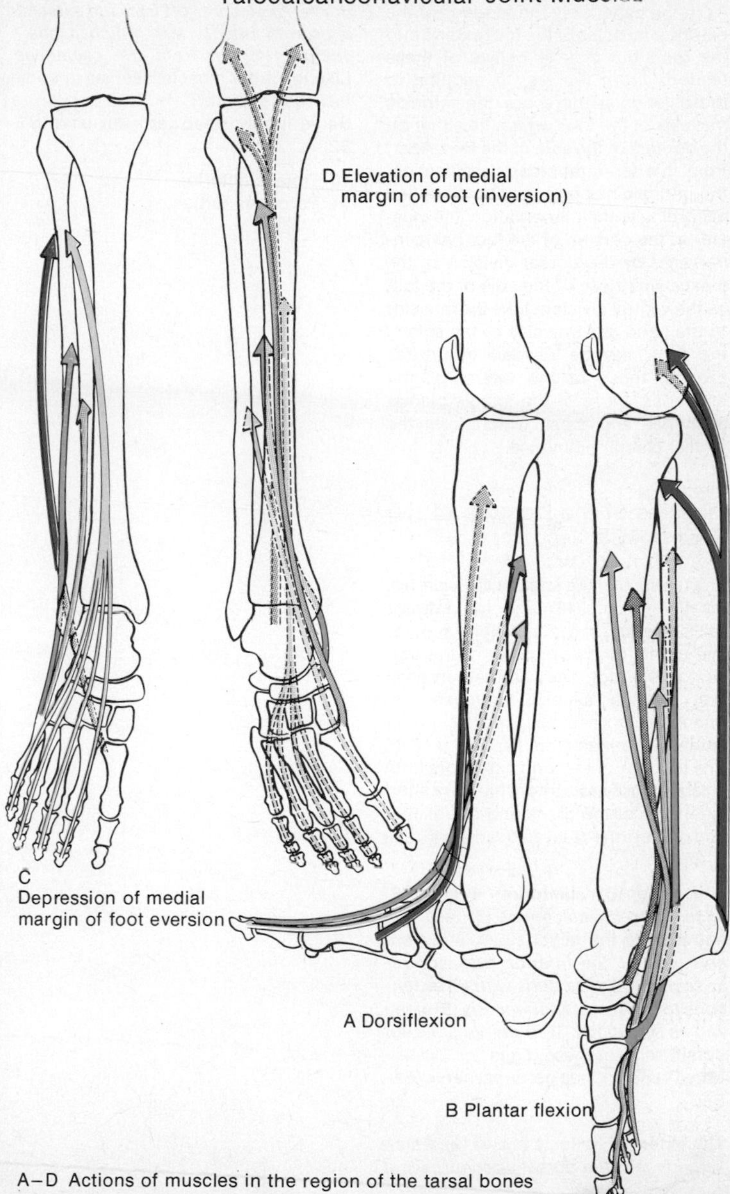

A–D Actions of muscles in the region of the tarsal bones

As in the hand, only the tendons of the extrinsic muscles of the foot extend into the foot; the muscle bellies of these tendons lie in the leg. In addition to these tendons there are the intrinsic muscles of the foot, which lie either on the dorsum or the sole of the foot. Apart from this topographical classification, the intrinsic muscles may be classified according to their innervation, the muscles of the dorsum of the foot being innervated by the dorsal division of the plexus and those of the sole of the foot by the ventral division. Like the muscles of the hand, the muscles of the sole of the foot may be divided into three groups; those of the lateral plantar eminence, those of the middle plantar eminence and those which form the medial plantar eminence.

Muscles of the Dorsum of the Foot (A–C)

The tendons of the **extensor digitorum longus** (**1**; see p. 246) and the **extensor hallucis longus** (**2**; see p. 246) lie superficial to the intrinsic muscles of the dorsum of the foot. They are held in position by the superior extensor retinaculum (**3**; see p. 264) and the inferior extensor retinaculum (**4**; see p. 264). The tendons of the long extensors form a **dorsal aponeurosis** into which the short extensors of the digits and the plantar and dorsal interossei also radiate (**5**; see p. 262).

The **extensor digitorum brevis** (**6**) *arises from the calcaneus* (**7**), near the entrance to the tarsal sinus, and *from one side of the inferior extensor retinaculum* (**4**). *It extends with three tendons to the dorsal aponeurosis* (**8**) *of the 2nd to 4th digits.* It is responsible for dorsiflexion of these digits.
Nerve supply: Deep peroneal nerve (S1–S2).

The **extensor hallucis brevis** (**9**), *which extends into the dorsal aponeurosis of the 1st digit, splits off from the extensor digitorum brevis, with which it has a common origin from the calcaneus.* Like the latter muscle it serves to dorsiflex the 1st digit.
Nerve supply: Deep peroneal nerve (S1–S2).

10 Tibialis anterior,
11 Peroneus tertius.

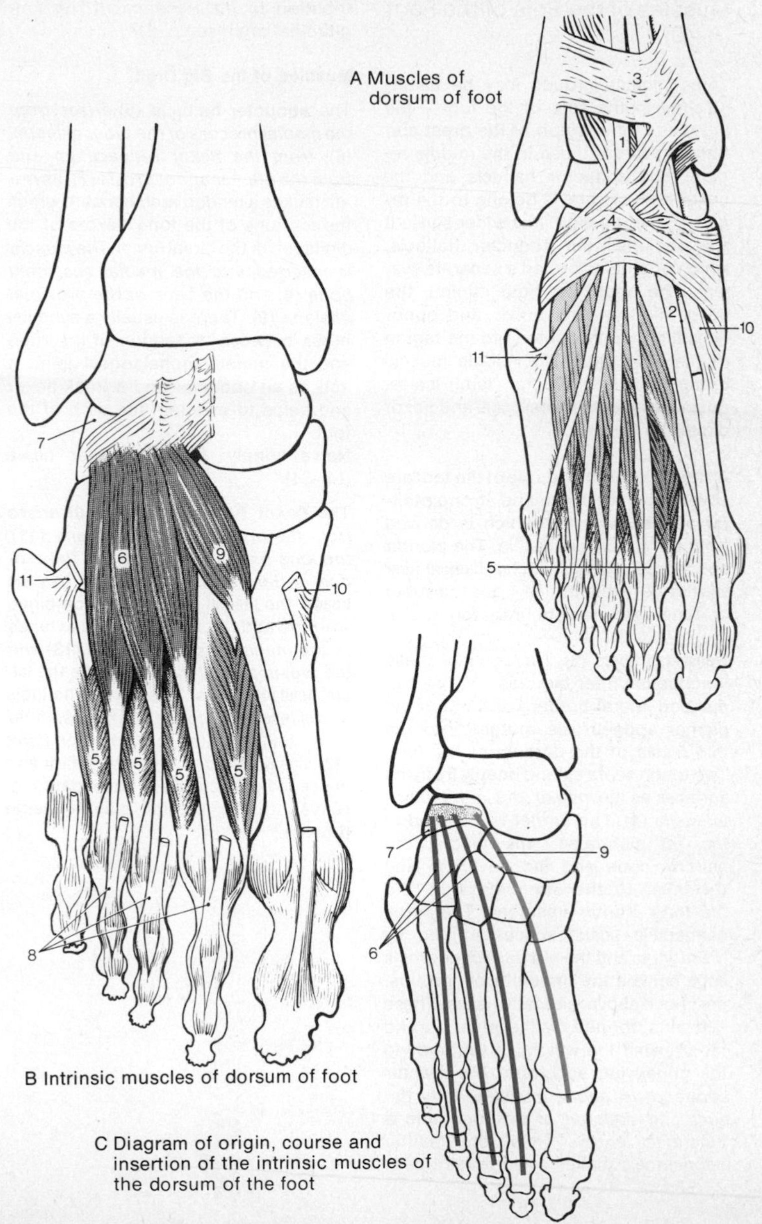

A Muscles of dorsum of foot

B Intrinsic muscles of dorsum of foot

C Diagram of origin, course and insertion of the intrinsic muscles of the dorsum of the foot

Muscles of the Sole of the Foot (A–C)

Three muscle groups may be distinguished in the sole of the foot – the muscles in the region of the great and little digits and those in the middle region. The abductor hallucis and the flexor hallucis brevis belong to the region of the big digit. In a wider sense it also includes the adductor hallucis, which originally formed a separate system. The abductor digiti minimi, the flexor digiti minimi brevis and opponens digiti minimi belong to the region of the little digit. The middle muscle group consists of the lumbricales, quadratus plantae, interossei and flexor digitorum brevis.

All the muscles of the sole of the foot are covered by the dense and strong **plantar aponeurosis** (**1**), which is derived from the superficial fascia. The plantar aponeurosis consists of **longitudinal fiber bundles** (**2**), which arise from the tuber calcanei and radiate into the digits.

Transverse fibers (**3**) interconnect these longitudinal fiber bundles. On the medial and lateral borders of the foot the plantar aponeurosis merges into the thin fascia of the dorsum of the foot. Two tough septa extend deeply from the surfaces as the *medial* and *lateral plantar septa* (**4**). The former is attached to the 1st metatarsal, the medial cuneiform bone and the navicular and the latter to the 5th metatarsal and the long plantar ligament. The three connective tissue spaces formed by these septa and the plantar aponeurosis each contain the three muscle groups, described above, and fatty tissue. These cushions, formed by the muscles and fat, transmit the weight of the body to the underlying substrate. *The plantar aponeurosis, septa, muscles, fatty tissues and skeleton of the foot form a functional entity*. Thus, the plantar aponeurosis makes an important contribution to maintenance of the longitudinal arch (see p. 214).

Muscles of the Big Digit

The **abductor hallucis** (**5**) *arises from the medial process of the tuber calcanei* (**6**), *from the flexor retinaculum and from the plantar aponeurosis* (**7**). Its origin makes a tendon arch beneath which the tendons of the long flexors of the digits run in the tarsal canal. *The muscle is inserted into the medial sesamoid bone* (**8**) *and the base of the proximal phalanx* (**9**). There is usually a synovial bursa between its tendon of insertion and the metatarsophalangeal joint. It acts as an abductor and a weak flexor and helps to maintain the arch of the foot.
Nerve supply: Medial plantar nerve (L5–S1).

The **flexor hallucis brevis** (**10**) *arises from the medial cuneiform bone* (**11**), *the long plantar ligament and the tendon of the tibialis posterior.* It has **two heads**; the **medial head** (**12**) is combined with the abductor hallucis and *extends to the medial sesamoid bone* (**13**) *and the proximal phalanx* (**14**), while the **lateral head** (**15**) joins the adductor hallucis and *is inserted into the lateral sesamoid bone* (**16**) *and the proximal phalanx* (**17**). It is an important plantar flexor and is needed particularly in ballet dancing.
Nerve supply: Medial plantar nerve (L5–S1).

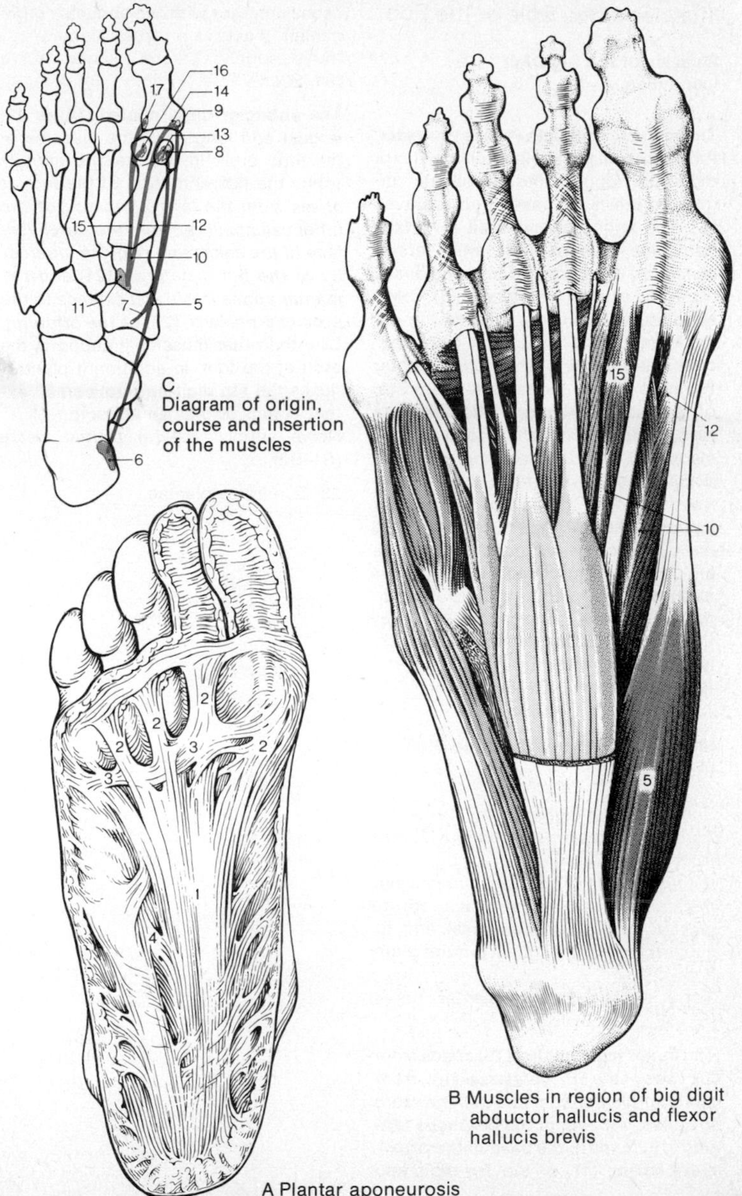

C
Diagram of origin, course and insertion of the muscles

B Muscles in region of big digit abductor hallucis and flexor hallucis brevis

A Plantar aponeurosis

Muscles of the Sole of the Foot

Muscles of the Big Digit (continued, A–C)

The **adductor hallucis** (**1**) has **two heads**. It only becomes visible after the flexor digitorum longus and the flexor digitorum brevis (**2**) have been removed (**A**). The strong **oblique head** (**3**) *arises from the cuboid* (**4**) and *lateral cuneiform* (**5**) *bones and from the bases of the 2nd and 3rd metatarsals* (**6**). Other surfaces of origin may include the 4th metatarsal, the plantar calcaneocuboidal ligament, the long plantar ligament (**7**) and the tendon sheath (**8**) of the peroneus longus. The **transverse head** (**9**) *arises from the capsular ligaments of the metatarsophalangeal joints of the 3rd–5th digits* (**10**) *and also from the deep transverse metatarsal ligament.* **Both heads** *are inserted into the lateral sesamoid bone* (**11**) *of the big digit.* The muscle acts especially as a tensor of the plantar arches. In addition it adducts the big digit and may then plantarflex the proximal phalanx.
Nerve supply: Deep branch of the medial plantar nerve (S1–S2).

Intrinsic Muscles of the Little Digit (A–C)

The **opponens digiti minimi** (**12**) *arises from the long plantar ligament* (**7**) *and from the tendon sheath of the peroneus longus* (**13**). *It is inserted into the 5th metatarsal* (**14**). Its functions are to plantarflex the 5th metatarsal and to support the plantar arch. It is quite often absent.
Nerve supply: Lateral plantar nerve (S1–S2).

The **flexor digiti minimi** (**15**) *arises from the base of the 5th metatarsal* (**16**), *from the long plantar ligament* (**7**) *and from the tendon sheath of the peroneus longus. It extends to the base of the proximal phalanx* (**17**) *of the 5th digit* and usually merges with the abductor digiti minimi. It acts as a plantar flexor.
Nerve supply: Lateral plantar nerve (S1–S2).

The **abductor digiti minimi** (**18**) is the largest and longest of the muscles of the little digit. In the main it actually forms the lateral margin of the foot. *It arises from the lateral process of the tuber calcanei* (**19**), *from the lower surface of the calcaneus* (**20**), *the tuberosity of the 5th metatarsal* (**21**) *and the plantar aponeurosis and extends to the proximal phalanx* (**22**) *of the 5th digit.* Like the other muscles it supports the arch of the foot. In addition it plantarflexes the 5th digit and, to a small extent, it acts also as an abductor.
Nerve supply: Lateral plantar nerve (S1–S2).

23 Quadratus plantae.

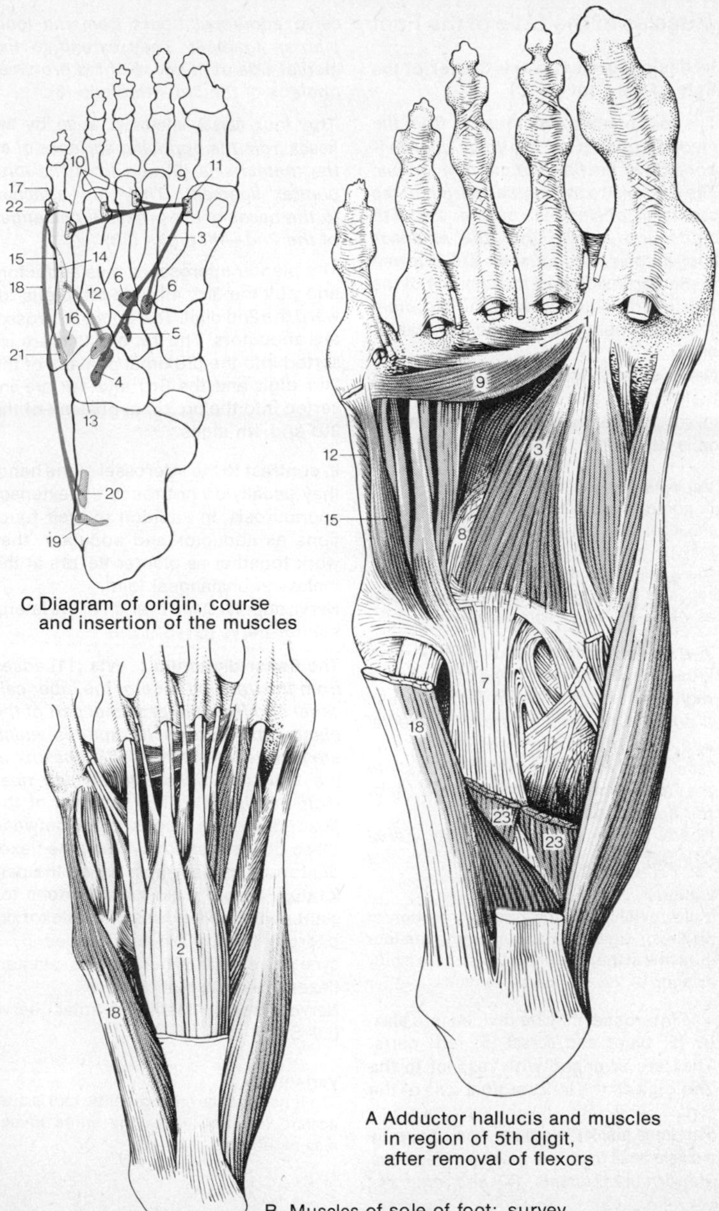

C Diagram of origin, course and insertion of the muscles

A Adductor hallucis and muscles in region of 5th digit, after removal of flexors

B Muscles of sole of foot; survey

Muscles of the Sole of the Foot

Intrinsic Muscles in the Center of the Sole of the Foot (A–C)

The **four lumbricales** (**1**) *arise from the medial surfaces of the individual tendons* (**2**) *of the flexor digitorum longus. They extend to the medial margin of the proximal phalanges of the 2nd–5th digits and radiate into the extensor aponeurosis.* The muscles are involved in plantarflexion and movements of the four lateral digits toward the big digit. They also help to reinforce the plantar arch.
Nerve supply: Medial plantar nerve to the 1st, 2nd and 3rd lumbricales, and lateral plantar nerve to the 4th lumbricalis (L5–S2).

Variants
In contrast to the lumbricales of the hand, those of the foot are quite variable. They may be absent or there may be more than four. They are inserted on the articular capsules of the metatarsophalangeal joints as well as to the proximal phalanges.

The **quadratus plantae** (**3**) is also known as the plantar head of the flexor digitorum longus (flexor accessorius). *It arises with two slips from the medial and lateral margins of the plantar surface of the calcaneus and projects into the lateral margin of the tendon* (**4**) *of the flexor digitorum longus.*
Nerve supply: Lateral plantar nerve (S1–S2).

Variants
It may extend into the common tendon of the flexor digitorum longus or into the four divisions of this tendon, in which case it only extends to the two lateral tendons.

The **interossei** may be divided into **plantar** (**5**; blue) and **dorsal** (**6**; red) parts. They are arranged with respect to the 2nd digit as the longitudinal axis of the foot.
The **three plantar interossei** each arise by a **single head** *from the medial side of the 3rd–5th metatarsals* (**7**) *and may receive additional fibers from the long plantar ligament. They extend to the medial side of the base of the proximal phalanx of the 3rd–5th digits* (**8**).

The four **dorsal interossei** arise by **two heads** *from the opposing surfaces of all the metatarsals* (**9**) *and from the long plantar ligament. They are attached to the bases of the proximal phalanges of the 2nd–4th digits* (**10**).

The plantar interossei act as adductors and pull the 3rd, 4th and 5th digits toward the 2nd digit. The dorsal interossei are abductors. The 1st and 2nd are inserted into the proximal phalanx of the 2nd digit and the 3rd and 4th are inserted into the proximal phalanx of the 3rd and 4th digits.

In contrast to the interossei of the hand, they usually do not reach the extensor aponeurosis. In addition to their functions as abductor and adductor, they work together as plantar flexors at the metatarsophalangeal joint.
Nerve supply: Deep branch of the lateral plantar nerve (S1–S2).

The **flexor digitorum brevis** (**11**) *arises from the undersurface of the tuber calcanei and from the proximal part of the plantar aponeurosis. Its tendons, which are inserted into the middle phalanx of the 2nd–4th digits, are divided near their termini* (**12**). The tendons of the flexor digitorum longus (**2**) run between these divided tendons. Thus, the flexor digitorum brevis is also called the perforatus. In this region the tendons together with the tendons of the flexor digitorum longus are surrounded by a synovial sheath. This muscle plantarflexes the middle phalanges.
Nerve supply: Medial plantar nerve (L5–S1).

Variants
The tendon to the 5th digit (little toe) is often absent. In some cases the entire muscle may be absent.

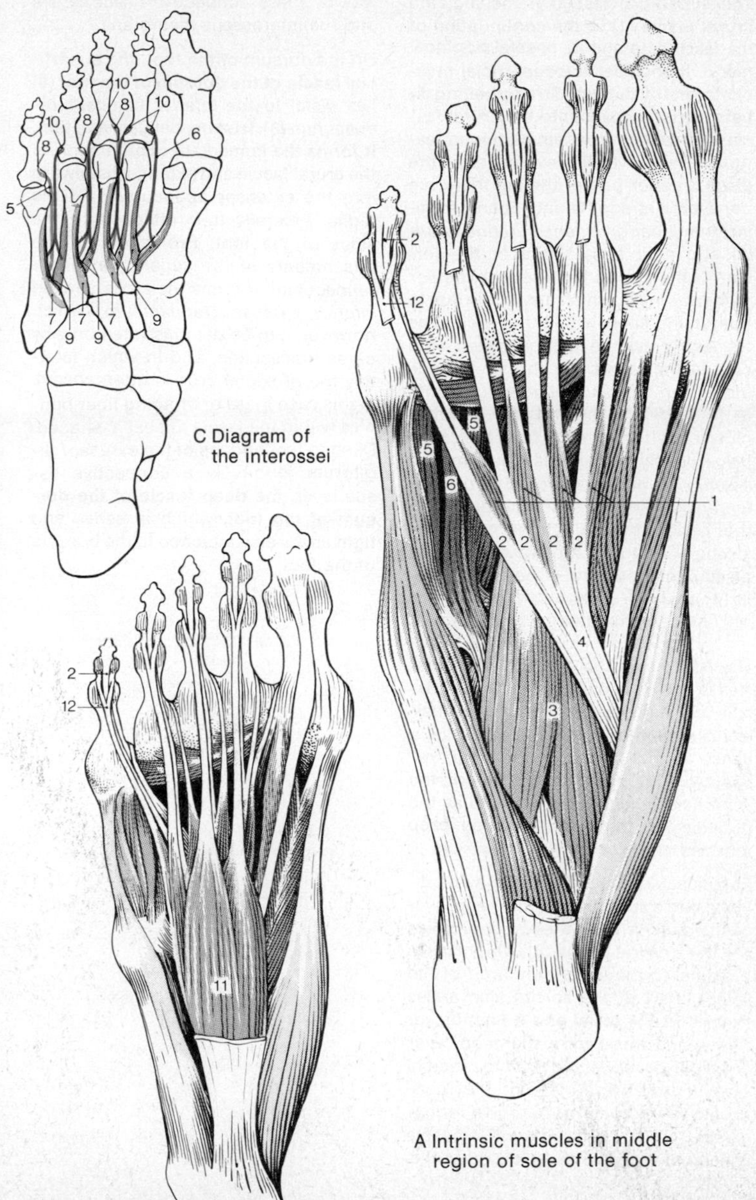

C Diagram of the interossei

A Intrinsic muscles in middle region of sole of the foot

B Flexor digitorum brevis

Fascias of the Leg (A–D)

The superficial fascia of the leg, the **crural fascia** (**1**), is the continuation of the fascia lata and its special popliteal fascia. It encloses the superficial muscle layers of the leg. Strengthening fibers are interwoven into the crural fascia and delineate certain particular features. Thus, over the extensors in the distal anterior part of the leg there are transverse strengthening fibers, forming the *superior extensor retinaculum* (**2**), and in the tarsal region on the dorsum of the foot as the *inferior extensor retinaculum* (**3**), which are visible due to reinforcing fibers within the fascia. The retinacula can be demonstrated with care in the fascia. On the lateral side there is an intermuscular septum, both in front of and behind the peroneal muscles, which extends from the crural fascia deeply to the fibula. These are the *anterior* (**4**) and *posterior* (**5**) *crural intermuscular septa*. At the distal end, in the region of the lateral malleolus, strong fiber tracts are woven into the fascia, and form the *superior* and *inferior peroneal retinacula* (**6**). Both can only be demonstrated by dissection.

The fascia over the dorsal crural muscles is thin. It is only strengthened distally, so that between the medial malleolus and the calcaneus there is a dense fibrous structure, the *flexor retinaculum* (**7**), or laciniate ligament, the superficial layer of which serves as the boundary of the tendons of the deep muscles of the tibia.

The musculature of the calf may be divided into a superficial and a deep layer of muscles. Between the two groups lies the **deep crural fascia** (**8**), which arises proximal to the *tendinours arch* of the *soleus*. Part of the soleus also arises from it. At the distal end it has thicker fibers, and these form the *deep layer of the flexor retinaculum* on the medial side, and on the lateral side they contribute to the *superior peroneal retinaculum*. The four different muscle groups in the leg are separated in this way by these connective tissue layers and the interosseus membrane.

On the dorsum of the foot, the superficial **fascia of the dorsum of the foot** (**9**) lies distal to the *inferior extensor retinaculum* (**3**). It is very delicate and thin. It forms the immediate continuation of the crural fascia and extends distalward into the extensor aponeurosis of the digits. Laterally it is attached to the sides of the foot. Proximally, at the attachments of the superior extensor retinaculum, it forms the cross-shaped *inferior extensor retinaculum,* which however, can be demonstrated only by careful dissection, and in which laterally the proximal crus is often absent. In this case these reinforcing fiber bundles within the fascia appear Y-shaped. Deep to the tendons of the extensor digitorum longus is a connective tissue layer, the **deep fascia of the dorsum of the foot,** which is dense and tight and is also attached to the borders of the foot.

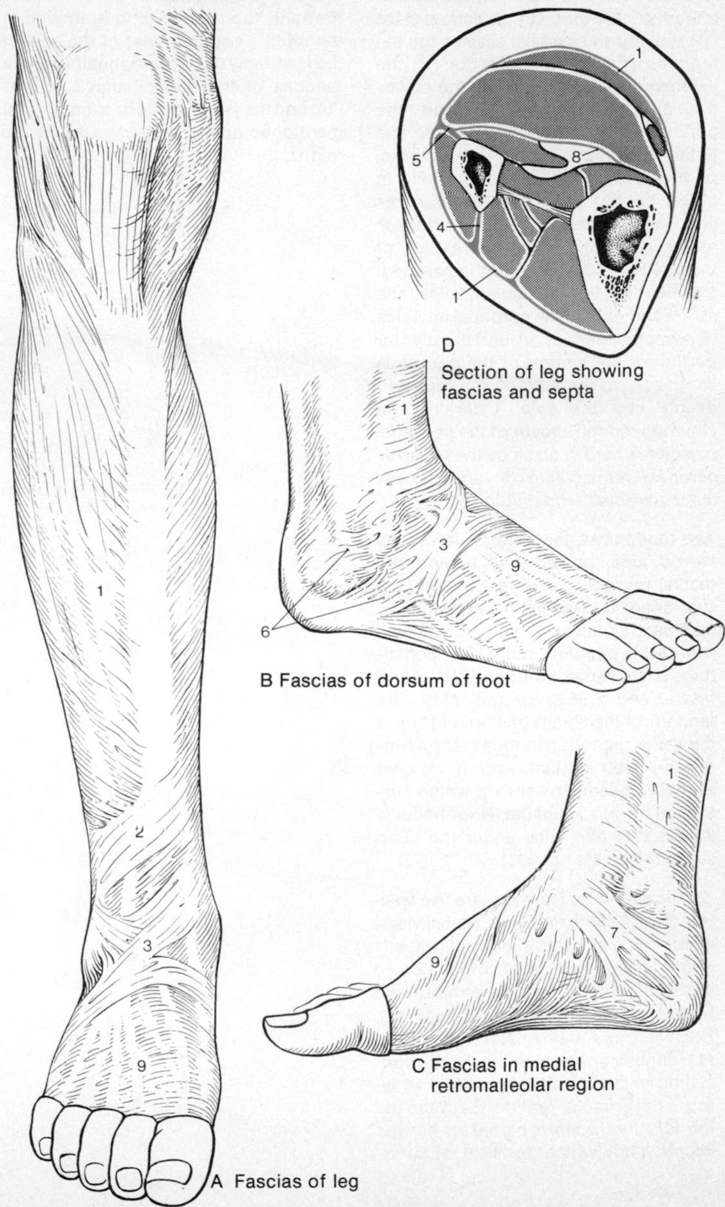

D
Section of leg showing fascias and septa

B Fascias of dorsum of foot

C Fascias in medial retromalleolar region

A Fascias of leg

As in the hand, there are various **tendon sheaths** in the foot. On the **dorsum of the foot** we find the **synovial sheaths** for the tendons of the tibialis anterior (**1**), the extensor hallucis longus (**2**), the extensor digitorum longus (**3**) and the peroneus tertius (when present). The tendons, or rather the tendon sheaths, on the dorsum of the foot, are held in place by the *superior extensor retinaculum* (**4**) and the *inferior extensor retinaculum* (**5**). On the lateral side of the tarsus, in the region of the peroneal trochlea of the calcaneus, lies the synovial sheath of the peroneal muscles (**6**), which continues around the plantar portion of the tendon of the peroneus longus (**7**) to the side of the foot and deeply into the sole. Laterally, the common tendon sheath of the peroneal muscles is held in place by the *superior peroneal retinaculum* (**8**) and the *inferior peroneal retinaculum* (**9**).

The tendons of the flexors lie on the medial side, immediately behind the medial malleolus. The tendon sheaths run deep to the *flexor retinaculum* (laciniate ligament). This consists of a *superficial stratum* (**10**), which constitutes a thickened portion of the crural fascia, and a *deep stratum* (**11**). The tendons of the tibialis posterior (**12**) and the flexor digitorum longus (**13**) run under the deep stratum, each in its own synovial sheath. The sheath which surrounds the tendon of the flexor hallucis longus (**14**) also runs under the deep stratum (see also p. 402).

On the **sole of the foot** there are **five synovial sheaths corresponding to the individual digits** (**15**), and these do not usually communicate with each other. These synovial tendon sheaths are reinforced by strong **fibrous sheaths of the digits** (**16**). Each fibrous sheath has an *annular part* (**17**, annular ligament of the digits), consisting of circular fiber bundles and lying in the articular regions. Between the joints is the *cruciform part of the fibrous sheath* (**18**), which consists of crisscross connective tissue fibers. Unlike in the hand, there are no tendon sheaths in the middle compartment of the sole of the foot. Only the tendon sheaths for the tendons of the flexor hallucis longus (**14**) and the flexor digitorum longus (**13**) mentioned above, extend as far as the midfoot.

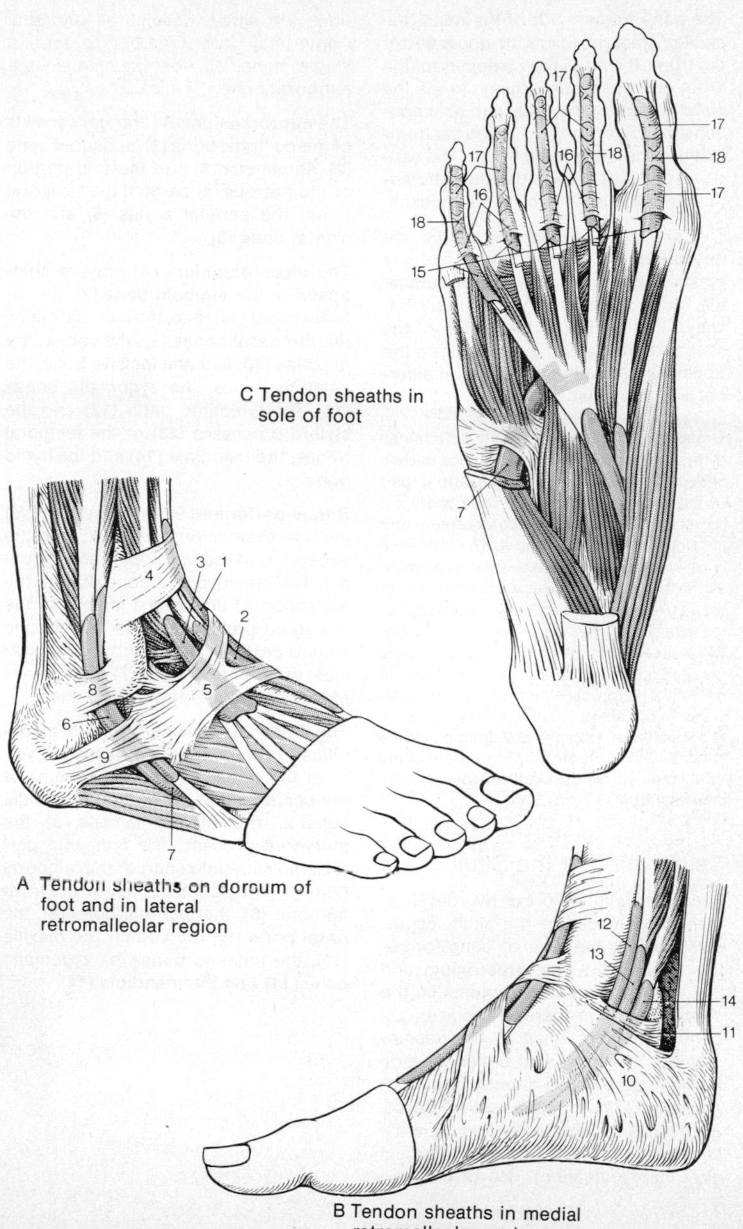

C Tendon sheaths in sole of foot

A Tendon sheaths on dorsum of foot and in lateral retromalleolar region

B Tendon sheaths in medial retromalleolar region

The bony frame-work of the head, the **skull** or cranium, forms the upper end of the trunk. It acts as the container for the brain and the sense organs, forms the substructure of the face, and also contains the initial portions of the gastrointestinal and respiratory tracts. The variety of its tasks determines the differentiation in the construction of the skull.

The skull consists of two parts, the **neurocranium** for the brain, and the **splanchocranium** or **viscerocranium**, the facial skeleton. The boundary between the two lies in the region of the root of the nose and extends along the upper margin of the orbits to the external auditory meatus.

The shape of the skull is partly determined by the muscles, which may produce certain changes due to their functions, and in part by the contents of the skull. Thus, there is a correlation between the neurocranium and the brain contained within it. The influence here is reciprocal, as excessive expansion of the brain may produce enlargement of the neurocranium, e. g., as in hydrocephalus (see p. 296). On the other hand, premature cessation of neurocranial growth may result in malformation of the brain. There is not only a reciprocal effect within the neurocranium but also a close relationship to the facial skeleton. Thus the development of the muscles and of the supporting system of the dura mater within the skull capsule are also interrelated.

Ossification of the Skull

Fundamentally there are two developmental processes in the skull, distinguishable by the type of bone formation. One is the **chondrocranium** and the other the **desmocranium**. In the chondrocranium there is replacement bone formation, while in the desmocranium, the individual bones develop as membrane bones directly from condensations in the connective tissue. Both types of development occur in the two functional parts (the neurocranium and viscerocranium). However, portions of either desmal or chondral origin may fuse together to form a single bone, as, for example, in the temporal bone.

The **neurocranium** (**A**; orange) consists of the occipital bone (**1**), sphenoid bone (**2**), squamous (**3**) and mastoid portion of the petrous (**4**) parts of the temporal bone, the parietal bones (**5**) and the frontal bone (**6**).

The **viscerocranium** (**A**; gray) is composed of the ethmoid bone (**7**), the inferior nasal conchae, the lacrimal bones (**8**), the nasal bones (**9**), the vomer, the maxillae (**10**) with the incisive bone, the palatine bones, the zygomatic bones (**11**), the tympanic parts (**12**) and the styloid processes (**13**) of the temporal bones, the mandible (**14**) and the hyoid bone.

Bones preformed in cartilage (**B**; blue) include the occipital bone (**1**; with the exception of the upper part of its squama, **15**), the sphenoid bone (**2**; with the exception of the medial lamella of the pterygoid process), the temporal bone with its petrous part (**4**) and the ear ossicles, the ethmoid bone (**7**), the inferior nasal concha and the hyoid bone.

The following bones are formed by **ossification in connective tissue** (**B**; yellow): the upper part of the squama of the occipital bone (**15**), the sphenoidal concha, the medial lamella of the pterygoid process, the tympanic part (**12**), the squamous part of the temporal bone (**3**), the parietal bone (**5**), the frontal bone (**6**), the lacrimal bone (**8**), the nasal bone (**9**), the vomer, the maxilla (**10**), the palatine bone, the zygomatic bone (**11**) and the mandible (**14**).

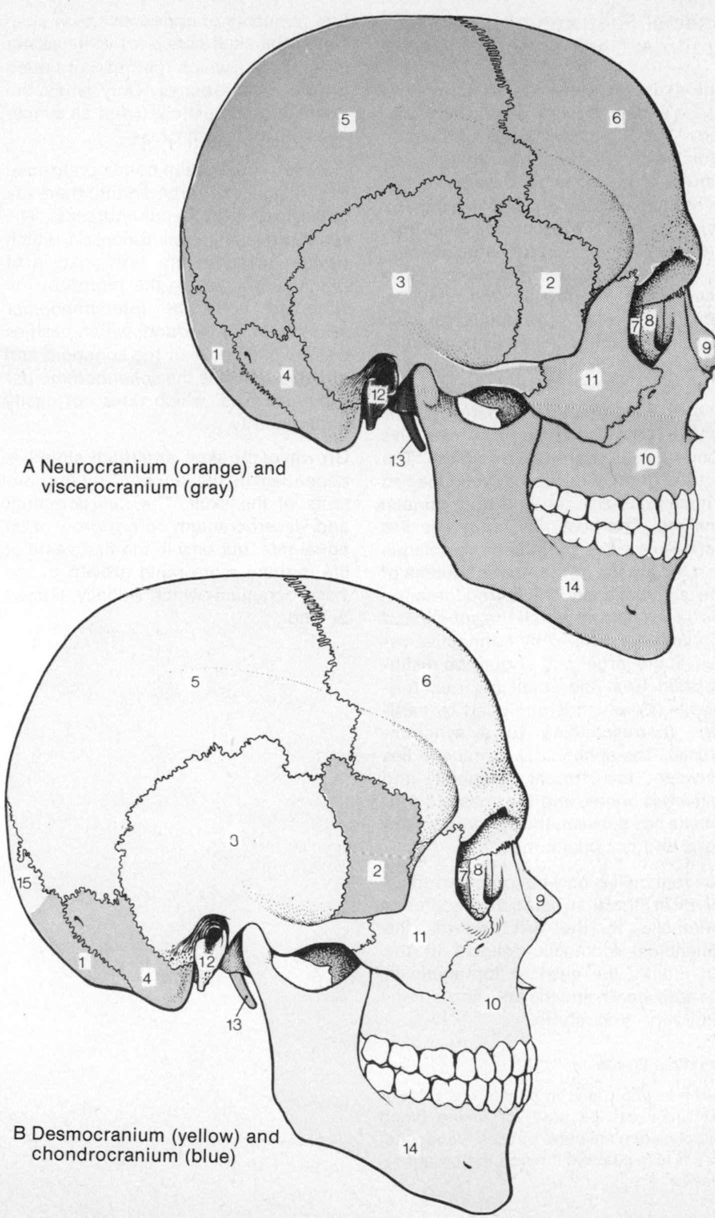

A Neurocranium (orange) and viscerocranium (gray)

B Desmocranium (yellow) and chondrocranium (blue)

Special Features of Intramembranous Ossification (A–D)

The skull cap develops in connective tissue and has several ossification centers from which bone formation radiates in all directions. In this way paired protuberances develop – two *frontal eminences* (**1**) and two *parietal eminences* (**2**). The bones develop from these eminences. At birth large connective tissue areas, the fontanelles or fonticuli, are still left between the individual bones. The *anterior fontanelle* (**3**) is an unpaired opening closed by connective tissue, which is almost square and at birth has a diagonal length of 2.5–3 cm. The smaller, unpaired *posterior fontanelle* (**4**) is also closed by connective tissue and is triangular in shape. The anterior fontanelle lies between the two frontal bone anlagen and both parietal anlagen. The posterior fontanelle lies between the two parietal bone anlagen and the anlage of the upper squama of the occipital bone. The paired fontanelles lie laterally, of which the *sphenoidal fontanelle* (**5**), closed by connective tissue, is the larger and should be distinguished from the small *mastoid fontanelle* (**6**), which is occluded by cartilage (corresponding to a synchondrosis). The sphenoidal fontanelle lies between the frontal, parietal and sphenoid bones, and the mastoid fontanelle lies between the sphenoid, temporal and occipital bones.

The fontanelles only become closed after birth, the first being the posterior fontanelle in the 3rd month, the sphenoidal fontanelle follows in the 6th month, the mastoid fontanelle in the 18th month and the anterior fontanelle in the 36th month.

Practical Points

In the newborn and in infants the anterior fontanelle can be used for taking blood samples from the dural sinuses. Venepuncture is also possible through the great fontanelle.

The remnants of connective tissue between the skull bones form the **sutures** (see p. 22), which permit continued growth of the bones. Only when the bones are completely fused as synostoses does growth cease.

Between some of the bones preformed in cartilage (chondrocranium) there are **cartilaginous areas** (synchondroses). The *spheno-occipital synchondrosis,* which ossifies at about the 18th year, is of practical interest. In the region of the sphenoid body the *intersphenoidal synchondrosis* is found, which ossifies early, while between the sphenoid and ethmoid bones is the *sphenoethmoidal synchondrosis*, which does not ossify until maturity.

Growth of the skull, as already stated, is dependent on the function and the contents of the skull. The neurocranium and viscerocranium do not grow at an equal rate, but only in the first years of life is there more rapid growth of the viscerocranium which initially lagged behind.

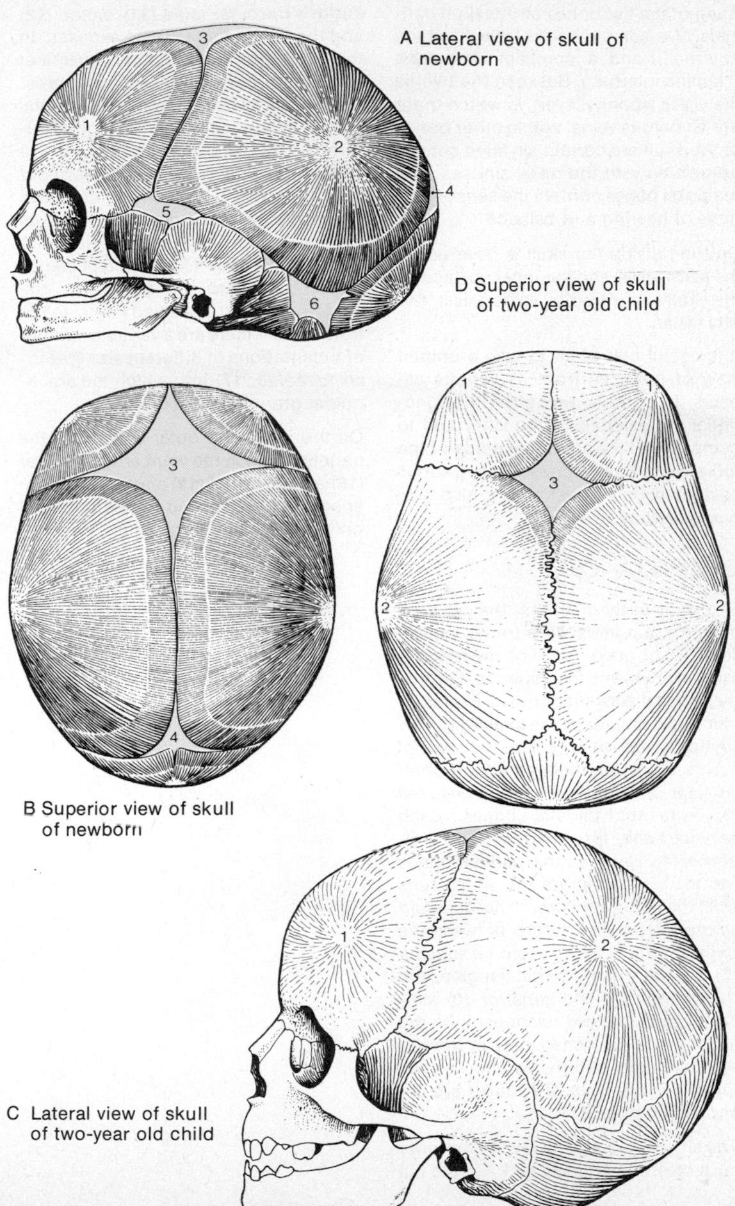

A Lateral view of skull of newborn

D Superior view of skull of two-year old child

B Superior view of skull of newborn

C Lateral view of skull of two-year old child

Each of the flat bones of the skull consists of a compact **outer table** ("lamina externa"), and a compact **inner table** ("lamina interna"). Between the two lie the **diploe** (spongy layer), in which there are numerous veins. Within other bones of the skull are certain air-filled spaces associated with the nasal sinuses. The temporal bones contain the sensory organs of hearing and balance.

On the outside the skull is covered by the **pericranium**, and the inner surface of the skull is covered by **endocranium**, the **dura mater**.

It is useful first of all to take a unified view of the skull from its various aspects, in order to recognise the functional associations of the latter and to comprehend the special features of the individual skull bones. The various cavities within the skull are also discussed below.

Calvaria (A–C)

The vault of the cranium, the calvaria, consists of a **frontal bone** (gray), **parietal bones** (light gray), parts of the **temporal bones** (brown) and the uppermost part of the **occipital bone** (dark gray). Examination of the outside of the skull will show first of all the sutures, i. e. the *coronal suture* (**1**) which separates the *frontal squama* (**2**) with the *frontal eminences* (**3**) from the parietal bones. Each parietal bone, too, has a *parietal eminence* (**4**). Between the parietal bones lies the *sagittal suture* (**5**), which runs from the coronal suture to the *lambdoid suture* (**6**), i. e., the suture between the parietal bone and the *occipital squama* (**7**). Laterally, in the parietal region, are the *inferior* (**8**) and *superior* (**9**) *temporal lines*. In close relationship to the sagittal suture, immediately in front of the lambdoid suture, lie the *parietal foramina* (**10**). Special features are described on page 276.

The sutures are also visible on the inner surface of the cranial vault. On the cut surface the *outer table* (**11**), *diploe* (**12**) and the *inner table* (**13**) are exposed. In the most anterior part of the squama of the frontal bone lies the *frontal crest* (**14**), which extends toward the parietal bones. In the region of the sagittal suture is the shallow *groove for the superior sagittal sinus* (**15**). The *arterial sulci* (**16**), which contain the branches of the middle meningeal artery and its accompanying vein, ascend from the lateral toward the midline and posterior areas. Lateral to the groove for the superior sagittal sinus and lateral to the frontal crest there are a variable number of indentations of different size (*granular foveolae;* **17**) into which the arachnoidal granulations extend.

On the inner and outer aspects of the parietal bone in the vault are the *frontal* (**18**) and *occipital* (**19**) *angles*, while the sphenoid and mastoid angles are found only at the base of the skull.

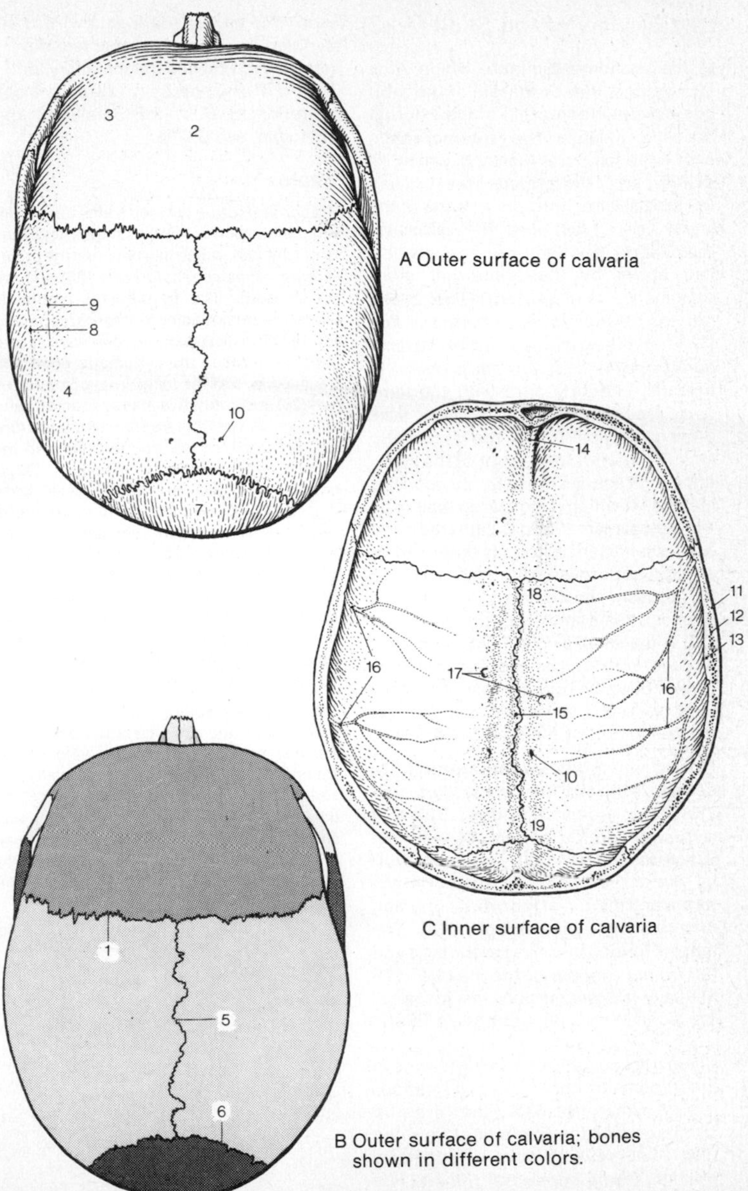

A Outer surface of calvaria

C Inner surface of calvaria

B Outer surface of calvaria; bones shown in different colors.

Lateral View of the Skull (A–C)

In the orbitomeatalplane, which runs through the inferior margin of the orbit and the superior margin of the external acoustic meatus, the **neurocranium** shows the temporal fossa (**1**), which includes part of the **temporal bone** (brown), the **parietal bone** (light gray), parts of the **frontal bone** (gray) and the **sphenoidal bone** (black). The temporal fossa is limited above by the somewhat more prominent *inferior temporal line* (**2**) and the less obvious *superior temporal line* (**3**). From the *squamous part of the temporal bone* (**4**) the *zygomatic process* (**5**) extends anteriorly, and with the *temporal process* (**6**) of the **zygomatic bone** (light yellow) it forms the *zygomatic arch* (**7**). Inferior to the root of the zygomatic process lies the *external acoustic meatus* (**8**) which is bordered mainly by the **tympanic part** (**9**, and **C**, light red), and to a lesser extent by the **squamous part** (**4**, and **C**, light brown) of the **temporal bone** (**B**, brown). Immediately above this there is often a small *suprameatal spine* (**10**) and a small cavity. Posterior to the external meatus lies the *mastoid process* (**11**), which originated as a muscular apophysis. The *mastoid foramen* (**12**) lies at the root of the mastoid process.

On examining the **viscerocranium** we see above the orbit the *supraciliary arch* (**13**) as a prominent ridge. Below it is the *supraorbital margin* (**14**) with the *supraorbital notch* (**15**). The supraorbital margin is continued over the anterolateral margin of the orbital opening into the *infraorbital margin* (**16**). The latter is formed by the **zygomatic bone** and the *frontal process of the maxilla* (**17**). Medially is a depression, the fossa for the lacrimal sac (**18**); orbit, see p. 292).

There are one (or two) small foramina in the zygomatic bone, the *zygomaticofacial foramen* (**19**). Below the infraorbital margin lies the *infraorbital foramen* (**20**). At the lowest point of the nasal opening the *anterior nasal spine* (**21**) is seen. The **maxilla** (dark yellow) has an *alveolar process* (**22**) directed downward, which carries the maxillary teeth. The *maxillary tuberosity* (**23**) *bulges out posterior to this* (for details of the mandible, see p. 288.)

Sutures

The *coronal suture* (**24**) separates the frontal and parietal bones. It meets the *sphenofrontal suture* (**25**), which lies between the *greater wing of the sphenoid bone* (**26**) and the frontal bone. The frontal and zygomatic bones are separated by the *frontozygomatic suture* (**27**). The *zygomaticomaxillary suture* (**28**) lies between the zygomatic bone and the maxilla, and the *temporozygomatic suture* (**29**) is found between the zygomatic and temporal bones. The *frontomaxillary suture* (**30**) lies between the frontal bone and the maxilla, and the *nasomaxillary suture,* (**31**) is between the maxilla and the nasal bone (light orange). The *sphenosquamous suture* (**32**) forms the boundary between the greater wing of the sphenoid bone and the temporal squama. The temporal bone (brown) joins the parietal bone at the *squamous suture* (**33**). It may extend into the mastoid process as the *petrosquanous suture* (**34**) between its squamous (**C**, dark pink) and petrous (**G**. dark brown) parts.

The *lambdoid suture* (**35**) separates the parietal from the occipital bone (dark gray). A small part of the greater wing of the sphenoid extends as far as the parietal bone. so that a *sphenoparietal suture* (**36**) can be described. Between the mastoid process and the parietal bone on the one hand and the occipital bone on the other lie the *parietomastoid* (**37**) and *occipitomastoid* (**38**) *sutures*.

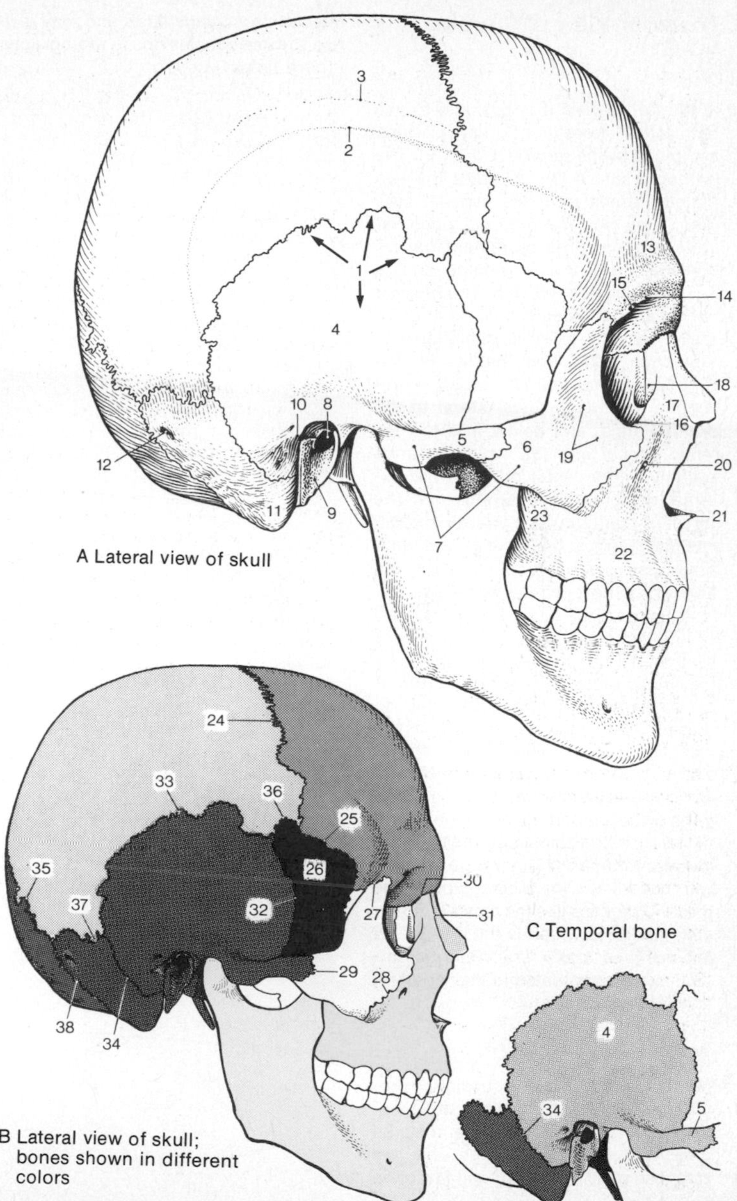

A Lateral view of skull

B Lateral view of skull; bones shown in different colors

C Temporal bone

Posterior View of the Skull (A–B)

In the dorsal view it is possible to see both **parietal bones** (light gray, **1**), which are joined by the *sagittal suture* (**2**). The *lambdoid suture* (**3**) separates the two parietal bones from the **occipital bone** (dark gray, **4**). The *external occipital protuberance* (**5**) is prominent on the occipital bone in the midline and is palpable through the skin. The *highest nuchal line* (**6**) extends upward and laterally from the external occipital protuberance. The line below is the *superior nuchal line* (**7**), which represents a transverse ridge lateral to the protuberance, and below it is the *inferior nuchal line* (**8**), which extends roughly in the center between the external occipital protuberance and the foramen magnum. The *inferior nuchal line* may begin at the more or less well-developed, *external occipital crest* (**9**). Lateral to the occipital bone lies the *mastoid process* (**11**), which is part of the temporal bone, but which is separated from the occipital bone by the *occipitomastoid suture* (**10**). A *petrosquamous suture* (**12**) may be present completely or in part in the mastoid process. This suture shows that the mastoid process is formed from both the squamous and the petrous parts of the temporal bone. In the region of the occipitomastoid suture (**10**) is the *mastoid foramen* (**13**), through which a vein passes. On the medial side of the mastoid process lies the *mastoid notch* (**14**), medial to which is the *groove for the occipital artery* (**15**). Parietal foramina (**16**) are situated in the region of the parietal bones.

Variants

Sometimes the external occipital protuberance is particularly well developed. The upper squama may be present as a separate bone, the **inca bone** (see p. 300). The parietal foramina may be particularly large and may give rise to false conclusions in radiographs ("bore holes").

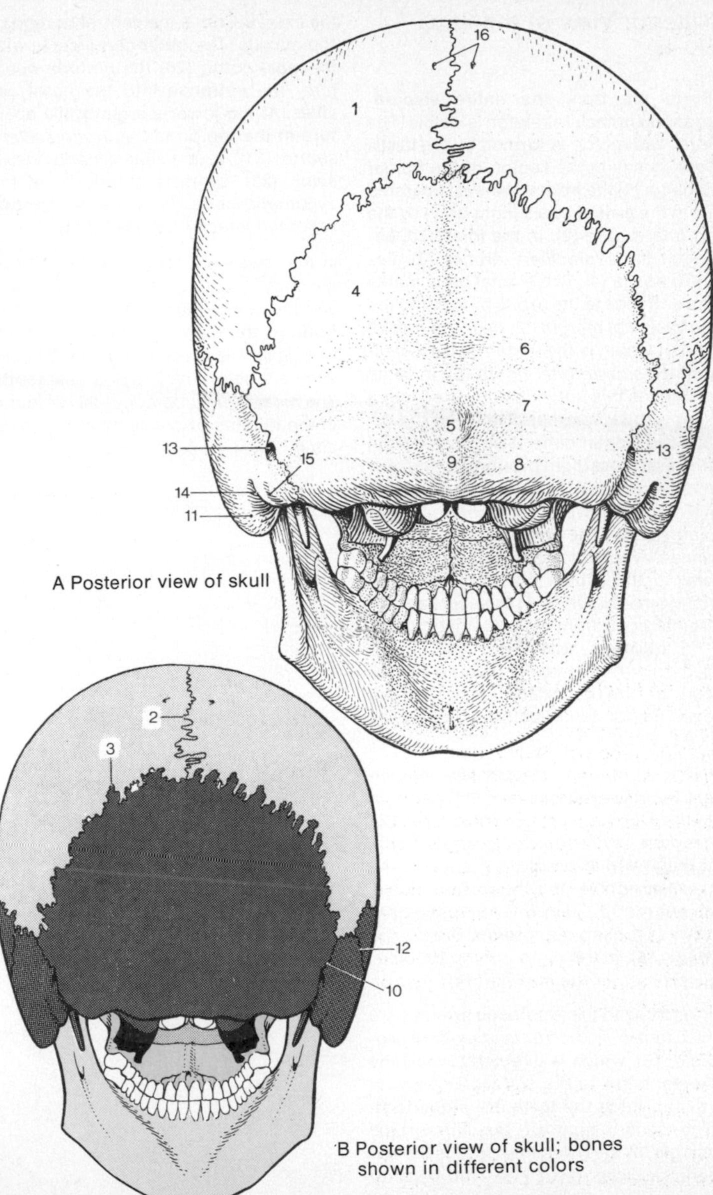

A Posterior view of skull

B Posterior view of skull; bones shown in different colors

Anterior View of the Skull (A–B)

From the front the entire **viscerocranium** or facial skeleton is visible. The forehead region is formed by the **frontal bone** (gray). In the region of the *frontal squama* (**1**) the frontal bone is separated from the **parietal bones** (light gray) by the *coronal suture* (**2**). In the forehead, between the *supraciliary arches* (**3**), lies the *glabella* (**4**). The frontal bone marks the entrance to the orbits by forming the *supraorbital margin* (**5**), near the medial end of which is the variably sized, well-defined *supraorbital notch* (**6**). In some instances this notch is converted into a supraorbital foramen. Between the orbits the frontal bone is separated from the **nasal bones** (light orange) by the *frontonasal sutures* (**7**), and from the **maxillae** (dark yellow) by the *frontomaxillary sutures* (**8**). The two nasal bones are joined by the *internasal suture* (**9**). Lateral to the orbital opening, the *frontozygomatic suture* (**10**) separates the frontal bone from the zygomatic bone. The **zygomatic bone** (light yellow) together with the maxilla forms a further part of the boundary of the orbital opening (for details of the orbital cavity, see p. 292).

In the region of the upper jaw, just below the *infraorbital margin* (**11**) and near to the *zygomaticomaxillary suture* (**12**), lies the *infraorbital foramen* (**13**), through which passes a branch of the maxillary nerve, the infraorbital nerve, an artery and a vein. Inferior to the orbit there is a deep depression, the *canine fossa* (**15**), in the region of the *zygomatic process of the maxilla* (**14**).

In addition to the zygomatic process, we distinguish also a *frontal maxillary process* (**16**), which is directed toward the frontal bone, and the *alveolar process* (**17**), in which the teeth are embedded. The continuation of the infraorbital margin on the frontal process is the *anterior lacrimal crest* (**18**). The *body of the maxilla* (**19**) is the central portion of the maxilla. The latter demarcates with its *nasal notch* (**20**) the *piriform aperture*, the entrance into the nasal cavities. At the lower margin of the aperture in the region of the *intermaxillary suture* (**21**), a spur, the *anterior nasal spine* (**22**), projects anteriorly. In the zygomatic bone there are one or two *zygomaticofacial foramina* (**23**).

In the lower jaw, the **mandible** (yellow), the *body* (**24**), the *alveolar process* (**25**) and the *ramus* (**26**) are visible from the front. In the region of the body of the mandible, the *mental foramen* (**27**) lies vertically below the 2nd premolar tooth. The *mental protuberance* (**28**) is found in the midline of the body of the mandible.

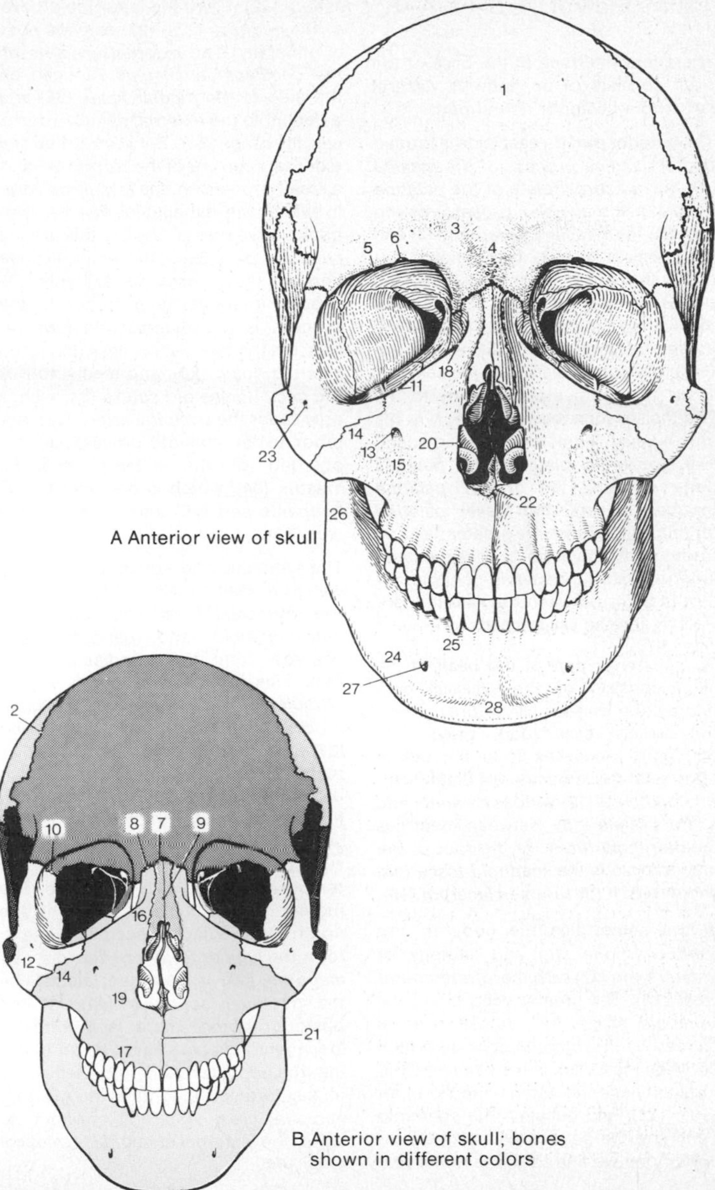

A Anterior view of skull

B Anterior view of skull; bones shown in different colors

Inferior View of the Skull (A–B)

The inferior surface of the base of the skull consists of an anterior visceral part and a posterior neural part.

The **anterior part** on each side is formed by the *palatine process of the maxilla* (**1**), the *horizontal plate of the palatine bone* (**2**), the *alveolar process, of the maxilla,* the *maxillary tuberosity* (**3**) and the **zygomatic bone** (**4**, light yellow). Medially the **vomer** (red) separates the posterior nasal apertures, the *choanae* (**5**). The palatine processes meet at the *median palatine suture* (**6**), whose anterior end is marked by the *incisive foramen* (**7**). From there laterally to the 2nd incisor runs the *incisive suture* (**8**), which may sometimes be evident. The horizontal plate of the palatine bone contains the *greater palatine foramen* (**9**) and the *lesser palatine foramina* (**10**). From the greater palatine foramen the *palatine grooves* extend anteriorly. The *transverse palatine suture* (**11**) lies between the **maxilla** (dark yellow) and the **palatine bone** (green).

The **posterior part** of the base of the skull consists of the **sphenoid bone** (black), the **temporal bones** (brown) and the **occipital bone** (dark gray). The pterygoid processes form the lateral borders of the choanae. We distinguish a *medial plate* (**12**) with its *hamulus* and a *lateral plate* (**13**). Between them lies the *pterygoid fossa*. At the root of the medial plate is the *scaphoid fossa* (**14**) and next to it the *foramen lacerum* (**15**).

In the center lies the *body of the sphenoid bone* (**16**) and laterally its *greater wing* (**17**) with the *infratemporal crest* (**18**). The greater wing bears the *sphenoid spine* (**19**), whose base is pierced by the *foramen* spinosum (**20**). Between the foramen spinosum and the foramen lacerum opens the *foramen ovale* (**21**), and between the sphenoid bone and the petrous part of the temporal bone we find the *sphenopetrosal fissure* (**22**). From the latter the groove of the *auditory tube* (**23**) extends posterolaterally. The *external aperture of the cochlear canaliculus* is found on the side of the *jugular fossa* (**25**) and adjacent to the *external aperture of the carotid canal* (**24**). Between it and the external aperture of the carotid canal is a small depression, the *fossula petrosa*, in which the canaliculus for the tympanic nerve opens. Next to this are the *tympanic part* (**26**) of the temporal bone and the *styloid process* (**27**) within its sheath. Immediately posterior to the process is the *stylomastoid foramen* (**28**). On the *mastoid process* (**29**) is the *mastoid notch* (**30**), and medial to it is the *occipitomastoid suture* (**31**) with a groove for the *occipital artery* (**32**). Anterior to the mastoid process lies the opening of the *external acoustic meatus* (**34**), which is bounded by the *tympanic part* (**26**) and the *squamous part* (**33**).

The tympanic and squamous parts, as well as a small ridge of the petrous part, the *tegmental crest* bounded by the *petrotympanic* and *petrosquamous fissures*, form the *mandibular fossa* (**35**). This is limited anteriorly by the *articular tubercle* (**36**). The *zygomatic process (zygoma) of the temporal bone* (**37**) extends anterolaterally. The *basilar part* (**38**) of the occipital bone, which bears the *pharyngeal tubercle* (**39**), fuses with the *body of the sphenoid bone* (**16**). The *petrooccipital fissure* runs between the petrosal part of the temporal and the occipital bone. The jugular fossa (**25**) is widened by the notch in the adjacent occipital bone to form the *jugular foramen*. The *foramen magnum* (**40**) is bounded laterally by the *occipital condyles* (**41**). At the posterior border there is a *condylar fossa* which is perforated by an opening, the *condylar canal* (**42**). Beginning at the foramen magnum, the *external occipital crest* (**43**) runs upwards toward the *external occipital protuberance* (**44**).

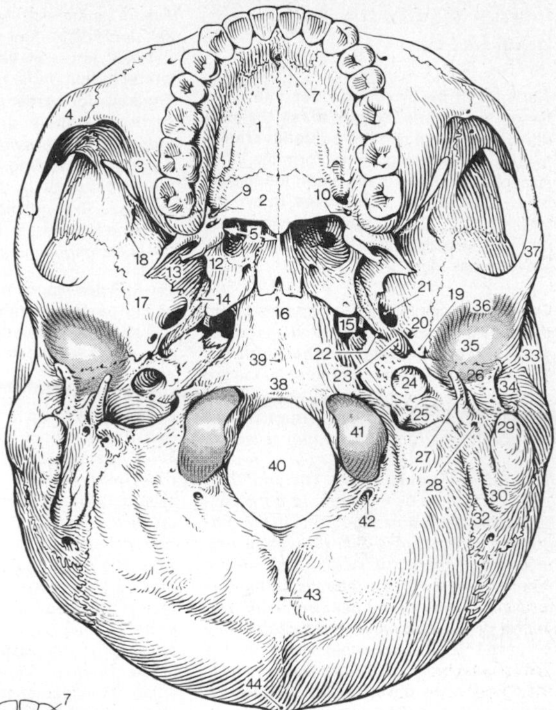

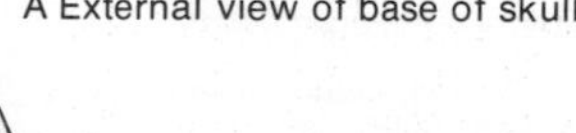

A External view of base of skull

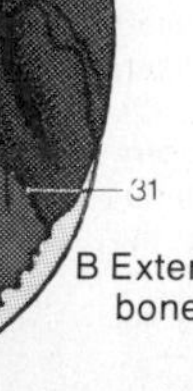

B External view of base of skull; bones shown in different colors

Interior View of the Base of the Skull (A–B)

The base of the skull is divided into three fossae, the **anterior cranial fossa**, the **middle cranial fossa** and the **posterior cranial fossa**. The following bones form the inner surface of the base of the skull: the **ethmoid bone** (orange), the **frontal bone** (gray) the **sphenoid bone** (black), the **temporal bones** (brown), the **occipital bone** (dark gray) and the **parietal bones** (light gray).

The anterior cranial fossa is separated from the middle fossa by the *lesser wings of the sphenoid* (**1**) and the *jugum sphenoidale* (**2**). The middle and posterior cranial fossae are separated from each other by the *superior borders* (**3**) of the petrosal portions of the temporal bones and the *dorsum sellae* (**4**).

The anterior cranial fossa. The *cribriform plate* (**5**) formed by the ethmoid bone contains many small holes and bears in the midline the vertical *crista galli* (**6**) with its *alar processes*. Anterior to the crista galli is the *foramen caecum* (**7**) and laterally lie the *orbital plates* (**8**) of the frontal bone with their *impressiones digitatae*. The cribriform plate is joined to the sphenoid bone by the *sphenoethmoidal suture* (**9**). In the middle, the *chiasmatic groove* (**11**) lies between the *optic canals* (**10**). The *anterior clinoid processes* (**12**) border the optic canals.

In the center of the **middle cranial fossa** there is the *sella turcica* with the *hypophysial fossa* (**13**) and laterally of the sella the *carotid groove* (**14**), which is the prolongation of the carotid canal. The carotid canal, which lies on the anterior wall of the petrous part of the temporal bone, is split open in its medial portion near the *foramen lacerum* (**15**). The medial end of the canal is bounded by the *lingula of the sphenoid bone* (**16**). Lateral to the carotid groove is the *foramen ovale* (**17**), in front the *foramen rotundum* (**18**) and lateral the *foramen spinosum* (**19**). The *groove for the middle meningeal artery* (**20**) runs laterally from the foramen spinosum. Near the apex of the petrous part the *trigeminal impression* (**21**) can be seen, and lateral and somewhat posterior to it is the *hiatus for the greater petrosal nerve* (**22**), which continues toward the sphenopetrosal fissure as the *groove for the greater petrosal nerve* (**23**). The *hiatus for the lesser petrosal nerve* (**24**) lies immediately anterolateral to that of the greater petrosal nerve. The *superior* border of the petrous part (**3**) carries the more or less well-developed *groove of the superior pretrosal sinus* (**25**). A priminent swelling, the *arcuate eminence* (**26**), is produced by the anterior semicircular canal. The squamous part of the temporal bone is joined to the sphenoid bone by the *sphenosquamous suture* (**27**).

The *foramen magnum* (**28**) lies in the middle of the **posterior cranial fossa**. The *clivus* (**29**) ascends anteriorly and ends in the *dorsum sellae* (**4**) and its *posterior clinoid processes* (**30**).

Between the occipital bone and the petrous part of the temporal lies the *groove of the inferior petrosal sinus* (**31**) and also the petrooccipital synchondrosis, which may be seen in the macerated skull as the *petrooccipital fissure* (**32**). The groove of the inferior petrosal sinus ends in the *jugular foramen* (**33**). The *opening of the internal acoustic meatus* (**34**) opens onto the posterior surface of the petrous part. Lateral to it, hidden under a small bony ridge, lies the *external opening of the vestibular aqueduct*. The jugular foramen (**33**) is formed by the apposition of the jugular notches in the temporal and occipital bones. The *jugular notch in the occipital bone* is limited anteriorly by the projection of the *jugular tubercle,* and the jugular foramen is partly divided by the *intrajugular process of the temporal bone* (**35**). On its lateral side the jugular foramen is reached by the *groove of the sigmoid sinus* (**36**) which continues posteriorly into the *groove of the transverse sinus* (**37**). This extends to the *internal occipital protuberance* (**38**), from which the *internal occipital crest* (**39**) runs toward the foramen magnum (**28**). On either side of the anterior rim of the foramen magnum is the opening of the *hypoglossal canal* (**40**). The clivus is formed by the body of the sphenoid bone and the basilar part of the occipital bone. During puberty they fuse (**os tribasilare**) but previously they are connected by the sphenooccipital synchondrosis.

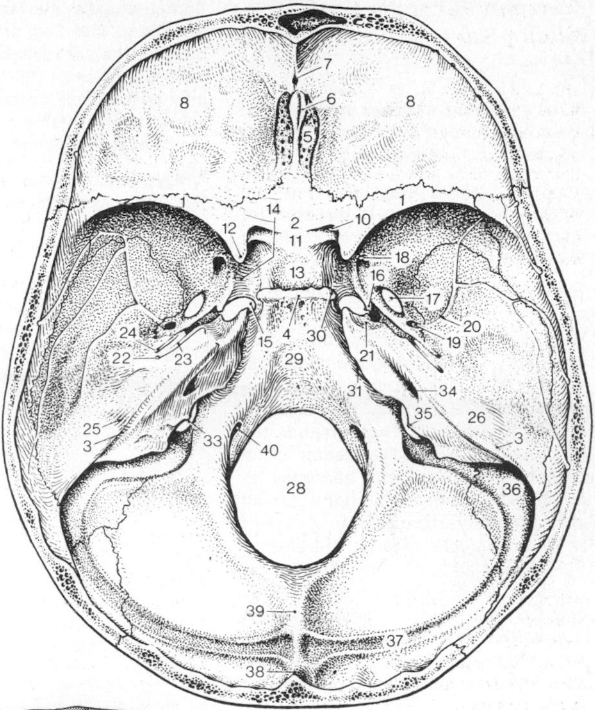

A Internal view of base of skull

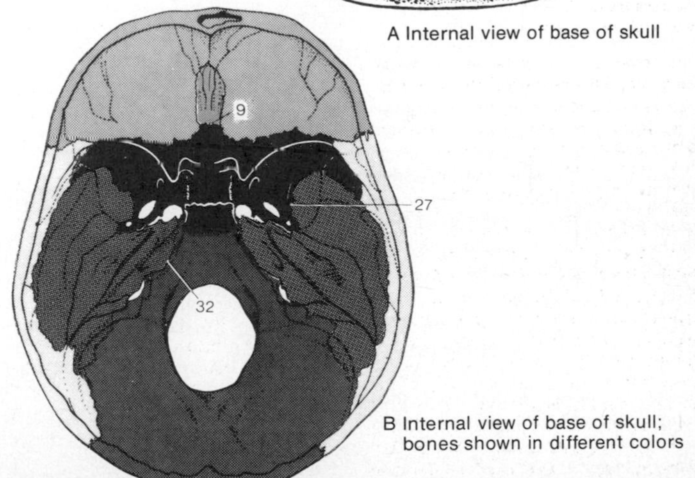

B Internal view of base of skull; bones shown in different colors

Common Variants of the Interior Surface of the Base of the Skull (A–E)

In the middle cranial fossa, in the region of the sella turcica, a number of variants can be seen in radiographs.

In some cases the *lingula* (**1**) of the sphenoid bone, which is directed toward the temporal bone, may be fused with it (**A**).

Between the anterior and posterior clinoid processes there may be an additional process, the *middle clinoid process* (**2**, **C**). The latter may then fuse with the anterior clinoid process (**C**), when it forms a special opening, the *caroticoclinoid* foramen (**3**). Through this, the carotid notch, which lies medial to the anterior clinoid process, becomes an opening surrounded by bone on all sides. Another variant is the presence of an *interclinoidal bridge* (**B**, **4**) between the anterior and posterior clinoid processes. This bony fusion of the two processes, when seen on radiographs, is termed the *sella bridge* (**4**). It may be present on one or both sides and can fuse with the middle clinoid process if it is present (**5**).

Between the foramen ovale and the body of the sphenoid bone there is sometimes an aperture (**D**), which serves as the exit for a vein. This opening, the foramen of Vesalius (**D**, **6**), is also called the *foramen venosum*. It is not very uncommon and it permits communication between the cavernous sinus and veins on the outside of the skull. The foramen of Vesalius may be present on one or both sides.

In some cases the dorsum sellae may be so eroded laterally by more extensive looping of the internal carotid artery that it no longer has any bony connection with the clivus. In that case, the dorsum sellae will be absent from the macerated skull (**D**).

Sometimes the internal occipital crest is divided into two and between the parts is the well-developed *groove of the occipital sinus* (**E**). This may extend into a marginal groove (**7**), running lateral to the foramen magnum (**8**), to the jugular foramen (**9**).

The jugular foramina may be unequal in size, more often the left being smaller than the right. *The hypoglossal canal may be divided into two* (**E, 10**).

The apex of the petrous part of the temporal bone may have a bony connection with the dorsum sellae. This bony bridge is also known as the *abducent bridge*, since the abducent nerve runs beneath it.

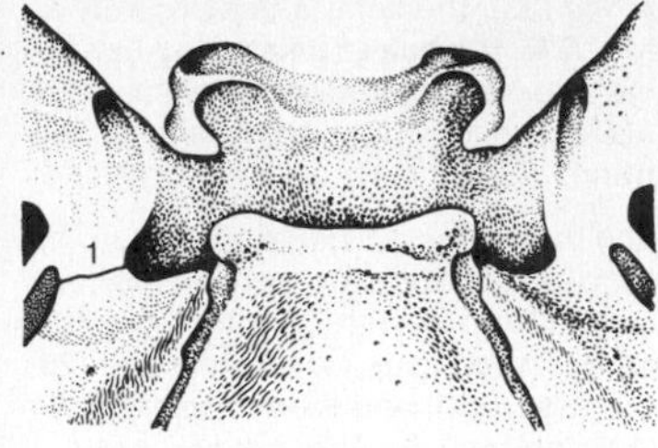

A
Sella turcica; right lingula of sphenoid bone fused with temporal bone

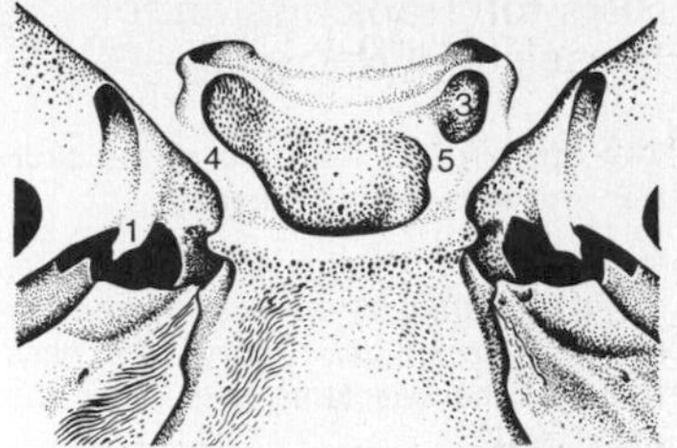

B
Sella turcica; interclinoid bridge, right caroticoclinoid foramen

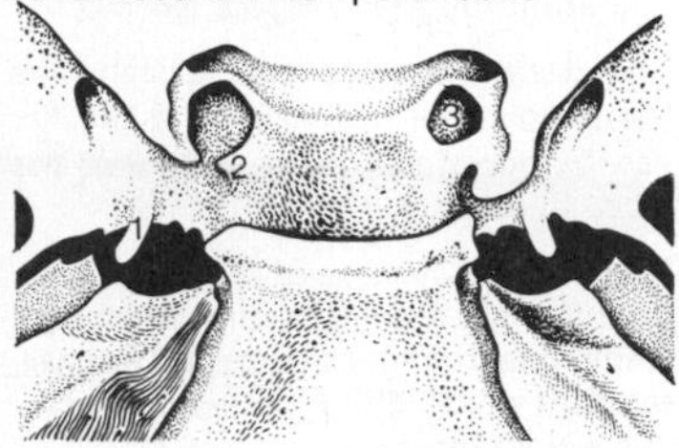

C
Sella turcica; left middle clinoid process, right caroticoclinoid foramen

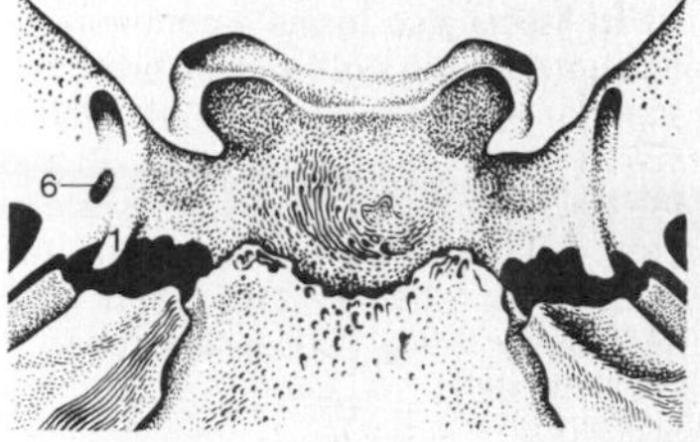

D
Sella turcica; absence of dorsum sellae, foramen of Vesalius

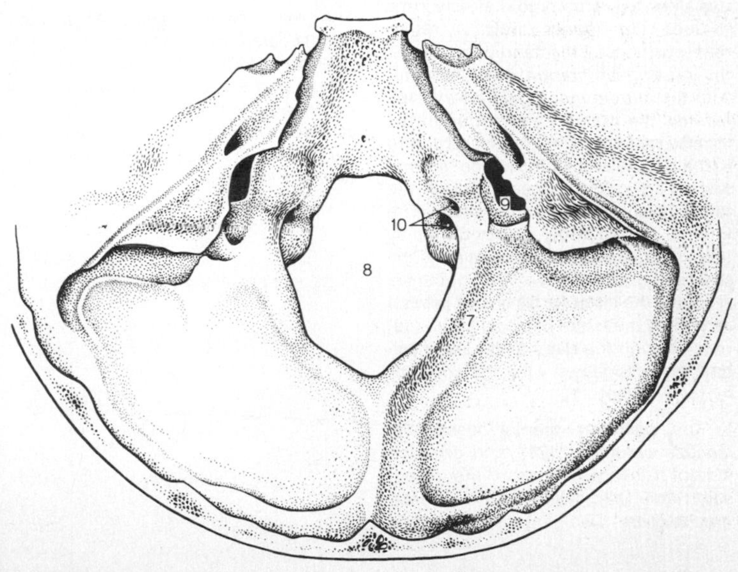

E Groove of right occipital sinus, divided canal for hypoglossal nerve

Sites for Transmission for Vessels and Nerves (A–B)

The openings in the base of the skull transmit vessels and nerves.

In the region of the anterior cranial fossa the *olfactory nerves* (**1**) and the *anterior ethmoidal artery* (**2**) pass through the **cribriform plate** from the nasal cavity.

The *optic nerve* (**3**) and the *ophthalmic artery* (**4**) run through the **optic canal**. Apart from the optic canal the **superior orbital fissure** also forms a communication between the skull and the orbit. The *superior ophthalmic vein* (**5**), the *lacrimal nerve* (**6**), the *frontal nerve* (**7**) and the *trochlear nerve* (**8**) run in its lateral part. The *abducent nerve* (**9**), the *oculomotor* nerve (**10**) and the *nasociliary nerve* (**11**) pass through it more medially.

The *maxillary nerve* (**12**) passes through the **foramen rotundum**, while the *mandibular nerve* (**13**), together with a *venous network* which joins the cavernous sinus to the pterygoid plexus, runs through the **foramen ovale**. A recurrent branch of the mandibular nerve, the *meningeal branch* (**14**), together with the *middle meningeal artery* (**15**), reaches the cranial cavity through the **foramen spinosum**. The largest structure in the middle cranial fossa, the *internal carotid artery* (**16**) passes through the **carotid canal** into the cranial cavity. The internal carotid artery is surrounded by the *sympathetic carotid plexus* (**17**). The *greater petrosal nerve* (**18**) becomes visible at the **hiatus for the greater petrosal nerve,** and the *lesser petrosal nerve* (**19**) runs through the **hiatus for the lesser petrosal nerve** together with the *superior tympanic artery* (**20**).

In the posterior cranial fossa, the *medulla oblongata* (**21**), and on each side of it the *spinal part of the accessory nerve* (**22**), pass through the **foramen magnum**. Two large *vertebral arteries* (**23**), the small *anterior spinal artery* (**24**), the paired small *posterior spinal arteries* (**25**) and the *spinal vein* (**26**) also pass through the foramen magnum.

The *hypoglossal nerve* (**27**) and the *venous network of the hypoglossal canal* (**28**) pass through the **hypoglossal canal**. The *glossopharyngeal nerve* (**29**), the *vagus* (**30**) and the *accessory nerve* (**31**), as well as the *inferior petrosal sinus* (**32**), the *internal jugular vein* (**33**) and the *posterior meningeal artery* (**34**) all pass through the **jugular foramen**.

The **internal acoustic meatus** transmits the *labyrinthine artery and vein* (**35**), the *vestibulocochlear nerve* (**36**) and the *facial* nerve (**37**).

On the *outer surface of the base of the skull* the facial nerve becomes visible as it emerges from the **stylomastoid foramen**, through which the *stylomastoid artery* (**38**) enters the skull.

The *chorda tympani* (**39**) and the *anterior tympanic artery* (**40**) traverse the **petrotympanic fissure.**

The *greater palatine artery* (**41**) and the *greater palatine nerve* (**42**) pass through the **greater palatine foramen** in the hard palate, and the *lesser palatine arteries and nerves* (**43**) run through the **lesser palatine foramina**. The *nasopalatine nerve* (**44**) runs through the **incisive canal** toward the palate.

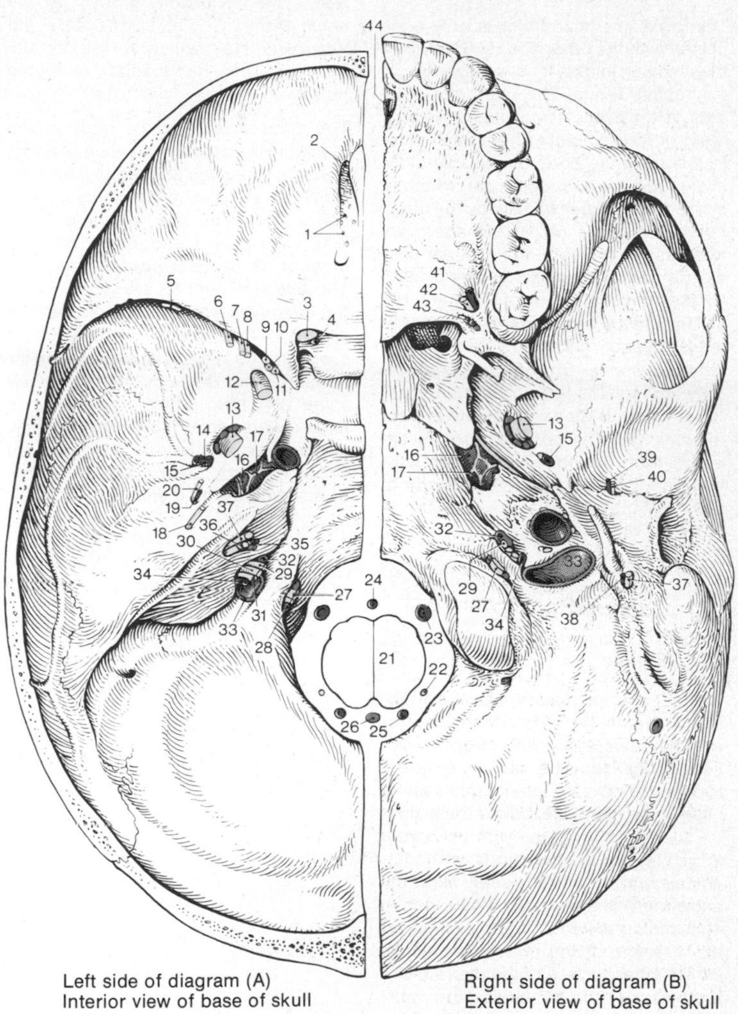

Left side of diagram (A)
Interior view of base of skull

Right side of diagram (B)
Exterior view of base of skull

Sites of transmission for vessels and nerves
in base of skull

Mandible (A–C)

The lower jaw (mandible) is only connected with the other bones of the skull by synovial joints. It is preformed in connective tissue. The mandible consists of the **body** (**1**) with its ascending **ramus** of the mandible (**2**) on each side. In the adult the body of the mandible bears the *alveolar process* (**3**), which is marked on its outer surface by the bulging *alveolar juga* (**4**). In old age, i. e., after loss of the teeth, the alveolar process undergoes regression (see p. 290). On the front of the body of the mandible lies the *mental protuberance* (**5**), which is elevated on each side to form the *mental tubercle*. On the outer surface, on a vertical line through the 2nd premolar, there is an opening, the *mental foramen* (**6**). The *oblique line* (7) ascends from the body to the ramus of the mandible. Posteriorly the body of the mandible merges at the *mandibular angle* (**8**) with the ramus.

The ramus of the mandible has two processes, the anterior *coronoid process* (**9**) for insertion of a muscle, and the posterior *condylar process* (**10**) for the joint surface.

Between the processes lies the *mandibular notch* (**11**). The condylar process has a *neck* (**12**) and supports the *head of the mandible* with its *articular surface* (**13**). On the inner aspect of the head of the mandible, below the articular surface, a small pit, the *pterygoid fovea* (**14**), for the insertions of the lateral pterygoid muscle is seen. Near the angle there is sometimes a roughened area, the *masseteric tuberosity* (**15**) for the insertion of the masseter muscle. On the inner surface of the mandible in the region of the ramus lies the *mandibular foramen* (**16**), which is the entrance to the mandibular canal. The opening is partly concealed by a delicate spur of bone, the *lingula of the mandible* (**17**). The *mylohyoid groove* (**18**) begins directly at the mandibular foramen and runs obliquely downward. Below the mylohyoid groove, at the angle of the mandible, is the *pterygoid tuberosity* (**19**), which serves for the insertion of the medial pterygoid muscle.

The inner surface of the body of the mandible is divided by an oblique ridge, the *mylohyoid line* (**20**). Below this line, from which the mylohyoid muscle arises, we find the *submandibular fossa* (**21**), while above it and somewhat more anterior, is the *sublingual fovea* (**22**). The alveoli or sockets are separated by the *interalveolar septa* (**23**). Within the alveoli of the molars, *interradicular septa* may be seen. Anteriorly, on the inner surface of the body, lies the *mental spine* (**24**) from which muscles arise (also called genial tubercles); laterally and somewhat inferiorly, there are the *paired digastric fossae* (**25**), the points of insertion of the digastric muscles.

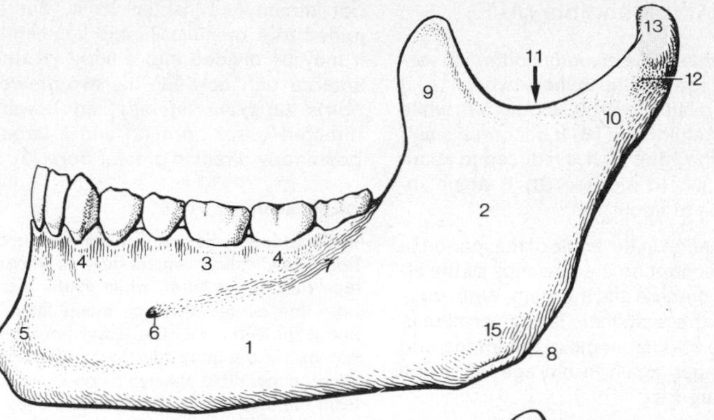

A Lateral view of mandible

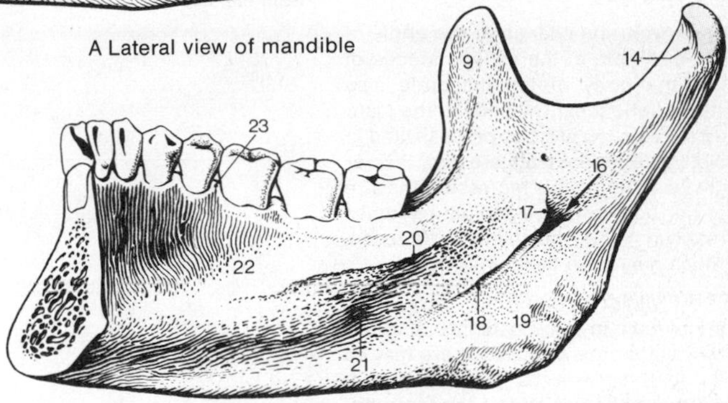

B Medial view of mandible

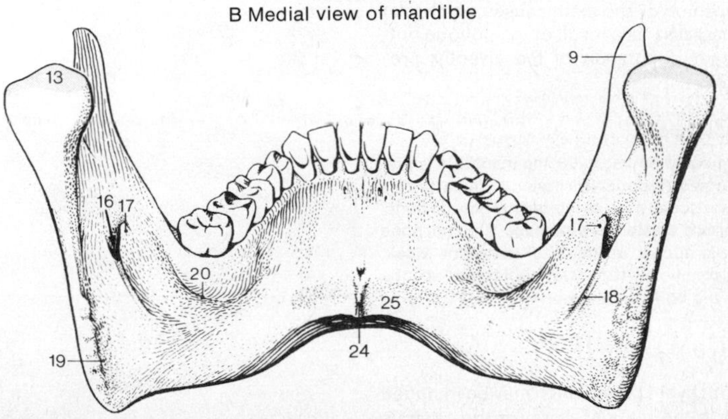

C Posterior view of mandible

Shape of Mandible (A–E)

The *angle of the mandible* differs at various stages of life. In the newborn (**A**) it is still relatively large, about 150°, while during childhood (**B**) it becomes smaller. In the adult (**C**) it is reduced to about 120–130°. In old age (**D**) it again increases to about 140°.

The change in the angle of the mandible is dependent on the presence of the alveolar process and the teeth. With eruption of the teeth there is an alteration in the mandibular angle of the infant, and it changes again in old age when the teeth are lost.

Apart from the change in the angle of the mandible at the various stages of life, the body of the mandible also shows variations. The body of the mandible bears the alveolar process, and in old age, after the teeth are lost, this regresses. During this regression the size of the body of the mandible becomes reduced and sometimes flattened, which may push the chin forward.

The alveolar process may vary in its orientation. In some instances, particularly among the primates, there may be an alveolar process protruding outward and the position of the teeth differs from that in modern man. This position of the teeth causes an **alveolar prognathia** as a result of the oblique outward orientation of the alveolar process.

Ossification

As noted on page 268, the mandible is preformed in connective tissue. It appears in the 1st visceral arch as intermembranous bone, formed on Meckel's cartilage. The first bone cells appear in the 6th intrauterine week. In common with the clavicle it is the 1st bone in the body to develop.

Hyoid Bone (F)

The hyoid bone, which may be included with the bony skeleton of the skull, is not directly connected to it, but is joined to it by muscles and ligaments. It may be divided into a *body* (**1**), the anterior part between the two *greater horns* (**2**) *lying laterally*, an upward directed *lesser horn* (**3**) and a larger, posteriorly directed *greater horn* (**2**).

Ossification

In the body and the greater horn of the hyoid bone, ossification centers develop in cartilage just before birth, while in the lesser horn the center develops much later, at about the 20th year. The lesser horn need not ossify but may remain cartilaginous. Like the mandible, the hyoid bone develops from the skeleton of the visceral arches.

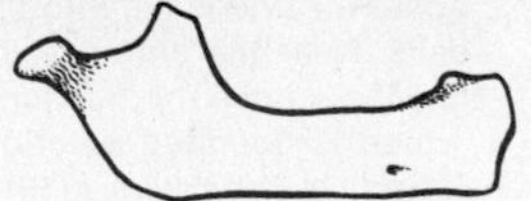

A Mandible in newborn

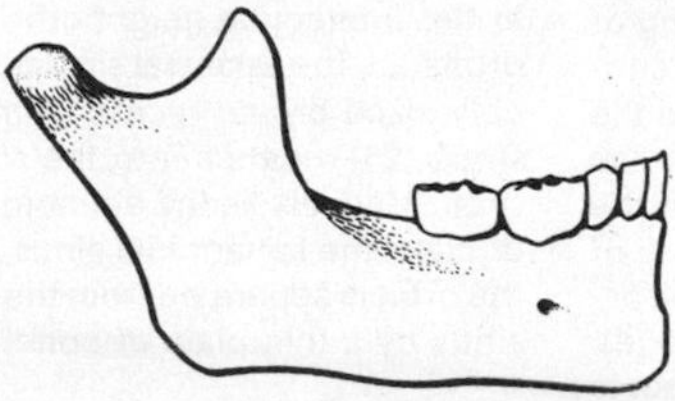

B Mandible of child (deciduous teeth)

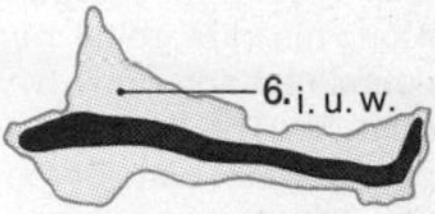

6. i. u. w.

E Medial view of mandible half, ossification

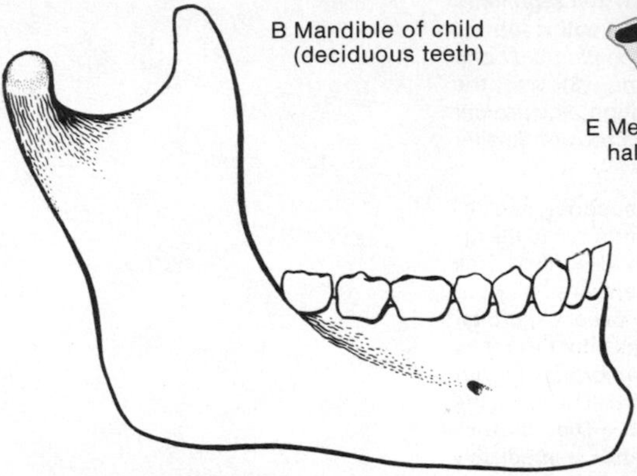

C Mandible of adult (permanent teeth)

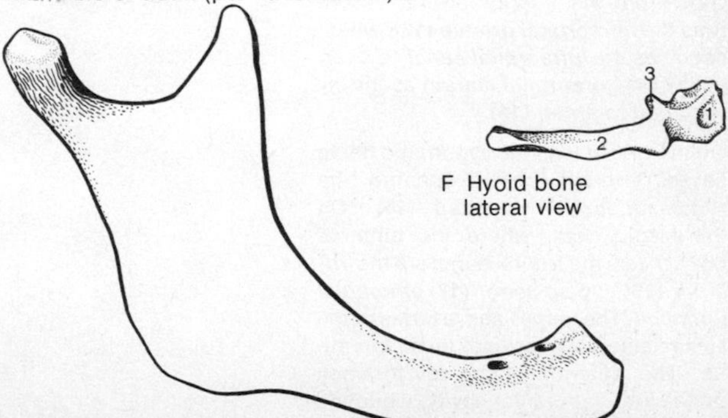

3
1
2

F Hyoid bone lateral view

D Mandible in old age

Orbital Cavity (A–B)

Each **orbit** is shaped like a four-sided pyramid, the apex lying deep inside and the base forming the orbital opening. It is demarcated by various bones.

The **roof of the orbit** is formed anteriorly by the *orbital plate of the frontal bone* (**1**) and posteriorly by the *lesser wing of the sphenoid* (**2**). The **lateral wall** consists of the *zygomatic bone* (**3**) and the *greater wing of the sphenoid* (**4**). The anterior part of the **floor** is formed by the orbital surface of the *orbital process of the maxilla* (**5**) and posteriorly by the *orbital process of the palatine bone* (**6**). Along the infraorbital margin the floor is completed anteriorly by the *zygomatic bone* (**3**). The thin **medial wall** is formed by the *orbital plate of the ethmoid bone* (**7**), the *lacrimal bone* (**8**) and the *sphenoid* (**9**). In addition, the *frontal bone* (**1**) and the *maxilla* provide smaller contributions to this wall.

Orbital Openings. The superior and inferior margins of the entrance to the orbit have already been described (see p. 278). Posteriorly there are two converging fissures, the *superior orbital fissure* (**10**) which opens into the cranial cavity, and the *inferior orbital fissure* (**11**) for the communication with the pterygopalatine fossa. The fissures converge medially and immediately above the junction lies the *optic canal* (**12**). From the inferior orbital fissure runs the *infraorbital groove* (**13**), which becomes the *infraorbital canal* to open below the infraorbital margin as the *infraorbital foramen* (**14**).

On the lateral wall the zygomatic nerve passes through a small opening, the *zygomaticoorbital foramen* (**15**). On the medial wall, where the ethmoid bone meets the frontal bone, are the *anterior* (**16**) and *posterior* (**17**) *ethmoidal foramina*. The nerves and arteries of the same name leave through these foramina. The anterior ethmoidal foramen opens into the cranial cavity, while the posterior one leads into the ethmoidal cells. Near the entrance into the orbit lies the *groove for the lacrimal sac* (**18**) which is bounded anteriorly and posteriorly by the *anterior* (**19**) and the *posterior* (**20**) *lacrimal crests*. It leads into the *nasolacrimal canal*, which opens into the nasal cavity (see p. 294).

In the immediate neighborhood of the orbits are the **paranasal sinuses**. The variably sized *orbital recess of the frontal sinus* (**21**) extends into the roof of the orbit. Medially lie the ethmoid cells and dorsally the sphenoidal sinus. Inferiorly the orbit is separated from the maxillary sinus by a thin plate of bone.

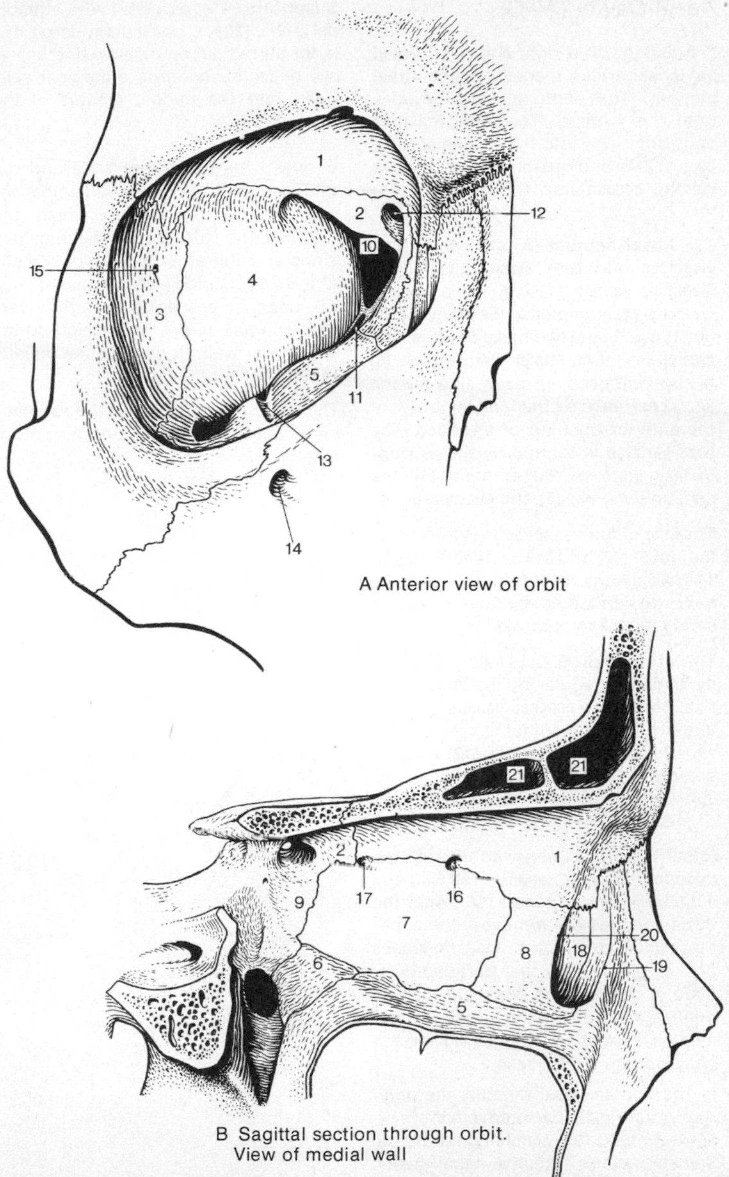

A Anterior view of orbit

B Sagittal section through orbit.
View of medial wall

Nasal Cavity (A–C)

We distinguish a right and a left **nasal cavity** separated medially by the **nasal septum**. The septum often deviates from the midline. The nasal cavities open anteriorly into the **piriform aperture** (see p. 278) and posteriorly each opens via the **choana** into the pharynx (see Vol. 2).

The **nasal septum** (**A**) consists of **cartilaginous** and **bony elements**. The **cartilaginous septum** (**1**) with its *posterior process* (**2**) completes the bony partition between the two nasal cavities. The **medial crus of the major alar cartilage** (**3**) is superimposed on each side on the septal cartilage as the medial border of the anterior opening of the nose. The **bony partition** is formed by the *perpendicular plate of the ethmoid* (**4**), the *sphenoidal crest* (**5**) and the *vomer* (**6**).

The **floor** of the nasal cavity is formed by the *maxilla* (**7**) and the *palatine bone* (**8**). The **roof** is formed anteriorly by the *nasal bone* (**9**), and then by the *cribriform plate* (**10**) *of the ethmoid.*

The **lateral wall (B, C)** of each nasal cavity is made irregular by the **three** turbinate bones, the **conchae nasales** and the underlying ethmoidal cells. The *superior* (**11**) and *middle* (**12**) *concha* belong to the ethmoid bone, while the *inferior concha* (**13**) is a separate bone of the skull.

Posterior to the superior concha lies the *sphenoethmoidal recess* (**14**) with the *sphenopalatine foramen* (**15**). After the three conchae are removed, the superior, middle and inferior nasal meatuses are revealed and the *perpendicular plate of the palatine bone* (**16**) can be completely seen. In the superior nasal meatus there are openings (**17**) into the posterior ethmoidal cells.

In the middle nasal meatus, the *uncinate process* (**18**) partly covers the *maxillary hiatus* (**19**), which connects the maxillary sinus with the nasal cavity. Superior to this process is the ethmoidal bulla (**20**), a particularly large anterior ethmoidal cell. Above and below the bulla the anterior ethmoidal cells open into the middle meatus of the nasal cavity.

Between the ethmoidal bulla and the uncinate process is the *ethmoidal infundibulum* (**21**), across which the *frontal sinus* (**22**), part of the maxillary sinus and the anterior ethmoidal cells (**23**) are connected with the nasal cavity. The uncinate process also partly covers the *lacrimal bone* (**24**) which forms the lateral wall along with the *maxilla* (**7**) and the ethmoid bone.

The *nasal opening* (**25**) *of the nasolacrimal duct* lies in the inferior nasal meatus.

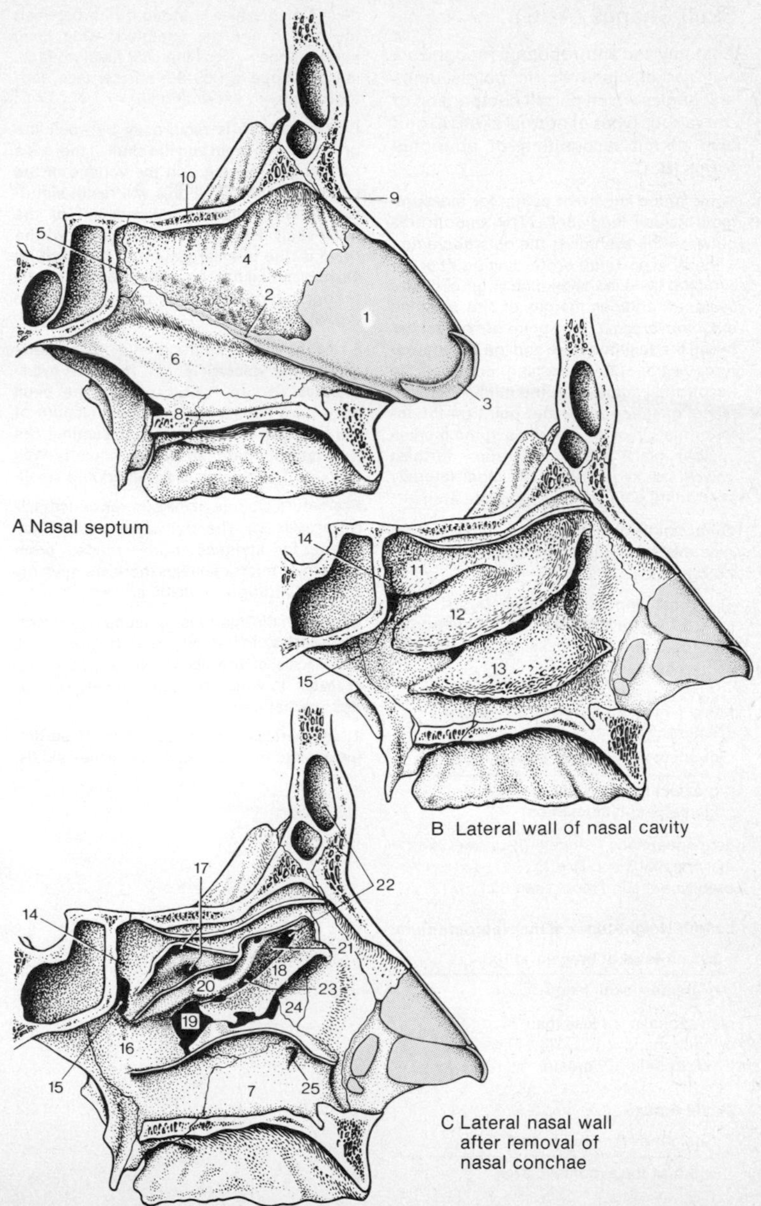

A Nasal septum

B Lateral wall of nasal cavity

C Lateral nasal wall after removal of nasal conchae

Skull Shapes (A–C)

Anatomy and anthropology recognize a number of craniometric points, lines and angles which permit comparison of the various types of normal skull (**A**) and also permit recognition of abnormal forms (**B, C**).

Some of the important points for measurement include: the *glabella* (**1**) = smooth area between the eyebrows; the *opisthocranion* = the most posterior protruding point of the occipital bone in the midline sagittal plane, *basion* = anterior margin of the foramen magnum; *bregma* (**2**) = point of contact between the sagittal suture and the coronal suture; *nasion* (**3**) = crossing point of the nasofrontal suture with the median sagittal plane; *gnathion* (**4**) = that point on the inferior margin of the mandible in the median sagittal plane which protrudes furthest downward; *zygion* (**5**) = the most laterally protruding point of the zygomatic arch.

Other points of measurement, lines and angles may be found in textbooks of anthropology.

The most important indices based on a comparison of the distances between the individual points of measurement are presented below.

Length-Breadth-Index of the Neurocranium:

$$\frac{\text{greatest width of the skull} \times 100}{\text{greatest length of the skull (glabella-opisthocranion)}}$$

dolichocephalic = index (I) under 75;
mesocephalic = I 75–80:
brachycephalic I more than 80.

Length-Height-Index of the Neurocranium:

$$\frac{\text{basion-level of bregma} \times 100}{\text{greatest skull length}}$$

platycephalic = I less than 70;
orthocephalic = 170–75;
hypsicephalic = I greater than 75.

Facial Index:

$$\frac{\text{height of the face} \times 100}{\text{width of the zygomatic arch}}$$

height of the face = straight line between the nasion and the gnathion; wide face, euryprosope = I less than 85; medium face, mesoprosope = I 85–90; narrow face, leptoprosope = I exceeding 90.

Basically there is reciprocity between the growth of the brain and the skull. If there is a pathological increase in the volume of the contents of the skull, this will result simultaneously in marked enlargement of the bony skull. Pathologic enlargement of the brain is due to enlargement of the cerebral cavities, and it may be associated with overproduction of cerebrospinal fluid (see also Vol. 3).

A relatively large neurocranium in comparison to the viscerocranium is called **hydrocephalus** (**B**). In hydrocephalus the skull bones are thin, there is delayed closure of the enlarged fontanelles and the eminences (frontal and parietal) are particularly well marked. The orbits are flattened and small.

Premature closure of the sutures causes **microcephalus** (**C**). The premature closure may result, for instance, from reduced brain growth. In microcephalus there are deep orbits and strong zygomatic arches.

Other malformations include the **scaphocephalus**, in which there is premature synostosis of the sagittal suture, and **oxycephalus**, in which the coronal suture ossifies prematurely.

These various malformations must be distinguished from artificially deformed skulls.

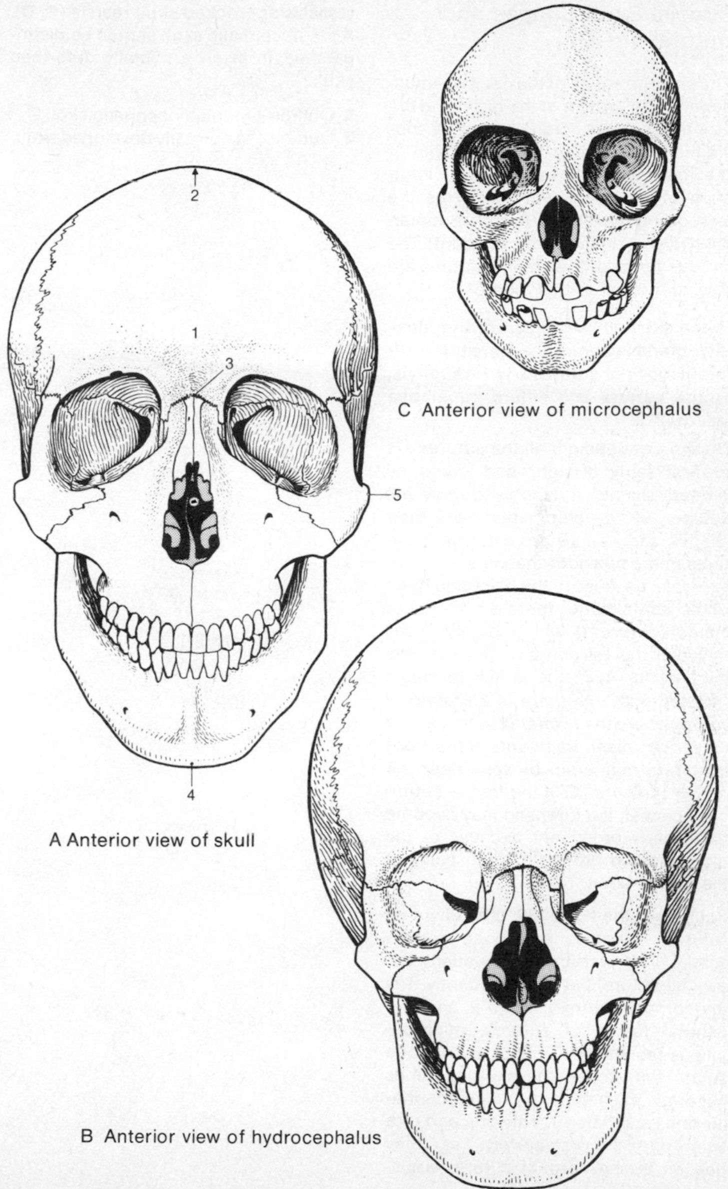

C Anterior view of microcephalus

A Anterior view of skull

B Anterior view of hydrocephalus

Special Skull Shapes and Sutures (A–D)

The size and shape of the neurocranium depends on growth of the brain and the size of the viscerocranium will be substantially influenced by the activity of the masticatory apparatus. The influence of other elements, such as the supporting system of the dura mater, must also be taken into account. The various forms of the cranial sutures are also of interest in this regard.

In the skull, in the region of the intermembranous bones, there are three different types of sutures – **sutura laevis, sutura serrata** and **sutura squamosa** (see p. 22).

During development all the sutures are at first fairly straight and could be termed simple. It is only during the course of development that their shapes alter. There are also more sutures in the newborn than in adults; for example, because of the paired anlagen of the frontal bones there is a *frontal* or *metopic suture* (**1**), which usually closes between the 1st and 2nd years of life. If it persists (**A, B**), the skull is termed a **"crossed skull"**, *as there is a cruciform suture where the frontal* (**2**) *and sagittal* (**3**) *sutures meet. Remnants of the frontal suture may often be seen near the root of the nose* (**4**). If the frontal suture does persist, the forehead may become particularly prominent because of the more marked growth of both parts of the frontal bone.

Roughly at the age of 30, the individual sutures synostose and bone growth ceases. The first to fuse is usually the sagittal suture, but less frequently it is the coronal suture. If there is an early general fusion of sutures, microcephalus results (see p. 296). If only one suture synostoses, the skull becomes abnormal in shape, e.g., scaphocephalus or oxycephalus. If only one part of a suture fuses prematurely, as may happen in the coronal suture, **plagiocephalus** or crooked skull results (**C, D**). A plagiocephalic skull should be distinguished from an artificially deformed skull.

5 Outline of a plagiocephalic skull,
6 Outline of a normally developed skull.

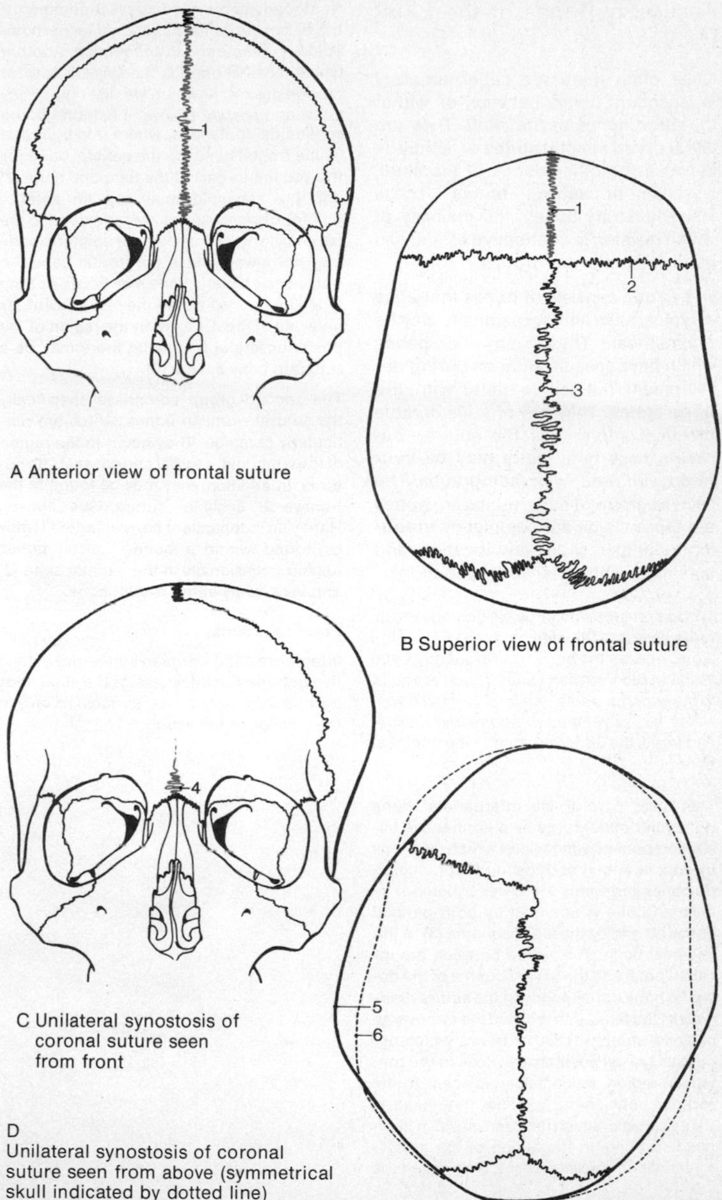

A Anterior view of frontal suture

B Superior view of frontal suture

C Unilateral synostosis of coronal suture seen from front

D
Unilateral synostosis of coronal suture seen from above (symmetrical skull indicated by dotted line)

Accessory Bones of the Skull (A–C)

Quite often there are supernumerary independent bones between or within the other bones of the skull. They are either called **epactal bones** or, if they lie between the other bones of the skull, wormian or **sutural bones**. These supernumerary bones, the majority of which develop in connective tissue, can be divided into two groups.

One group consists of bones that arise at typical sites and occasionally may be symmetrical. These may be bones which have specific anlagen during development but fail to unite with the other bones. They are of considerable practical interest, as the sutures between these bony parts may be confused with fissures in radiographs. The second group of supernumerary bones are those which are completely irregular in number, shape and location, and commonly show individual variations.

To the first group belongs particularly the **incarian bone** (**1**). This term is derived from the word Inca, as the bone has frequently been found in old Peruvian skulls. *It corresponds to the superior part of the interparietal bone, which has developed in connective tissue*, and forms the upper squama of the occipital bone.

The lower part of the interparietal bone (triangular plate) fuses as a connective tissue component with the part which develops by endochondral ossification (supraoccipital bone) and forms the lower squama. The incarian bone is bounded by both parietal bones (**2**) and by the lower squama (**3**) of the occipital bone. The suture between the incarian bone and the lower squama of the occipital bone corresponds to the *sutura mendosa* of the fetus, and is called the *transverse occipital suture* (**4**). Other bones which occur in a typical position are those in the fontanelle region. Immediately adjacent to the incarian bone, in the posterior fontanelle, is the **apical bone**, which may persist as an independent bone. In the region of the greater fontanelle the **bregmatic bone**, also called the frontoparietal bone, occurs less commonly. It is an epactal bone, either circular or rhomboidal in shape, and is uncommon. Another typical epactal bone is the **epipteric bone** or pterion ossicle, in which we distinguish *anterior* and *posterior parts*. It is found in the sphenoidal fontanelle, where it is bounded by the frontal bone (**6**), the parietal bone (**2**), the squamous part of the temporal bone (**7**) and the sphenoid bone (**8**). An anterior epipteric bone may not always extend to the parietal bone, and a posterior epipteric bone may not always reach the frontal bone. An undivided epipteric bone may occur, or both types mentioned above may be present, or only one of them. Lastly, in the region of the posterior lateral fontanelle there may be a separate bony anlage (**9**).

The second group comprises specifically the sutural wormian bones, which are particularly common. They occur in the region of the lambdoid, sagittal and coronal (**10**) sutures. In addition, they may be found in the transverse occipital suture (see above). Rarely an independent bony anlage (**11**) may be found within a bone. Epactal bones appear occasionally in the parietal bone (**2**) and very rarely in the frontal bone.

Practical Points

Intercalated and wormian bones may extend through the full thickness of the skull, they may be seen only on the surface, or only in the interior of the vault.

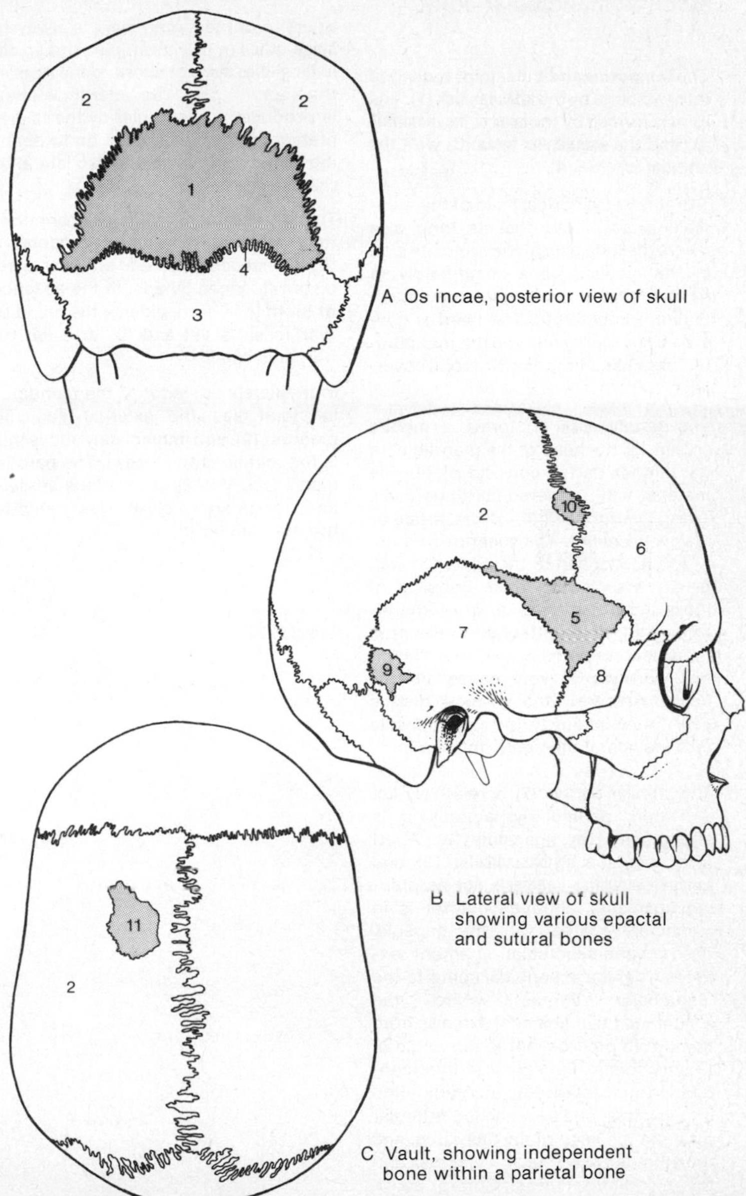

A Os incae, posterior view of skull

B Lateral view of skull showing various epactal and sutural bones

C Vault, showing independent bone within a parietal bone

Temporomandibular Joint (A–B)

The **temporomandibular joint** is divided into two parts by the **articular disk** (**1**). The joint is formed by the **head of the mandible** (**2**) and the **mandibular fossa** (**3**) with the **articular tubercle** (**4**).

The almost cylindrical head of the mandible is so placed that its long axis meets the long axis of the opposite side in the median plane immediately in front of the foramen magnum at an angle of about 160°. The head is covered by fibrocartilage and the mandibular fossa has a fibrocartilaginous covering.

The **articular disk** (**1**) forms a mobile socket for the head of the mandible. In its anterior part it consists of fibrous material with scattered cartilage cells. The *posterior part* (**5**) *of the articular disk is bilaminar.* The superior portion, which is attached to the posterior wall of the mandibular fossa, consists of loose, fibroelastic tissue, while the inferior portion (**6**), **attached** to the posterior margin of the head of the mandible, consists of very dense fibrous tissue. Anteriorly the articular disk is very firmly bound to the joint capsule and the lateral pterygoid muscle.

The **articular capsule** (**7**) is relatively lax and thin, particularly laterally it is strengthened by ligaments (**8**). Apart from this, the **stylomandibular** (**9**) and **sphenomandibular ligaments** act as guiding ligaments, although neither is in immediate contact with the capsule. The sphenomandibular ligament extends from the sphenoidal spine to the mandibular lingula, while the stylomandibular ligament extends from the styloid process (**10**) to the angle of the mandible. Functionally the mandibular joint represents a combination of two joints: one between the articular disk and the head of the mandible, and the other between the articular disk and the mandibular fossa. During active opening of the mouth there is always a **hinge action** in the lower joint and an **anterior gliding movement** toward the front in the superior part. The latter movement is produced in particular by the lateral pterygoid muscle. In addition to opening movements there are also lateral or **chewing movements**.

The temporomandibular joint, or rather its articular surfaces are dependent on the dental occlusion and are, therefore, also influenced by age. In the absence of teeth (newborn, elderly) the mandibular fossa is flat and the articular tubercle is small.

Immediately posterior to the mandibular joint lies the external acoustic meatus (**12**), and immediately above this is the middle cranial fossa. The parotid gland (see Vol. 2) and various vessels and nerves are in close relationship to the mandibular joint.

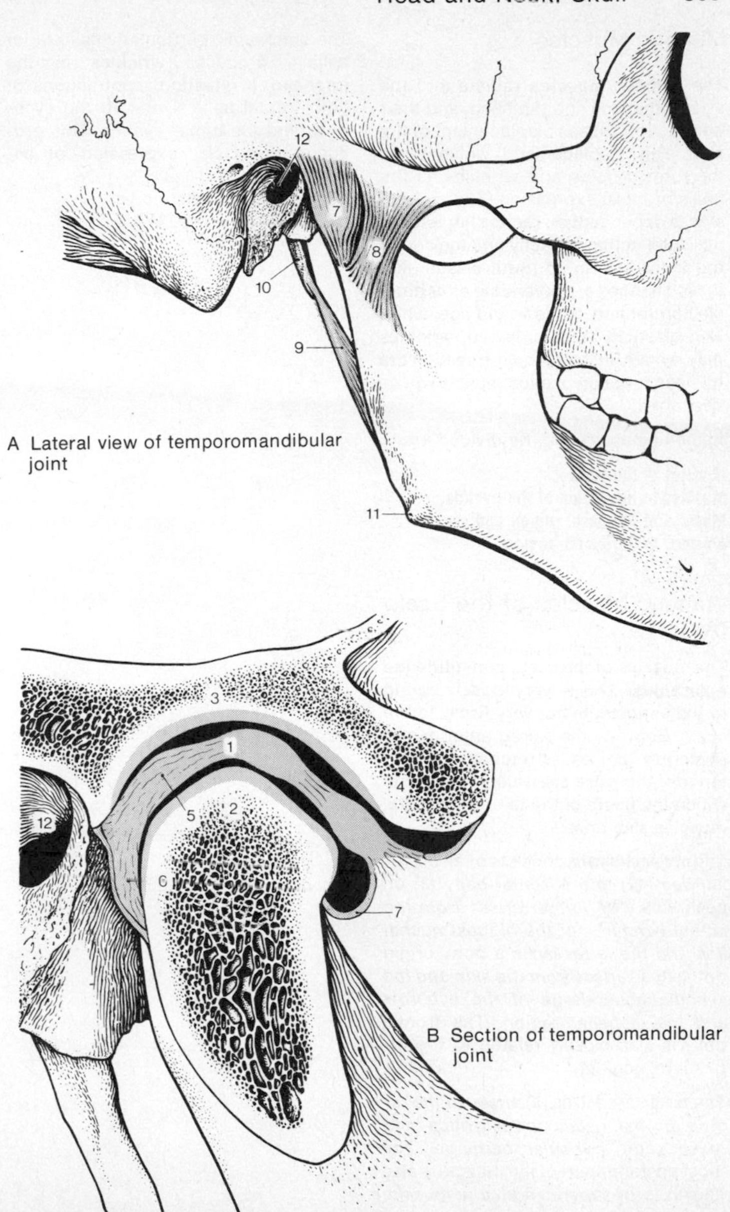

A Lateral view of temporomandibular joint

B Section of temporomandibular joint

Mimetic Muscles

The **mimetic muscles** radiate into the skin of the face and the head, and their contraction causes displacement of the skin. This displacement, which takes the form of folds and wrinkles, is the basis of facial expression. The expression is dependent on racial characteristics, intellectual capacity and the age of the individual. In youthful elastic skin these changes are reversible after muscle contraction, while in old age, when skin elasticity is deminished, wrinkles may remain. In the following section the mimetic function of each muscle will be described.

Mimetic muscles can be divided into:

Muscles of the scalp,
Muscles in the region of the eyelids,
Muscles of the nasal region and
Muscles of the mouth region.

Mimetic Muscles of the Scalp (A–B)

The muscles of the scalp constitute the **epicranius**. This is very loosely bound to the periosteum but very firmly to the scalp. Between the paired anterior and posterior bellies stretches a taut tendon, the **galea aponeurotica** (**1**), from which the fibers of the temporoparietal muscles also arise.

The **occipitofrontalis** consists of an *occipital belly* (**2**) and a *frontal belly* (**3**) on each side. *The former arises from the lateral twothirds of the highest nuchal line and the latter* lacks a bony origin but instead *arises from the skin and the subcutaneous tissue of the eyebrow and the glabellar region.* The frontal belly is also closely related to the orbicularis oculi (**4**).

The **temporoparietalis** (**5**) *arises in the region of the galea aponeurotica and reaches the auricular cartilage.* The most posterior part of the muscle is also known as the *superior auricular muscle.*

The epicranius, particularly its anterior bellies, produces wrinkles in the forehead. In addition, contractions of both frontal bellies may lift the eyebrows and the upper eyelids. This produces the facial expression of astonishment.

Nerve supply: Facial nerve

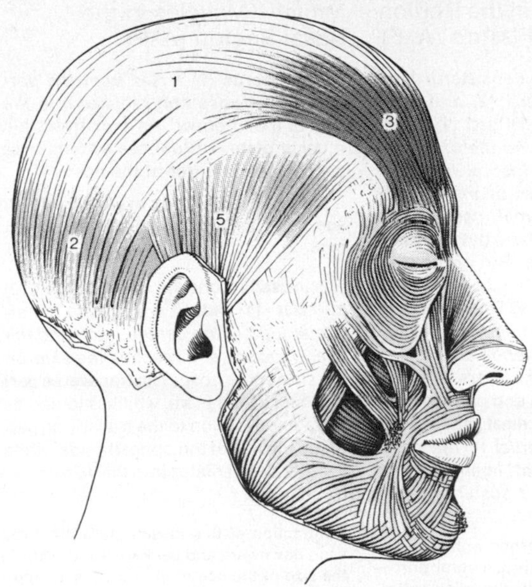

A Lateral view of mimetic muscles of scalp

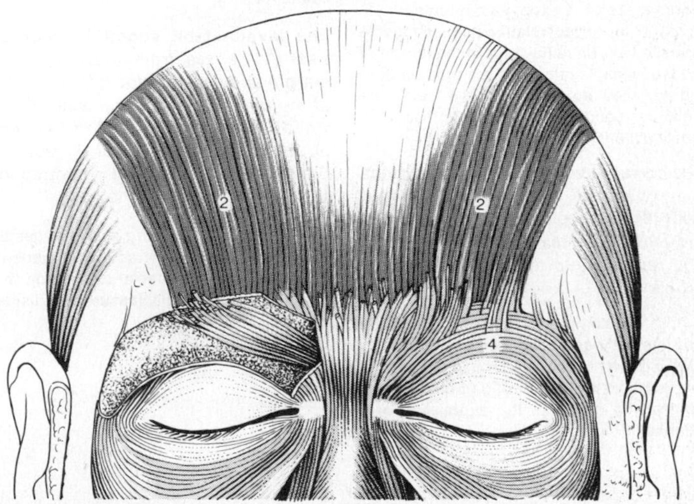

B Anterior view of mimetic muscles of forehead

Mimetic Muscles in the Region of the Palpebral Fissure (A–F)

The **orbicularis oculi** consists of **three parts–orbital** (**1**), **palpebral** (**2**) and **lacrimal** (**3**). The thick **orbital part** (**1**) *is arranged circularly around the orbit and is attached to the palpebral ligament* (**4**), *the frontal process of the maxilla and the anterior lacrimal crest.* In the upper lid the medial fibers of the orbital part fan out in the direction of the eyebrows. These fibers are also known as the *depressor supercilii.* The more delicate **palpebral part** (**2**) *lies immediately on the eyelids and extends also to the palpebral ligament.* The fibers lie partly on the tarsal plates (**5**) and partly on the orbital septum. the **lacrimal part** (**3**; Horner's muscle) *lies medial to the deep crus of the palpebral ligament and arises chiefly from the posterior lacrimal crest* (**6**).

The orbital part is concerned with firm closure of the lid, while the palpebral part is primarily concerned with the blink reflex. The function of the lacrimal part is not fully understood. It is thought to expand the lacrimal sac or to expel its contents.
Through the close relationship of muscle fibers to the skin radial folds in the region of the lateral angle of the eye are produced; in old age they are called "crow's feet". The orbicularis oculi produces an expression of worry (**C**) and concern.

The **corrugator supercilii** (**7**) penetrates the orbicularis oculi and the frontal belly (**8**) of the epicranius. *It arises from the glabella and the supraorbital margin and radiates into the skin of the eyebrows.*

It pulls the skin of the eyebrows downward and medially and produces a vertical furrow. It has a protective action in bright light and is called the muscle of pathetic pain. Its contraction produces the expression of a "thinker's brow" (**D**).

Mimetic Muscles in the Nasal Region (A–F)

The **procerus** (**9**) *arises from the dorsum of the nose and radiates into the skin of the forehead.* As a relatively thin muscle plate it produces a transverse fold across the root of the nose.

It produces a menacing expression. In old age these folds normally become permanent.

The **nasalis** consists of **transverse** (**10**) and **alar** (**11**) **parts**. *It arises from the alveolar juga of the canine tooth and the lateral incisor, and reaches the skin on the side of the nose.* The transverse part is a thin, broad plate, which is joined by a flattened tendon to the transverse part of the muscle of the opposite side, while the alar part radiates into the skin on the nasal wing.

Contraction of this muscle pulls the nasal wing downward and backward and reduces the size of the nostril. It produces a happy, astonished expression and gives the impression of desiring, demanding and sensuousness (**E**).

The **levator labii superioris alaeque nasi** (**12**) *arises from the infraorbital margin and extends down into the skin of the upper lip and nasal wing.* It elevates not only the skin of the nasal wing but also that of the upper lip upward. Simultaneous bilateral contraction slightly lifts the tip of the nose.

It elevates the nasal wing and enlarges the nostrils. Stronger contractions produce a fold in the skin. The facial expression thus produced is one of displeasure and discontent (**F**).

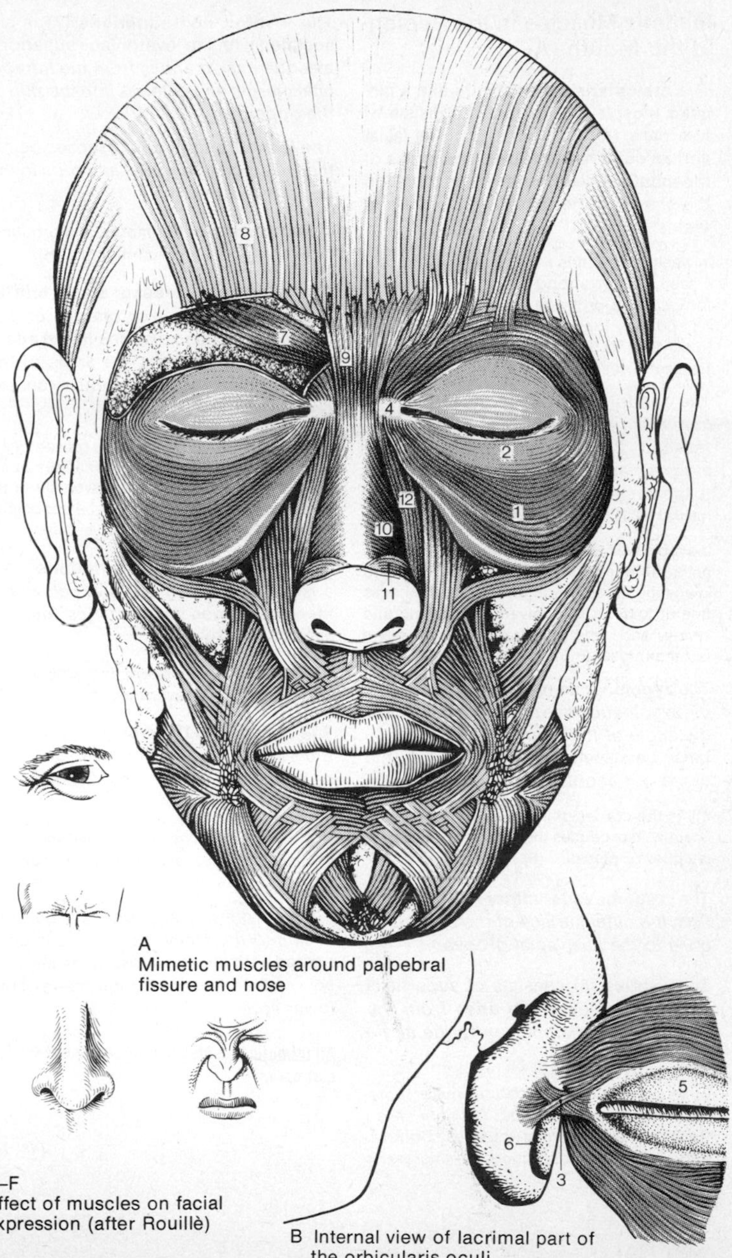

A
Mimetic muscles around palpebral fissure and nose

C–F
Effect of muscles on facial expression (after Rouillè)

B Internal view of lacrimal part of the orbicularis oculi

Mimetic Muscles in the Region of the Mouth (A–L)

The **orbicularis oris** appears like a circular muscle, but in fact it consists of four parts (**A**). It also has an inner **labial** and an outer **marginal part**. The shape of the mouth is determined by its tone and the shape of the underlying bone and teeth.

In weak contraction the lips are in contact or closed, while in strong contraction they pout forward and protrude in a sucking shape. The primary function of this muscle is seen in eating and drinking. Mimetically its contraction gives an expression of reserve (**D**).

The quadrilateral **buccinator** (**2**) *arises from the mandible in the region of the 1st and 2nd molars and from the pterygomandibular raphe* (**3**). It extends to the angle of the mouth and forms the lateral wall of its vestibule.

It enables air to be blown out of the mouth, pulls the angle of the mouth laterally and keeps the mucous membrane of the cheeks free of folds. It is involved in laughing and crying, and, when contracted, produces a facial expression of satisfaction (**E**).

The **zygomaticus major** (**4**) *arises from the zygomatic bone and extends toward the angle of the mouth.* Some of its fibers decussate with those of the depressor anguli oris.

It lifts the corner of the mouth upward and laterally. It produces the facial expression of laughter or pleasure (**F**).

The **zygomaticus minor** (**5**) *extends from the outer surface of the zygomatic bone to the nasolabial groove.*

The **risorius** (**6**) consists of superficial muscle bundles which *arise from the masseteric fascia and run to the angle of the mouth*

Together with the zygomaticus major it produces the nasolabial folds. They are called, therefore, the laughing muscles. Contraction of the muscle produces an expression of action (**G**).

The **levator labii superioris** (**7**) is associated with the levator labii superioris alaeque nasi. *It arises from the infraorbital margin and extends into the skin of the upper lip.*

The **levator anguli oris** (**8**) *arises below the infraorbital foramen and runs to the angle of the mouth.*

It lifts the angle of the mouth and produces an expression of self-confidence (**H**).

The triangular **depressor anguli oris** (**9**) *arises from the lower margin of the mandible and also extends to the angle of the mouth.* It pulls the angle of the mouth downward to produce an expression of sadness (**1**).

The **transversus menti** is only present as a specialization of the depressor anguli oris, a few fibers of which run transversely in the region of the chin and may be associated with the formation of a double chin.

The **depressor labii inferioris** (**10**) *arises from the mandible below the mental foramen and radiates into the skin of the lower lip.*

It pulls the lower lip down and produces an expression of perseverance (**K**).

The **mentalis** (**11**) *arises from the mandible in the region of the alveolar jugum of the lateral incisor and radiates into the skin of the chin.*

It produces the chin-lip furrow and is responsible for an expression of doubt and indecision (**L**).

The **platysma** (**12**) *radiates from the neck into the facial region* and is connected with the risorius and the depressors of the angle of the mouth and of the lower lip.

All mimetic muscles are innervated by the facial nerve.

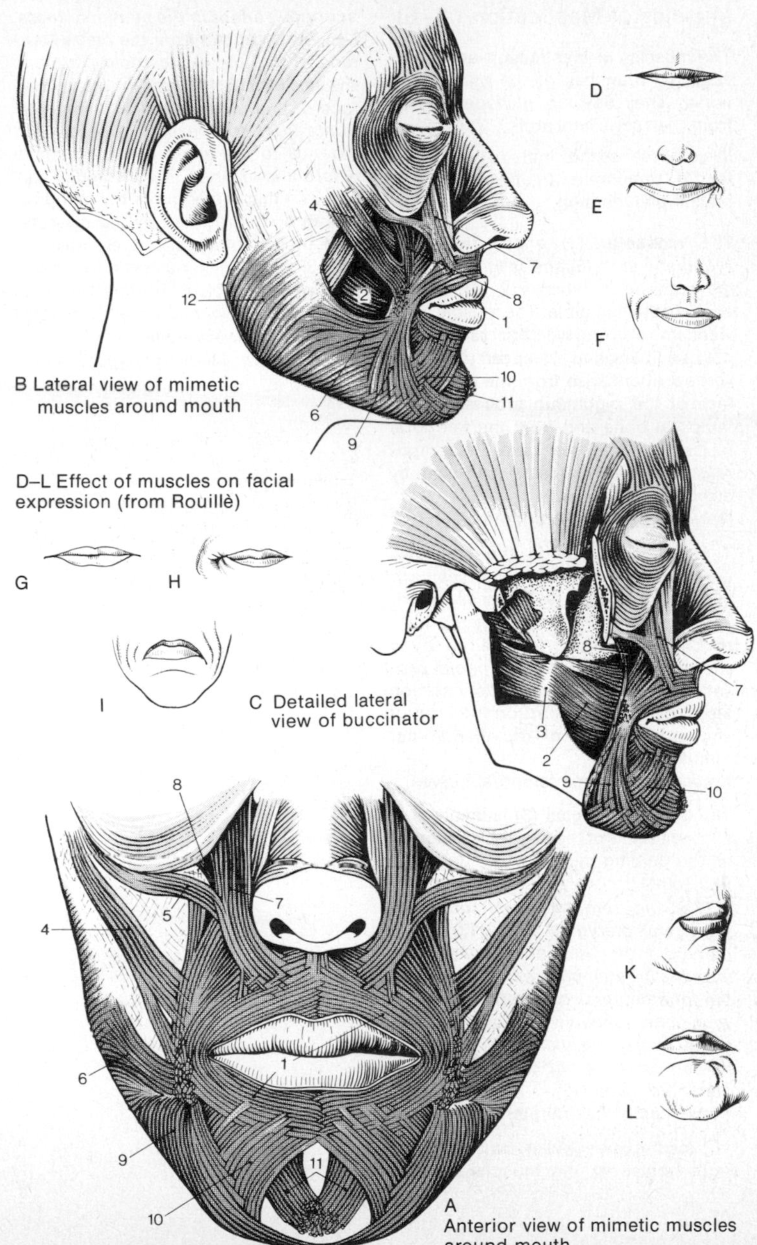

B Lateral view of mimetic muscles around mouth

D–L Effect of muscles on facial expression (from Rouillè)

C Detailed lateral view of buccinator

A Anterior view of mimetic muscles around mouth

Muscles of Mastication (A–E)

The muscles of mastication are innervated by branches of the mandibular nerve. They develop phylogenetically from the 1st visceral arch.

In a strict sense they include the masseter (**1**), temporalis (**2**), lateral (**3**) and medial pterygoid (**4**).

The **masseter** (**1**) *arises from the zygomatic arch* (**5**) *and is inserted into the masseteric tuberosity* (**6**) on the angle of the mandible. The muscle is divided into a strong **superficial part** (**7**) with oblique fibers, and a **deep part** (**8**) whose vertical fibers arise from the inner surface of the zygomatic process of the temporal bone and from the temporal fascia. The masseter, like the temporalis, powerfully closes the jaws by elevating the mandible.
Nerve supply: Masseteric nerve.

The **temporalis** (**2**) is the strongest elevator of the lower jaw, *It arises from the temporal fossa* (**9**) *as far as the inferior temporal line and from the temporal fascia* (**10**). *It is inserted by a strong tendon into the coronoid process of the mandible* (**11**). Its insertion also extends downward on the interior and anterior side of the mandibular ramus.
Nerve supply: Deep temporal nerves.

The **lateral pterygoid** (**3**) is involved in all movements of the mandible. It serves as the guiding muscle of the mandibular joint. It consists of **two parts, one** (**12**) *arising from the lateral surface of the lateral pterygoid plate* (**13**) *of the pterygoid process* and the **other** (**14**) *from the infratemporal surface* (**15**) *and the infratemporal crest of the greater wing of the sphenoid. The latter part extends to the articular disk, while the former part is inserted into the pterygoid fovea* (**16**).
Nerve supply: Lateral pterygoid nerve.

The **medial pterygoid** (**4**) runs almost at right angles to the muscle just described. *It arises in the pterygoid fossa, i.e., the* **larger part** *from the medial surface of the lateral pterygoid plate* and the **smaller part** (**17**) *from the lateral surface of that plate as well as with a few fibers from the maxillary tuberosity. It extends to the angle of the mandible where it is inserted into its medial surface,* so that the angle of the mandible lies in a sling formed by the masseter and medial pterygoid. It elevates the mandible and also pushes it forward. It may also be involved in lateral displacement of the lower jaw and participate in rotational movements.
Nerve supply: Medial pterygoid nerve.

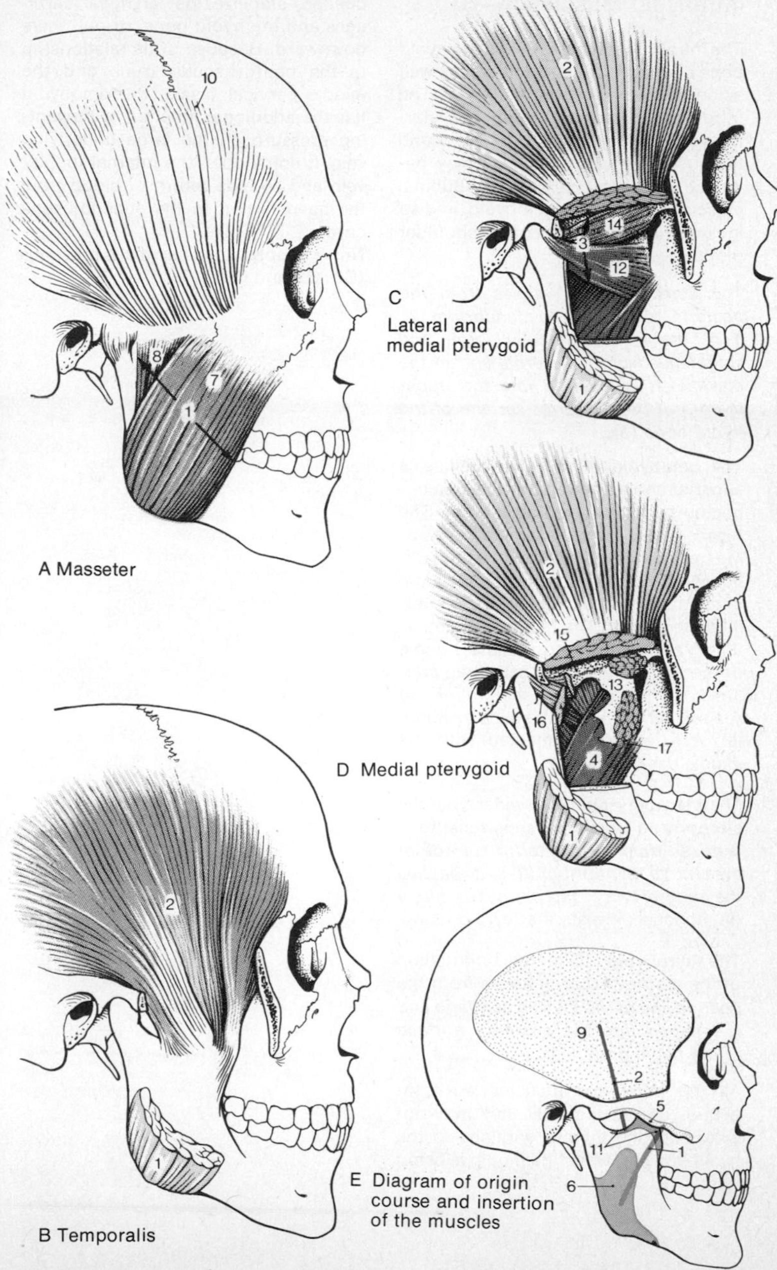

A Masseter

B Temporalis

C Lateral and medial pterygoid

D Medial pterygoid

E Diagram of origin course and insertion of the muscles

Infrahyoid Muscles (A–B)

The infrahyoid muscles act on the hyoid bone and thus on the mandible, as well as on the cervical vertebral colum. The infrahyoid muscles include the sternohyoid, omohyoid, sternothyroid and thyrohyoid. Phylogenetically, they belong to the great ventral longitudinal muscle system. The omohyoid is also included in the muscles of the shoulder girdle (see p. 142).

The **sternohyoid** (**1**) *arises from the posterior surface of the manubrium* (**2**), *from the sternoclavicular joint, and sometimes from the sternal end of the clavicle. It is inserted into the upper margin of the posterior surface of the hyoid bone* (**3**).

The **omohyoid** (**4**) has two bellies, a superior and an inferior, which are connected by an intervening tendon. The **superior belly** *arises from the body of the hyoid bone* (**5**); its fibers extend obliquely downward into the lateral region of the neck, where they end in the intermediate tendon. The tendon lies superficially across the neurovascular bundle of the neck. The **inferior belly** then *continues to the superior margin of the scapula adjacent to the scapular notch* (**6**). It is closely connected with the middle cervical fascia.

The **sternothyroid** (**7**) is wider than the sternohyoid which lies superficial to it. *It arises from the posterior surface of the sternal manubrium* (**8**) *and reaches the oblique line of the thyroid cartilage* (**9**). It closely invests the thyroid gland.

The **thyrohyoid** (**10**) is the continuation of the sternothyroid. *It arises from the oblique line of the thyroid cartilage and is inserted into the posterior surface of the hyoid bone* (**11**).

All the infrahyoid muscles work together, and specifically they may approximate the thyroid cartilage to the hyoid bone or, when the mouth is being opened, stabilize the laryngeal cartilages and the hyoid bone, or pull them downward. Because of its relationship to the neurovascular trunk and the middle cervical fascia, the omohyoid has the additional function of preventing pressure on the large underlying vein. It holds open the internal jugular vein and so aids return of blood from the head region to the superior vena cava.

Nerve supply: Ansa cervicalis profunda (C1, C2 and C3).

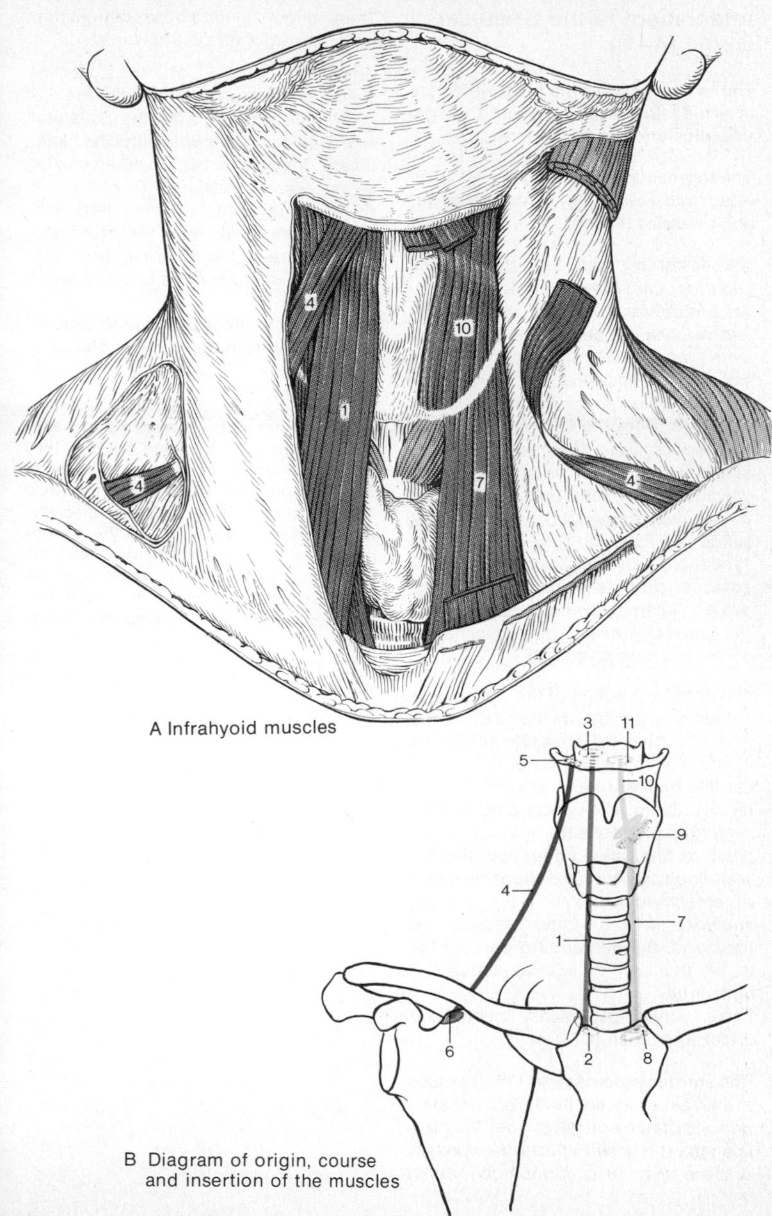

A Infrahyoid muscles

B Diagram of origin, course and insertion of the muscles

Attachment to the Shoulder Girdle (A–C)

The two muscles of the head which are inserted into the shoulder girdle are the trapezius and sternocleidomastoid.

The **trapezius** (**1**; see also p. 142) is divided into **descending** (**2**), **transverse** (**3**) and **ascending** (**4**) **parts**.

The descending part *arises from the superior nuchal line, the external occipital protuberance* (**5**) *and the ligamentum nuchae* (**6**; see p. 56) *and is inserted into the lateral third of the clavicle* (**7**). The **transverse part** *arises from the 7th cervical to the 3rd thoracic vertebrae* (**8**; from the spinous processes and supraspinous ligaments) *and is inserted into the acromial end of the clavicle* (**9**), *the acromion* (**10**) *and part of scapular spine* (**11**). The **ascending part** *arises from the 2nd or 3rd to the 12th thoracic vertebrae* (**12**); from the spinous processes and the supraspinous ligaments) *and is inserted onto the spinal trigone and the adjacent part of the scapular spine* (**13**).

The primary function of the trapezius is a static one: it supports the scapula and thus stabilizes the shoulder girdle. Its contraction pulls the scapula and the clavicle backward and toward the vertebral column. The descending and ascending parts rotate the scapula. In addition to producing adduction, the descending part produces slight elevation of the shoulder, assisting the serratus anterior. If the latter muscle is paralyzed, the descending part is able to lift the arm to a little above the horizontal.
Nerve supply: Accessory nerve and trapezius branch (C2–C4).

The **sternocleidomastoid** (**14**; see also p. 142) *arises by* **one head** *from the sternum* (**15**) *and by the* **other** *from the clavicle* (**16**). *It is inserted into the mastoid process and the superior nuchal line.* There it has a tendinous connection with the origin of the trapezius.

Unilateral action of the sternocleidomastoid turns the head to the opposite side and bends it to the ipsilateral side. Bilateral contraction lifts the head. Finally, the sternocleidomastoid can be an accessory muscle of respiration if the head is fixed and the intercostal muscles are paralyzed. If the intercostal muscles are still functioning, however, the sternocleidomastoid is not brought into action.
Nerve supply: Accessory nerve and fibers C1–C2 from the cervical plexus.

Variants

Since the sternocleidomastoid and trapezius develop from the same material, they sometimes remain in a close relationship. The insertion of the trapezius to the clavicle may be considerably extended medially, and conversely the origin of the sternocleidomastoid may be displaced laterally. In this case the greater supraclavicular fossa, which is bordered by these two muscles and the clavicle, is reduced in size.

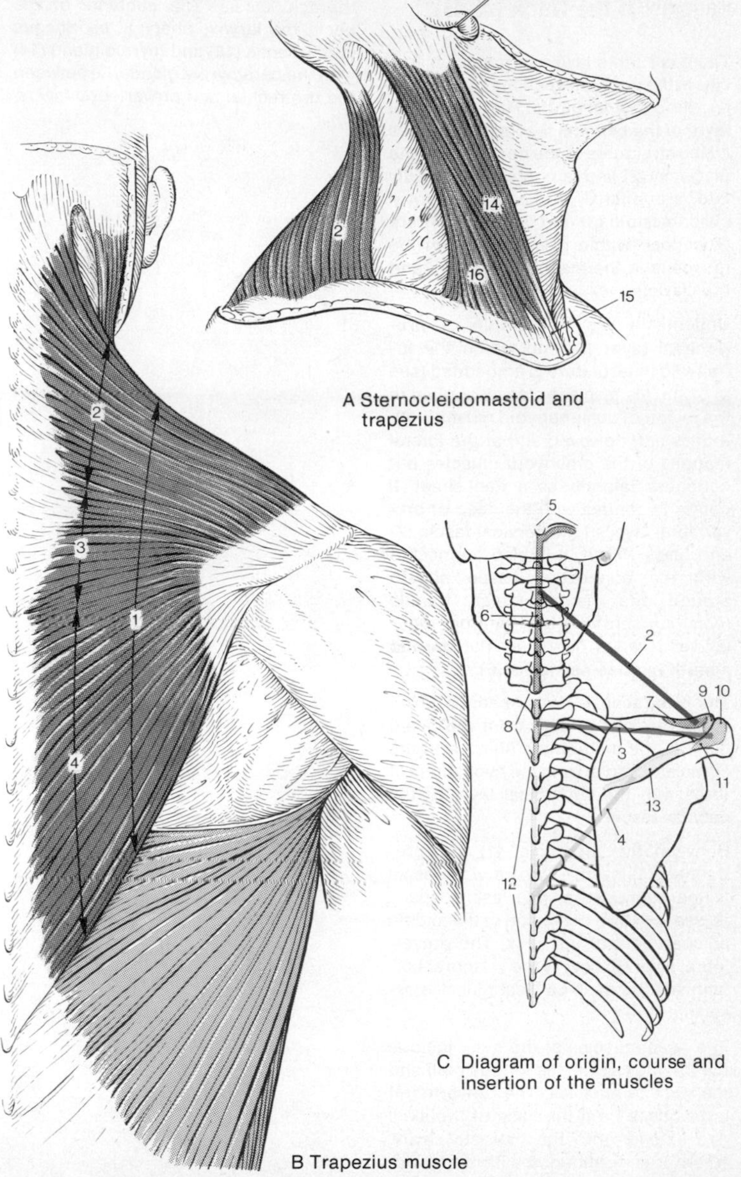

A Sternocleidomastoid and trapezius

B Trapezius muscle

C Diagram of origin, course and insertion of the muscles

Fascias of the Neck (A–B)

There are three layers of muscular fascias in the neck between the hyoid bone and the shoulder girdle. The **superficial layer of the cervical fascia** (**1**) encloses all the structures of the neck except the platysma (**2**) and is continued dorsally into the nuchal fascia. The sternocleidomastoid (**3**) and trapezius (**4**) are embedded within. It extends from the mandible to the manubrium sterni and the clavicles.

Underneath lies the **middle** or **pretracheal layer** (**5**) into which the infrahyoid musculature is embedded (see p. 312). This fascia is closely applied in the region of the infrahyoid muscles (**6**). It does not, however, end at the lateral margins of the omohyoid muscles but continues laterally as a thin sheet. It comes in contact with the deep or prevertebral layer of the cervical fascia (**7**) and fuses with it. It is also connected with the connective tissue sheath around the neurovascular bundle (common carotid artery, internal jugular vein, vagus nerve) as the **carotid sheath** (fasciae cervicalis; **8**).

The pretracheal layer extends in a craniocaudal direction from the hyoid bone to the manubrium sterni and the clavicles. Cranial from the hyoid bone, it fuses with the superficial layer of the cervical fascia.

Between the superficial (**1**) and pretracheal (**5**) layers of the cervical fascia is the suprasternal interfascial space (**9**; see p. 340) in the region of the middle compartment of the neck. The prevertebral layer (**7**) covers the vertebral column and the deep cervical muscles associated with it.

The deep muscles of the neck include the longus capitis, the longus colli and the scalene muscles. The prevertebral layer arises from the base of the skull and extends into the thoracic cavity, where it is continuous with the endothoracic fascia. The contents of the neck, the larynx, pharynx, esophagus (**12**), trachea (**13**) and thyroid gland (**14**) with the parathyroid glands, lie between the pretrachial and prevertebral layers.

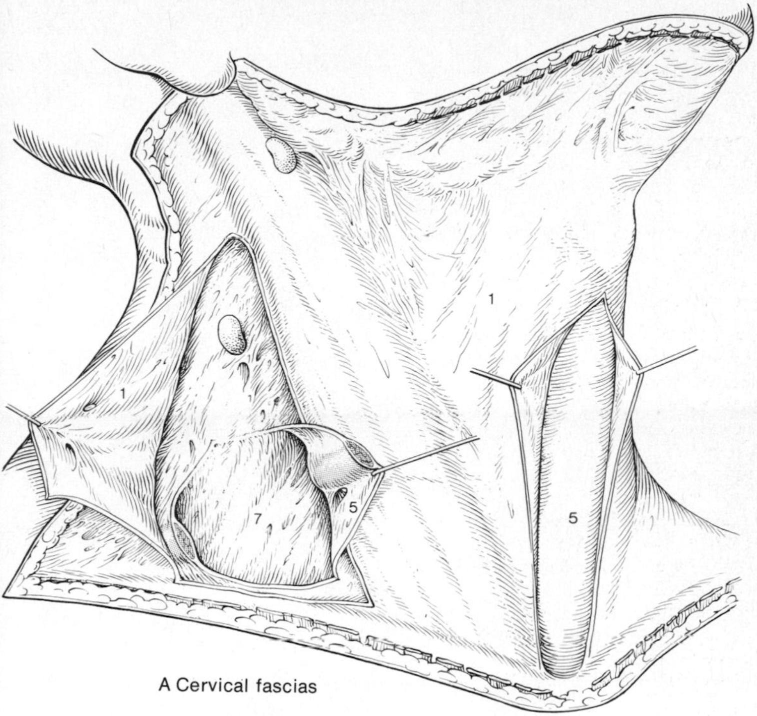

A Cervical fascias

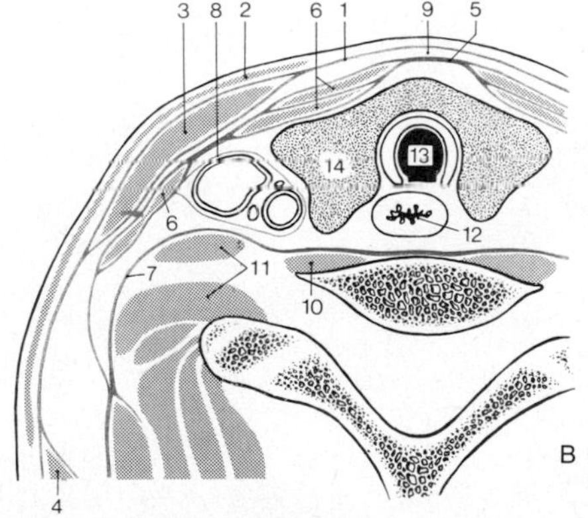

B Section through the neck to show the cervical fascias

Topography of Peripheral Pathways

Regions (A–B)

The head is separated from the neck by a line beginning at the chin continuing over the angle of the mandible, the mastoid process and the superior nuchal line to reach the external occipital protuberance.

The neck is separable from the trunk by the jugular notch of the sternum and the clavicles. Dorsally no precise boundary line can be defined.

Regions of the Head

The **frontal region** (**1**) comprises the forehead up to the coronal suture. Adjacent to it over the parietal bone on each side, is the **parietal region** (**2**), and over the temporal squama lies the **temporal region** (**3**). The **infratemporal region** (**4**) is covered by the zygomatic arch. Dorsally the **occipital region 5**) lies over the occipital bone.

The various regions of the face are the **nasal region** (**6**), the **oral region** (**7**) and the **chin or mental region** (**8**). The **orbital region** (**9**) lies around the eyes, the **infraorbital region** (**10**) is the area lateral to the nose, and the **buccal region** (**11**) is lateral to the oral region. The **zygomatic region** (**12**) lies about the zygomatic bone, and the **parotid-masseteric region** (**13**) contains the masseter muscle and the parotid gland.

Regions of the Neck

The **neck** is divided into a **posterior region** (**14**) and ventrolateral regions. The latter is divided by the **sternocleidomastoid region** (**15**) into an unpaired **anterior neck region** and the paired lateral regions of the neck. The anterior neck region includes the area between the lower jaw and the anterior margins of both sternocleidomastoids. It can be further subdivided. In the center lies the **middle neck region** (**16**), which is limited by the hyoid bone, the omohyoids and sternocleidomastoids, and inferiorly by the jugular notch of the sternum. The depressed part of the middle neck region, which lies just above the sternal jugular notch, is designated the *suprasternal fossa* (**17**). The **suprahyoid region** (**18**) extends between the hyoid bone and the chin region. Laterally it is separated from the **submandibular triangle** (**19**) by the anterior belly of the digastric muscle. This triangular area is limited cranially by the mandible. It might be helpful to use the angular tract of the cervical fascia to separate the submandibular triangle from its superoposterior part, the **retromandibular fossa** (**20**), which contains the cervical part of the parotid gland and the trunk of the facial nerve. The **carotid triangle** (**21**) is of great practical importance as it contains the bifurcation of the common carotid artery. It is limited cranially by the posterior belly of the digastric muscle, anteriorly by the superior belly of the omohyoid and dorsally by the sternocleidomastoid.

The **lateral region of the neck** (**22**) or **posterior triangle of neck** ends anteriorly at the sternocleidomastoid, posteriorly at the trapezius and inferiorly at the clavicle. The omoclavicular triangle, or *greater supraclavicular fossa or triangle* (**23**), deserves special mention in this area. It is limited by the sternocleidomastoid, the inferior belly of the omohyoid and the clavicle. In thin individuals it may also be possible to see the *lesser supraclavicular (triangle) fossa* (**24**) between the two heads of the origin of the sternocleidomastoid.

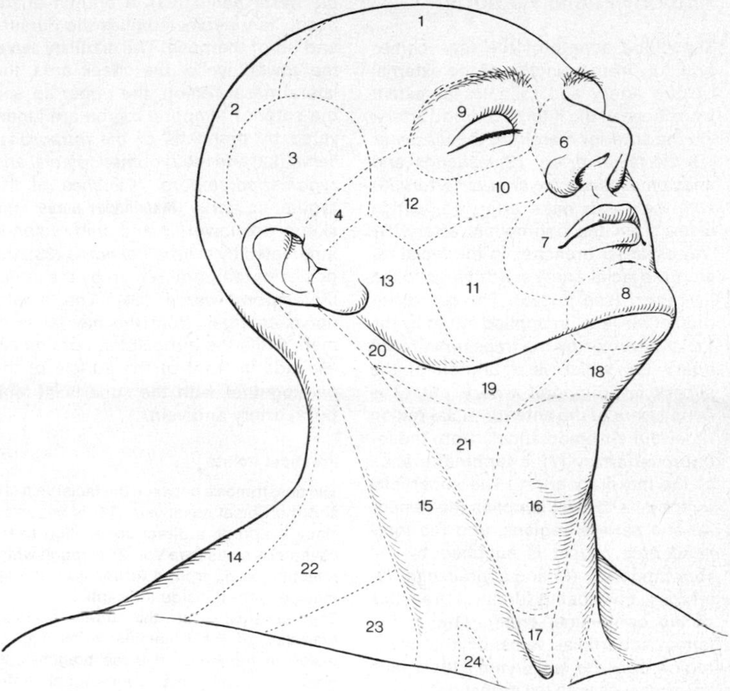

A Lateral view of regions of head and neck

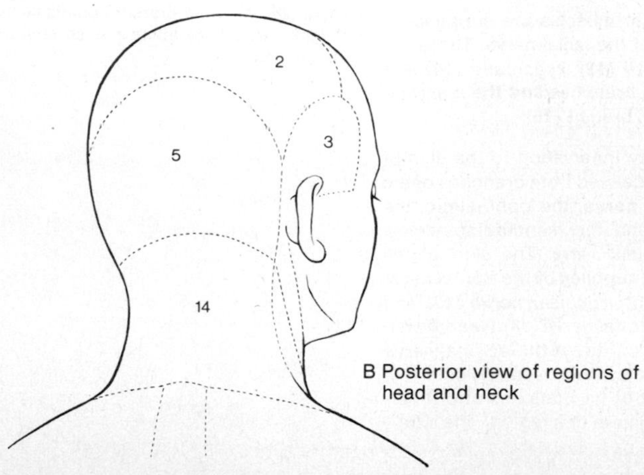

B Posterior view of regions of head and neck

Anterior Facial Regions

The blood supply of the face comes primarily from branches of the external carotid artery and to a lesser extent from those of the internal carotid artery. On the anterior margin of the *masseter* (**1**), the *facial artery (***2**) ascends and anastomoses via the *angular artery* (**3**) with the *dorsal nasal artery* (**4**), which stems from the ophthalmic artery. By way of larger branches in the facial region, the facial artery sends twigs to the lip-region (see p. 326). The lateral region of the face is supplied either by the facial artery or by the *transverse facial artery* (**5**), which is a branch of the *superficial temporal artery* (**6**). The deep layers of the anterior facial region receive their blood supply from the *infraorbital artery* (**7**), a terminal branch of the maxillary artery. The superficial temporal artery (**6**) supplies the temporal and parietal regions, and the forehead area proper is supplied by the *supratrochlear* (**8**) and *supraorbital* (**9**) *arteries*, both being terminal branches of the ophthalmic artery. Among the larger superficial veins of the facial region only the *facial vein* (**10**), which anastomoses with the *dorsal nasal vein* (**11**) and the *superficial temporal vein* (**12**) lie superficially.

The mimetic muscles are supplied by branches of the facial nerve. These are the *temporal* (**13**), *zygomatic* (**14**) and *buccal* (**15**) branches and the *marginal mandibular branch* (**16**).

The sensory innervation to the skin of the face is derived from branches of the **trigeminal nerve**, the ophthalmic, the maxillary and the mandibular nerves. The **ophthalmic nerve:** The skin of the forehead is supplied by the frontal nerve with its *supratrochlear nerve* (**17**) and the *supraorbital nerve* (**18**). Near the lateral corner of the eye the *lacrimal nerve* (**19**) penetrates the orbicularis oculi (**20**) with a few of its branches and innervates the skin in this region. The *external nasal nerve* (**21**), a branch of the nasociliary nerve, supplies the dorsum and tip of the nose. The **maxillary nerve:** the lower eyelid, the cheek area, the lateral nasal region, the upper lip and the anterior temporal region are innervated by branches of the *infraorbital nerve* (**22**) and the *zygomaticofacial* and *zygomaticotemporal branches* of the zygomatic nerve. **Mandibular nerve:** the skin of the lower lip and chin region is innervated by the *mental nerve* (**23**), the posterior temporal region by the *auriculotemporal nerve* (**24**). The mental nerve emerges from the mental foramen, while the auriculotemporal nerve ascends in front of the auricle of the ear together with the superficial temporal artery and vein.

Practical Points

The anastomosis between the facial vein (**10**) and the dorsal nasal vein (**11**) is important since it affords a direct connection to the cavernous sinus (see Vol. 2), through which infection, e. g., from a furuncle on the lip, may be carried inside the skull.

The sensitivity of the three principal branches of the trigeminal nerve can be tested in the twigs of these branches. As pressure points the supraorbital notch serves for the supraorbital nerve (**18**), the infraorbital foramen for the infraorbital nerve (**22**) and the mental foramen for the mental nerve (**23**). All three pressure points lie in a roughly vertical line, about 2–3 cm lateral to the midline.

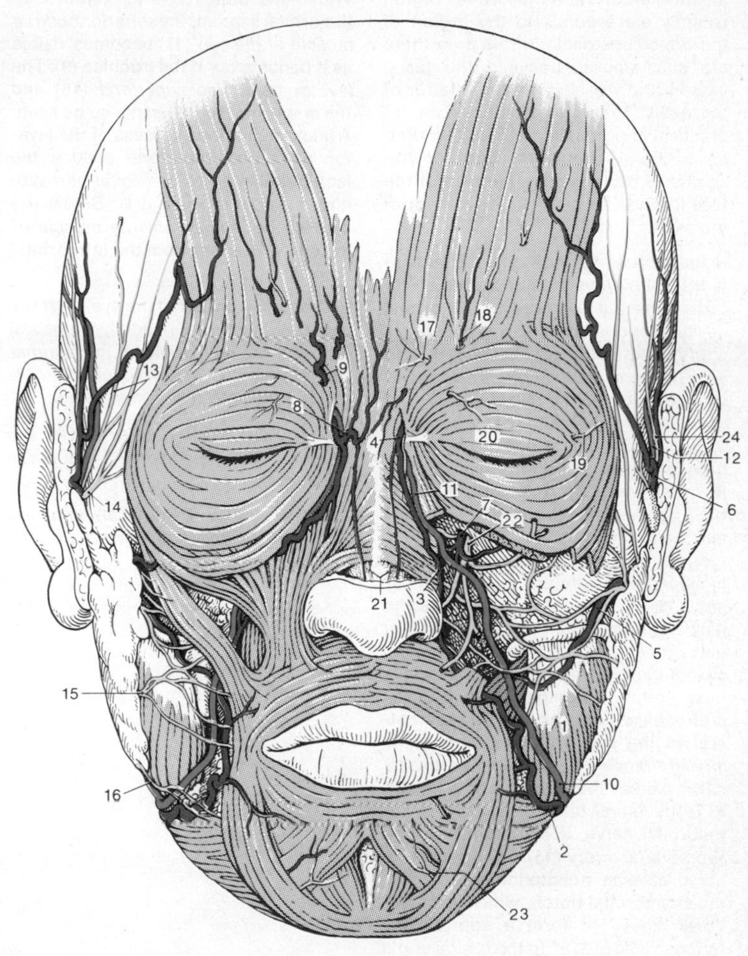

A Anterior view of facial region

Orbital Region (A–B)

In an anterior view the orbital region roughly corresponds to the region of the orbicularis oculi. In this area there are anastomoses between the facial vessels and vessels from the interior of the skull. These anastomoses are of practical importance, both as a source of collateral circulation and for the spread of bacteria from the skin of the face through the veins to the interior of the skull.

In the **orbital region** (**A**) the *orbital septum* (**1**) separates the superficial structures from the contents of the orbital cavity. Superficially the vessels are a continuation of the *facial artery and vein* (**2**), namely the *angular artery and vein* (**3**). The *dorsal nasal artery and vein* (**5**) lie in front of the *palpebral ligament* (**4**). The dorsal nasal artery may branch from the *supratrochlear artery* (**6**) outside (see figure) or within the orbit. Together with the dorsal nasal artery, the *infratrochlear nerve* (**7**) also pierces the orbital septum. It often anastomoses with the *supratrochlear nerve* (**8**), which is only separated from it by the *trochlea* (**9**). The supratrochlear nerve innervates the skin of the medial part of the forehead and the root of the nose and is accompanied by the *supratrochlear artery and veins* (**10**). Lateral to the supratrochlear nerve, the *medial branch* (**11**) of the supraorbital nerve pierces the septum and adjacent to it the *lateral branch* (**12**) of the supraorbital nerve, accompanied by the *supraorbital artery* (**13**). This artery and nerve leave an indentation in the bone, the supraorbital notch, which is sometimes closed to form a supraorbital foramen (see p. 278). In the lateral angle of the eye, branches of the *lacrimal nerve* (**14**) pierce the orbital septum. The upper eyelid is innervated by these nerves and by branches of the frontal nerve. The lower eyelid is innervated by branches of the *infraorbital nerve* (**15**), which emerges from the infraorbital foramen together with the *infraorbital artery* (**16**).

Within the **orbit** (**B**), after removal of the orbital septum, the *superior oblique muscle of the eye* (**17**) becomes visible as it bends around the trochlea (**9**). The *levator palpebrae superioris* (**18**) and the *tarsal muscle* (**19**) can also be seen. A lateral tendinous process of the levator palpebrae superioris divides the lacrimal gland into an *orbital part* (**20**) and a *palpebral part* (**21**). Below the eyeball the *inferior oblique muscle of the eye* (**22**) arises from the infraorbital margin.

In the medial corner of the eye, after the outer limb of the (medial) palpebral ligament has been divided, the *lacrimal sac* (**23**) with the *lacrimal canaliculi* (**24**) which open into it become visible.

25 Cut edge of the lateral part of the tendon of the levator palpebrae superioris,

26 Outer limb of the (medial) palpebral ligament, divided and reflected.

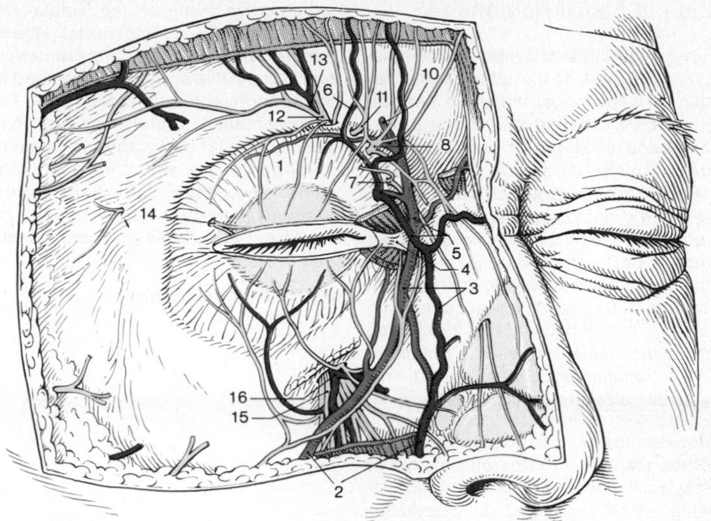

A Orbital region, orbital septum

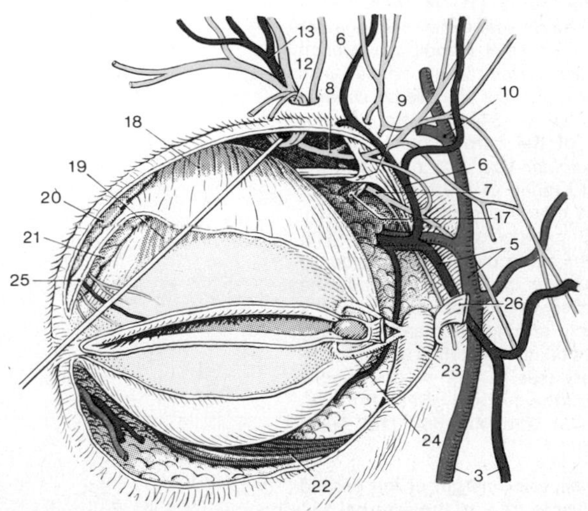

B Orbital region, lacrimal apparatus, vessels and nerves in the orbit

Lateral Facial Regions (A)

The **parotidomasseteric region** is the most important part of the lateral facial region. In it lies the parotid gland (see Vol. 2) which is differentiated into a superficial and a deep part. Anteriorly the *parotid gland* (**1**) lies on the *masseter muscle* (**2**) and posteriorly it occupies the retromandibular fossa. At the anterior margin of the parotid gland the *parotid* or *Stensen's duct* (**3**) leaves the gland and turns deeply down in front of the *buccal fat pad* (**4**). It is accompanied by the somewhat variably developed *transverse facial artery* (**5**), a branch of the *superficial temporal artery* (**6**). This supplies blood to parts of the face.

Between the superficial and deep parts of the gland lies the parotid plexus of the facial nerve, whose branches, as *temporal* (**7**) *zygomatic* (**8**), *buccal* (**9**) and *marginal mandibular* (**10**) *become visible on the superior and anterior border of the gland and run to the mimetic muscles.* At the inferior border of the parotid gland the *cervical branch of the facial nerve* (**11**) is seen, which sometimes runs for a distance together with the marginal mandibular branch and which forms the superficial ansa cervicalis with the transverse cervical nerve (see p. 344). At the inferior margin of the parotid gland the *retromandibular vein* (**12**) runs with the cervical branch of the facial nerve or with the marginal mandibular branch. This vein is joined by the *facial vein* (**13**) as it runs along the anterior border of the masseter muscle (**2**). Usually the *facial* artery (**14**) passes in front of the facial vein around the mandible (bony pressure point). It extends as the angular artery (see p. 322) to the medial corner of the eye and gives off the *inferior* (**15**) and *superior* (**16**) *labial arteries.*

On the superior margin of the parotid gland, just in front of the external ear, runs the superficial temporal artery (**6**), which, after giving off the middle temporal artery, divides into *frontal* (**17**) and *parietal* (**18**) *branches*. It may run a very tortuous course and is accompanied by the *superficial temporal vein* (**19**). The parietal branch (**18**) follows a branch of the mandibular nerve, the *auriculotemporal nerve* (**20**), which innervates the skin of the posterior temporal region. *Superficial parotid lymph nodes* (**21**) are found in variable numbers, usually just in front of the auricle.

22 Great auricular nerve,
23 Platysma.

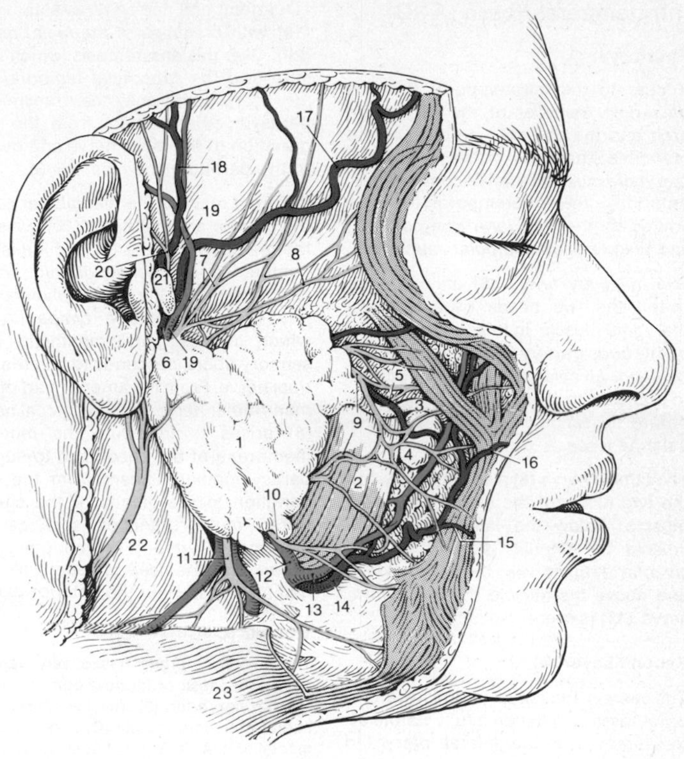

A Parotidomasseteric region

Infratemporal Fossa (A–G)

First Layer (A)

Access to the infratemporal fossa is gained by removal of the zygomatic arch and the coronoid process of the mandible. The *lateral* (**1**) and *medial* (**2**) *pterygoid muscles* then become visible. Anteriorly, the infratemporal fossa is limited by the *maxillary tuberosity* (**3**) and the *pterygomandibular raphe* (**4**).

The *maxillary artery* (**5**) may run between the two heads of the lateral pterygoid muscle. In this region it gives off the *buccal artery* (**6**) and the *superior posterior alveolar artery* (**7**) in addition to branches to the masticatory muscles, before descending into the pterygopalatine fossa.

The *buccal nerve* (**8**) also runs between the two heads of the lateral pterygoid muscle. Below the lateral pterygoid muscle the *lingual* (**9**) and *inferior alveolar* (**10**) *nerves* become visible, and above the muscle the *masseteric nerve* (**11**) is seen.

Second Layer (B)

The vessels and nerves of the infratemporal fossa only become fully visible after removal of the lateral pterygoid muscle and the condylar process of the mandible. The maxillary artery (**5**) lies lateral to the *sphenomandibular ligament* (**12**) and to the large branches of the *mandibular nerve* (**13**) and may be followed throughout its entire length. In its mandibular part it gives off the *anterior tympanic artery* (**14**), the *deep auricular artery* (**15**) and the *middle meningeal artery* (**16**), which reaches the interior of the skull through the foramen spinosum.

The middle meningeal artery is surrounded by the two roots of the *auriculotemporal nerve (***17**), which often receives additional fibers (**18**) from the inferior alveolar nerve (**10**). The auriculotemporal nerve (**17**) anastomoses (**19**) with branches of the *facial nerve* (**20**). Over this anastomosis, which may surround the *superficial temporal artery* (**21**), there may be transmitted parasympathetic fibers from the otic ganglion to the facial nerve and over it to the parotid gland (see Vol. 3).

Before it reaches the mandibular canal the inferior alveolar nerve (**10**) gives off the *mylohyoid nerve* (**22**), which is accompanied by the *mylohyoid artery* (**23**), a branch of the *inferior alveolar artery* (**24**). The *chorda tympani* (**25**), which carries parasympathetic and sensory fibers, descends to join the lingual nerve. From the anterior part of the mandibular nerve (**13**), the buccal nerve (**8**) arises to innervate the mucous membrane of the cheek and to supply parasympathetic fibers from the otic ganglion to the glands of the cheek. Purely motor branches, such as the masseteric nerve (**11**), the pterygoid nerves and the *deep temporal nerves,* (**26**) arise also from the anterior part.

Variants (C–G)

The maxillary artery has a very variable course because of its development. Thus, the maxillary artery (**5**) often lies lateral to the lateral pterygoid muscle (**C**) and less often medial to it (**A, D**). When it does lie medially, the artery usually runs to the pterygopalatine fossa, lateral (**E**) to the inferior alveolar nerve (**10**) and the lingual nerve (**9**), but medial to the buccal nerve (**8**). However, the artery may run between the branches (**F**) or, more rarely, medial to the trunk of the mandibular nerve (**G**).

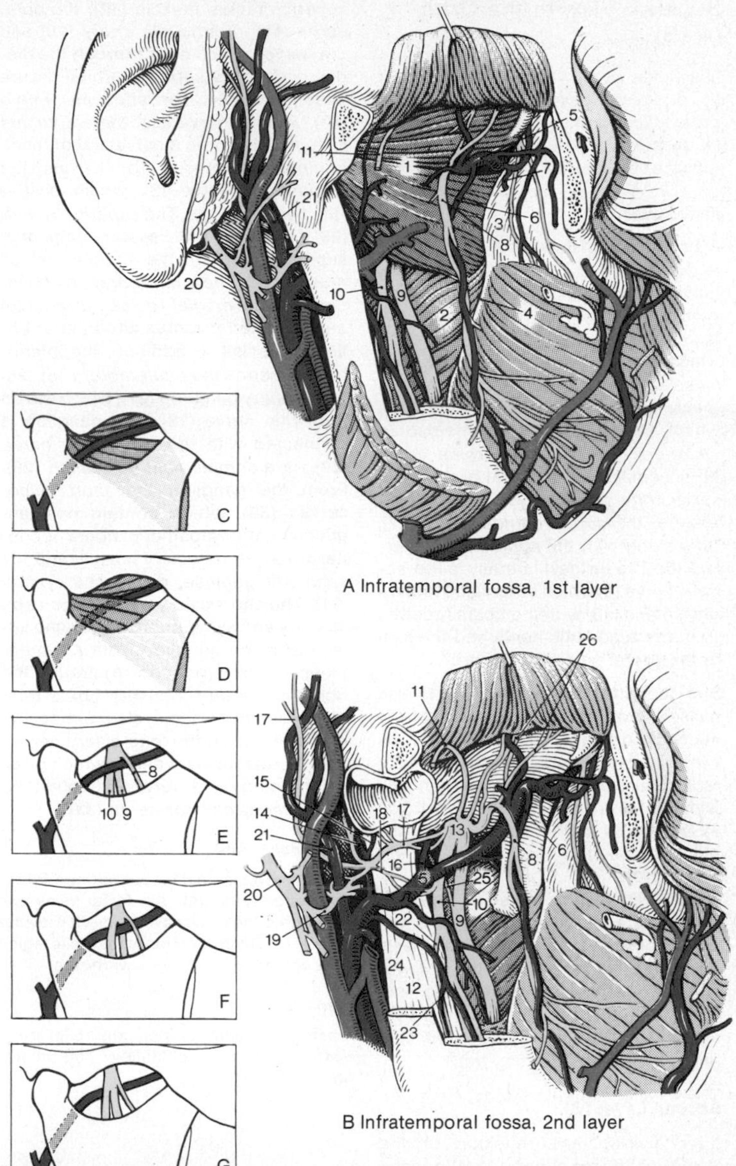

A Infratemporal fossa, 1st layer

B Infratemporal fossa, 2nd layer

C–G Variants of maxillary artery

Superior View of the Orbit (A–B)

Only a few of the vessels and nerves of the orbit can be seen in an anterior approach and a clear view of their relationships can be gained only by removal of the roof of the orbit.

First Layer (A)

After removal of the orbital roof and the periorbita, it is possible to see the nerves which run through the lateral part of the superior orbital fissure; the most medial is the *trochlear nerve* (**1**), which innervates the *superior oblique muscle of the eye* (**2**). Alongside runs the relatively thick *frontal nerve* (**3**), which lies on the *levator palpebrae superioris* (**4**). The *supraorbital artery* (**5**) accompanies its lateral branch, the *supraorbital nerve* (**6**), while the medial branch, the *supratrochlear* nerve (**7**), runs along with the *supratrochlear artery* (**8**). The furthest laterally is the *lacrimal nerve* (**9**) which innervates the *lacrimal gland* (**10**) with the fibers received from the zygomatic nerve and the skin at the lateral corner of the orbit.

The superior *opthalmic vein* (**11**) also passes through the lateral part of the superior orbital fissure. One of its tributaries crosses below the *superior rectus muscle* (**12**) having anastomosed with the external facial veins (see p. 322) in the region of the *trochlea* (**13**); the other branch runs together with the *lacrimal artery* (**14**), which may give off small branches to muscles, and the *short posterior ciliary arteries* (**B, 15**). Covered by the superior oblique muscle (**2**) on the medial side lie the *anterior ethmoidal artery and nerve* (**16**), and superior to this muscle and more posteriorly run the *posterior ethmoidal artery and nerve* (**17**).

Second Layer (B)

After division and reflexion of the levator palpebrae superioris (**4**) and the superior rectus muscle (**12**), the *optic nerve* (**18**), *ophthalmic artery* (**19**) and the nerves which pass through the medial part of the superior orbital fissure become visible. The *abducens nerve* (**20**), which innervates the *lateral rectus muscle* (**21**), is the most lateral of them. Immediately medial to it runs the *oculomotor nerve* (**2**), which divides into two branches. The *superior branch* (**23**) supplies the levator palpebrae superioris (**4**) and the superior rectus muscle (**12**). The *inferior branch (***24**) innervates the *medial rectus muscle* (**25**) and the inferior rectus and inferior oblique muscles. In addition, the inferior branch sends the *oculomotor root* (**26**) to the *ciliary ganglion* (**27**), which lies on the optic nerve (**18**). The ganglion is connected with the *nasociliary nerve* (**29**) via a *communicating branch* (**28**). From the ganglion the *short ciliary nerves* (**30**), which contain postganglionic parasympathetic fibers for innervation of the ciliary muscle and the sphincter pupillae, run to the *eyeball* (**31**). The short ciliary nerves also carry sensory and sympathetic fibers, the latter reach the ganglion from a sympathetic network (not shown) around the ophtalmic artery. Sensory fibers from the nasociliary nerve also run to the eyeball through the *long ciliary nerves* (**32**). The nasociliary nerve, which gives off the ethmoidal nerves, is continued as the *infratrochlear nerve* (**33**).

Practical Points

The superior ophthalmic vein is important as it anastomoses with the facial veins and opens into the sinus cavernosus. It provides a route by which infection in the facial region may spread to the sinus cavernosus.

Variants

There is sometimes a *meningoorbital artery* (**34**) joining the ophthalmic and middle meningeal arteries.

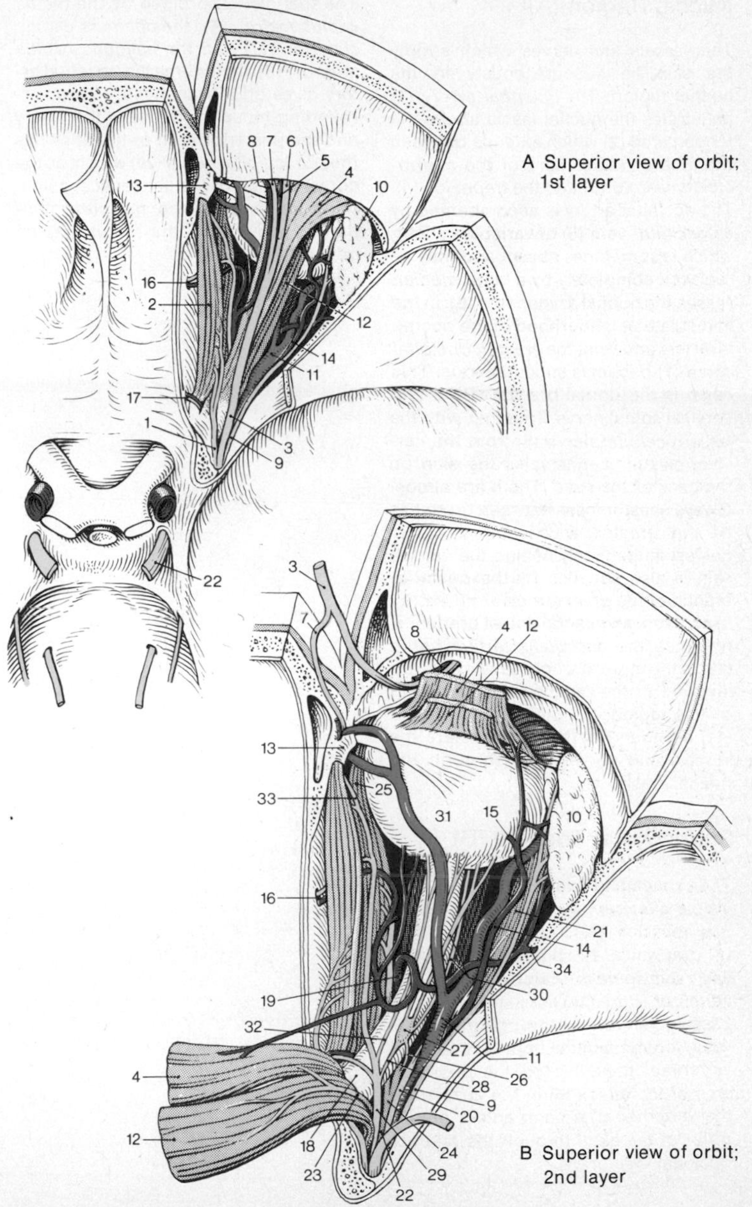

A Superior view of orbit; 1st layer

B Superior view of orbit; 2nd layer

Nuchal Region (A)

The vessels and nerves which supply the skin lie subcutaneously in the nuchal region. The *occipital artery* (**1**) penetrates the nuchal fascia above the tendon arch (**2**) which extends between the area of attachment of the *sternocleidomastoid* (**3**) and the *trapezius* (**4**). The occipital artery is accompanied by an *occipital* vein (**5**) of variable caliber, which is sometimes absent and may be replaced completely by a *large median vessel*, the nuchal azygos vein (**6**). In the immediate neighborhood of the occipital artery and vein, the *greater, occipital nerve* (**7**) becomes subcutaneous. This nerve is the dorsal branch of the 2nd cervical spinal nerve. Together with the *lesser occipital nerve* (**8**) from the cervical plexus, it innervates the skin on the back of the head. There are almost always anastomoses between branches of the greater and lesser occipital nerves. Immediately behind the ear the skin is also supplied by the posterior branch of the *great auricular nerve* (**9**). In addition, segmental dorsal branches, of which the *occipitalis tertius nerve* (**10**) is the more strongly developed, are involved in the cutaneous innervation of this region. *Occipital lymph nodes* (**11**) are found at the points where the vessels and nerves pass through the nuchal fascia.

Suboccipital Triangle (B)

The suboccipital triangle only becomes visible after removal of all the superficial muscles (A; sternocleidomastoid [**3**], trapezius [**4**], *splenius capitis* [**12**] and *semispinalis* **capitis** [**13**]). The *vertebral artery* (**14**) lies in this region. It passes cranialward through the transverse foramina of the upper six cervical vertebrae, then lies on the *posterior arch of the atlas* (**15**) in the groove for the vertebral artery and enters the interior of the skull through the atlanto-occipital membrane.

The triangle is bordered by the *rectus capitis major* (**16**), the *obliquus capitis superior* (**17**) and the *obliquus capitis inferior* (**18**). In this area the vertebral artery gives off a branch (**19**) to the surrounding muscles. Between the artery and the posterior arch of the atlas lies the *suboccipital nerve* (**20**) which, as the dorsal branch of the 1st cervical spinal nerve, innervates the muscles mentioned above and the *rectus capitis minor* (**21**).

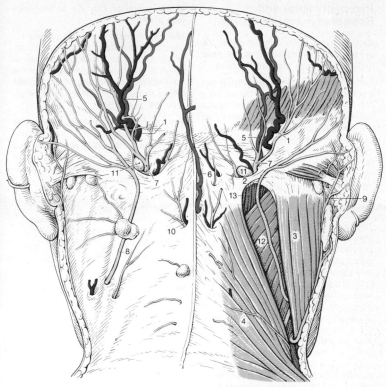

A Nuchal region; left: subcutaneous layer
right: subfascial layer

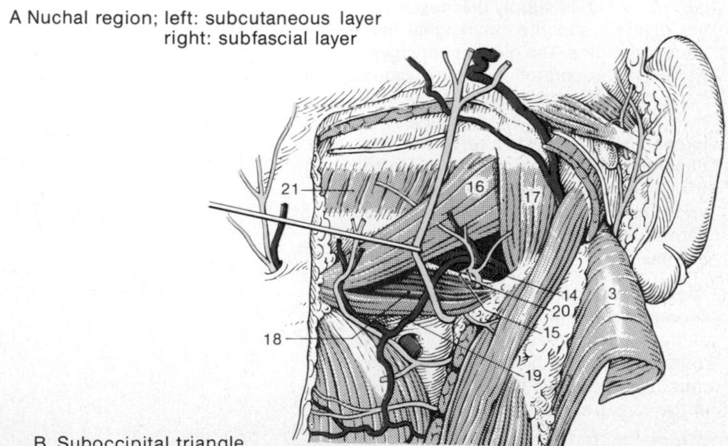

B Suboccipital triangle

Parapharyngeal and Retropharyngeal Spaces (A)

Lateral to and behind the pharynx, the vessels and nerves between the head and the trunk run through the neck.

Furthest dorsally lies the *sympathetic trunk* (**1**), which divides at the *superior cervical ganglion* (**2**), into the *jugular nerve* (**3**) and the *internal carotid nerve* (**4**). While the carotid nerve follows the *internal carotid artery* (**5**), the jugular nerve turns toward the *inferior ganglion* (**6**) of the *vagus nerve* (**7**). In addition, there are connections to the *hypoglossal nerve* (**8**) and to the *carotid body* (**9**), which also receives fibers from the *nerve to the carotid sinus* (**10**).

The vagus nerve (**7**) passes through the jugular foramen and developes a superior and inferior ganglion. It descends between the internal carotid artery (**5**) and the *internal jugular vein* (**11**). In addition to small branches and anastomoses, the vagus nerve running medial to the internal carotid artery gives off the *superior laryngeal nerve* (**12**) which divides into an *external* (**13**) and an *internal* (**14**) *branch*. Other branches include the *pharyngeal rami* (**15**), which run along with the *pharyngeal branches* (**16**) of the *glossopharyngeal nerve* (**17**) to supply the muscles of the pharynx and the pharyngeal mucous membrane. The glossopharyngeal nerve (**17**), separated from the vagus nerve (**7**) and the *accessory nerve* (**19**) by a bridge of dura (**18**), transverses the jugular foramen and, after giving off pharyngeal branches and the nerve to the carotid sinus (**10**), runs caudalward and anteriorly between the internal carotid (**5**) and *external carotid* (**20**) arteries.

The accessory nerve (**19**) usually takes a course dorsal to the *superior bulb* (**21**) of the internal jugular vein (**11**). Then it runs laterally and passes through the *sternocleidomastoid* (**22**), or medial to it in the lateral region of the neck, also called posterior triangle of the neck (see p. 346).

The hypoglossal nerve (**8**) passes toward the front lateral to both carotid arteries. Immediately below the base of the skull it receives fibers (**23**) from the 1st and 2nd cervical segments. It gives off the *superior root of the ansa cervicalis* (**24**; see p. 348).

The external carotid artery gives off its dorsal branch, the *ascending pharyngeal artery* (**25**) which ascends alongside the pharynx, and reaches the base of the skull by its branch, the posterior meningeal artery.

26 Pharyngobasilar membrane,
27 Pharyngeal raphe,
28 Constrictor pharyngis superior,
29 Constrictor pharyngis medius,
30 Constrictor pharyngis inferior,
31 Stylopharyngeus,
32 Facial nerve,
33 Thyroid gland,
34 Superior parathyroid gland (right).

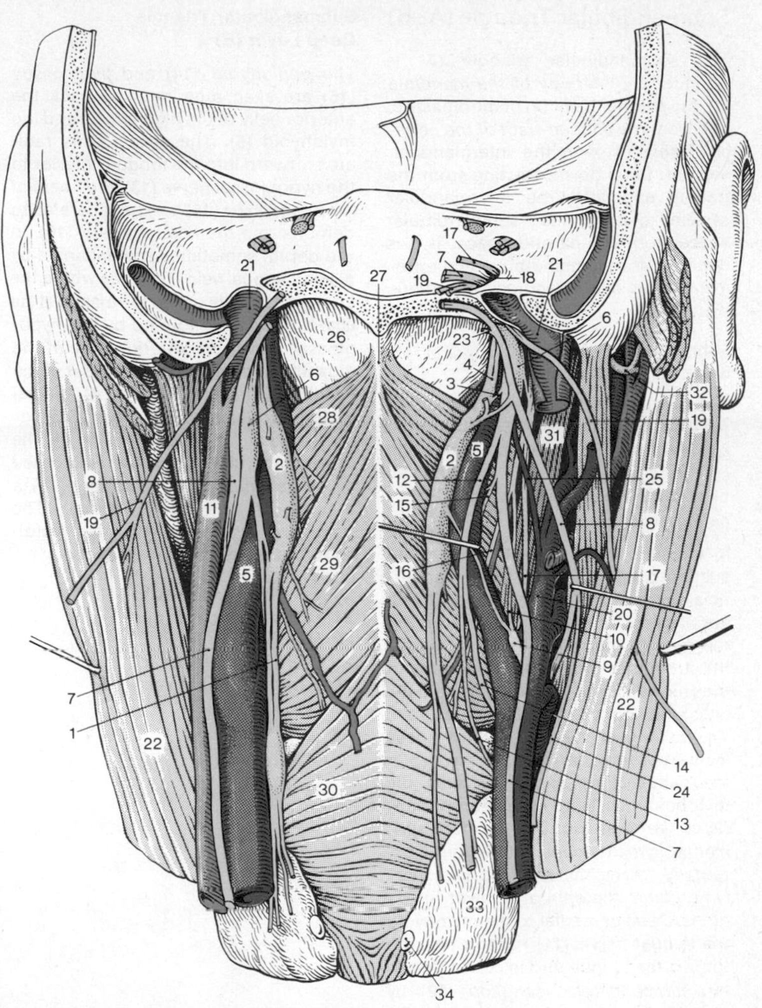

A Retropharyngeal and parapharyngeal space

Submandibular Triangle (A–B)

The submandibular triangle (**A**) is bounded by the *body of the mandible* (**1**), the *anterior belly* (**2**) of the *digastric*, and from the *angular tract of the cervical fascia* (**3**) with the interglandular septum. Deep down, starting from the tractus angularis, the interglandular system divides the submandibular space from the parotid space. If it is removed, the submandibular and retromandibular fossa become continuous (**B**).

Submandibular Triangle Superficial Layer (A)

The *submandibular gland* (**4**) lies superficial to the *mylohyoid* (**5**), around the posterior margin of which winds the *submandibular duct* (**6**) accompanied by a more or less well developed *uncinate (deep) process.*

In addition, the mylohyoid divides the submandibular triangle into a superficial and a deep compartment. The *facial artery and vein* (**7**) pass through the gland. The facial artery gives off the *submental artery* (**8**), which runs to the chin superficial to the mylohyoid (**5**), accompanied by the submental vein. The *mylohyoid nerve* (**9**), which arises from the inferior alveolar nerve lies in the same plane and innervates the mylohoid muscle and the anterior belly (**2**) of the digastric. One or more *submental lymph nodes* (**10**) adhere externally to the mylohyoid and collect lymph from the chin and lower lip regions. Deep or medial to the mylohyoid the *lingual nerve* (**11**) runs in an arch toward the tongue and is connected to the *submandibular ganglion* (**12**) by *ganglionic branches. Glandular branches* run from the ganglion to the submandibular gland. The submandibular duct (**6**) runs in the immediate vicinity of the ganglion together with the *hypoglossal nerve* (**13**) and a *vena comitans* (accompanying vein) *of the hypoglossal nerve.*

Submandibular Triangle Deep Layer (B)

The *geniohyoid* (**14**) and *hyoglossus* (**15**) are seen after bending back the anterior belly of the digastric (**2**) and the mylohyoid (**5**). The styloglossus radiates forward into the tongue. Inferior to the hypoglossal nerve (**13**), the fibers of the *hyoglossus* (**15**) may be separated to demonstrate the *lingual artery* (**16**), in the depth, sometimes accompanied by a small lingual vein. The area where the artery is found is called the **triangle of the lingual artery**. It is formed by the hypoglossal nerve, the anterior belly of the digastric and the posterior border of the mylohyoid muscle (see Fig. **A**). Medial to the hyoglossus, the *glossopharyngeal nerve* (**17**) descends from the retromandibular fossa and is crossed by the *ascending palatine artery* (**18**), a branch of the facial artery. The *stylohyoid ligament* (**19**) runs parallel to the glossopharyngeal nerve.

20 External carotid artery,
21 Facial nerve,
22 Masseter,
23 Sternocleidomastoid,
24 External jugular vein.

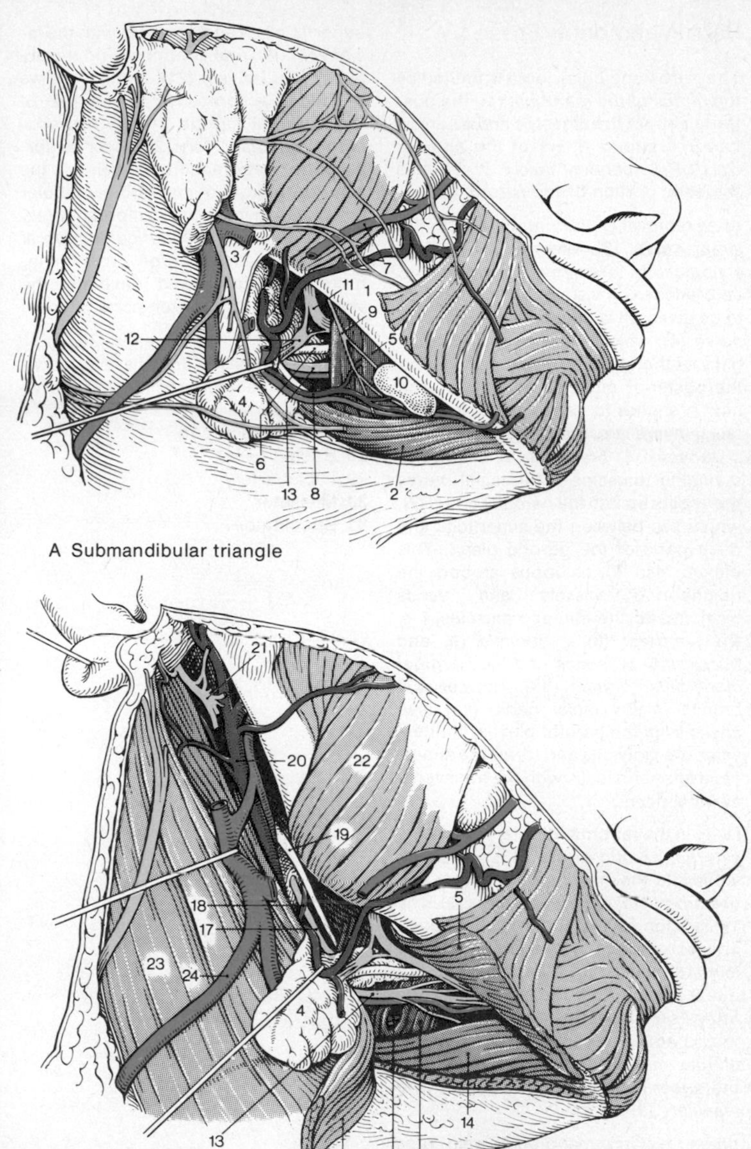

A Submandibular triangle

B Submandibular triangle (deep layer) and retromandibular fossa

Retromandibular Fossa (A)

The retromandibular fossa is limited by the *ramus of the mandible* (**1**), the posterior belly of the digastric and a narrow band of strong fibers of the *angular tract of the cervical fascia*. It contains the deep portion of the parotid gland.

After removal of the parotid gland, the *facial nerve* (**3**), emerging from the stylomastoid foramen and dividing into its branches, is visible. The 1st branch to be given off is the *posterior auricular nerve* (**4**), which supplies the occipital belly of the occipitofrontal muscle and the posterior muscles of the ear. The next branches to leave the trunk of the facial nerve are the *digastric* (**5**) and *stylohyoid* (**6**) *branches* to the corresponding muscles. The facial nerve then splits up into the *parotid plexus* (**7**), which lies between the superficial and deep parts of the parotid gland. This plexus also forms loops around the neighboring vessels and sends branches to the mimetic muscles, i. e. the *temporal* (**8**), *zygomatic* (**9**) and *buccal* (**10**) *branches* and the *marginal mandibular branch* (**11**). The *cervical branch of the facial nerve* (**12**) also arises from the parotid plexus. It innervates the platysma and forms the superficial ansa cervicalis with the transverse cervical nerve.

Deep in the retromandibular fossa is the *external carotid artery* (**13**), which divides into the *maxillary artery* (**14**) and the *superficial temporal artery* (**15**). The 1st branch of the superficial temporal artery is usually the *transverse facial artery* (**16**), which, however, may arise as a direct branch from the external carotid artery (see Fig.). The external carotid artery is accompanied by the *retromandibular vein* (**17**), which is formed from the *superficial temporal* (**18**) and *the maxillary* (**19**) *veins*.

When the retromandibular vein runs superficially, it anastomoses with the *facial vein* (**20**) and continues into the *external jugular vein* (**21**). In this case we find deep accompanying veins (**22**) of the external carotid artery. The *posterior auricular artery* (**23**) ascends dorsal to the retromandibular vein. At the superior margin of the retromandibular fossa, the superficial temporal artery and vein cross the *auriculotemporal nerve* (**24**), which emerges from the infratemporal fossa and innervates the skin of the posterior temporal region.

25 Great auricular nerve,
26 Anastomosis with transverse cervical nerve (superficial ansa cervicalis),
27 Parotid duct (cut),
28 Buccal nerve,
29 Facial artery,
30 Masseter
31 Buccinator

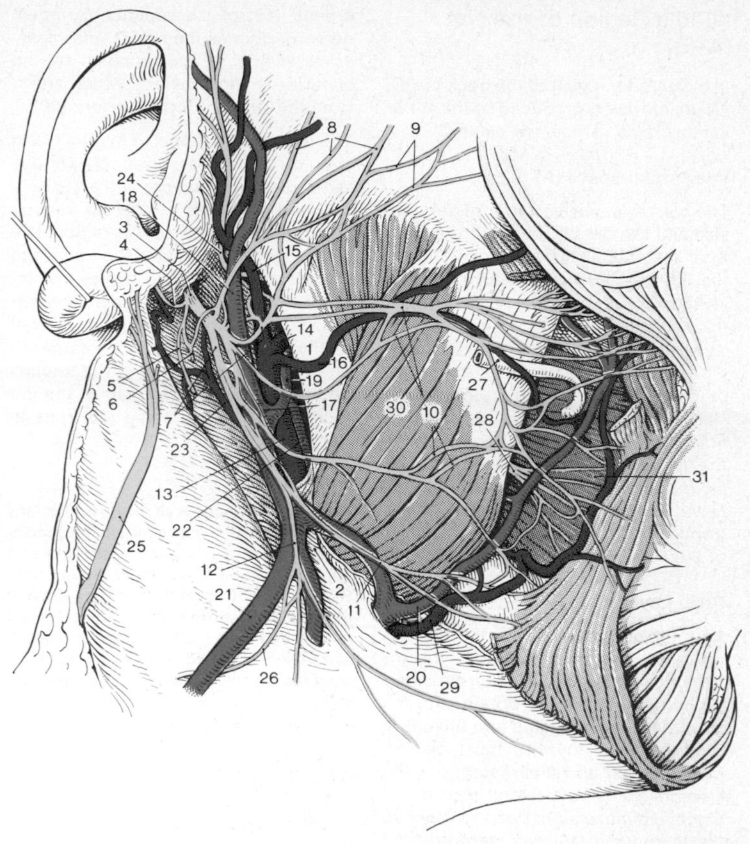

A Retromandibular fossa

Middle Region of the Neck (A–B)

In the anterior region of the neck the division into layers produced by the cervical fascias is particularly clear.

Interfascial Space (A)

The *platysma muscle* (**1**) is of variable size and lies directly beneath the skin. After this integumentary muscle is removed, the *superficial layer of the cervical fascia* (**2**) becomes visible, and if this is divided it reveals the *pretracheal layer of the cervical fascia* (**3**) covering the infrahyoid muscles. Caudally the region is limited by the *sternocleidomastoids* (**4**). Just above the jugular notch, the *jugular venous arch* (**5**) joins the *right anterior* (**6**) to the left *anterior jugular vein.* These veins may also receive blood from deep structures through the middle or pretracheal layer of the cervical fascia (**3**).

Deep Layer (B)

After the pretracheal layer of the cervical fascia has been removed, the infrahyoid muscles and the *thyroid gland* (**7**) become visible. To obtain a better view of the thyroid gland and the entire region, certain muscles must be cut. Most medially and superficially lies the *sternohyoid* (**8**) and lateral to it is the *omohyoid muscle* (**9**). Deep to them lie the *thyrohyoid* (**10**) and *sternothyroid* (**11**). All the infrahyoid muscles are innervated on their respective sides by the *deep ansa cervicalis* (**12**).

The thyroid gland (**7**) lies in front of the cricoid cartilage and the *trachea* (**13**). Its lateral lobes (see p. 342) reach the *thyroid cartilage* (**14**). Between the thyroid and the cricoid cartilages extends the *cricothyroid ligament* (**15**), which is covered laterally by the *cricothyroid muscles* (**16**). On each side these muscles are innervated by the *external branch* (**17**) of the *superior laryngeal nerve* (**18**). The *internal branch* (**19**) of the superior laryngeal nerve perforates the *thyrohyoid membrane* (**21**). It is accompanied by the superior laryngeal artery, which arises from the *superior thyroid artery* (**20**).

The blood return from the thyroid gland (see p. 342) passes through various veins, of which the *superior thyroid vein* (**22**) and the unpaired *thyroid venous plexus* (**23**) are visible in this region. The plexus extends in front of the trachea to the left brachiocephalic vein as the "inferior thyroid vein". The *brachiocephalic trunk* (**24**), which lies directly in front of the trachea, rises obliquely upward and to the right. Lateral to the trachea and in front of the esophagus, the left *recurrent laryngeal nerve* (**25**) runs to the larynx.

Variants

The jugular venous arch may occur at any level between the hyoid bone and the jugular notch. In one position, just below the hyoid bone, it is called the subhyoid venous arch. Rarely, a vein ascends from the thyroid gland to perforate the middle cervical fascia and to end in the anterior jugular vein. In some cases a thyroidea ima artery may arise from the brachiocephalic trunk or from the aorta.

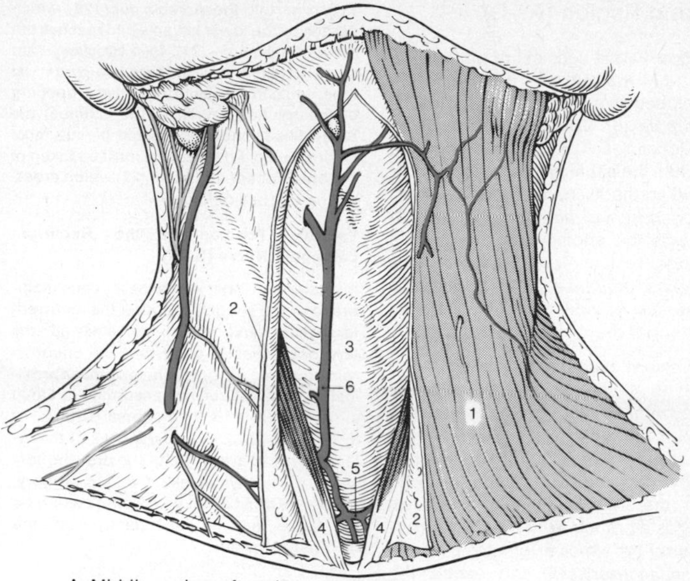

A Middle region of neck;
interfascial space

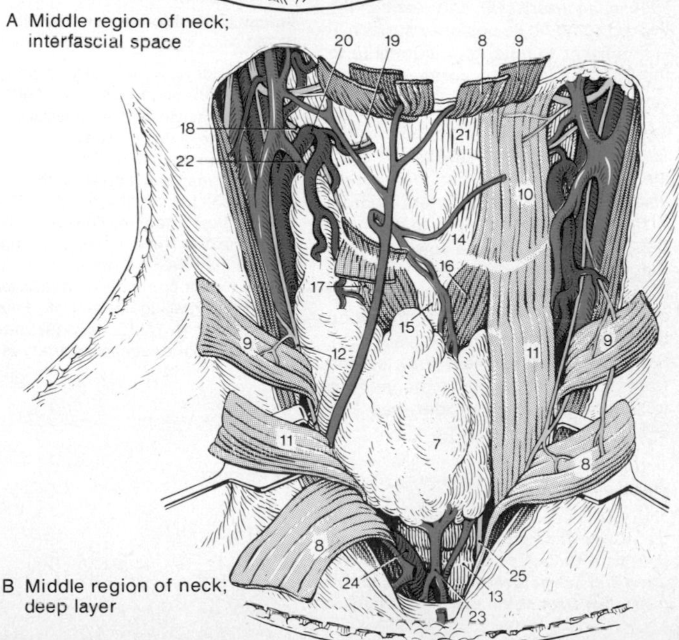

B Middle region of neck;
deep layer

Thyroid Region (A–G)

The **thyroid gland** consists of an *isthmus* (**1**), a *right lobe* (**2**) and a *left lobe* (**3**). Each lobe has a *superior* (**4**) and an *inferior pole* (**5**). The superior poles of both lobes reach the *thyroid cartilage* (**6**), while the isthmus lies in front of the cricoid cartilage and the trachea. Thus, the *cricothyroid ligament* (**7**), which connects the cricoid with the thyroid cartilage, remains free, provided there is no *pyramidal lobe*. Such a lobe may sometimes ascend from the isthmus (remnant of the thyroglossal duct).

The thyroid gland receives its blood supply on each side from the *superior* (**8**) and *inferior* (**9**) *thyroid arteries*. The superior thyroid artery arises from the *external carotid artery* (**10**) and reaches the thyroid gland at its superior pole, while the inferior thyroid artery (**9**) arises as a branch from the *thyrocervical trunk* (**11**), which originates from the *subclavian artery* (**12**), and reaches the thyroid gland on its posterior surface. It is important to note its relationship to the *recurrent laryngeal nerve* (**13, B–D**).

The blood returns through the *superior thyroid veins* (**14**), which open into the *internal jugular* veins (**16**) by the *common facial veins* (**15**). A *middle thyroid vein* (**17**) runs from the lateral margin of the thyroid gland directly to the internal jugular vein. At the lower end of the thyroid gland is the unpaired *thyroid venous plexus* (**18**) which, as the "inferior thyroid vein", sends blood to the *left brachiocephalic vein* (**19**). Sometimes another vein may extend from the cranial margin of the isthmus to the anterior jugular vein (see Fig. 341 B).

Practical Points

The close relationship of the thyroid gland to the vessels and nerves of the neck endangers them during operations on the thyroid gland and in emergency operations on the respiratory tract. Great care must be taken with regard to the *thoracic duct* (**20**), which passes by the lower left pole and reaches the *left venous angle* (**21**). In a **coniotomy** care must be taken in case there is a pyramidal lobe, while in an **inferior tracheotomy** (opening of the trachea caudal to the isthmus) the blood-filled, unpaired thyroid plexus must be preserved. Equally, care must be taken of the *brachiocephalic trunk* (**22**) which crosses the trachea obliquely.

Variable Position of the Recurrent Laryngeal Nerve (B–D)

In addition to innervating the mucous membrane of the subglottic space, the recurrent laryngeal nerve (**13**) innervates all the laryngeal muscles other than the cricothyroid muscle. Its position is with approximately equal frequency (according to Lanz) either ventral to (**B**, 27%), dorsal (**C**, 36%) or in between (**D**, 32%), the branches of the inferior thyroid artery (**9**). In the drawing forward of the thyroid gland during surgery, great care must be taken, as even pulling on the nerve may produce paralysis of the laryngeal muscles.

Variants of the Inferior Thyroid Artery (E–G)

The inferior thyroid artery is particularly variable both as to its site of origin and its course. Because of the importance of the vessel some of its more uncommon variants will be mentioned here. The inferior thyroid artery (**9**) may run dorsal to the *vertebral artery* (**23**) toward the middle (**E**). Sometimes (**F**) the artery may divide immediately after it leaves the thyrocervical trunk. One branch may then lie ventral and the other dorsal to the *common carotid artery* (**24**) and the internal jugular vein (**16**). Finally (**G**), the inferior thyroid artery (**9**) may arise directly from the subclavian artery as the 1st branch.

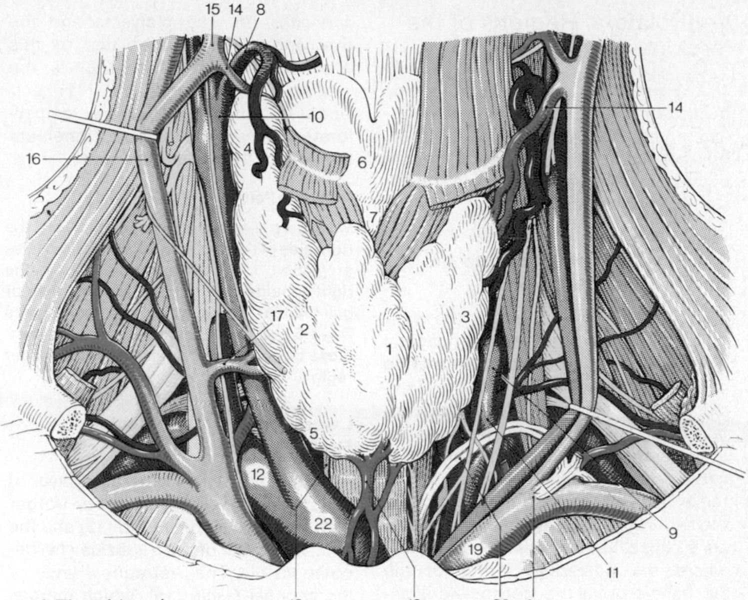

A Thyroid region

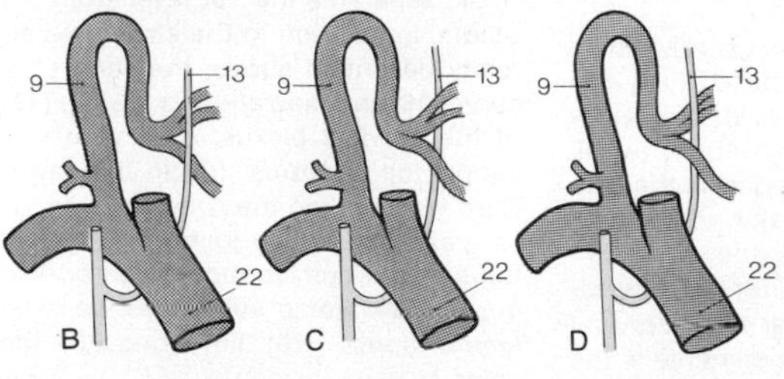

B–D

Variation in relationship of recurrent laryngeal nerve to inferior thyroid artery (after Lanz-Wachsmuth)

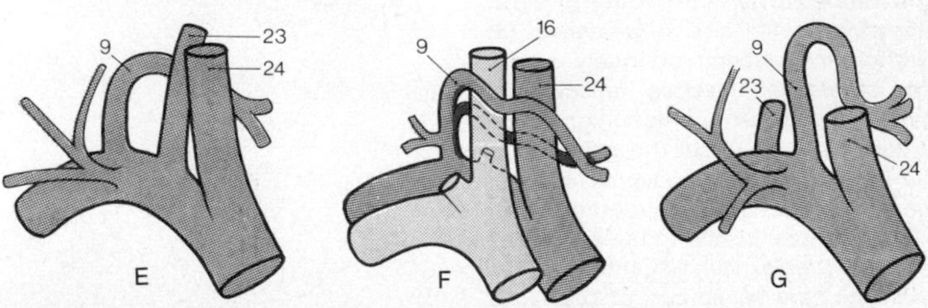

E–G Variants of branches of subclavian artery (personal observations)

Ventrolateral Regions of the Neck (A–B)

The ventrolateral cervical regions may be divided into a superficial subcutaneous region with the nerve point, the lateral cervical region (posterior triangle of the neck), the carotid triangle and the sternocleidomastoid region.

The Ventrolateral Subcutaneous Region of the Neck (A)

Its boundaries are superiorly the *mandible*, anteriorly the median sagittal plane, posteriorly the palpable margin of the *trapezius* and inferiorly the *clavicle* (**1**). The subcutaneous layer contains a cutaneous muscle, the platysma, large veins and the cutaneous branches of the cervical plexus. The area in which these cutaneous branches penetrate the superficial layer of the cervical fascia is called the **nerve point**. It lies roughly where the posterior border of the platysma crosses the sternocleidomastoid. After the platysma has been removed all the superficial vessels and nerves become visible.

The lesser *occipital nerve* (**2**), which runs subcutaneously parallel to the posterior border of the sternocleidomastoid muscle, is the most cranial. This nerve, which takes part in the sensory innervation of the skin of the back of the head, may divide into two branches immediately after it has perforated the superficial layer of the cervical fascia. The largest caliber nerve is the *great auricular nerve* (**3**), which gives off an *anterior* (**4**) and a *posterior* (**5**) *branch* that ascend obliquely across the sternocleidomastoid muscle and take part in sensory innervation of the external ear. At about the same place as this nerve, the *transverse cervical nerve* (**6**) perforates the superficial layer of the cervical fascia, runs deep to the *external jugular vein* (**7**) and, together with the *cervical branch of the facial nerve* (**8**), forms the *superficial ansa cervicalis* (**9**). The platysma and the overlying skin are innervated by this ansa. Caudally, at different levels, the *medial* (**10**), *intermediate* (**11**) and *lateral* (**12**) *supraclavicular nerves* perforate the cervical fascia to innervate the skin of the shoulder region.

Practical Points

Eiselsberg's phenomenon occurs on the right side of the shoulder as a so-called false projection, i. e. pain may radiate into the right shoulder due to disease of the liver or gall bladder. Pain spreads into dermatomes C3–C5 (see Vol. 3). Diseases of the pancreas may produce pain in the left shoulder region.

Lateral Region of the Neck, First Layer (B)

After removal of the superficial layer of the cervical fascia, the posterior border of the *sternocleidomastoid* (**13**) and the anterior border of the *trapezius* (**14**) become visible. The *pretracheal layer of the cervical fascia* (**15**), which merges with the prevertebral layer of the cervical fascia in the lateral region of the neck, separates the 1st layer from the others. In addition to the structures already described above, the *accessory nerve* (**16**) and the *trapezius branch* (**17**) of the cervical plexus, both of which supply the trapezius, run in this layer. Here we also find the *superficial cervical vein* (**18**), which joins the external jugular vein, and the *superficial cervical artery* (**19**). Some *superficial cervical lymph nodes* (**20**) lie alongside the veins.

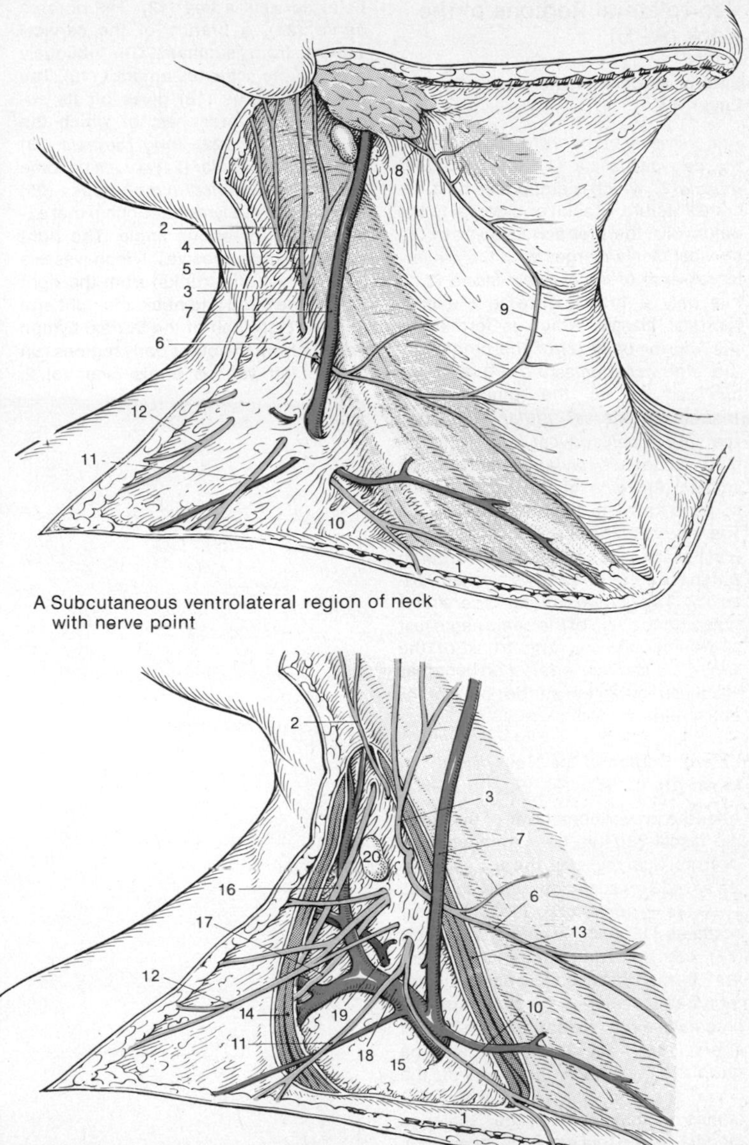

A Subcutaneous ventrolateral region of neck with nerve point

B Lateral region of neck, 1st layer

Ventrolateral Regions of the Neck (A–B)

Lateral Region of the Neck, Second Layer (A)

After removal of the *pretracheal layer of the cervical fascia* (**1**), the *omohyoid muscle* (**2**), which is embedded by it, becomes visible. Cranial and dorsal to the omohyoid, the pretracheal layer of the cervical fascia merges with the *prevertebral layer of the cervical fascia* (**3**). It has only a firm texture in the **omoclavicular triangle**, which is formed by the *inferior belly* (**2**) *of the omohyoid,* the *sternocleidomastoid* (**4**) and the *clavicle* (**5**). In the omoclavicular triangle the *external jugular vein* (**6**) and the *superficial cervical vein* (**7**) combine with the *subclavian* (**8**) and *internal jugular* (**9**) *veins* at the *right* venous angle to form the brachiocephalic vein. The *suprascapular vein* (**10**) also reaches the venous angle. The order in which the veins join shows marked variability. The *suprascapular artery* (**11**) runs with the vein of the same name just above the clavicle. The trunk of the *superficial cervical artery* (**12**) becomes visible cranial to the inferior belly of the omohyoid.

Lateral Region of the Neck, Third Layer (B)

After the prevertebral layer of the cervical fascia (**3**) has been removed, the deep cervical muscles, the *scalenus anterior* (**13**), *scalenus medius* (**14**), *scalenus posterior* (**15**), *levator scapulae* (**16**) and the *splenius cervicis* (**17**), can be seen. Within the "**scalene gap**" formed between the scalenus anterior and scalenus medius runs the *brachial plexus* (**18**) and the *subclavian artery* (**19**). In the area of the scalene gap the subclavian artery gives off the *dorsal scapular artery* (**20**), which becomes visible behind the scalenus medius. When this artery is absent, it is replaced by a deep branch of the superficial cervical artery (**12**). The *phrenic nerve* (**21**), a branch of the cervical plexus from segment C4, obliquely crosses the scalenus anterior (**13**). The brachial plexus (**18**) gives off its supraclavicular branches, of which the *suprascapular* (**22**), *long thoracic* (**23**) and *dorsal scapular* (**24**) *nerves* become visible. The *cervical lymph nodes* (**25**) together form a lymphatic chain that extends to the venous angle. The right venous angle receives lymph vessels (right lymphatic trunks) from the right half of the head and neck, the right arm and the right half of the thorax. Lymph vessels from the other body regions run to the left venous angle (see Vol. 2, p. 80).

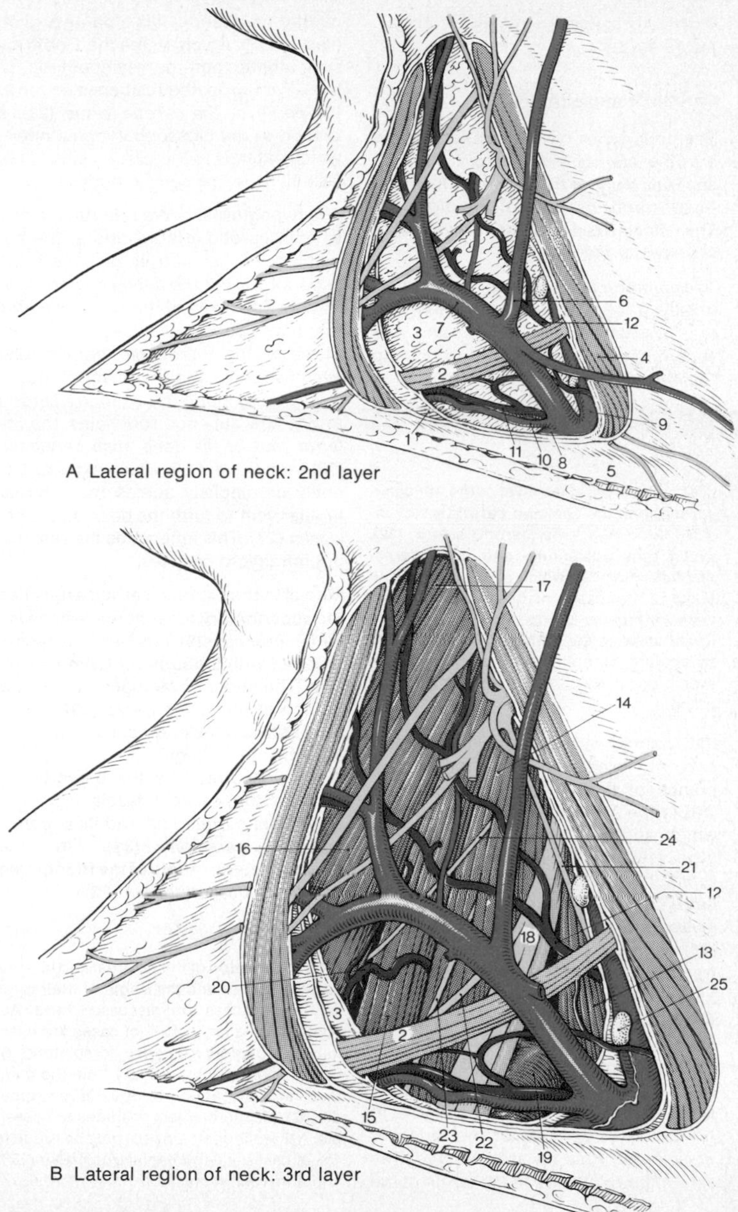

A Lateral region of neck: 2nd layer

B Lateral region of neck: 3rd layer

Ventrolateral Regions of the Neck (A–F)

Carotid Triangle (A)

The boundaries of the carotid triangle are the *sternocleidomastoid* (**1**), the *superior belly* of the *omohyoid* (**2**) and the *posterior belly* (**3**) of the *digastric*. The latter is fixed by the *stylohyoid* (**4**) to the *hyoid bone* (**5**).

The *common facial vein* (**6**) runs superficially; it receives the *vena comitans of the hypoglossal nerve* (**7**) and the *superior thyroid vein* (**8**) before joining the *internal jugular vein* (**9**). Ventral to the latter lies the *common carotid artery* (**10**) with the *carotid sinus* (**11**) see Vol. 2).

In 67% of cases, at the level of the 4th cervical vertebra, the common carotid artery divides into the *internal carotid artery*, (**12**), which runs posteriorly, and the *external carotid artery* (**13**), which runs anteriorly. In about 20% of cases the division occurs one vertebra higher, and in 11% one vertebra lower, while in the remaining 2% there are particularly high or low divisions, perhaps even completely outside the carotid triangle.

The internal carotid artery (**12**) has as a rule no branches. The 1st ventral branch of the external carotid artery (**13**) is the *superior thyroid artery* (**14**) which supplies blood to the *thyroid gland* (**15**) and to the larynx through the *superior laryngeal artery* (**16**). Sometimes the superior thyroid artery also gives off a *sternocleidomastoid artery* (**17**), which more often arises directly from the external carotid artery and loops over the *hypoglossal nerve* (**18**). The *lingual artery* (**19**) is another ventral branch which extends to the tongue, medial to the *hyoglossus* (**20**). The last branch within the carotid triangle is the *facial artery* (**21**), which arises medial to the posterior belly (**3**) of the digastric muscle and runs toward the face. The *carotid body* (**22**) lies in the angle of the carotid bifurcation. It is a paraganglion (see Vol. 2) which is reached both by sympathetic and parasympathetic fibers. Parasympathetic fibers also run in the *nerve of the carotid sinus* (**23**), a branch of the glossopharyngeal nerve, which extends to the carotid sinus (**11**), as well as to the carotid body.

The hypoglossal nerve (**18**) runs lateral to both carotid arteries and at the beginning of its arch it gives off the *superior root of the deep ansa cervicalis* (**24**). The fibers of this root arise from the first two cervical segments, like those of the *thyrohyoid branch* (**25**) which supplies the thyrohyoid muscle. Descending along the common carotid artery, the superior root joins the *inferior root of the deep ansa cervicalis* (**26**) from C2 and C3, which extends laterally or medially across the internal jugular vein to form the *deep ansa cervicalis* (**27**). This innervates the remaining infrahyoid muscles.

Medial to the external carotid artery lies the *superior laryngeal nerve*, whose *internal branch* (**28**) reaches the larynx together with the *superior laryngeal artery*. The superior laryngeal nerve is a branch of the *vagus nerve* (**29**), which runs between the internal carotid artery and the internal jugular vein and which is only separated by the prevertebral layer of the cervical fascia from the *sympathetic trunk* (**30**) and its *superior cervical ganglion* (**31**). In the superoposterior angle of the triangle we find the *accessory nerve* (**32**).

Variants (B–F)

Only the position of the external and internal carotid arteries and the origin of their three ventral branches are discussed here. According to Faller, in 49% of cases the internal carotid artery may arise dorsolateral (**B**) to the external carotid artery from the common carotid artery, and in 9% it is ventromedial (**C**). All intermediate positions are possible. A thyrolingual trunk (**D**) may be found in 4% of cases, a linguofacial trunk (**E**) in 23% and a thyrolinguofacial trunk (**F**) in 0.6%.

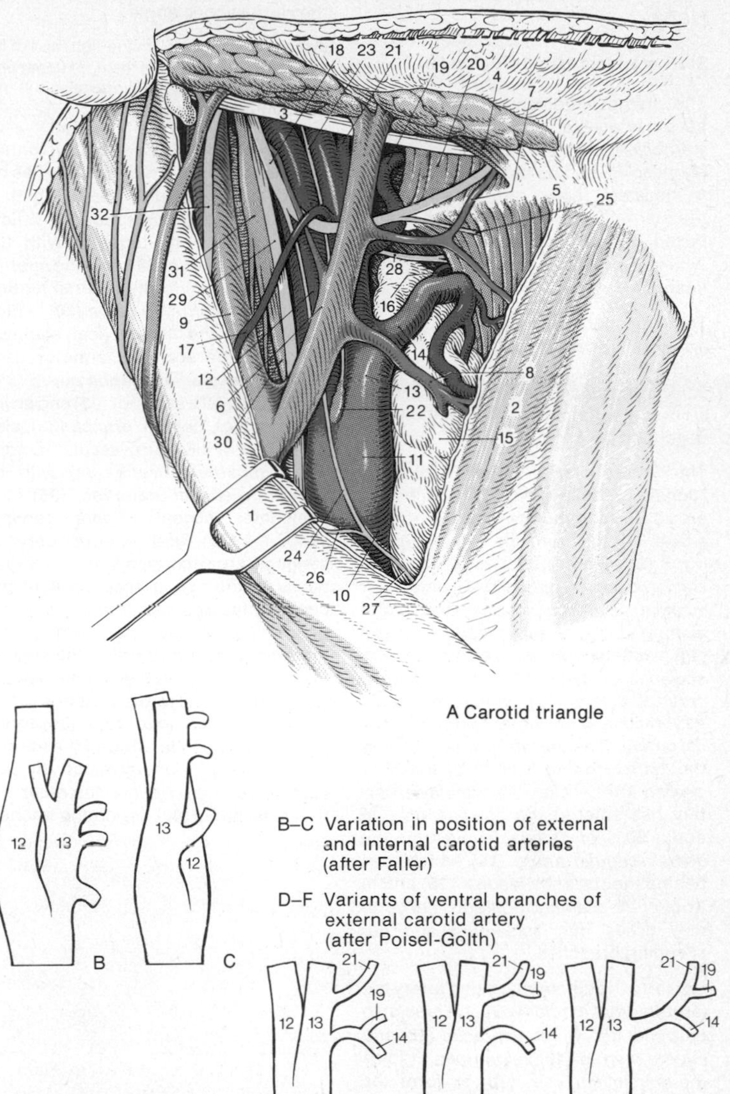

A Carotid triangle

B–C Variation in position of external and internal carotid arteries (after Faller)

D–F Variants of ventral branches of external carotid artery (after Poisel-Golth)

Ventrolateral Regions of the Neck

Sternocleidomastoid Region (A)

The sternocleidomastoid region only becomes visible after removal of the *sternocleidomastoid* (**1**) and *omohyoid* (**2**) muscles. It joins the carotid triangle to the lateral region of the neck. When the sternocleidomastoid region is exposed, the large vessels and nerves which run through the neck can be seen.

The largest artery, the *common carotid artery* (**3**), ascends obliquely. It divides into the *external* (**4**) and *internal* (**5**) *carotid arteries.* The level of the division and variations in its position are described on page 348.

The arched *inferior thyroid artery* (**6**) running to the *thyroid gland* (**7**) is covered by the common carotid artery. This artery arises from the *thyrocervical trunk* (**8**), which branches off the *subclavian artery* (**9**) just before it enters the scalene gap. The thyrocervical trunk also gives off the *suprascapular artery* (**11**), which crosses ventral to the *scalenus anterior* (**10**), the *superficial cervical artery* (**12**), which lies quite superficially, and the *ascending cervical artery.* The *vertebral artery* (**13**) is the 1st ascending branch of the subclavian artery. After the subclavian artery has entered the scalene gap, in about 60% of people it gives off the *dorsal scapular artery* (**14**), which runs behind the *scalenus medius* (**15**) and in front of the *scalenus posterior* (**16**), and may divide into ascending and descending branches.

Dorsal to the common carotid artery the large *internal jugular vein* (**17**) is seen to descend, into which the *facial* (**18**) and *middle thyroid* (**19**) *veins* open. It joins the *subclavian vein* (**20**) to form the right brachiocephalic vein (**21**). The *external jugular vein* (**22**), which joins the *superficial cervical vein* (**23**), and the *suprascapular vein* (**24**) also reach the right venous angle.

Lymph vessels (**25**) from the right half of the head and neck and from the right upper limb and the right half of the thorax also run into the right venous angle.

The *deep cervical ansa* (**26**), which innervates the infrahyoid muscles, lies on the common carotid artery (**3**). It is formed from a *superior root* (**27**) which, at its origin, runs together with the *hypoglossal nerve* (**28**), and the *inferior root* (**29**). Dorsal to the internal jugular vein runs the *phrenic nerve* (**30**), which stems from the 4th cervical segment and uses the scalenus anterior as a guiding muscle. The *vagus nerve* (**31**), which gives off a superior (**32**) and an *inferior cervical cardiac branch* (**33**), also forms part of the neurovascular bundle. The *sympathetic trunk* (**34**) with its *superior cervical ganglion* (**35**), the sometimes absent *middle cervical ganglion* (**36**) and *inferior cervical ganglion* are separated from the vagus nerve by the prevertebral layer of the cervical fascia. The inferior cervical ganglion is usually fused with the 1st thoracic ganglion, forming the *stellate ganglion* (**37**), which lies on the head of the 1st rib medial to the vertebral artery (**13**). The sympathetic trunk (**34**) forms the *thyroid loop* (**38**) around the inferior thyroid artery (**6**) and gives off the *cardiac nerves* (**39**). Deeply, the *recurrent laryngeal nerve* (**40**) lies on the trachea.

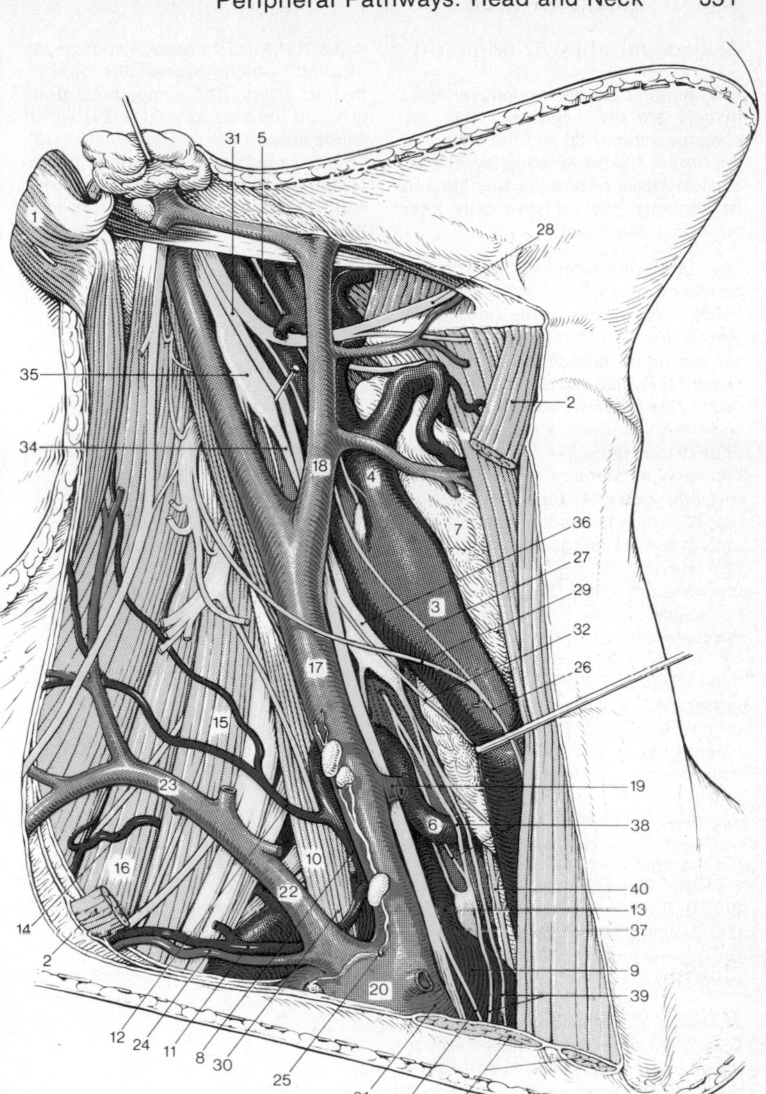

A Sternocleidomastoid region

Scalenovertebral Triangle (A)

The margins of the scalenovertebral triangle are the *longus colli* (**1**), the *scalenus anterior* (**2**) and the cupula of the pleura. The prevertebral layer of the cervical fascia covers the triangle and its contents can be seen only after removal of the fascia.

The *subclavian artery* (**3**) lies on the cupula of the pleura, from which connective tissue fiber bands (the costopleural ligament) run to the 1st rib. Its 1st ascending branch is the *vertebral artery* (**4**), which crosses ventrally the roots of the *brachial plexus from Th 1* (**5**) *and C8* (**6**), to reach the vertebral column at the transverse foramen of the 6th cervical vertebra. Dorsal to the *vertebral artery* (**4**) runs the *vertebral vein* (**7**) which leaves the vertebral column at the transverse foramen of the 7th cervical vertebra. Adjacent to the vertebral artery, the *thyrocervical trunk* ascends (see p. 350), followed by the *costocervical trunk* (**8**), which gives off the *deep cervical artery* (**9**), the *highest intercostal artery* and, rarely, a dorsal *scapular artery* (**10**) of abnormal origin. The *internal thoracic artery* (**11**) extends caudally running parasternally with the *internal thoracic vein* (**12**) to reach the sternocostal triangle.
Ventrally, the subclavian artery and its branches on the left side are crossed by the *thoracic duct* (**13**), which forms a cranially convex arch. The thoracic duct opens into the *left venous angle* (**14**), which is formed by the junction of the *internal jugular* (**15**) and *subclavian veins* (**16**).

The roots of the brachial plexus out of C5–C7 run deep down, while the *sympathetic trunk* (**17**) runs superficial to them. At the level of the 6th cervical vertebra, the sympathetic trunk often contains a *middle cervical ganglion* (**18**) lying on the scalenus anterior (**2**). Caudal to the ganglion, the sympathetic trunk together with the *superior cardiac nerve* (**19**), form the *ansa thyroidea* (**20**), through which passes the inferior thyroid artery. The sympathetic trunk gives off the *ansa subclavia* (**21**), which winds around the subclavian artery (**3**). This ansa subclavia extends to the inferior cervical ganglion which fuses with the 1st thoracic ganglion to form the *stellate (cervicothoracic) ganglion* (**22**). The latter lies on the head of the 1st rib. The *inferior cardiac nerve* (**23**) arises from it. Medially, the *recurrent laryngeal nerve* (**24**) ascends to the larynx. It runs in a groove formed by the *trachea* (**25**) and the *esophagus* (**26**).

27 Phrenic nerve,
28 Left brachiocephalic vein,
29 Scalenus medius,
30 Scalenus posterior,
31 Levator scapulae,
32 Trapezius,
33 Clavicular part of the pectoralis major.

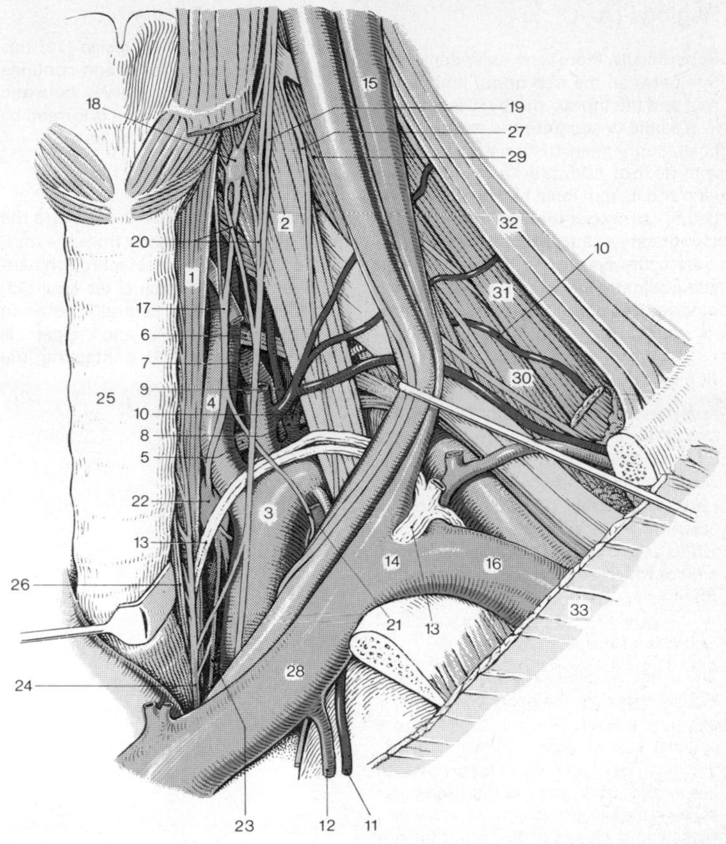

A Scalenovertebral triangle

Regions (A–C)

Superficially, there is no clear demarcation between the free upper limb or its root and the thorax, but by dissection it is possible to separate the mainly muscular connection of the arm together with its root from the thorax. The free limb and its root must be considered together for proper understanding of the topography of the peripheral neurovascular pathways. The following regional subdivisions are made for practical purposes and are not founded on development.

Regions around the Shoulder

Anteriorly there is the **infraclavicular region** (**1**) with the *deltopectoral triangle* (**2**) through which the peripheral pathways extend to the arm, i.e., the central part of the **axilla** (**3**) with the *axillary fossa* (**4**). Lateral to the shoulder joint is the **deltoid region** (**5**), onto the dorsal side of which adjoins the **scapular region** (**6**).

Regions of the Arm

The arm is divided into an **anterior brachial region** (**7**), the basic components of which are the flexor muscles, and a **posterior brachial region** (**8**) with the extensors. The *medial bicipital groove* (**9**) lies in front of the medial intermuscular septum and is the main track for the vessels and nerves of the arm that run from the axilla to the cubital fossa. It is prominent within the anterior brachial region.

Regions of the Elbow

The **anterior cubital region** (**10**), the center of which is represented by the cubital fossa, adjoins the anterior brachial region on the flexor side. Within the cubital fossa the vascular and nerve bundles divide. The **posterior cubital region** (**11**), which lies dorsally, contains muscles and only smaller vascular networks.

Regions of the Forearm

The **anterior antebrachial region** (**12**) lies distal to the cubital fossa and contains the large vessels and nerves between the flexors. The dorsal part is formed by the **posterior antebrachial region** (**13**).

Regions of the Hand

In the wrist, there is the transition to the **palm** (**14**), which extends from the midcarpal joint to the metacarpophalangeal joints. The **dorsum of the hand** (**15**) has the same limits. Laterally, between the dorsum of the hand and the palm is the **radial foveola** (**16**) containing the radial artery.

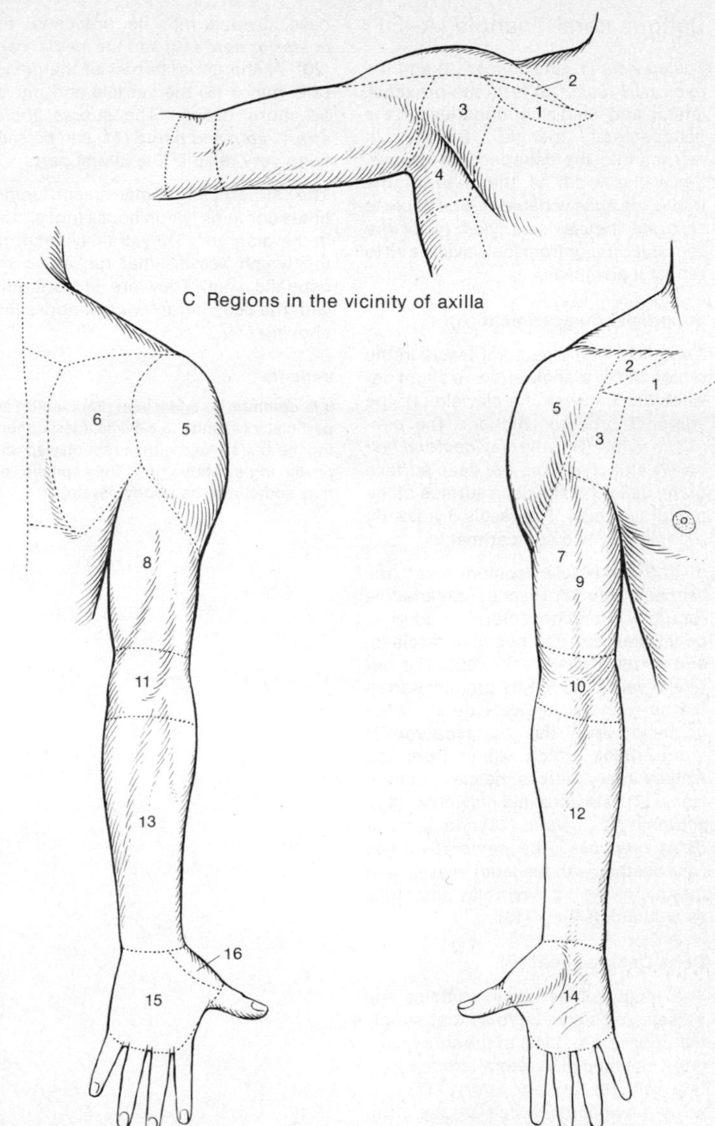

C Regions in the vicinity of axilla

B Posterior view of regions of upper limb

A Anterior view of regions of upper limb

Deltopectoral Triangle (A–B)

The *clavicle* (**1**), the *deltoid* (**2**) and the *pectoralis major* (**3**) form the proximal, lateral and medial boundaries of the deltopectoral triangle. Distally, it merges into the deltopectoral groove. Since the width of the base of the triangle is quite variable, it is possible to separate the *clavicular part* (**4**) *of the pectoralis major* from the clavicle and to reflect it downward.

Superficial Compartment (A)

Superficially, the pectoral fascia in the region of the triangle shows a slight depression. Between the clavicle (**1**), the *coracoid process* (**B5**) and the *pectoralis minor* (**B6**), the *clavipectoral fascia* (**7**) stretches from the deep surface of the deltoid to the deep surface of the pectoralis major. This fascia divides the triangle into two compartments.

In the superficial compartment the *cephalic vein* (**8**) reaches the triangle through the deltopectoral groove. It penetrates the clavipectoral fascia to end in the *axillary vein* (**B9**). The cephalic vein is joined by branches from the surrounding areas. Lateral to the cephalic vein, the *thoracoacromial artery* (**B10**), which stems from the axillary artery pierces the clavipectoral fascia (**7**). It divides into *clavicular* (**11**), *acromial* (**12**), *deltoid* (**13**) and *pectoral* (**B14**) *branches*. The *pectoral nerves* run together with the latter vessels and may penetrate the fascia clavipectoralis as a common trunk (**15**).

Deep Compartment (B)

The deep compartment contains the vessels and nerve bundles that supply the upper limb. Distal to the *subclavius* (**16**) from medial to lateral are the axillary vein (**9**), *axillary artery* (**17**) and three nerve cords, which are the infraclavicular portion of the brachial plexus. They are the superficially situated *lateral cord* (**18**), which may already have divided into its branches, the *posterior cord* (**19**) and the *medial cord* (**20**). At the upper border of the pectoralis minor (**6**) the vessels and nerves lie more deeply. The *suprascapular artery, vein and nerve* (**21**) can be seen lying very deep in the lateral part.

The superficial compartment sometimes contains lymph nodes (not shown in the diagram). They drain lymph from the lymph vessels that run along the cephalic vein. They are in continuity with the deep infraclavicular nodes (not shown).

Variants

It is common to find a vein (**22**) looping superficially around the clavicle interconnecting the axillary vein with the subclavian vein, producing a venous ring. The cephalic vein may sometimes be poorly developed.

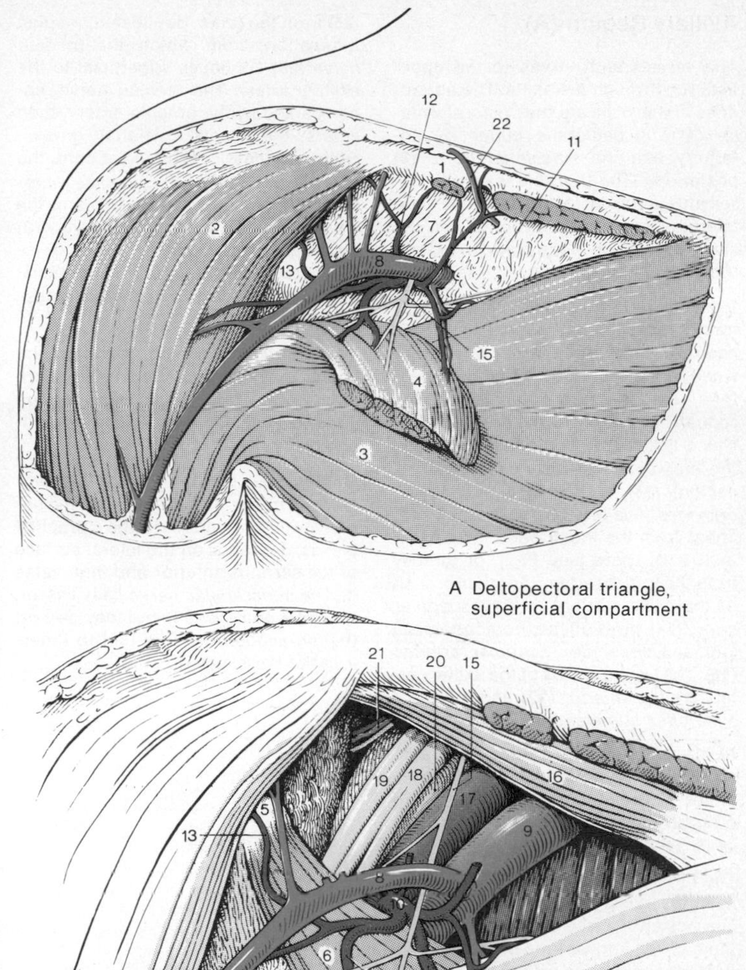

A Deltopectoral triangle, superficial compartment

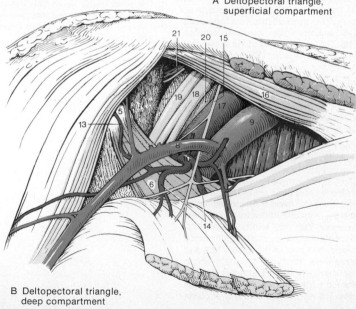

B Deltopectoral triangle, deep compartment

Axillary Region (A)

The vessels and nerves to the upper limb run through the axilla. The boundaries of the axilla are the *pectoralis major* (**1**) and *pectoralis minor* (**2**) anteriorly and the *latissimus dorsi* (**3**) posteriorly. The thoracic wall with the *serratus anterior* (**4**) lie medially, and laterally there is the humerus with the short *head of the biceps brachii* (**5**) and the *coracobrachialis* (**6**).

Most medial of all is the *axillary vein* (**7**) formed from the brachial veins. It runs centrally, receiving a larger number of small veins. It is joined in the deltopectoral triangle (see p. 356) by the *cephalic vein* (**8**). The *axillary artery* (**9**), which lies lateral to the vein, gives off the *thoracoaomial artery* (**10**) with its *pectoral* (**11**), *acromial* (**12**) and *deltoid branches.* A *lateral thoracic artery* (**13**) arises from the thoracoacromial artery in 10% of cases (see Fig.), or directly from the axillary artery. Another branch of the axillary artery, the *subscapular artery* (**14**), gives off the *thoracodorsalis* (**15**) and *circumflex scapular arteries* (**16**). The last branches of the axillary artery are the *anterior* (**17**) and *posterior circumflex humeral arteries* (**18**).

At the tendinous insertion of the latissimus dorsi (**3**), the axillar artery continues as the *brachial artery* (**19**) and gives off the profunda brachii artery (**20**) as its 1st branch.

The three cords of the brachial plexus lie in the axillary region medial, lateral and posterior to the axillary artery, and there divide into various branches. The posterior cord gives off the *axillary* (**21**) and *radial* (**22**) *nerves*. Accompanied by the posterior circumflex humeral artery and vein (**18**), the axillary nerve (**21**) passes through the quadrangular space (see p. 360) toward the *deltoid* (**23**) and *teres minor*. The radial nerve (**22**) runs in the sulcus for the radial nerve accompanied by the profunda brachii artery (**20**). The *medial* (**24**) and *lateral cords* (**25**) form the (often duplicated) median bifurcation, from which the *median nerve* (**26**) continues superficial to the axillary artery. The median nerve, accompanied by the brachial artery, then enters the medial bicipital groove. Other branches of the medial cord, the *ulnar nerve* (**27**), the *medial antebrachial cutaneous nerve* (**28**) and the *medial brachial cutaneous nerve* (**29**) also reach this groove. Branches of intercostal nerves 1–3 join the medial cutaneous brachial nerve as *intercostobrachial nerves* (**30**).

The lateral cords give off, apart from the lateral root of the median nerve (here duplicated), the *musculocutaneous nerve* (**31**), which pierces the coracobrachialis.

On the wall of the thorax, the *long thoracic nerve* (**32**), arising from the supraclavicular part of the brachial plexus, descends on the lateral surface of the serratus anterior and innervates it. The *subscapular nerve* (**34**) lies on the *subscapularis* (**33**) and may give off the *thoracodorsal nerve* (**35**) to innervate the latissimus dorsi (**3**).

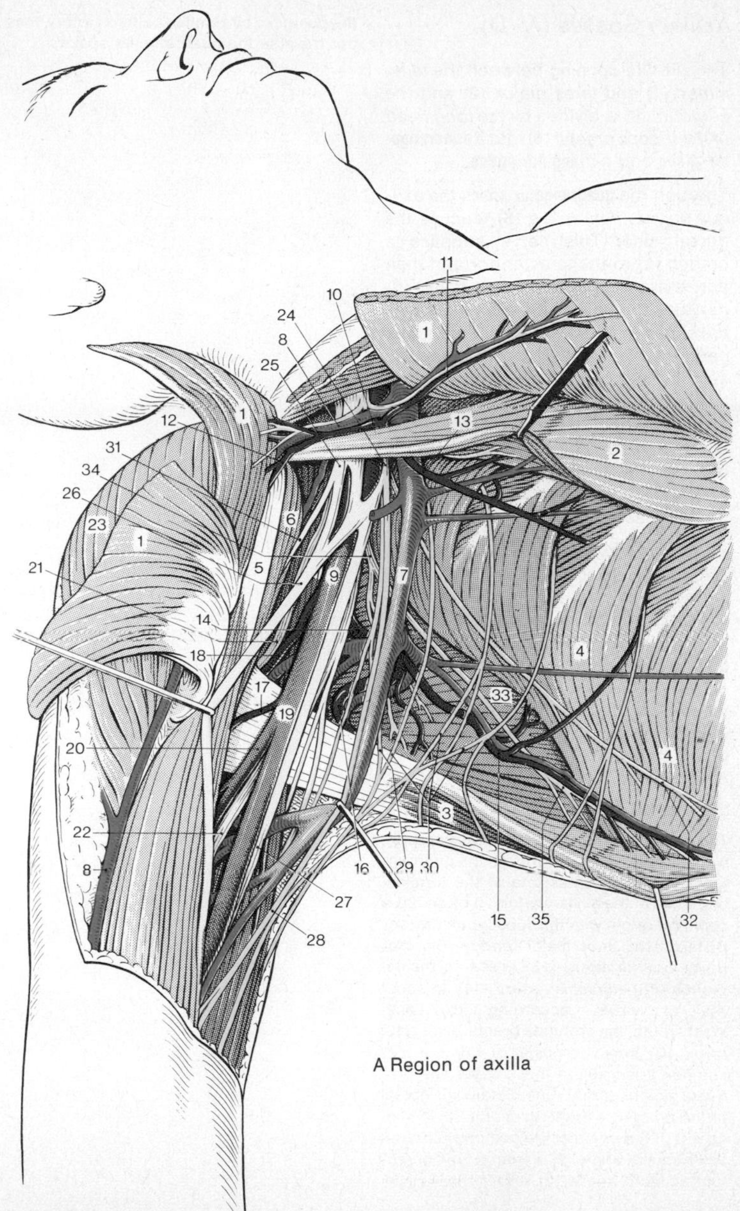

A Region of axilla

Axillary Spaces (A–D)

The slit-like opening between the *teres minor* (**1**) and *teres major* (**2**) and the *humerus* (**3**) is divided by the *long head of the triceps brachii* (**4**) into a **quadrangular space** and a **triangular space**.

Through the **quadrangular space** the *axillary (circumflex) nerve* (**5**) reaches the dorsal side. This nerve supplies a branch (**6**) to the teres minor and then buries itself in the *deltoid* (**7**). It also innervates the upper lateral skin area via the *superior lateral brachial cutaneous nerve* (**8**). The axillary nerve is usually accompanied by the *posterior circumflex humeral artery* (**9**), and the commonly paired *posterior circumflex humeral veins*. The artery supplies the deltoid, the long head of the triceps brachii (**4**) and the *lateral head of the triceps brachii* (**10**).

The *circumflex scapular artery* (**11**) runs through the **triangular space** to the dorsal surface of the scapula on which it anastomoses with the suprascapular artery. The artery is accompanied by the *circumflex scapular vein.* Deeply a twig (**12**) from the subscapular nerve, which innervates the teres major (**2**) can be seen. It does not run through the triangular space.

Variants (B–D)

The posterior circumflex humeral artery (**9**), which usually (**B**) runs through the quadrangular space, arises as one of the terminal branches of the axillary artery. It often has a common origin with the subscapular artery. Distal to the teres major tendon, the *profunda brachii artery* (**13**) arises as the 1st branch of the *brachial artery* (**14**). In about 7% of cases, according to Lanz-Wachsmuth, the profunda brachii artery (**13**) arises (**C**) from the posterior humeral circumflex artery (**9**). In these cases the profunda brachii artery runs distalward dorsal to the tendon of the teres major. In 16% of cases (**D**) the origin of the posterior circumflex humeral artery (**9**) is from a typical profunda brachii artery (**13**), and in those cases the posterior circumflex humeral artery does not traverse the quadrangular space.

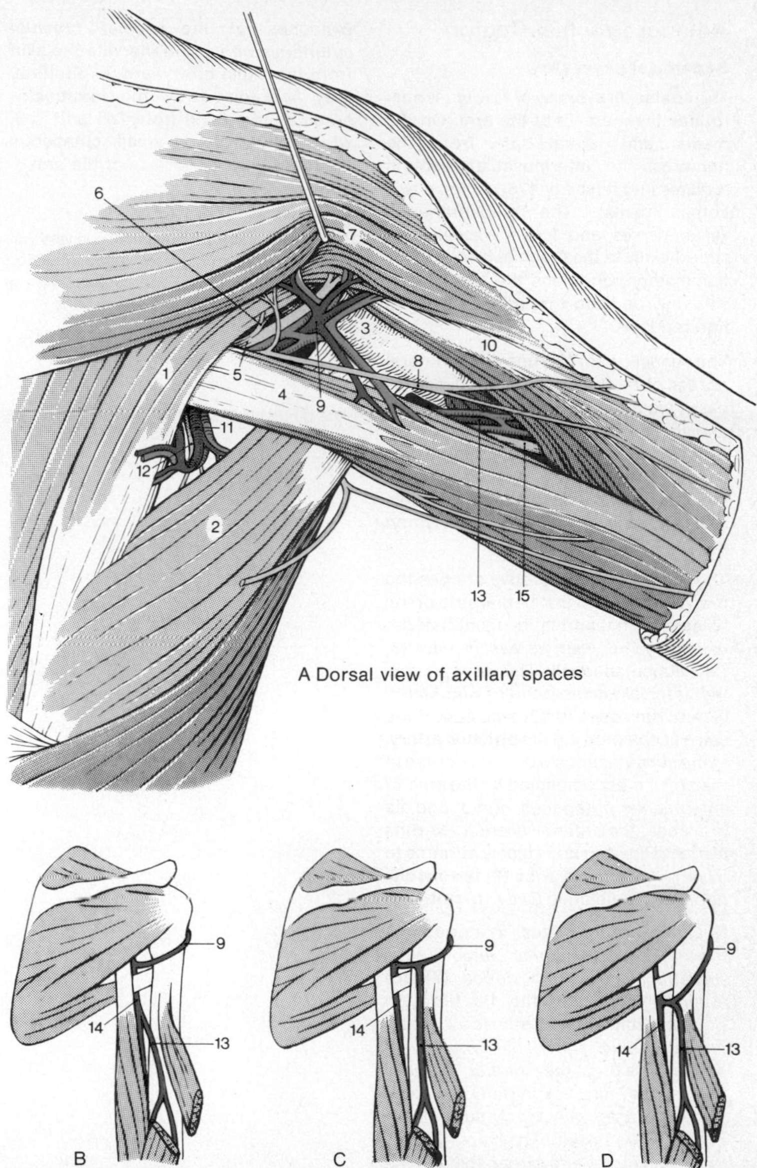

A Dorsal view of axillary spaces

B–D Variants of arteries (after Lanz-Wachsmuth)

Anterior Brachial Region

Superficial Layer (A)

The coarse, firm *brachial fascia* (**1**) surrounds the muscles of the arm. On the medial and lateral side from the humerus, the intermuscular septum radiates into it (see p. 176) to form two compartments. The subcutaneous veins, nerves and lymph vessels run superficially to the brachial fascia. In inflammatory conditions the lymph vessels may be seen through the skin as fine red lines.

The *cephalic vein* (**2**) runs on the lateral border of the biceps brachii. It carries blood from the radial side of the hand and the forearm via the deltopectoral groove to the deltopectoral triangle (see p. 356). The veins are accompanied by the *lateral superficial lymph vessels* (not shown) which transport lymph from the two radial digits.

The medial bicipital groove shapes the brachial fascia on the medial side of the biceps brachii, and in its distal half the usually well-developed *basilic vein* (**3**) runs subcutaneously. This vein pierces the brachial fascia at the *basilic hiatus* (**4**) and runs deep to become one of the veins accompanying the brachial artery. In the subcutaneous part of its course in the arm it is accompanied by the *medial antebrachial cutaneous nerve* and its branches; the *anterior branch* (**5**) runs lateral to the vein and closely adheres to it, while the *ulnar branch* (**6**) lies medial and a short distance away from it.

Near the basilic hiatus, in about one third of cases, *cubital* (also called *supratrochlear*) *lymph nodes* (**7**) are found which act as the 1st filtration point for lymph from the three ulnar digits. The *medial superficial lymph vessels* run along the medial bicipital groove; they may accompany the basilic vein, or they may reach subcutaneously to the axilla. They are usually more numerous and larger than those that accompany the cephalic vein.

Branches of the *medial brachial cutaneous nerve* (**8**) innervate the skin from the axilla downward. In addition, they are joined by the *intercostobrachial nerves* (**9**) from Th1 and Th3, which innervate a small cutaneous area on the inner surface of the arm.

Variants

The position of the basilic hiatus is very variable. It may lie immediately at the transition to the cubital region. The cephalic vein is sometimes absent.

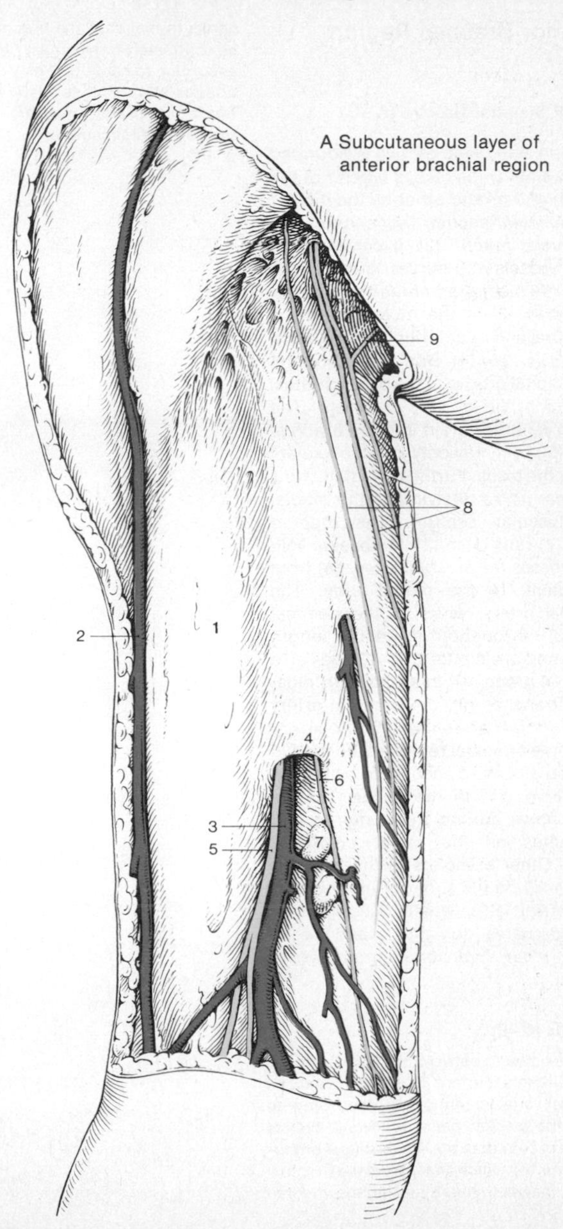
A Subcutaneous layer of anterior brachial region
9
8
2
1
4
6
3
5
7

Anterior Brachial Region (A–E)

Medial Bicipital Groove (A–B)

The medial bicipital groove is bounded on one side by the *biceps brachii* of the arm (**1**) and on the other by the *medial intermuscular septum* (not shown) and the *triceps brachii* (**2**). It contains the blood vessels and nerves to the upper limb. The *medial antebrachial cutaneous nerve* (**3**) is the most superficial structure, and its anterior branch lies on the *basilic vein* (**4**). Both leave the medial bicipital groove at the basilic hiatus, which may lie at various levels. The basilic vein may drain into the *brachial veins* (**5**), or it may only join the axillary vein in the axilla. Furthest medially runs the *ulnar nerve* (**6**), lying on the medial intermuscular septum. The *median nerve* (**7**) runs lateral to the basilic vein and crosses the *brachial artery* (**8**) from the lateral to the medial side. The brachial artery, which is the deepest structure throughout the entire length of the medial bicipital groove, gives off a series of branches. In addition to muscular branches (**9**), the brachial artery gives off the *profunda brachii artery* (**10**) in the proximal region of the medial bicipital groove. It accompanies the *radial nerve* (**11**) in the sulcus for the radial nerve around the humerus and terminates as the *radial collateral artery*. Other branches of the brachial artery include the *superior ulnar collateral artery* (**12**), which accompanies the ulnar nerve (dorsal to it) and the *inferior ulnar collateral artery* (not visible).

Variants (C–E)

The relationship between the median nerve (**7**) and brachial artery (**8**) and its branches may be variable. Although, according to Lanz, the median nerve follows a typical course in 74% of cases, a *superficial brachial artery* (**13**), which arises from the brachial artery, may run superficial to the median nerve. In that case the brachial artery may be completely rudimentary (in 12% of cases according to Lanz), or it may divide into two arteries at variable levels (14%). The profunda brachii artery may arise together with the posterior circumflex humeral artery (see p. 360).

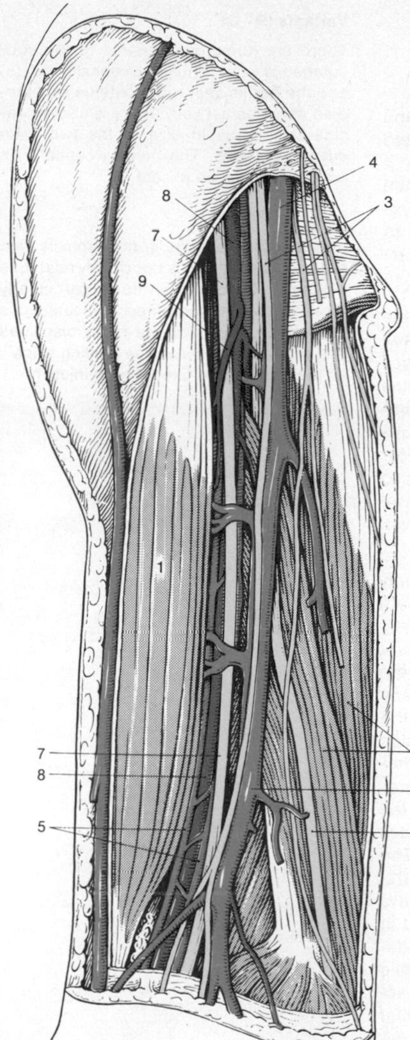

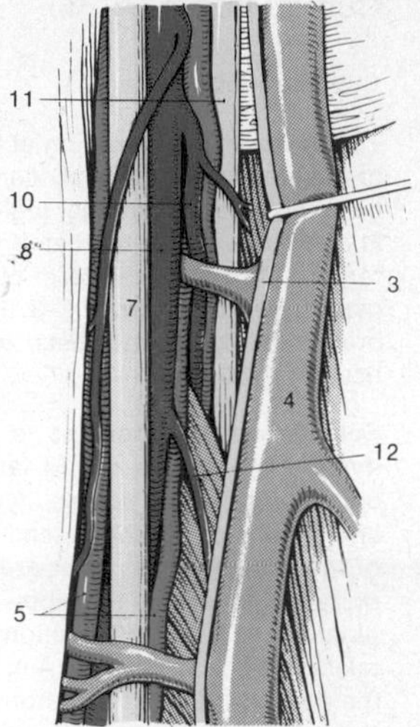

B Detailed view, basilic vein displaced medially

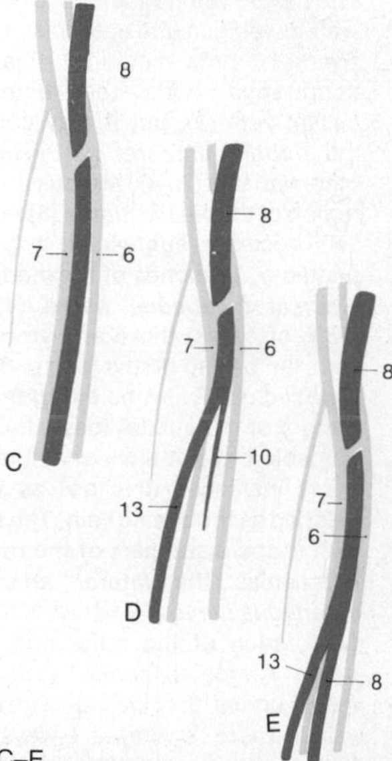

A Anterior brachial region, medial bicipital groove

C–E
Arteries and nerves in medial bicipital groove (after Lanz-Wachsmuth)

Cubital Fossa (A–G)

Subcutaneous Layer (A)

The anterior cubital region at the bend of the elbow is not sharply demarcated from the anterior brachial region and it is just as poorly demarcated from the forearm. Normally the term cubital region refers to an area 2–3 fingers in breadth proximal and distal to the articular space.

Subcutaneously there is a variable amount of well-developed fatty tissue containing veins, nerves, lymphatics and lymph nodes. The cutaneous veins of the subcutaneous layer are very important clinically, as the elbow is the region for intravenous injections and for taking blood sample etc. According to the development of the venous system, the course taken by the veins as well as their caliber, fluctuate widely.

The *basilic vein* (**1**), which is commonly well-developed and easy to see beneath the skin, runs medially. It is usually continuous with the *antebrachial basilic vein* (**2**), but it may come from the *middle antebrachial vein*. Many other variants (**B – G**) are possible. In the region of the *basilic hiatus* (**3**) the basilic vein becomes subfascial. It is accompanied by branches of the *medial antebrachial cutaneous nerve* (**4**). Often (33% of cases) there are lymph nodes near the basilic hiatus (see p. 362). The *cephalic vein* (**5**) runs along the lateral margin of the cubital fossa. It is always palpable but not always visible, and in many instances it is not as well developed as the basilic vein. The cephalic vein in the distal part of the region accompanies the *lateral antebrachial cutaneous nerve* (**6**), which is the terminal branch of the musculocutaneous nerve. A *median cubital vein* (**7**) normally unites the basilic and cephalic veins. There is almost always a *deep median cubital vein* (**8**), which joins the superficial and deep veins.

Variants (B – G)

There are numerous variants of the subcutaneous veins. Thus, the cephalic vein (**5**) and the basilic vein may continue as a median antebrachial vein. There is also a considerable range in size of the two main cutaneous veins. The median cubital vein may sometimes be absent (**E**).

Practical Points

Intravenous injections in the cephalic vein are less painful, as it is not closely related to any nerve. In some individuals, particularly those with poorly developed subcutaneous fatty tissue, the veins are easily displaced and are known clinically as "rolling veins", as they have to be fixed during injection.

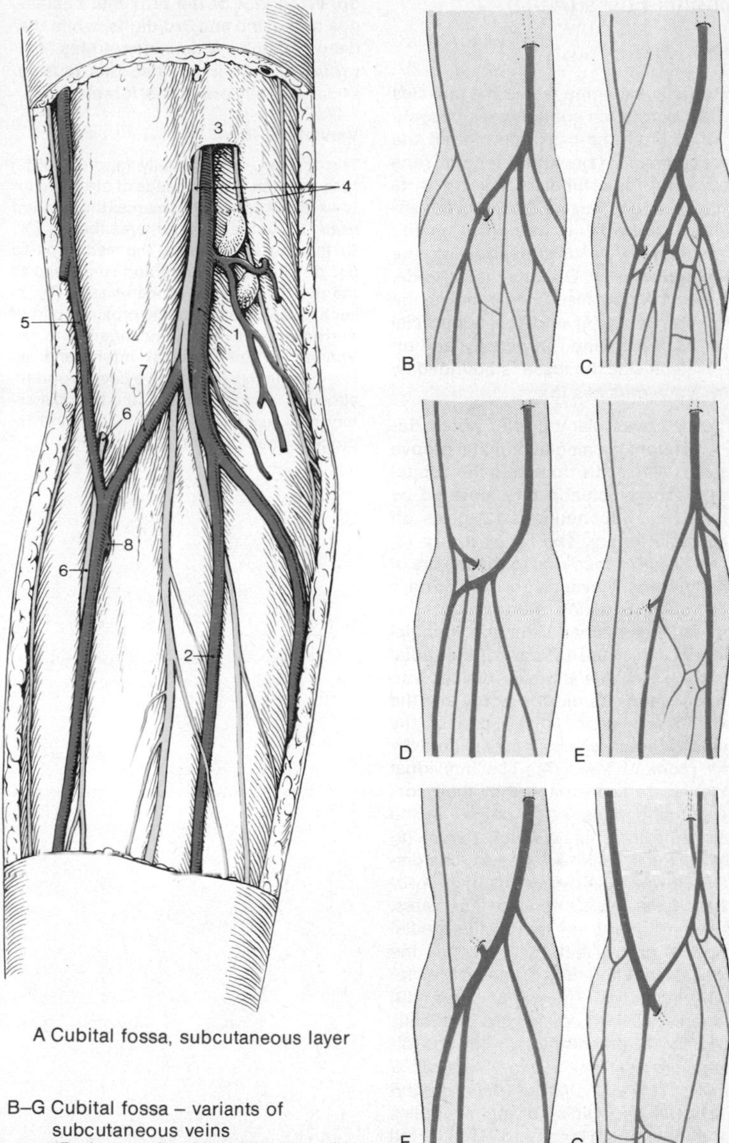

A Cubital fossa, subcutaneous layer

B–G Cubital fossa – variants of subcutaneous veins (Redrawn after Lanz-Wachsmuth)

Cubital Fossa (A–D)

Deep Layer (A)

After removal of the fascia the muscles which border the cubital fossa become visible. From the proximal margin the *biceps brachii* (**1**) with its tendon runs toward the radial tuberosity, and with its *bicipital aponeurosis* (**2**) toward the antebrachial fascia. It partly covers the *brachialis* (**3**), which is inserted into the ulnar tuberosity. On the medial side, arising from the medial epicondyle, the *pronator teres* (**4**) and the superficial flexors of the hand run distally, and on the lateral side the fossa is bounded by the *brachioradialis* (**5**).

The neurovascular bundle, which descends from the medial bicipital groove (see p. 364), splits up within the cubital fossa. The brachial artery, covered by the bicipital aponeurosis (**2**) gives off the radial artery. The *radial artery* (**6**) runs distally superficial to the flexors of the forearm. The *recurrent radial artery* (**7**), which ascends along the radial nerve, arises either from the brachial artery or from the 1st part of the radial artery. The *brachial artery* divides into the *common interosseus artery* and the *ulnar artery* in the distal part of the cubital fossa, where it is covered by the pronator teres (**4**). The individual arteries are accompanied by their corresponding veins, often paired. In the cubital fossa the *median nerve* (**8**) leaves the brachial artery and runs distally between the two heads of the pronator teres, which it also innervates. The *ulnar nerve* (**9**) leaves the medial bicipital groove before it reaches the cubital fossa and runs dorsal to the medial epicondyle. The *radial nerve* (**10**) becomes visible between the brachialis (**3**) and the brachioradialis (**5**) and divides into a smaller, sensory, *superficial branch* (**11**) and a larger, *deep branch* (**12**). The superficial branch supplies cutaneous fibers to the radial half of the dorsum of the hand, the thumb and the dorsal surface of the proximal phalanges of the 2nd and 3rd digits, while the deep branch, which penetrates the *supinator* (**13**), innervates this muscle and the extensors of the forearm.

Variants (B–D)

The median nerve usually (approx. 95%) runs between the two heads of the pronator teres (**B**). Occasionally it pierces the *humeral head* (**14**) of the pronator teres (barely 2%; **C**). In about 3% of cases, the median nerve lies directly on the bone and runs deep to the two heads of the pronator teres (**D**). In such cases a fracture of the proximal part of the radius and ulna may endanger the nerve. Variants of the brachial artery and its branches in this region have been reported, although infrequently, e. g., the brachial artery may run dorsal to the supracondylar process when present.

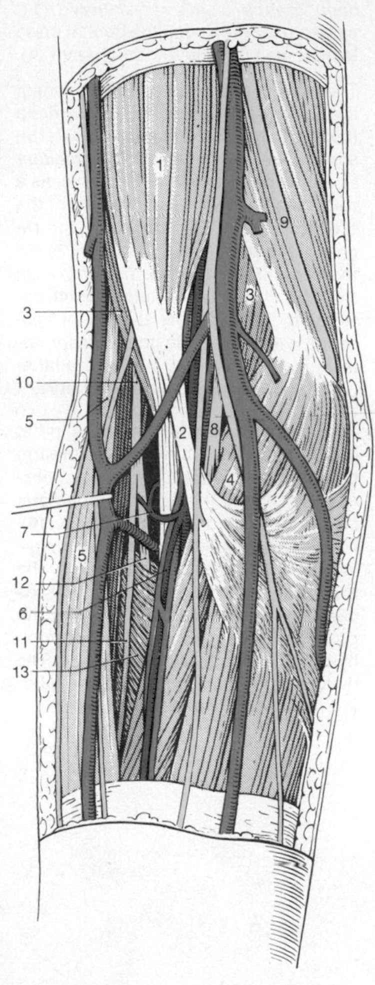

A Deep layer of cubital fossa

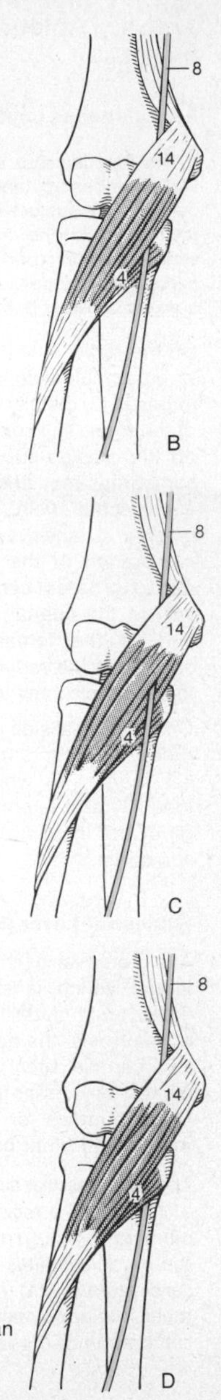

B–D. Variation in relationship of median nerve to pronator teres (after Lanz-Wachsmuth)

Anterior Antebrachial Region (A–B)

Subcutaneous Layer (A)

In the subcutaneous adipose tissue are the well-developed cutaneous veins, which, to be sure, are subject to great variations in their courses. The cutaneous arteries are small and unimportant. The cutaneous nerves run independently of the veins and are very constant both in location and size.

On the radial side there is the *cephalic antebrachial vein* (**1**), which *anastomoses* (**2**) distally with the other veins of the forearm. Proximally it often gives off the *median cubital vein* (**3**), which sometimes may arise from the median antebrachial vein. The *lateral antebrachial cutaneous nerve* (**4**), the terminal branch of the musculocutaneous nerve, crosses beneath the cephalic vein in the cubital fossa. In the distal part of the forearm the *superficial branch of the radial nerve* (**5**) is lying in close proximity to the cephalic vein.

On the medial side of the anterior antebrachial region runs the *antebrachial basilic vein* (**6**), which is accompanied medially and laterally by the branches (**7**) of the *medial antebrachial cutaneous nerve.*

Subfascial Layer (B)

After removal of the firm antebrachial fascia, which is strengthened proximally and medially by the bicipital aponeurosis, the deep nerves and vessels can be seen. These vessels and nerves are essentially arranged into three bundles or tracts, the radial, middle and ulnar bundles.

The **radial vascular bundle**, which consists of the *radial artery* (**8**) and its *accompanying veins* (**9**), runs distally between the *brachioradialis* (**10**) and the *flexor carpi radialis* (**11**). In the proximal segment it is accompanied by the *superficial branch of the radial nerve* (**12**). The *deep branch of the radial nerve* (**13**) passes deeply through the cubital fossa to become buried in the *supinator* (**14**).

The **middle neurovascular bundle**, which lies between the superficial and deep flexors, contains the *median nerve* (**15**), sometimes accompanied by a *median artery* (variant). The median nerve, as a rule, runs between the two heads of the *pronator teres* (**16**) and lies, in the region of the wrist, radial to the tendons of the *flexor digitorum superficialis* (**17**). In a deeper stratum of the middle tract, between the deep flexors and the interosseous membrane, lie the *anterior interosseous artery and nerve*, the latter being a branch of the median nerve.

The **ulnar neurovascular bundle** lies in the middle and distal thirds of the forearm between the *flexor digitorum superficialis* (**17**) and the *flexor carpi ulnaris* (**18**). It consists of the *ulnar nerve* (**19**), the *ulnar artery* (**20**) and its *accompanying veins* (**21**). After its origin from the brachial artery, the ulnar artery crosses deep to the median nerve (**15**), the pronator teres (**16**) and the common head of the superficial flexors. The flexor carpi ulnaris (**18**) serves as a guiding muscle for the ulnar nerve (**19**).

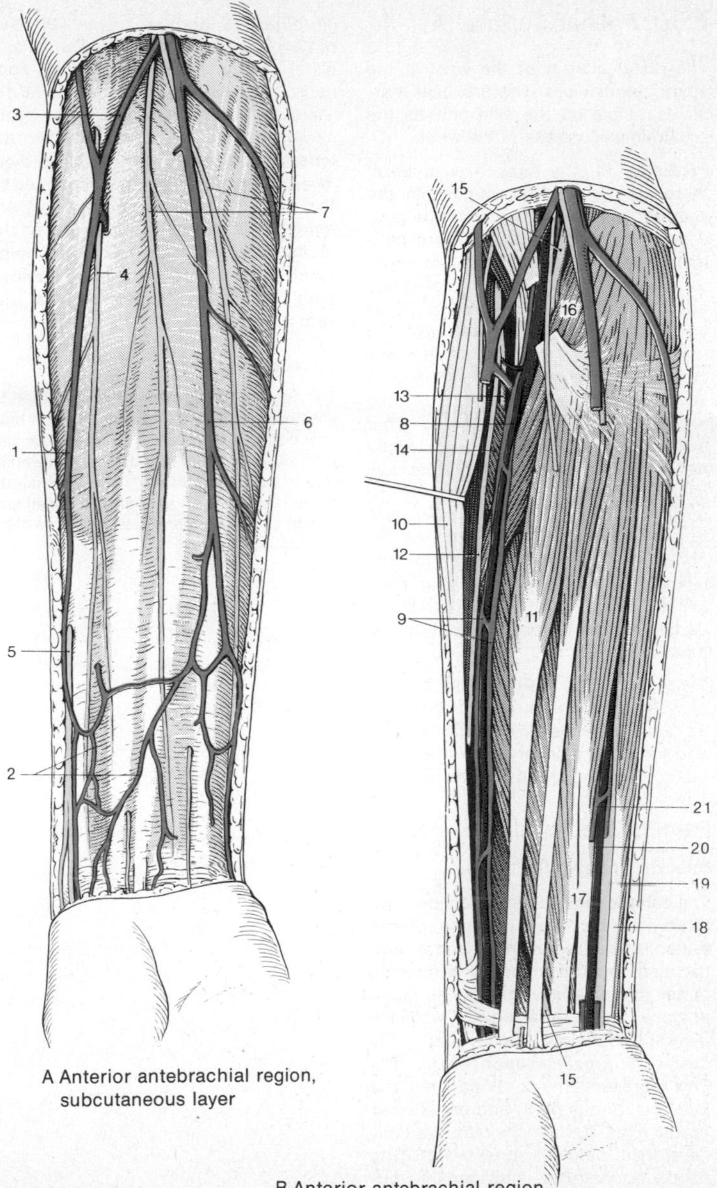

A Anterior antebrachial region, subcutaneous layer

B Anterior antebrachial region, subfascial layer

Wrist, Palmar Surface (A)

The distal margin of the wrist is the flexor retinaculum. The proximal margin is visible on the skin only as the proximal skin crease of the wrist.

Proximal to the *flexor retinaculum* there are strong fiber strands in the *antebrachial fascia* (**1**), which also form a deep layer (**2**) and which are connected to the bones of the forearm. Superficially run the veins and nerves as described previously on page 370, as well as the tendon of the *palmaris longus* (**3**). Deeply, the most radial structure is the *radial artery* (**5**) and its accompanying veins lying on the *pronator quadratus* (**4**). On the ulnar side of the artery lies the tendon of the *flexor carpi radialis* (**6**) within its own synovial sheath, followed nect by the tendon sheath of the *flexor pollicis longus* (**7**). Between this muscle and the common tendon sheath (**8**) for the *flexor digitorum superficialis* and the *flexor digitorum profundus*, the *median nerve* (**9**) runs toward the palm of the hand.

The *ulnar artery* (**10**) with its accompanying veins and the *ulnar nerve* (**11**) lie radial to the *flexor carpi ulnaris* (**12**) and run to the palm of the hand superficial to the flexor retinaculum.

Palm of the Hand

Superficial Layer (B)

The palm of the hand is subdivided into three regions: the eminence of the thumb (thenar region), the central compartment and the eminence of the little finger (hypothenar region). The fascia encloses these lateral regions, while the central compartment is covered by the coarse, firm *palmar aponeurosis* (**13**). This represents the continuation of the palmaris longus (**A, 3**) and on its ulnar border it radiates into the rather variably developed palmaris brevis (**14**). The palmar aponeurosis is divided into *longitudinal* (**15**) and *transverse* (**16**; see p. 174) *fascicles*. At the radial, ulnar and distal margins of the palmar aponeurosis the *common palmar digital arteries* (**17**) and the nerves of the same name become subcutaneous. The arteries divide into the proper *palmar digital arteries* (**18**), which, accompanied by the proper *palmar digital nerves,* extend to the terminal phalanges of the digits. The *proper palmar digital veins* reach the *superficial palmar venous arch,* which lies superficially at the root of the digits.

Practical Point

The nerves at the sides of the digits can be anesthetized by the Oberst method of local injection. It is important to remember that the skin of the middle and terminal phalanges of the thumb, index and middle digits is innervated also on the dorsal surface by proper *palmar* digital branches of the median nerve.

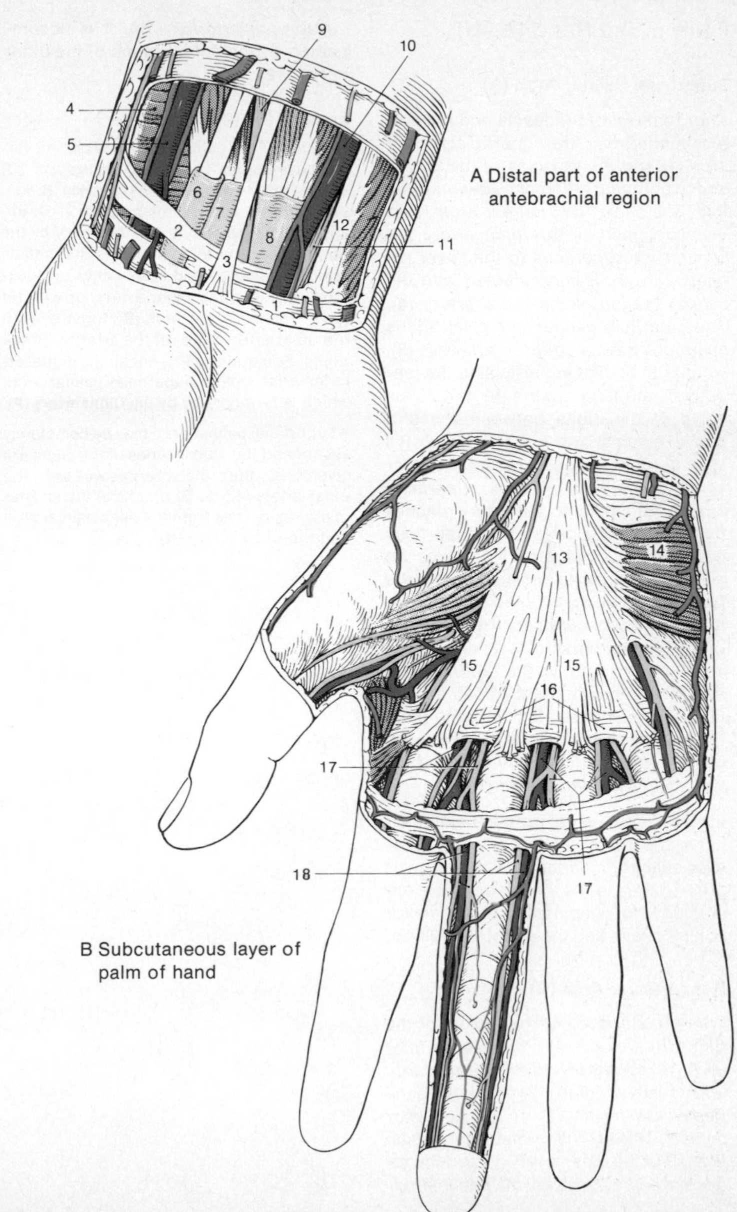

A Distal part of anterior antebrachial region

B Subcutaneous layer of palm of hand

Palm of the Hand (A–H)

Superficial Palmar Arch (A)

After removal of the fascia and the palmar aponeurosis, the superficial palmar arch (**1**) and the muscles of the thenar and hypothenar eminences become visible. The *superficial palmar arch* (**1**) is mainly formed by the *ulnar artery* (**2**), which runs superficial to the *flexor retinaculum* (**3**). It is connected with the *palmar branch of the radial artery* (**4**). The superficial palmar arch gives off the *common palmar digital arteries* (**5**), which run at first superficial to the tendons of the long flexors (**6**) and at the roots of the digits between the tendons. The ulnar artery, which gives off a *deep branch* (**7**), accompanies the *ulnar nerve* (**8**), which with its *superficial branch* (**9**) medial to the artery reaches the palm of the hand. The superficial branch of the ulnar nerve innervates the skin of the ulnar half of the palm of the hand and normally two and a half digits. It is often connected to the branches of the *median nerve* (**11**) by an *anastomotic branch* (**10**). In the region of the flexor retinaculum (**3**), the *deep branch* (**12**) becomes separated from the ulnar nerve and penetrates deeply between the *abductor digiti minimi* (**13**) and the *flexor digiti minimi brevis* (**14**).

Already in the carpal tunnel the median nerve has often divided into the *common palmar digital nerves* (**15**). It gives off branches to the thenar muscles, excluding the deep head of the flexor pollicis brevis and the adductor pollicis.

Deep Palmar Arch (B)

When the tendons of the flexors of the digits (**6**) are removed, the *deep palmar arch* (**18**) appears lying on the *interossei* and usually running (**16**) proximal to the *transverse head* (**17**) *of the adductor pollicis*. This arch is formed by the deep branch of the ulnar artery (**7**) and the radial artery and gives off the *palmar metacarpal arteries* (**19**). It is accompanied by the deep branch of the ulnar nerve (**12**).

Variants (C–H)

The superficial palmar arch may be very variably developed. The typical palmar arch (**C**) is present in only 27% of cases (Lanz-Wachsmuth). In the same proportion of subjects (27%) the arch is formed solely by the ulnar artery (**D**). In some cases the median artery is retained and may, either by anastomosing with the ulnar artery, or without the formation of the arch (**E**), together with the ulnar artery, give off the arteries for the digits. Sometimes (6%) not all the digital arteries arise from a superficial palmar arch, which is formed only by the ulnar artery (**F**).

A superficial palmar arch may be completely absent and then the arteries of the digits are given off by the radial artery as well as by the ulnar artery (4.5%, **G**) or, (12%) the arteries of the digits arise from the deep palmar arch and the ulnar artery (**H**).

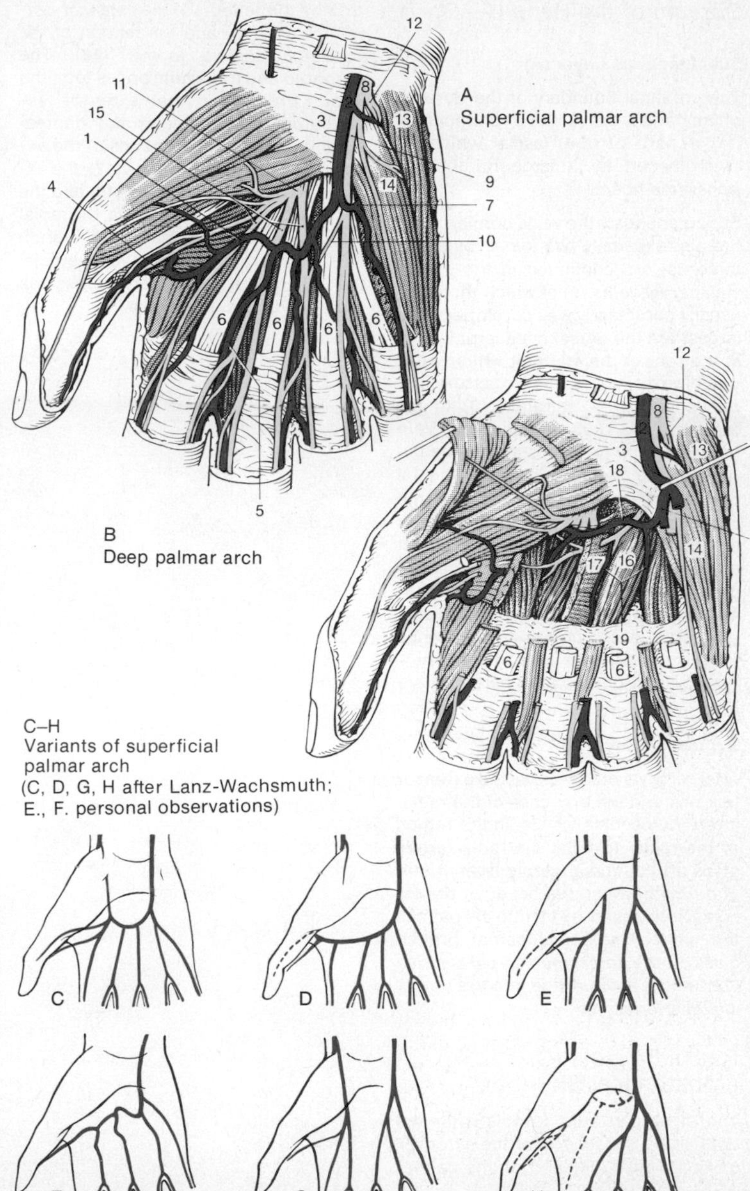

A
Superficial palmar arch

B
Deep palmar arch

C–H
Variants of superficial palmar arch
(C, D, G, H after Lanz-Wachsmuth; E., F. personal observations)

Dorsum of the Hand (A–B)

Subcutaneous Layer (A)

The proximal boundary of the dorsum of the hand is the *extensor retinaculum* (**1**), a part of the fascia which is strengthened by a large number of transverse fibers.

Subcutaneously the veins coming from the digits (usually two joined by anastomoses) are continued in the *dorsal metacarpal veins* (**2**) of which three are usually particularly well developed. The largest are the dorsal metacarpal veins at the root of the 4th digit which, after combining, run as the *accessory cephalic vein* (= v. salvatella, **3**) to the forearm. The *dorsal metacarpal vein of the 5th digit* (**4**) represents the beginning of the basilic vein, while the 1st dorsal metacarpal vein is called the *cephalic vein of the thumb* (**5**). A large number of anastomoses interconnect all the veins to form the *venous network of the dorsum of the hand* (**6**). On the ulnar side, covered by veins, runs the *dorsal branch of the ulnar nerve* (**7**), while radially the terminal parts of the *superficial branch of the radial nerve* (**8**) are found.

Subfascial Layer (B)

After removal of the fascia, the extensor tendons and the branches of the *radial artery* (**9**) become visible. In the region of the radial foveola, the radial artery gives off the *dorsal carpal branch* (**10**) and runs between the heads of the *1st dorsal interosseous* (**11**) into the palm of the hand. The dorsal carpal branch gives off the *dorsal metacarpal arteries* (**12**), which again divide into the *dorsal digital arteries* (**13**).

Radial Foveola (C) ("Anatomical Snuffbox")

The triangular radial foveola is limited dorsally by the tendon of the *extensor pollicis longus* (**14**) and on the palmar side by the tendon of the *extensor pollicis brevis* (**15**) and the tendon of the *abductor pollicis longus* (**16**). The scaphoid and trapezium bones form the floor. Proximally the extensor retinaculum (**1**) completes the depression. It contains the tendons of the *extensor carpi radialis longus* (**17**), the *extensor carpi radialis brevis* (**18**) and the radial artery (**9**). In the foveola, the radial artery gives off its dorsal carpal branch (**10**). The branches of the superficial part (**8**) of the radial nerve cross the radial foveola superficially.

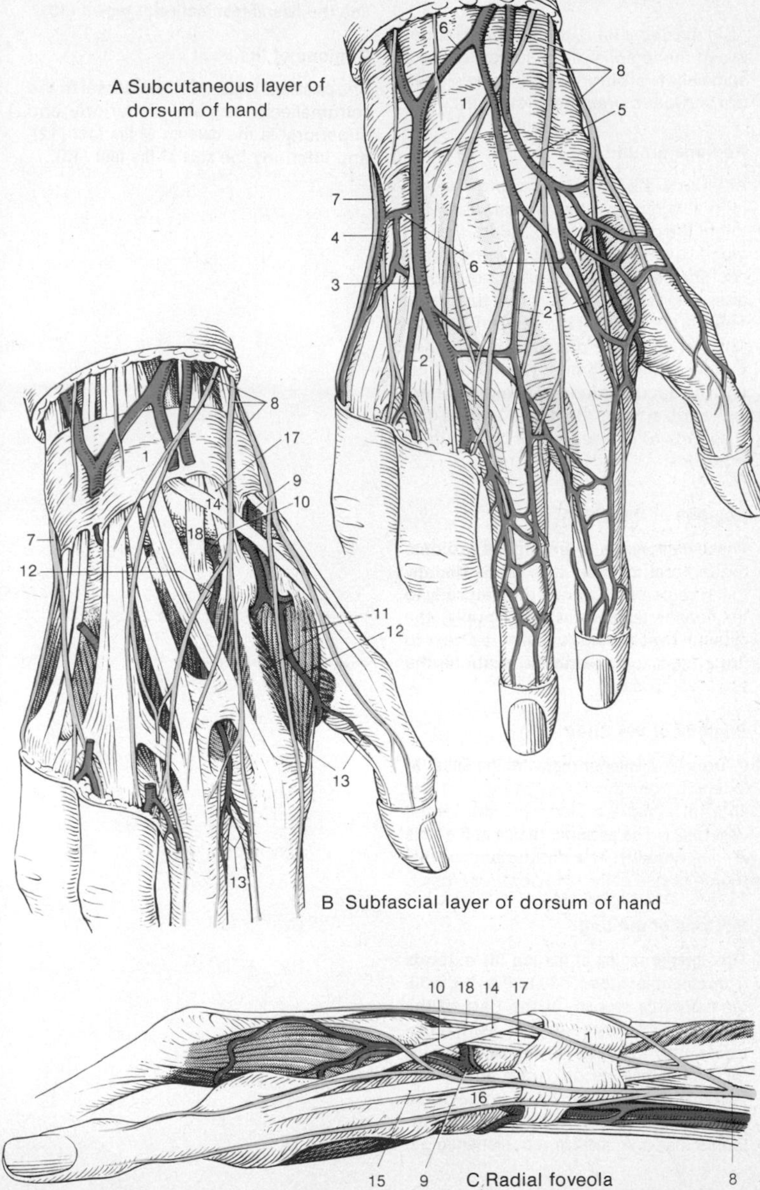

A Subcutaneous layer of dorsum of hand

B Subfascial layer of dorsum of hand

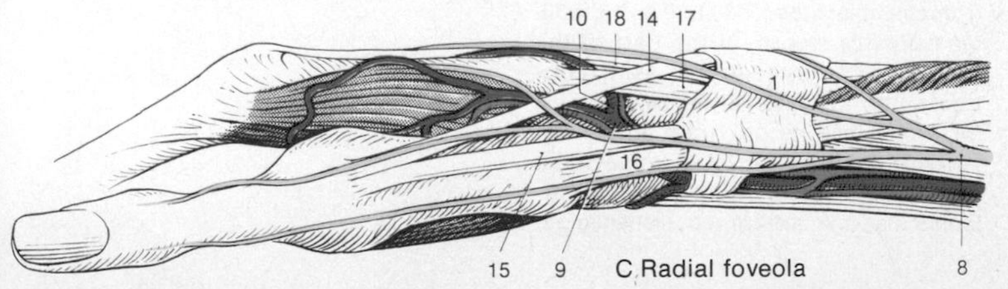

C Radial foveola

Regions (A–B)

As in the upper limb, the boundaries between the regions of the lower limb are somewhat arbitrary and have been drawn from a practical viewpoint.

Regions around the Hip

Anteriorly the regions around the hip joint also represent subdivisions of the thigh. We distinguish a *subinguinal region* (**1**), which is bounded by the inguinal ligament, the sartorius and pectineus muscles as part of the large femoral triangle. The **femoral triangle** (**2**) extends further distally and is limited by the inguinal ligament, the sartorius and the adductor longus. Dorsally there is the **gluteal region** (**3**), which almost corresponds to the region of the gluteus maximus.

Regions of the Thigh

The **anterior region of the thigh** (**4**) adjoins the femoral triangle. It extends distally to the region of the knee and laterally to the tensor fasciae latae. Dorsally, the **posterior region of the thigh** (**5**) lies next to the gluteal region and ends above the popliteal fossa.

Regions of the Knee

In front, the **anterior region of the knee** (**6**) extends from the lower margin of the anterior thigh region to the tibial tuberosity. The **posterior region of the knee** (**7**) lies dorsally. The middle part of this region is also called the *popliteal fossa.*

Regions of the Leg

The **anterior region of the leg** (**8**) extends from the tibial tuberosity to the malleoli. Medially this region, at the part of the tibia palpable through the skin, continues into the **posterior region of the leg** (**9**), which has its proximal and distal borders at the same level as those of the anterior region. Behind the medial malleolus lies the **medial retromalleolar region**, and behind the lateral malleolus lies the **lateral retromalleolar region** (**10**).

Regions of the Foot

The **calcaneal region** (**11**) lies dorsal to the retromalleolar regions. Anteriorly and superiorly is the **dorsum of the foot** (**12**), and inferiorly the **sole of the foot** (**13**).

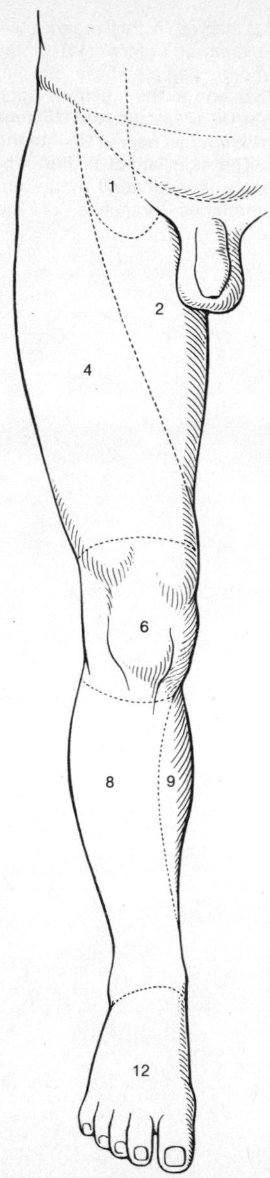

A Anterior view of regions of lower limb

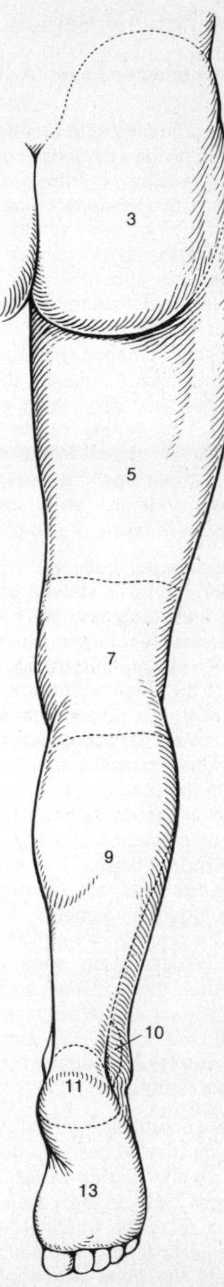

B Posterior view of regions of lower limb

Subinguinal Region

Subcutaneous Layer (A–B)

The abundant subcutaneous fatty tissue is divided by dense *connective tissue lamellae* (**1**) into two layers. The connective tissue lamellae, which were formerly known as the superficial femoral fascia or Scarpa's fascia, partly cover the subcutaneous vessels and nerves and extend below the saphenous hiatus. Only after removal of all the subcutaneous fatty tissue and connective tissue lamellae the *fascia lata* (**2**) can be seen. Most of the fascia lata is generally of an aponeurotic character, except in the region of the saphenous opening, where there is a looser, reticular structure, called the *cribriform fascia* 3; see p. 242).

The subcutaneous veins, which reach this region in a stellate pattern, pierce the cribriform fascia. The largest and the most regularly occurring vessel is the *great saphenous vein* (**4**). It runs from the thigh to the cribriform fascia (**3**). Often a *lateral accessory saphenous vein* (**5**) accompanies it. The superficial *external pudendal veins* (**6**) run from the pubic region and the *superficial epigastric vein* (**7**) runs from the umbilical region of the abdomen to the cribriform fascia. The *superficial circumflex iliac vein* (**8**) runs parallel to the inguinal ligament. The junction of all these veins is very variable and will be discussed on page 382. Smaller arteries, the *external pudendal artery* (**9**), the *superficial epigastric artery* (**10**) and the *superficial circumflex iliac artery* (**11**) accompany the veins of the same names.

The superficial inguinal lymph nodes, which may be divided into two groups, lie on the cribriform fascia. The *horizontal limb on proximal set* (**12**) lies parallel to the inguinal ligament, and the *vertical limb or distal set* (**13**), parallels the great saphenous vein. The cutaneous nerves in this region stem from the *femoral branch* (**14**) of the *genitofemoral nerve.* Above the inguinal ligament, in the inguinal region in the male, the *spermatic cord* (**15**) runs with the *ilioinguinal nerve* (**16**) into the scrotum. The skin lateral to the cribriform fascia is innervated by the anterior cutaneous branches of the femoral nerve.

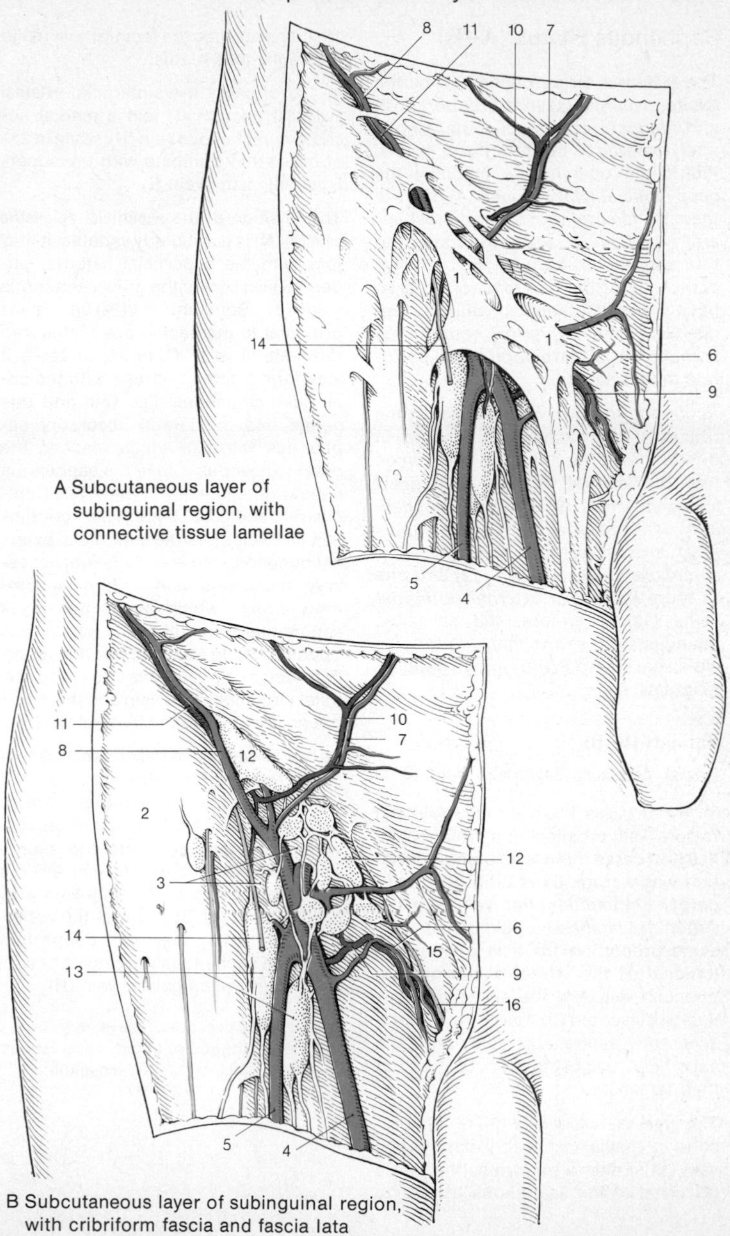

A Subcutaneous layer of subinguinal region, with connective tissue lamellae

B Subcutaneous layer of subinguinal region, with cribriform fascia and fascia lata

Saphenous Hiatus (A–R)

The **saphenous hiatus**, delineated by the *falciform margin* (**1**) with its *superior* (**2**) and *inferior* (**3**) *cornua*, becomes visible after removal of the cribriform fascia. Within the opening lie medially the *deep inguinal lymph nodes* (**4**), next to them the *femoral vein* (**5**) and most laterally the *femoral artery* (**6**). Lateral to the saphenous hiatus, the *femoral branch* (**7**) of the *genitofemoral nerve* becomes subcutaneous. Still further laterally, the *anterior cutaneous branches* (**8**) of the *femoral nerve* perforate the fascia lata.

According to Lanz-Wachsmuth, in the region of the saphenous opening in 37% of cases the following veins open into the femoral vein (**A**): the *great saphenous vein* (**9**), the *lateral accessory saphenous vein* (**10**), the *superficial circumflex iliac vein* (**11**), the *superficial epigastric vein* (**12**) and one or more *superficial external pudendal veins* (**13**). Therefore, the so-called "**venous star**" shows many variations, which are shown in the various detailed diagrams.

Variants (B–R)

Lateral Accessory Saphenous Vein (B–E)

In 1% of cases this vein may join the femoral vein proximal to the hiatus (**B**). In 9% of cases there is a common junction with a trunk consisting of the superficial circumflex iliac vein and the superficial epigastric vein (**C**). In the same proportion there is a common terminal of the lateral accessory saphenous vein and the superficial circumflex iliac vein (**D**). Rarely, the lateral accessory saphenous vein and the superficial epigastric vein (**E**) join at their termination.

The **great saphenous vein** (**F–G**) may receive a medial accessory saphenous vein (**14**). Either it perforates the fascia (**F**) distal to the saphenous hiatus (in 1%), or it reaches the femoral vein (**G**) in the saphenous hiatus.

In 1% of cases the superficial **external pudendal veins** (**H–I**) join a medial accessory saphenous vein (**H**), while in 2% of cases they combine with the superficial epigastric vein (**I**).

The position of the **superficial epigastric vein** (**J–N**) is particularly variable. It may join with the superficial external pudendal vein before the great saphenous vein (**J**). Sometimes (1%) it opens proximal to the saphenous hiatus into the femoral vein (**K**). In 9% of cases it may form a common trunk with the superficial circumflex iliac vein and this opens into the lateral accessory saphenous vein (**L**), which reaches the great saphenous vein in the saphenous hiatus. Sometimes the superficial epigastric and the superficial circumflex iliac veins join the superficial external pudendal vein and the lateral accessory saphenous vein to form a common trunk, which joins the great saphenous vein within the saphenous opening (**M**). In 6% of cases, the superficial epigastric vein runs into the superficial circumflex iliac vein and this trunk opens directly into the femoral vein (**N**).

As has already been described, in 9% of cases the **superficial circumflex iliac vein** (**O–R**) may open with the superficial epigastric vein and the lateral accessory saphenous vein into the saphenous vein (**O**), and in a further 9% the lateral accessory saphenous vein also opens into it (**P**). Sometimes the superficial circumflex iliac vein opens into the great saphenous vein together with the superficial epigastric vein (**R**).

The variants described above represent a summary of the author's many observations, as well as those of Lanz-Wachsmuth.

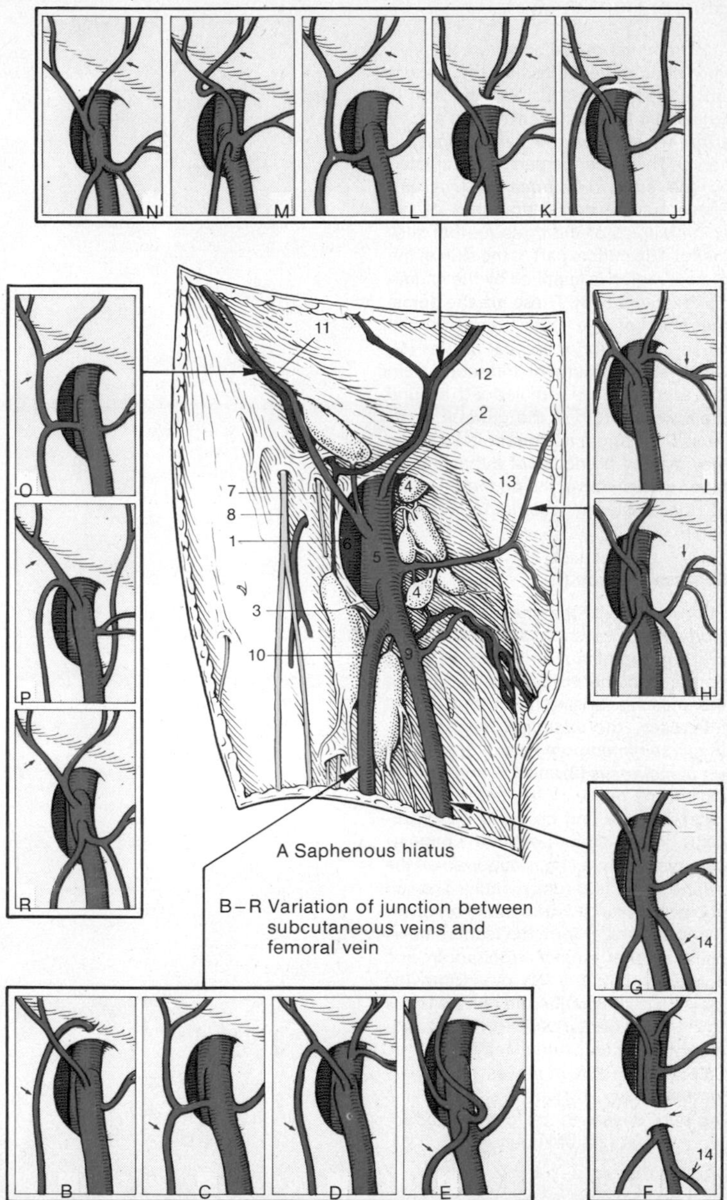

A Saphenous hiatus

B–R Variation of junction between subcutaneous veins and femoral vein

Gluteal Region (A–B)

After removal of the skin and the very fatty subcutaneous tissue, the *gluteal fascia* (**1**) becomes visible. The skin is innervated by the cluneal nerves and by a *branch* (**2**) *of the iliohypogastric nerve*. The superior part is innervated by the *superior cluneal nerves* (**3**). These are the dorsal branches of the spinal nerves of the three lumbar segments. The middle part of the skin of the gluteal region is supplied by the *middle cluneal nerves* (**4**). These are the dorsal branches of the three sacral spinal nerves. The *inferior cluneal nerves* (**5**), which stem directly or indirectly from the sacral plexus, are looped around the lower margin of the gluteus maximus. Their origin is indirect in so far as they may be branches of either the inferior gluteal nerve, the pudendal nerve or the posterior cutaneous femoral nerve.

Subfascial Layer (B)

After removal of the gluteal fascia, the *gluteus maximus* (**6**) and the ischiocrural group of muscles below its lower border become visible. These include the muscles arising from the ischial tuberosity, the *adductor magnus* (**7**), the *semimembranosus* (**8**) and *semitendinosus* (**9**) and the *long head of the biceps femoris* (**10**). Lateral to the latter muscle and crossing it superficially, runs the *posterior femoral cutaneous nerve* (**11**). Deeper down the *sciatic nerve* (**12**) runs distally. The sciatic nerve may be found relatively easily if a line is drawn from the ischial tuberosity to the greater trochanter and divided into thirds. By extending the junction of the medial and middle thirds to the lower border of the gluteus maximus, the sciatic nerve may be seen. Lateral to the sciatic nerve, the *1st perforating artery* (**13**) with its accompanying veins descends to cross the *adductor minimus* (**14**) obliquely.

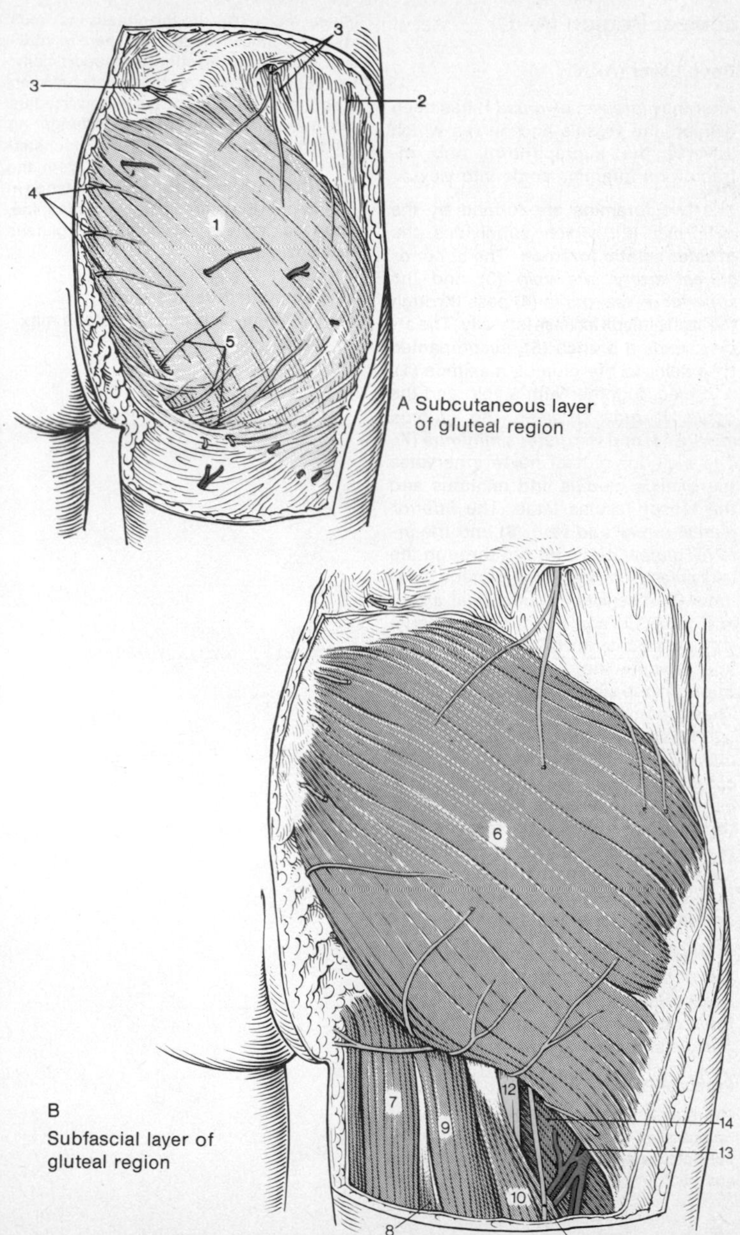

A Subcutaneous layer of gluteal region

B
Subfascial layer of gluteal region

Gluteal Region (A–C)

Deep Layer (A)

After the *gluteus maximus* (**1**) has been divided, the vessels and nerves which traverse the suprapiriform and infrapiriform foramina come into view.

The two foramina are formed by the *piriformis* (**2**), which subdivides the **greater sciatic foramen**. The *superior gluteal artery and vein* (**3**) and the *superior gluteal nerve* (**4**) pass through the **suprapiriform foramen** laterally. The artery sends a branch (**5**), accompanied by a vein, to the gluteus maximus (**1**), and then, together with a vein and the nerve, it runs between the *gluteus medius* (**6**) and the *gluteus minimus* (**7**). The superior gluteal nerve innervates the gluteus medius and minimus and the tensor fasciae latae. The *inferior gluteal artery and vein* (**8**) and the *inferior gluteal nerve* (**9**) run through the **infrapiriform foramen** to the gluteus maximus (**1**). The *internal pudendal artery and vein* (**10**) and the *pudendal nerve* (**11**) arch posterior to the ischial spine and reach the ischiorectal fossa through the lesser sciatic foramen. They run dorsal to the *superior gemellus* (**12**) and then adhere to the *obturator internus* (**13**). The *posterior femoral cutaneous nerve* (**14**) and the *sciatic nerve* (**15**) leave the lesser pelvis through the infrapiriform foramen and reach the thigh by passing dorsal to the *superior gemellus* (**12**), the *obturator internus* (**13**), the *inferior gemellus* (**16**) and the *quadratus femoris* (**17**).

The posterior femoral cutaneous nerve (**14**) then runs superficial to the *long head of the biceps femoris* (**18**), while the sciatic nerve (**15**) runs between this muscle and the *adductor magnus* (**19**).

Practical Points

The gluteal region is an ideal site for intramuscular injections. Intragluteal injections are usually given into the superolateral quadrant (cross hatched in blue) of the gluteal region (**B**), into the gluteus maximus (**1**) or the gluteus medius (**6**). There is, however, danger of injecting too superficially, i. e., subcutaneously, or too deeply between the gluteus maximus and the gluteus medius into the intermuscular fat, thus endangering the superior gluteal nerve (**4**). A. v. Hochstetter has recommended injecting from the side (**C**) in a triangular field (cross hatched in red), behind the anterior superior iliac spine, into the gluteus medius and gluteus minimus.

20 Sacrotuberous ligament,
21 Trochanteric bursa of gluteus maximus.

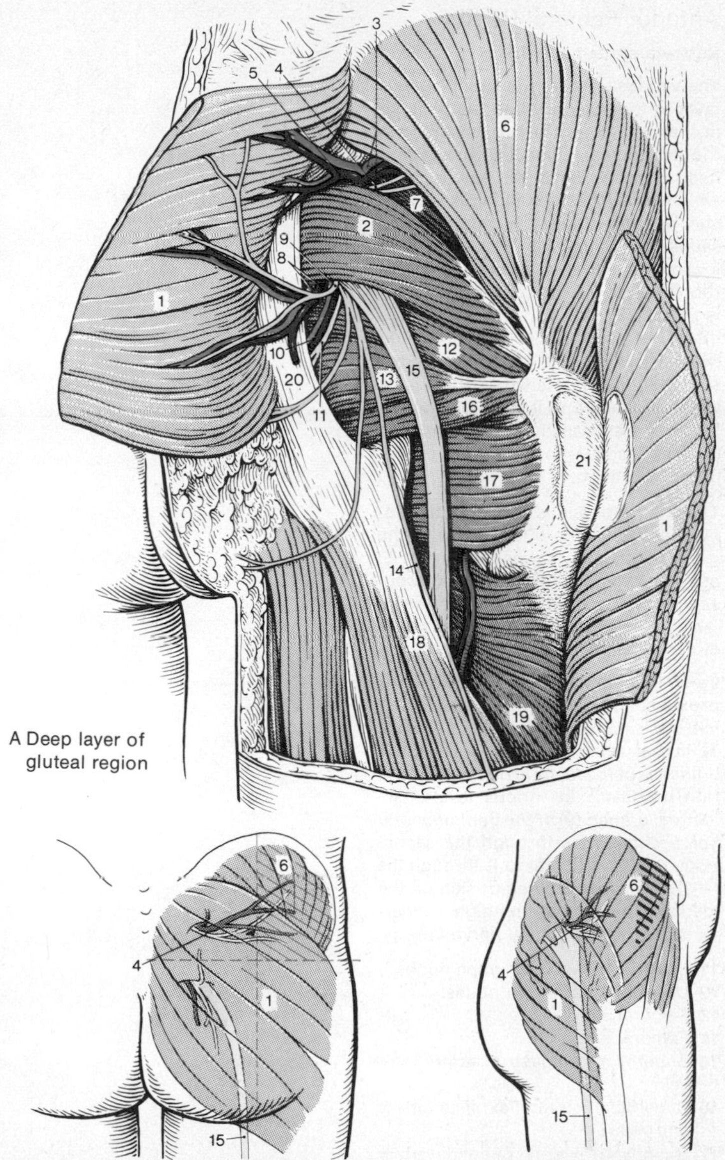

A Deep layer of gluteal region

B Diagram of vessels and nerves potentially endangered by intragluteal injections

C Intragluteal injection site as recommended by A. v. Hochstetter

Anterior Femoral Region

Subcutaneous Layer (A)

The various areas of the subcutaneous layer of the anterior thigh region differ in their structure. The proximal part, in the subinguinal region, has strong connective tissue lamellae (see p. 380), which divide the subcutaneous fatty tissue into two layers. In addition, the *saphenous hiatus* (**1**) is covered by a loose connective tissue layer, the cribriform fascia. The *fascia lata* (**2**), which is complete but for the saphenous hiatus, is also variable in structure. In the lateral thigh it is taut and kept stretched by the tensor faciae latae which radiates into it. This part of the fascia is also called the *iliotibial tract* (**3**). The fascia is looser in the medial part of the thigh.

The *great saphenous vein* (**4**) runs subcutaneously and is often joined by the *lateral accessory saphenous vein* (**5**) and less often by the *medial accessory saphenous vein* (**6**). The other veins which enter the saphenous hiatus have already been described on page 382.

Laterally, near the junction between the proximal and middle thirds, the *lateral femoral cutaneous nerve* (**7**) becomes epifascial, while the *anterior cutaneous branches of the femoral nerve* (**8**) perforate the fascia at various levels. The *femoral branch* (**9**) *of the genitofemoral nerve* either runs through the saphenous hiatus or lateral to it through the fascia lata. A small area of skin on the medial upper side of the thigh is innervated by the *ilioinguinal nerve* (**10**).

11 Superficial inguinal lymph nodes,
12 Deep inguinal lymph nodes,
13 Femoral vein,
14 Femoral artery,
15 Superficial epigastric artery and vein,
16 Superficial circumflex iliac artery and vein,
17 Superficial external pudendal artery and vein.

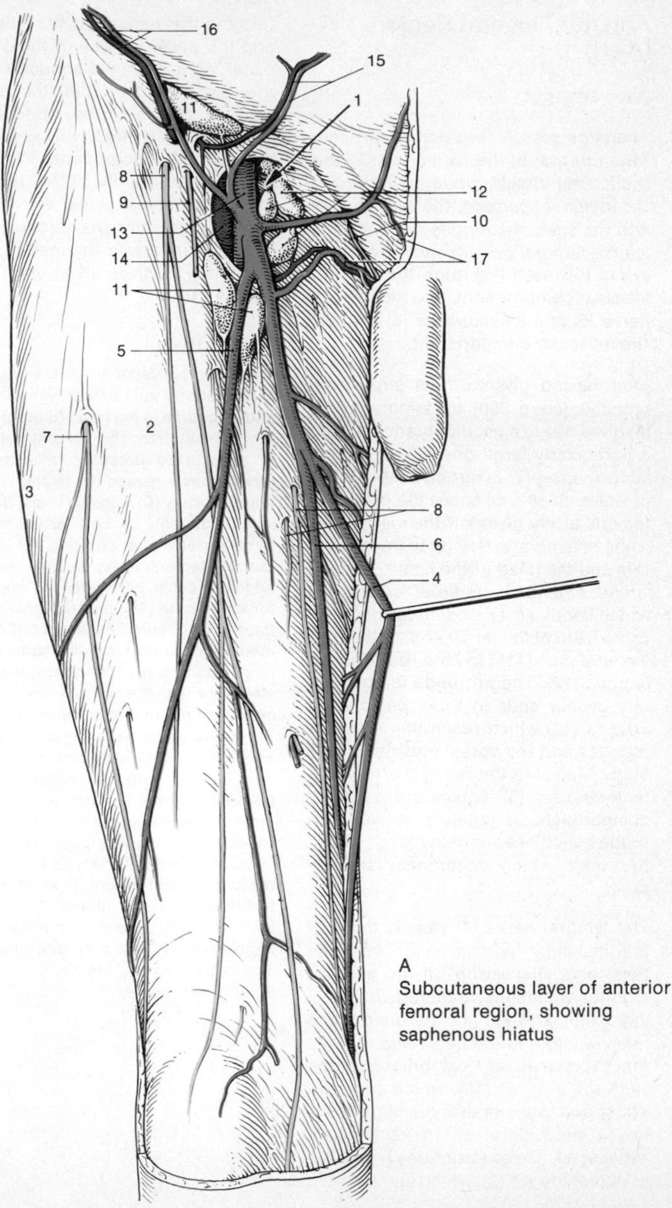

A
Subcutaneous layer of anterior femoral region, showing saphenous hiatus

Anterior Femoral Region (A–H)

Deep Layer (A)

The large vessels and nerves are seen after removal of the fascia lata. Within the **femoral triangle**, which is limited by the *inguinal ligament*, the *sartorius* (**1**) and the *adductor longus* (**2**), lymphatics, the *femoral vein* (**3**) and the *femoral artery* (**4**) reach the thigh through the vascular compartment, and the *femoral nerve* (**5**) and the *iliopsoas* (**6**) through the muscular compartment.

After having given off its superficial branches (see p. 380), the femoral artery (**4**) gives rise to muscular branches, and a particularly large one, the *profunda femoris artery* (**7**), is buried deeply in the muscles. In 58% of cases the profunda femoris artery gives off the *medial circumflex femoral artery* (**8**) to the adductors and the head of the femur, and the *lateral circumflex femoral artery* (**9**), which sends an *ascending branch* (**10**) to the head of the femur and a *descending branch* (**11**) to the *quadriceps femoris* (**12**). The profunda femoris artery usually ends in three *perforating arteries* (**13**) which reach the adductor muscles and the dorsal muscles of the thigh. Medial to the femoral artery, the femoral vein (**3**) enters the vascular compartment. It collects, in addition to the subcutaneous veins (see p. 382), the veins which accompany the arteries.

The femoral nerve (**5**) passes through the muscular compartment into the thigh and, after giving off the anterior femoral cutaneous branches, it innervates the sartorius (**1**), the quadriceps femoris (**12**) and the *pectineus* (**14**). Its longest, purely sensory branch is the *saphenous nerve* (**15**), which runs lateral to and together with the femoral artery (**4**) and femoral vein to reach the **adductor canal.** These structures lie on the adductor longus (**2**), which takes part in forming the vastoadductor membrane, and the posterior wall of the adductor canal. Apart from the adductor longus, the *vastus medialis* (**16**), the *adductor magnus* (**17**) and the *vastoadductor membrane* (**18**) are involved in formation of the adductor canal. The saphenous nerve usually (62%) perforates this membrane together with the *descending genicular artery* (**19**) to extend onto and innervate the medial surface of the leg. It gives off an *infrapatellar branch* (**20**).

Variants (B–H)

There is great variability in the origin of the saphenous nerve (**15**) from the femoral nerve and its course in the thigh (Sirang). Very often it arises from the femoral nerve (**5**, B) proximal to the lateral circumflex femoral artery. It may embrace the lateral circumflex femoral artery (**C**) with two roots. Somewhat less commonly it only arises from the femoral nerve after crossing the lateral circumflex femoral artery (**D**, **E**). It reaches the adductor canal, perforates the vastoadductor membrane (**18**) and may give off its infrapatellar branch, either lateral (**B**, **C**) or medial (**D**) to or through the sartorius (**E**). In rare instances (**E**) the infrapatellar branch also receives fibers from the *superficial branch of the obturator nerve* (**21**).
The branches from the femoral artery (**4**) are also very variable. Most commonly (58% according to Lippert) the medial (**8**) and lateral (**9**) circumflex femoral arteries arise from the profunda femoris artery (**F**, **7**). In 18% of cases (according to Lippert, **G**) the lateral circumflex femoral artery (**9**) arises from the profunda femoris artery (**7**), while, according to the same author, the medial circumflex femoral artery (**8**) arises from the profunda femoris artery (**7**) in only 15% of cases (**H**). The remaining 8% are distributed among much rarer variants.

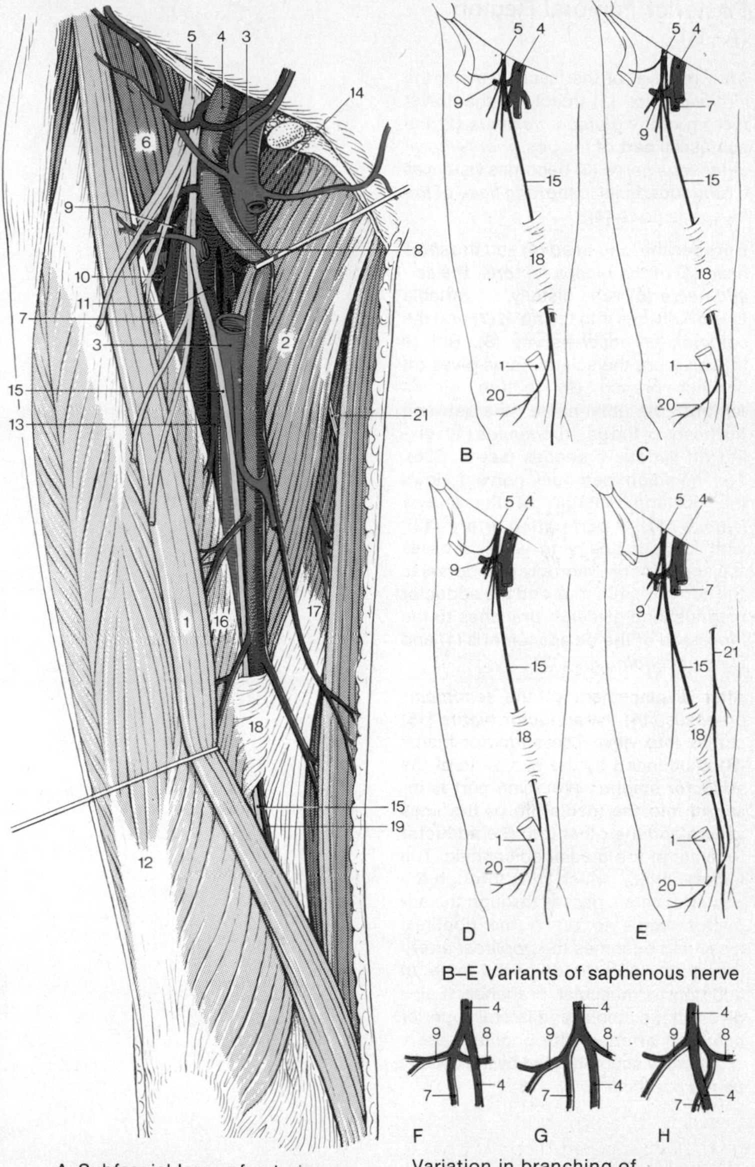

A Subfascial layer of anterior femoral region femoral artery displaced medially

B–E Variants of saphenous nerve

Variation in branching of femoral artery in subinguinal region (after Lanz-Wachsmuth)

Posterior Femoral Region (A–B)

After removal of the fascia, leaving the *iliotibial tract* (**1**) intact, at the lower margin of the *gluteus maximus* (**2**) the subfascial part of the *posterior femoral cutaneous nerve* (**3**) becomes visible as it runs superficial to the *long head of the biceps femoris* (**4**).

Between the *long head* (**4**) and the *short head* (**5**) *of the biceps femoris*, the *sciatic nerve* (**6**) runs distally. At variable levels it divides into the *tibial* (**7**) and the *common peroneal nerves* (**8**). Before this division, the sciatic nerve gives off another branch (**9**) to the biceps femoris. The tibial nerve runs between the heads of the *gastrocnemius* (**10**) giving off various branches (see p. 396). The common peroneal nerve follows the posterior margin of the *biceps femoris* (**11**). A *perforating artery* (**12**), with its accompanying veins, crosses the sciatic nerve ventrally (but dorsal to the adductor minimus and the adductor magnus) and gives off branches to the long head of the biceps femoris (**4**) and the *semitendinosus* (**13**).

After displacement of the *semimembranosus* (**14**) the *adductor hiatus* (**15**) comes into view. The addcutor hiatus (**B**) is bounded by the two parts of the *adductor magnus* (**16**). One part is inserted into the medial lip of the linea aspera and the other into the adductor tubercle of the medial epicondyle. The femoral artery, which runs through the adductor canal, passes through the adductor hiatus to reach the popliteal fossa and becomes the *popliteal artery* (**17**) on the dorsal side of the thigh. In addition to muscular branches, it also gives off the medial and lateral superior genicular arteries. The popliteal artery is generally accompanied by the usually paired *popliteal veins* (**18**).

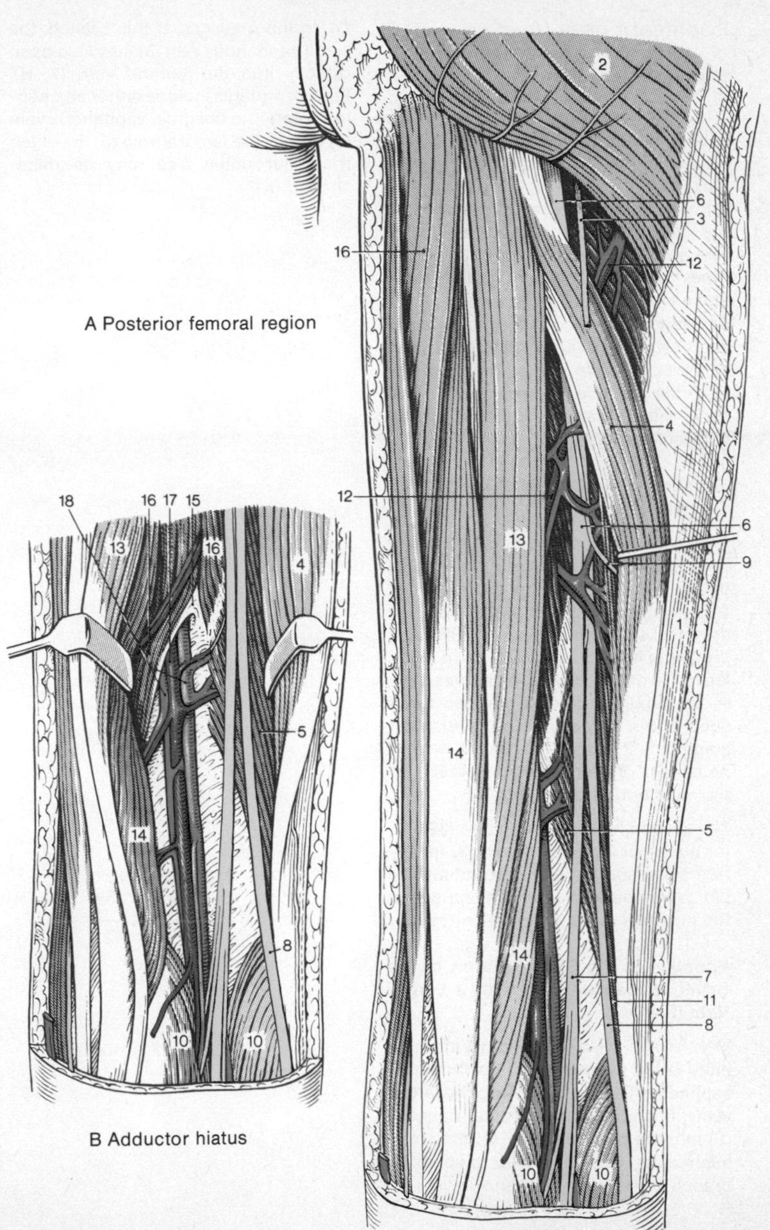
2
6
3
16
12
A Posterior femoral region
4
18
16 17 15
12
13
16
4
6
13
9
1
5
14
14
5
8
14
7
11
8
10 10
10 10
B Adductor hiatus

Popliteal Fossa (A–K)

Subcutaneous Layer (A)

The *great saphenous vein* (**1**) lies in the subcutaneous layer at the medial margin of the popliteal fossa. In the leg it is accompanied by the *saphenous nerve* (**2**), which becomes subcutaneous at the lower margin of the popliteal fossa. The *small saphenous vein* (**3**) sometimes (see below) perforates the fascia at the lower margin of the popliteal fossa. It is accompanied by the *medial sural cutaneous nerve* (**4**) which is continued as the sural nerve (see p. 400). In addition, the *posterior femoral cutaneous nerve* with its branches (**5**) terminates in the popliteal fossa.

Variation in the Course of the Small Saphenous Vein (B–E)

The small saphenous vein, which is very important in phlebology, runs a variable course in relation to the crural fascia. According to Moosmann and Hartwell the small saphenous vein (**3**) perforates the crural fascia in the distal third of the leg in 7% of cases (**B**), runs subfascially to the popliteal fossa and then turns deep to join the *popliteal vein* (**6**). Most commonly (51,5%) the small saphenous vein (**3**) perforates the fascia in the middle third of the leg (**C**).

The second most common site (32.5%) for the small saphenous vein (**3**) to perforate the fascia is in the proximal third (**D**). It only perforates the fascia within the popliteal fossa (**E**) in 9% of cases.

Variation in the Site of Union of the Small Saphenous Vein with a Larger Vein (F–K)

Mercier et al. also reported great variability in the manner in which the small saphenous vein (**3**) opens into the larger veins. In addition to its typical opening (**F**) into the popliteal vein (**6**), the small saphenous vein may also give off a branch to the great saphenous vein (**1**, **G**). In the presence of this branch, the small saphenous vein (**3**) may also open directly into the *femoral vein* (**7, H**). Further variants include either an opening solely into the great saphenous vein (**1**) or into the femoral vein (**J**), in which the latter union also may be delta-shaped (**K**).

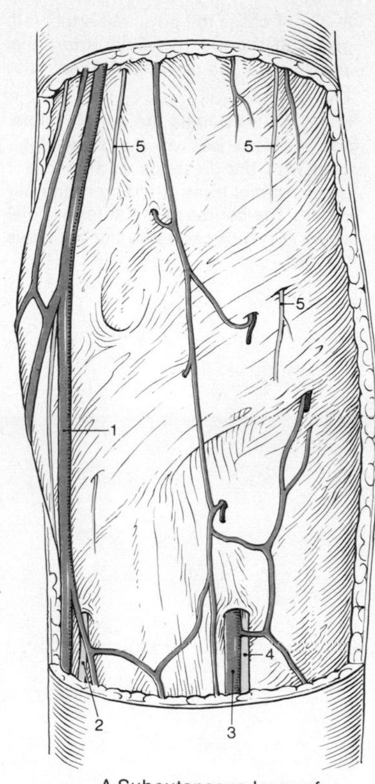

A Subcutaneous layer of popliteal fossa

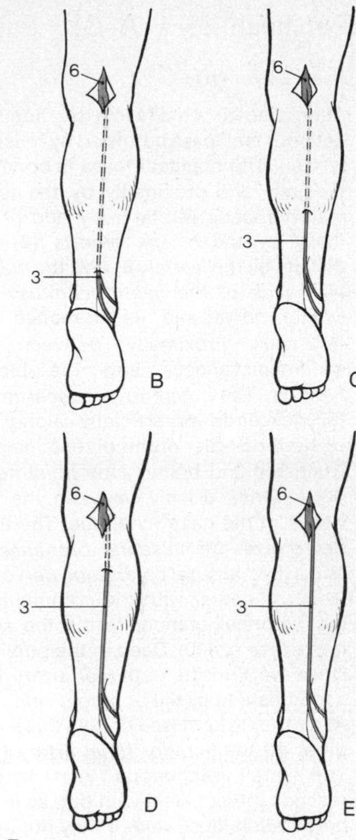

B–E
Sites of perforation of fascia by small saphenous vein (after Moosmann and Hartwell)

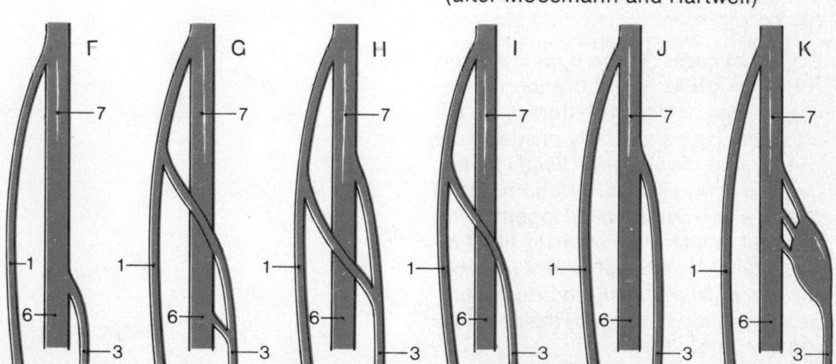

F–K Various ways in which small saphenous vein opens into larger vein (after Mercier et al.)

Popliteal Fossa (A–G)

Deep Layer (A)

After removal of the fascia the rhomboidal popliteal fossa bounded by muscles is seen. The popliteal fossa is bounded medially and proximally by the *semimembranosus* (**1**), laterally and proximally by the *biceps femoris* (**2**) and distally by the *lateral* (**3**) and the *medial* (**4**) *heads of the gastrocnemius.* The sciatic nerve and its branches can be seen proximally between the semimembranosus and the biceps femoris. The *common peroneal nerve* (**5**) descends superficially along the posterior border of the biceps femoris, while the 2nd branch, the *tibial nerve* (**6**), extends distally between the two heads of the gastrocnemius. The tibial nerve gives off *muscular branches* (**7**) and a *medial sural cutaneous nerve* (**8**), which, together with the communicating peroneal branch, forms the sural nerve (see p. 400). Deep in the popliteal fossa we find the *popliteal artery* (**10**) accompanied by the *popliteal veins* (**9**). At a variable level (see below) this artery gives off the *anterior tibial artery* (**11**). The small saphenous vein usually reaches the popliteal vein but, as in the preparation illustrated, it may not open into a larger vein until it is proximal to the popliteal fossa.

Variants of the Arterial Branches (B–G)

In 90% of cases (**B**) the popliteal artery (**10**) gives off as its 1st branch the anterior tibial artery (**11**) dorsal to the *popliteus* (**12**), and it only divides more distally into the *posterior tibial* (**13**) and *peroneal* (**14**) *arteries*. In about 4% of cases (**C**) the arteries arise together. It is unusual (1%) for the anterior tibial artery and the peroneal artery (*anterior peroneotibial trunk;* **15**) to originate together at the distal edge of the popliteus (**D**).

In 3% of cases the popliteal artery (**10**) gives off the anterior tibial artery just proximal to the popliteus (**E**, see also Fig. **A**).

In 1% of individuals the anterior tibial artery (**11**) arises at the same high level with the presence of an anterior peroneotibial trunk (**F**, **15**), or, another variant, the course of the anterior tibial artery (**11**) runs ventral to the popliteus (**12**, **G**).

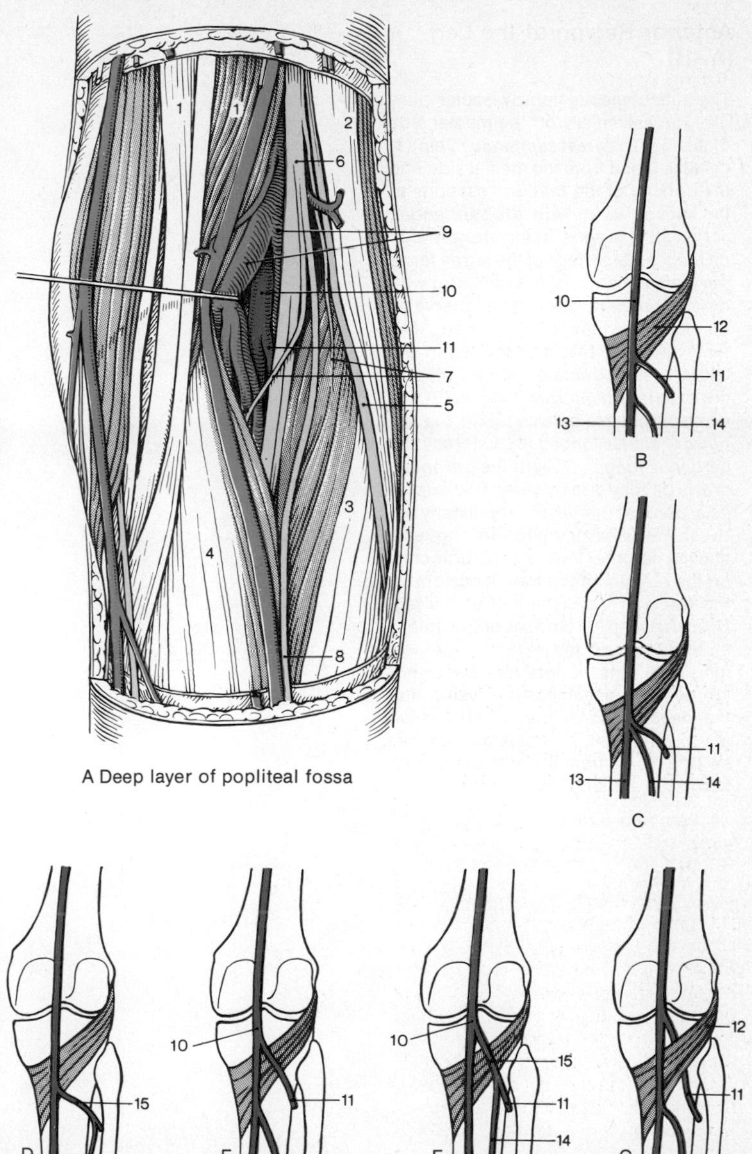

A Deep layer of popliteal fossa

B–G Variants of arterial branches of popliteal artery (after Lanz-Wachsmuth)

Anterior Region of the Leg (A–B)

The subcutaneous neurovascular bundles run essentially on the medial side of the leg. The *great saphenous vein* (**1**) collects blood from the medial side and the dorsum of the foot and ascends to the triceps surae with the *saphenous nerve* (**2**). This nerve innervates the skin on the medial surface of the leg as far as the medial margin of the foot, and with its *infrapatellar branch* (**3**) it innervates the skin of the infrapatellar region. After removal of the fascia of the leg in the lateral area, the *tibialis anterior* (**4**) and the *extensor digitorum longus* (**5**) become visible and between them the *extensor hallucis longus* (**6**). Laterally the *peroneus longus* (**7**) and the *peroneus brevis* (**8**) may also be seen. The *superficial peroneal nerve* (**9**) runs distally between the extensor digitorum longus (**5**) and the peroneal muscles and branches on the dorsum of the foot. It perforates the fascia in the distal half of the leg. Deep between the tendons of the tibialis anterior (**4**) and the extensor hallucis longus (**6**) runs the *anterior tibial artery* (**10**) with its accompanying veins and the deep *peroneal nerve* (**11**), which along with its motor fibers also carries sensory fibers from the area of skin between the 1st and 2nd digits.

12 Peroneus tertius.

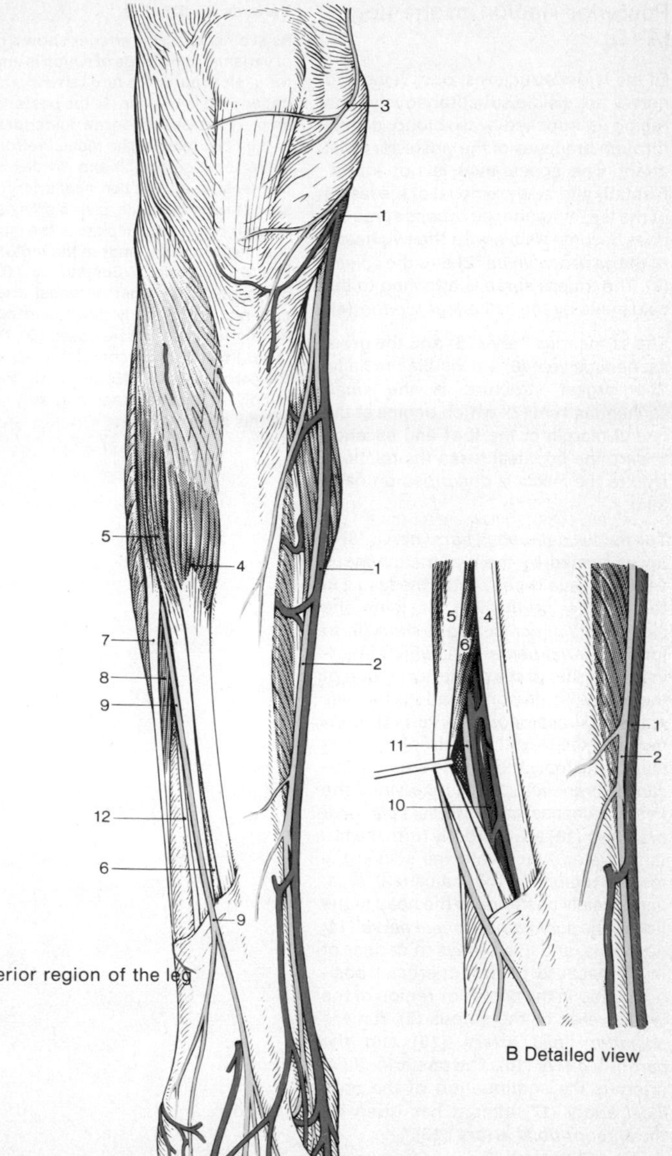

A Anterior region of the leg

B Detailed view

Posterior Region of the Leg (A–D)

Of the larger structures, only veins and nerves are visible subcutaneously. The region is supplied with blood deeply through branches of the posterior tibial artery. The appearance is not fundamentally altered by removal of the fascia of the leg, although the *triceps surae* (**1**) does become visible with the two heads of the *gastrocnemius* (**2**) and the *soleus* (**3**). The triceps surae is attached to the calcaneus by the *calcaneal tendon* (**4**).

The *saphenous nerve* (**5**) and the *great saphenous vein* (**6**) are visible medially. The largest structure is the *small saphenous vein* (**7**), which begins at the lateral margin of the foot and ascends toward the popliteal fossa (its relationship to the fascia is described on page 394).

The *medial cutaneous sural nerve* (**8**) is accompanied by the small saphenous vein and usually perforates the fascia in the middle of the leg. It joins the *peroneal communicating branch* (**9**) to form the *sural nerve* (**10**), which innervates the skin of the posterior region of the leg. With its continuation, the *lateral dorsal cutaneous nerve* (**11**), it innervates the lateral margin of the dorsum of the foot, and with the *lateral calcaneal branches* (**12**) it innervates the lateral calcaneal area. *Medial calcaneal branches* (**13**) arise directly from the tibial nerve and innervate the skin in the medial region of the calcaneal area. Immediately posterior to the head of the fibula, the *common peroneal nerve* (**14**) descends, and it is always in danger of injury because of its superficial position. Deep in the posterior region of the leg, covered by the soleus (**3**), run the *posterior tibial artery* (**15**) and the *peroneal artery* (**16**). The posterior tibial artery is the continuation of the *popliteal artery* (**17**) after it has given off the *anterior tibial artery* (**18**).

Variants (B–D)

As at other sites, the arteries show a number of variants, knowledge of which is important for clinical purposes (e. g. arteriography, ligations etc.). As a rule (**B**) the posterior tibial artery (**15**) descends on the posterior surface of the tibia, reaches the medial retromalleolar region (see p. 402) and divides into the plantar arteries. The peroneal artery (**16**) descends near the fibula, giving off a *perforating branch* (**19**) which pierces the interosseous membrane and ends in the region of the lateral malleolus. Sometimes (**C**) the phylogenetically older peroneal artery (**16**) may replace a poorly developed posterior tibial artery (**15**). In rare cases (**D**), the posterior tibial artery is completely absent and the peroneal artery (**16**) takes over the blood supply for the entire region usually supplied by this artery.

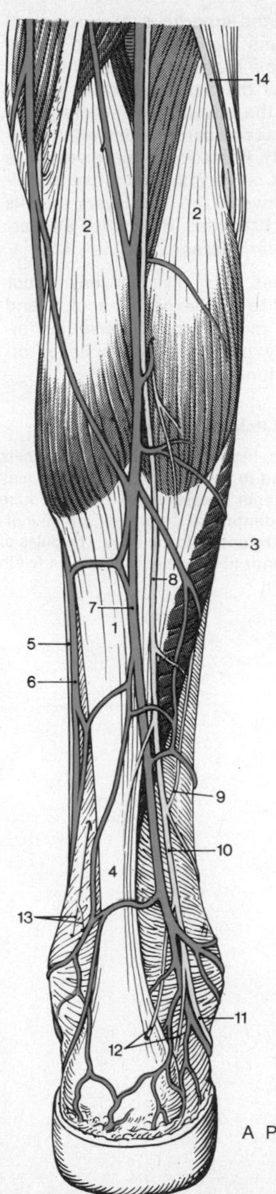

A Posterior region of the leg

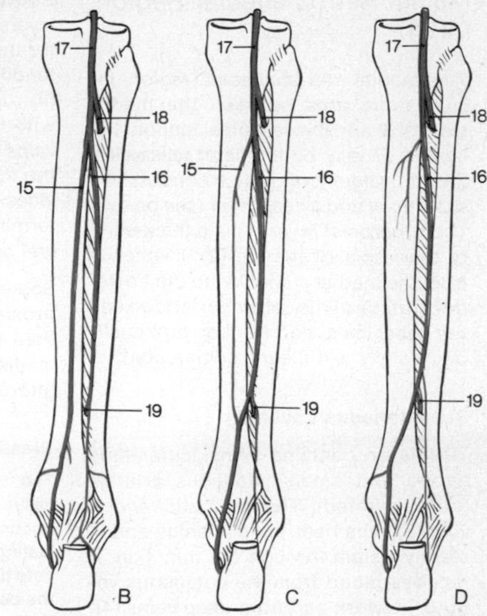

B–D Variants of posterior tibial artery and peroneal artery (Redrawn after Lanz-Wachsmuth)

Medial Retromalleolar Region (A–B)

The medial retromalleolar region includes the area between the medial malleolus and the calcaneal tendon. It is limited distally by the **flexor retinaculum** (laciniate ligament), which consists of a *superficial* and a *deep layer* (see below). The *superficial layer* (**1**) is a thickening of the *fascia* of the leg (**2**). It extends from the medial malleolus to the posterior surface of the calcaneal tendon and the tuber calcanei. Neither proximally nor distally is it clearly demarcated.

Subcutaneous Layer (A)

This layer contains veins, cutaneous nerves and small cutaneous arteries (not illustrated). The *great saphenous vein* (**3**) runs near the malleolus and is readily visible through the thin skin. It receives blood from the cutaneous venous network and from deep veins (**4**). The *saphenous nerve* (**5**) branches in this region to supply sensory innervation to the skin.

Subfascial Layer (B)

After removal of the fascia of the leg, the neurovascular bundle and the long muscles of the sole to the foot can be seen proximal to the flexor retinaculum. Also visible is the *deep layer* (**6**) of the flexor retinaculum, which extends from the medial malleolus to the calcaneus and provides the osteofibrous canal for the long muscles of the foot.

Immediately behind the medial malleolus runs the tendon of the *tibialis posterior* (**7**) and adjacent to it the tendon of the *flexor digitorum longus* (**8**). The tendon of the *flexor hallucis longus* (**9**) lies deeper and is displaced somewhat backward by the medial tubercle of the posterior process of the talus. All three muscles have their own tendon sheaths (see p. 267), which are not illustrated here.

Between the superficial (**1**) and deep (**6**) layers runs the neurovascular bundle for the sole of the foot. Adjacent to the tendon of the flexor digitorum longus (**8**) runs the *posterior tibial artery* (**10**) with its accompanying *posterior tibial veins* (**11**). Posterior to these veins lies the *tibial nerve* (**12**), which usually divides between the two layers into its terminal branches, the *medial* and *lateral plantar nerves.*

Sometimes this division may occur proximal to the flexor retinaculum and then the medial plantar nerve lies immediately posterior to the flexor digitorum longus.

Practical Points

The loose, highly mobile skin here permits tissue fluid to accumulate, and edema may occur. Finger pressure will then produce lasting indentations ("pitting"), which indicate fluid retention in the body. The pulse of the posterior tibial artery may also be felt in this region.

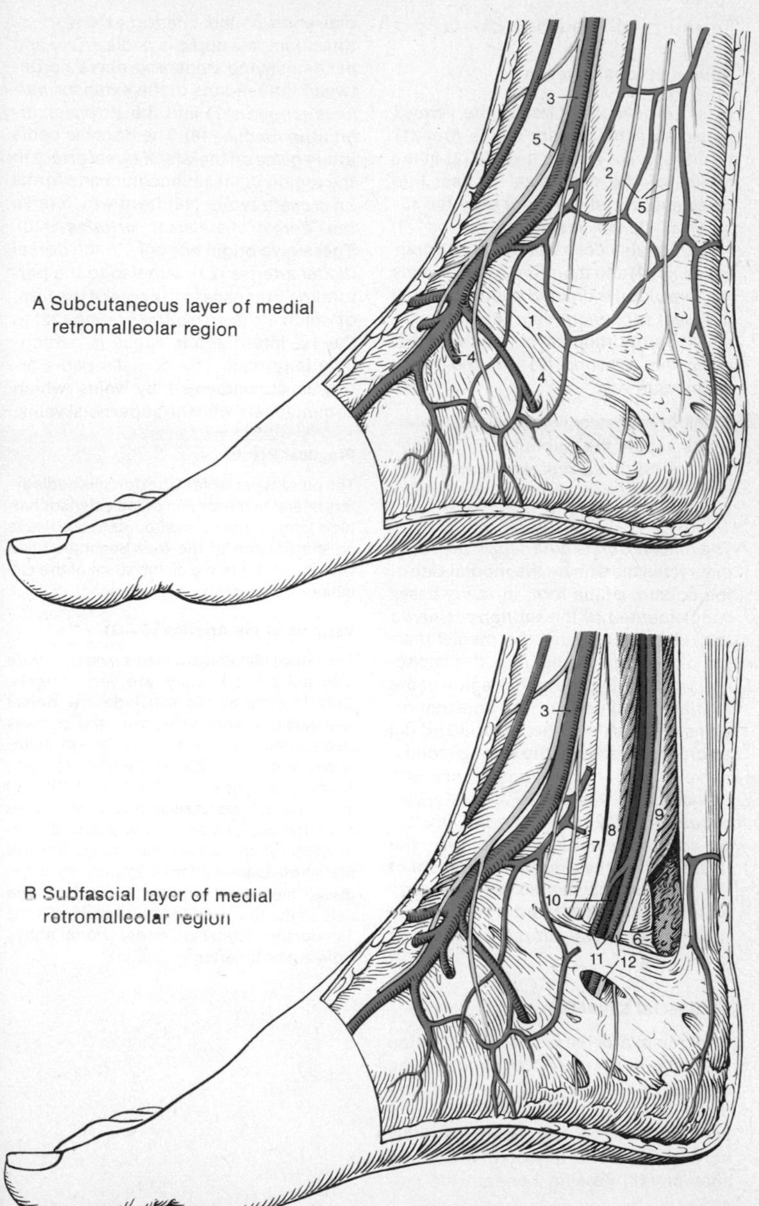

A Subcutaneous layer of medial retromalleolar region

B Subfascial layer of medial retromalleolar region

Dorsum of the Foot (A–G)

Subcutaneous Layer (A)

A dense network of veins, the *venous network of the dorsum of the foot* (**1**), forms a *dorsal venous arcade* (**2**) in the region of the metatarsal bones. Into these superficial veins not only the *superficial dorsal metatarsal veins* (**3**) open, but also deep veins, the *perforating veins* (**4**) and the *intercapitular veins* (**5**). The blood is drained mainly through the *great saphenous vein* (**6**) and only a smaller proportion travels via the *lateral malleolar network* (**7**) to the small saphenous vein.

Small branches only from the deep arteries reach the subcutaneous layer, and the *1st dorsal metatarsal artery* (**8**), which has a variable origin (see below), is the only one that is visible.

The *medial dorsal cutaneous nerve* (**9**) innervates the skin on the medial side of the dorsum of the foot, in many cases supplemented by the *saphenous nerve* (**10**), which innervates the medial margin of the foot. Sometimes the saphenous nerve (**10**) ends in the region of the medial malleolus. Only the adjacent regions of the skin of the 1st and 2nd dig its are innervated by the *deep peroneal nerve* (**11**), which may *anastomose* with branches of the *medial dorsal cutaneous nerve* (**12**). The *intermediate dorsal cutaneous nerve* (**13**) supplies the lateral half of the skin of the dorsum of the foot, supplemented at its lateral margin by the final branch of the sural nerve, the *lateral dorsal cutaneous nerve* (**14**).

Subfascial Layer (B)

After removal of the fascia and retention of the inferior extensor retinaculum, the *dorsalis pedis artery* (**15**) becomes visible. It runs onto the dorsum of the foot, accompanied by the deep peroneal nerve (**11**). With the tendon of the *tibialis anterior* (**16**) passing beneath the medial ends of the inferior extensor retinaculum, the dorsalis pedis artery and accompanying veins and nerve lie between the tendons of the *extensor hallucis longus* (**17**) and the *extensor digitorum longus* (**18**). The dorsalis pedis artery gives off the *lateral tarsal artery* in the region of the retinaculum and forms an *arcuate artery* (**19**) from which arise the *dorsal metatarsal arteries* (**20**). These give origin not only to the *dorsal digital arteries* (**21**), but also to the perforating branches to the sole of the foot, of which the *deep plantar branch* (**22**) to the 1st interosseous space is particularly important. The dorsalis pedis artery is accompanied by veins which communicate with the superficial veins.

Practical Points

The pulse is palpable in the dorsalis pedis artery lateral to the tendon of the extensor hallucis longus. The loose subcutaneous tissue on the dorsum of the foot becomes filled with fluid if there is a disturbance of the circulation, thus producing edema.

Variants of the Arteries (C–G)

The dorsal metatarsal arteries, and therefore also the arcuate artery, are very variable. Only in 20% of cases (**C**) do the dorsal metatarsal arteries arise from the dorsalis pedis artery while in 6% (**D**) the 4th metatarsal artery is supplied by a perforating branch from the sole of the foot in 40% (**E**) only the 1st metatarsal artery originates from the dorsalis pedis artery, and the remainder of the dorsal metatarsal arteries stem from plantar arteries. In 10 % (**F**) all the dorsal metatarsal arteries come from the sole of the foot, and in 5% of cases (**G**) the 1st dorsal metatarsal artery alone arises from a plantar artery.

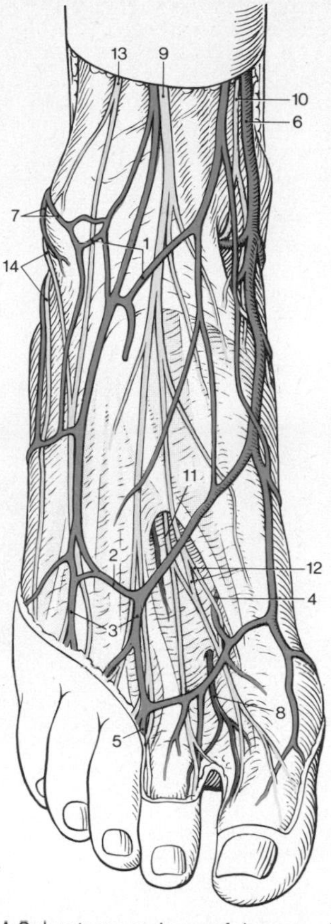

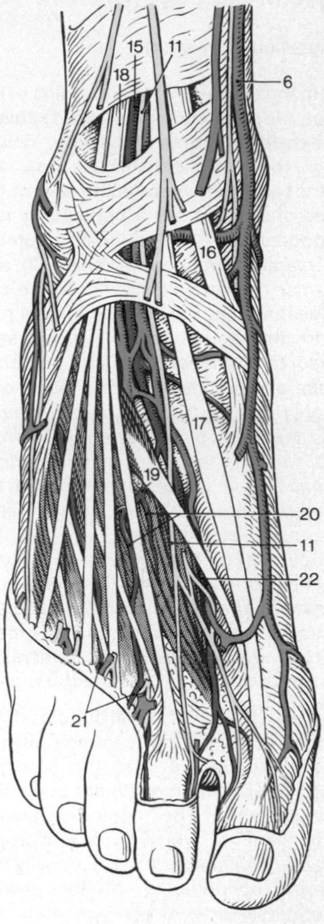

A Subcutaneous layer of dorsum of foot

B Subfascial layer of dorsum of foot

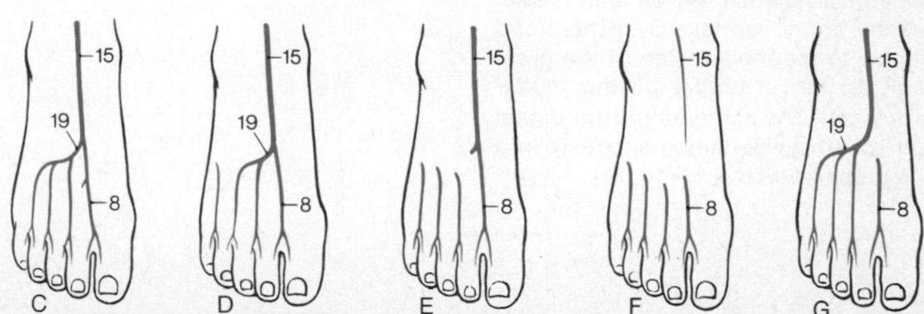

C–G Variants of arteries of dorsum of foot (after Lippert)

Sole of the Foot (A)

Superficial Layer (A)

With the exception of the margins of the foot, the *plantar aponeurosis* (**1**) covers the deep structures of the sole, including the principal trunks of the peripheral pathways. As the skin of the sole of the foot has a particularly rich blood supply, there are a large number of *plantar cutaneous arteries* (**2**) and *plantar cutaneous veins* (**3**). In the calcaneal region, the arteries form a network, the *rete calcaneum*, which is supplied by branches from the *posterior tibial* and *peroneal arteries*. Additional branches stem from the *medial plantar* and the *lateral plantar arteries*. The *medial plantar artery* gives off a *superficial branch* (**4**), which becomes visible at the medial margin of the plantar aponeurosis, accompanied by the *1st proper plantar digital nerve* (**5**). Lateral to the aponeurosis there is often a subcutaneous *branch* (**6**) *of the lateral plantar artery* accompanied by the *proper plantar digital nerve* (**7**) for innervation of the outer margin of the little digit.

Between the longitudinal bundles of the aponeurosis (**1**), the *common plantar digital arteries* (**8**) and the *common plantar digital nerves* (**9**) are becoming sucutaneous. The common plantar digital arteries, which divide into *proper plantar digital arteries* (**10**), usually represent continuation of the plantar metatarsal arteries (see p. 408), but may (very uncommonly) arise from a **"superficial" plantar arch.** Often the superficial branch (**4**) of the medial plantar artery can take over the blood supply to the medial side of the great digit as the *1st proper plantar digital artery* (**11**). The common plantar digital nerves (**9**) divide subcutaneously into the *proper digital nerves* (**12**).

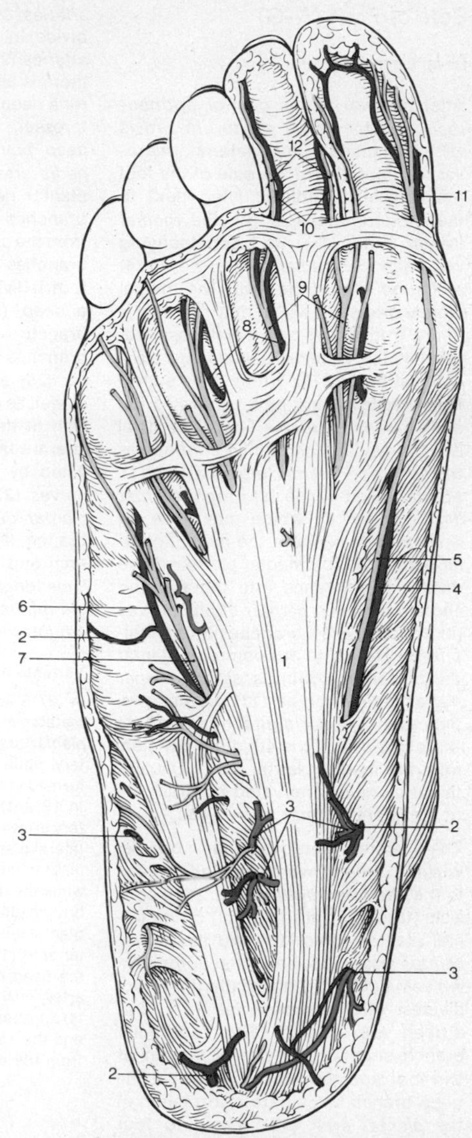

A Superficial layer of sole of foot

Sole of Foot (A–G)

Deep Layer (A)

After removal of the *plantar aponeurosis* and the *flexor digitorum brevis* (**1**), the medial and lateral neurovascular bundles of the sole of the foot are revealed. Medially, lying next to the *abductor hallucis* (**2**), the *medial plantar artery* (**3**), its accompanying veins and the *medial plantar nerve* (**4**) reach the sole of the foot. The medial plantar artery (**3**), which may run lateral (more frequently) or medial (less frequently) to the nerve, divides into a *superficial branch* (**5**), which runs superficially to the *flexor hallucis brevis* (**6**), and a *deep branch*. The superficial branch may (uncommonly) continue as the *1st proper plantar digital artery* (**7**), accompanied by the *1st proper plantar digital nerve* (**8**), which may have divided proximally from the medial plantar nerve (**4**). The medial plantar nerve divides in sequence into the *1st, 2nd and 3rd common plantar digital nerves* (**9**), which give off branches to the lumbricals. The 1st to 3rd common plantar digital nerves continue as the *proper planar digital nerves* (**11**). Sometimes, the *proper plantar digital nerve* (**12**) to the lateral side of the 4th digit may stem from the medial plantar nerve. Usually, this regions is innervated by branches of the *lateral plantar nerve* (**13**).

The lateral neurovascular bundle, which extends toward the digits medial to the *abductor digiti minimi* (**14**), consists (from medial to lateral) of the lateral plantar nerve (**13**) and the *lateral plantar artery* (**15**) and its *accompanying veins* (**16**). The lateral plantar artery divides into a *superficial* (**17**) and a *deep* (**18**) *branch*. The superficial branch supplies the lateral margin of the foot and the little digit, while the deep branch takes part in formation of the *plantar arch* (**19**). Three to four *plantar metatarsal arteries* (**20**), which usually give off *common plantar digital arteries* (**21**), arise from the arch and divide into the *proper plantar digital arteries* (**22**). The **plantar arch** (**"deep"**, if there is also a superficial plantar arch) runs deeply, closely adhering to the interossei, and anastomoses with the *deep plantar branch of the dorsalis pedis artery* (see p. 404). The lateral plantar nerve (**13**) gives off muscular branches to the muscles which arise from the calcaneus, and also cutaneous branches to the lateral margin of the foot. It divides into a *superficial* (**23**) and a *deep* (**24**) *branch*. The superficial branch innervates via muscular branches the *flexor digiti minimi Brevis* (**25**) and the *4th lumbricalis* (**26**), as well as areas of skin above them. The skin of the little digit and usually the lateral surface of the 4th digit are innervated by the *common plantar digital nerves* (**27**), which divide into *proper plantar digital nerves* (**28**). The deep branch (**24**) accompanies the plantar arch and innervates the *adductor hallucis longus* (**29**) and the *opponens digiti minimi* as well as the *2nd, 3rd and 4th interossei.*

Variants of the Plantar Arch (B–G)

In 27% of cases (**B**) the four plantar metatarsal arteries are supplied by the *deep plantar branch* (**30**) of the dorsalis pedis artery, while in 26% (**C**) the plantar arch (**19**) is formed entirely by the deep plantar branch. In 19% (**D**), the 4th plantar metatarsal artery arises from the deep branch (**18**) of the lateral plantar artery, and in 13% (**E**) the 3rd plantar metatarsal artery does so as well, while the others stem from the deep plantar branch (**30**). In only 7% of cases (**F**) do all the plantar metatarsal arteries arise from a plantar arch (**19**), which is formed entirely from the deep branch (**18**) of the lateral plantar artery. In 6% (**G**) the 2nd to 4th plantar metatarsal arteries arise from a plantar arch (**19**) and the 1st plantar metatarsal artery arises from the deep plantar branch (**30**).

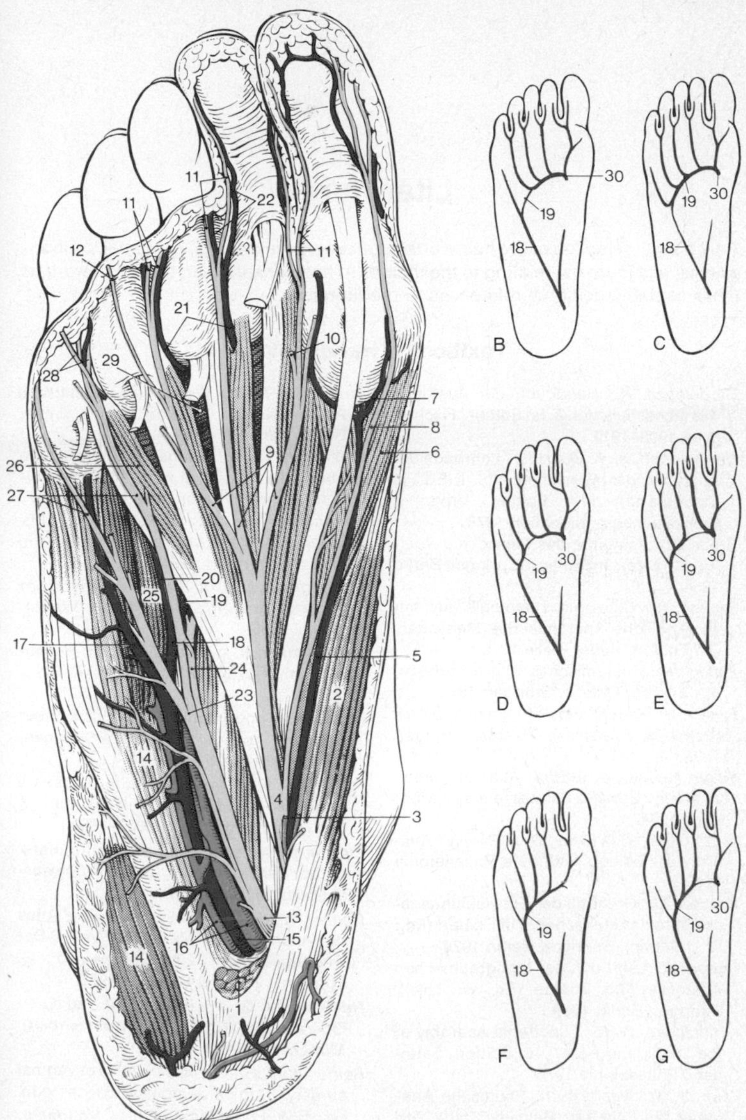

A Deep layer of sole of foot

30
19
18
B
30
19
18
C
30
19
18
D
30
19
18
E
19
18
F
30
19
18
G

B–G Variants of arteries of sole of foot (after Lippert)

Literature

Only a small selection of the numerous publications (textbooks, handbooks, monographs, and journals) relating to the themes of each chapter can be cited here, and these contain additional references to the literature.

Textbooks, Handbooks

Bardeleben, K.: Handbuch der Anatomie des Menschen. Vol. 2. 1st Edition. Fischer, Jena 1908–1912

Benninghoff, A., K. Goerttler: Lehrbuch der Anatomie des Menschen. Vol. I (Ed.: J. Staubesand). 11th Edition. Urban & Schwarzenberg, München 1975

Braus, H.: Anatomie des Menschen. Vol. I (Ed.: C. Elze). 3rd Edition. Springer, Berlin 1954

Bucher, O.: Cytologie, Histologie und mikroskopische Anatomie des Menschen. 7th Edition. Huber, Bern 1970

Feneis, H.: Anatomisches Bildwörterbuch. 4th Edition. Thieme, Stuttgart 1974

Feneis, H.: Pocket atlas of human anatomy (transl. H. E. Kaiser), Thieme, Stuttgart 1976

Figge, F. H. J., W. J. Hild: Atlas of Human Anatomy. Urban & Schwarzenberg, München 1974

Gardner, E., J. D. Gray, R. O'Rahilly: Anatomy. 3rd Edition. Saunders, Philadelphia 1969

Grosser, O.: Grundriß der Entwicklungsgeschichte des Menschen. 7th Edition (Ed.: R. Ortmann). Springer, Berlin 1970

Hafferl, A.: Lehrbuch der topographischen Anatomie. 3rd Edition (Ed. W. Thiel). Springer, Berlin 1969

Hollinshead, W. H.: Functional Anatomy of the Limbs and Back. 4th Edition. Saunders, Philadelphia 1976

Lang, J., W. Wachsmuth: Praktische Anatomie. Vol. I, 4th Part: Bein und Statik. 2nd Edition. Springer, Berlin 1972

Langman, J.: Medizinische Embryologie. Thieme, Stuttgart 1970

von Lanz, T., W. Wachsmuth: Praktische Anatomie. Vol. I, 2nd Part: Hals. Springer, Berlin 1955

von Lanz, T., W. Wachsmuth: Praktische Anatomie. Vol. I, 3rd Part: Arm. 2nd Edition. Springer, Berlin 1959

Leonhardt, H.: Histologie, Zytologie und Mikroanatomie des Menschen. 4th Edition. Thieme, Stuttgart 1974

McGregor, A. L., J. du Plessis: A Synopsis of Surgical Anatomy. 3rd Edition. Wright, Bristol 1969

Montgomery, R. L., M.C. Singleton: Human Anatomy Review. Pitman Medical, London 1975

Nishi, S.: Topographical Atlas of Human Anatomy. Vols. I–IV. Kanehara Shuppan, Tokyo 1974–1975

Pernkopf, E.: Topographische Anatomie des Menschen. Vols. I–IV. Urban & Schwarzenberg, Berlin 1937–1960

Platzer, W.: Anleitung für Präparierübungen an der ganzen Leiche. Urban & Schwarzenberg, München 1971

Rauber, A., F. Kopsch: Lehrbuch und Atlas der Anatomie des Menschen. Vol. I: Bewegungsapparat. 20th Edition (Ed.: G. Töndury). Thieme, Stuttgart 1968

Reiffenstuhl, G., W. Platzer: Die vaginalen Operationen. Urban & Schwarzenberg, München 1974

Reiffenstuhl, G., W. Platzer: Atlas of vaginal surgery. Surgical anatomy and technique. Ed.: E. A. Friedman. Volume I, Volume II. Saunders, Philadelphia and London 1975

Saegesser, M.: Spezielle chirurgische Therapie. 8th Edition. Huber, Bern 1972

Starck, D.: Embryologie. 3rd Edition. Thieme, Stuttgart 1975

Töndury, G.: Angewandte und topographische Anatomie. 4th Edition. Thieme, Stuttgart 1970

Warwick, R., P. L. Williams: Gray's anatomy. 35th Edition. Longman, Edinburg 1973

General Anatomy

Barnett, C. H.: The structure and functions of synovial joints. In: Clinical Surgery (Eds.: Rob, C., R. Smith). pp. 328–344. Butterworths, London 1966

Barnett, C. H., D. V. Davies, M. A. MacConaill: Synovial Joints, their Structure and Mechanics. Longmans, London 1961

Basmajian, J. V.: Muscles Alive. 3rd Edition. Williams & Wilkins, Baltimore 1974.

Bernstein, N.: The Coordination and Regulation of Movements. Pergamon Press, Oxford 1967

Bourne, G. H.: Biochemistry and Physiology of Bone. 2nd Edition. Vol. 1: Structure. Academic Press, New York 1972

Bourne, G. H.: The Structure and Function of Muscle. 2nd Edition. Vol. 1: Structure. Academic Press, New York 1972

Brookes, M.: The Blood Supply of Bone. Butterworths, London 1971

Dowson, D., V. Wright, M. D. Longfield: Human joint lubrication. Biomed. Eng., 4, (1969) 8–14, 160–165, 517–522

Freeman, M. A. R.: Adult Articular Cartilage. Pitman Medical, London 1973

Haines, R. W., A. Mohiudin: The sites of early epiphyseal union in the limb girdles and major long bones of man. J. Anat. (Lond.) 101, (1967) 823–831.

Hancox, N. M.: Biology of Bone. Cambridge University Press, London 1972

Jonsson, B., S. Reichmann: Reproducibility in kinesiologic EMG-investigation with intramuscular electrodes. Acta Morphol. Neerl. Scand. 7 (1968), 73–90

Joseph, J.: Man's Posture: Electromyographic Studies. Thomas, Springfield 1960

Kapandji, I. A.: The Physiology of Joints. 2nd Edition. Vols. 1–3. Longman: London 1970/71/74

MacConaill, M. A., J. V. Basmajian. Muscles and Movements. Williams & Wilkins, Baltimore 1969

McLean, F. C., M. R. Urist: Bone: Fundamentals of Physiology of Skeletal Tissue. 3rd Edition. Chicago University Press, Chicago 1968

Meschan, I. An Atlas Basic to Radiology. Saunders, Philadelphia 1974

Mysorecar, V. R.: Diaphyseal nutrient foramina in human long bones. J. Anat. (Lond.) 101 (1967) 813–822

Rasch, P. J., R. K. Burke: Kinesiology and Applied Anatomy. 5th Edition. Lea & Febiger, Philadelphia 1974

Serratrice, G., J. Eisinger: Innervation et circulation osseuses diaphysaires, Rev. Rhum. Mal. Osteo-Articulaires 34 (1967) 505–519

Smith, D. S.: Muscle. Academic Press, New York 1972

Trunk

Ankel, F.: Morphologische Spézialisationen der menschlichen Wirbelsäule. Bull. Schweiz. Ges. Anthropol. Ethnol. 43 (1967) 70–81

Anson, B. J., E. H. Morgan, C. B. MacVay: Surgical anatomy of the inguinal region based upon a study of 500 body halves. Surg. Gynecol. Obstet. 111 (1960) 707–725

Beck, A., J. Kilius: Mathematisch-statistische Methoden zur Untersuchung der Wirbelsäulenhaltung mittels Computer. Biomed. Tech. 19 (1974) 72–74

Bowden, R., H. El-Ramli: The anatomy of the oesophageal hiatus. Br. J. Surg. 54 (1967) 983–989

Boyd, W., H. Blincoe, J. C. Hayner. Sequence of action of the diaphragm and quadratus lumborum during quiet breathing. Anat. Rec. 151 (1965) 579–582

Cavallotti, C.: Morfologia dei trigoni lombocostali del diaframma umano. Acta Med. Roma 6 (1968) 21–29

Condor, R. E.: Surgical anatomy of the transversus abdominis and transversalis fascia. Ann. Surg. 173 (1971) 1–5

Danbury, R.: Functional anatomy and kinesiology of the cervical spine. Man. Med. 9 (1971) 97–101

Davis, P. R.: Some effects of lifting, pulling and pushing on the human trunk. Ergonomics 6 (1963) 303–304

Diaconescu, N., C. Veleanu: Die Wirbelsäule als formbildender Faktor. Acta anat. (Basel) 73 (1969) 210–241

Donisch, E. W., W. Trapp: The cartilage endplates of the human vertebral column (some considerations of postnatal development). Anat. Rec. 169 (1971) 705–716

Doyle, J. F.: The superficial inguinal arch. A reassessment of what has been called the inguinal ligament. J. Anat. (Lond.) 108 (1971) 297–304

Drexler, L.: Röntgenanatomische Untersuchungen über Form und Krümmung der Halswirbelsäule in den verschiedenen Lebensaltern. Hippokrates-Verlag, Stuttgart 1962

During, J., H. Goudfrooy, T. H. W. Beeker: Function of the lower back in man. Institute of Medical Physics, TNO Progress Report No Pr 4 (1974) 30–39

Epstein, B. S.: The Vertebral Column. Year Book Medical, Chicago 1974

Helmy, I. D.: Congenital diaphragmatic hernia. (A study of the weakest points of the diaphragm by dissection and a report of a case of hernia through the right foramen of Morgagni. Alexandria Med. J. 13 (1967) 121–132

Johnson, R. M., E. S. Crelin, A. A. White et al.: Some new observations on the functional anatomy of the lower cervical spine. Clin. orthop. (Phila.) 111 (1975) 192–200

Kapandji, A.: L'Anatomie fonctionelle du rachis lombo sacre. Acta Orthop. Belg. 35 (1969) 543–566

Krmpotic-Nemanic, J., P. Keros: Funktionale Bedeutung der Adaption des Dens axis beim Menschen. Verh. Anat. Ges. (Jena), 67 (1973) 393–397

Langenberg, W.: Morphologie, physiologischer Querschnitt und Kraft des M. erector spinae im Lumbalbereich des Menschen. Z. Anat. Entwicklungsgesch. 132 (1970) 158–190

Lewit, K., L. Krausová: Mechanismus und Bewegungsausmaß in den Kopfgelenken bei passiven Bewegungen. Z. Orthop. Ihre Grenzgeb. 103 (1967) 323–333

Liard, A. R., M. Latarjet, F. Crestanello: Precisions anatomiques concernant la partie superieure du muscle grand droit de l'abdomen et de sa gaine. C. R. Assoc. Anat. 148 (1970) 532–542

Ludwig, K. S.: Die Frühentwicklung des Dens epistrophei und seiner Bänder beim Menschen. Morph. Jb. 93 (1953) 98–112

Ludwig, K. S.: Die Frühentwicklung des Atlas und der Occipitalwirbel beim Menschen. Acta anat. (Basel) 30 (1957) 444–461

Lytle, W. J.: The inguinal and lacunar ligaments. J. Anat. (Lond.). 118 (1974) 241–251

MacVay, C. B.: The normal and pathologic anatomy of the transversus abdominis muscle in inguinal and femoral hernia. Surg. Clin. North Am. (1971) 51, 1251–1261

Mambrini, A., M. Argeme, J. P. Houze, H. Isman: A propos de l'orifice aortique du diaphragme. C. R. Assoc. Anat. 148 (1970) 433–441

Menárguez Carretero, L., M. Campo Muñoz: E studio radiólogico y tipos morfológicos de costillas cervicales en el sexo femenino. Enferm. Tórax Tuberc. 16 (1967) 285–308

Nathan, H., B. Arensburgh: An unusual variation in the fifth lumbar and sacral vertebrae; a possible cause of vertebral canal narrowing. Anat. Anz. 132 (1972) 137–148

Okada, M., K. Kogi, M. Ishii: Endurance capacity of the erectores spinae muscles in static work. J. Anthropol. Soc. Nippon 78 (1970) 99–110

Pierpoint, R. Z., A. W. Grigoleit, M. K. Finegan. The transversalis fascia. A practical analysis of an enigma. Am. Surg. 35 (1969) 737–740

Putz, R.: Zur Manifestation der hypochordalen Spangen im cranio-vertebralen Grenzgebiet beim Menschen. Anat. Anz. 137 (1975) 65–74

Putz, R., A. Pomaroli: Form und Funktion der Articulatio atlanto-axialis lateralis. Acta anat. (Basel) 83 (1972) 333–345

Radojevic, S., E. Stolic, S. Unkovic: Le muscle cremaster de l'homme (Variations morphologiques et importance partique). C. R. Assoc. Anat. 143 (1969) 1383–1386

Reichmann, S., E. Berglund, K. Lundgren: Das Bewegungszentrum in der Lendenwirbelsäule bei Flexion und Extension, Z. Anat. Entwicklungsgesch. 138 (1972) 283–287

Shimaguchi, S.: Tenth rib is floating in Japanese. Anat. Anz. 135 (1974) 72–82

de Sousa, O. M., J. Furlani: Electromyographic study of the m. rectus abdominis. Acta anat. (Basel) 88 (1974) 281–298

Steubl, R.: Innervation und Morphologie der Mm. levatores costarum. Z. Anat. Entwicklungsgesch. 128 (1969) 211–221

Taylor, A.: The contribution of the intercostal muscles to the effort of respiration in man. J. Physiol. (Lond.) 151 (1960) 390–402

Töndury, G.: Entwicklungsgeschichte und Fehlbildungen der Wirbelsäule. Hippokrates-Verlag, Stuttgart 1958

Veleanu, C., U. Grun, M. Diaconescu, E. Cocota: Structural peculiarities of the thoracic spine. Their functional significance. Acta Anat. (Basel) 82 (1972) 97–107

Vitale, V., Giuntini: Rara anomalia delle vertebre lombari. Rass. Arch. Chir. 5 (1967) 20–26

Vitti, M., M. Fujiwara, J. V. Basmajian, M. Iida: The integrated roles of longus colli and sternocleidomastoid muscles: an electromyographic study. Anat. Rec. 177 (1973) 471–484

Wassilev, W.: Veränderungen im Halsteil der Wirbelsäule bei vertikaler Belastung. Anat. Anz. 121 (1967) 453–467

Waters, R. L., J. M. Morris: Electrical activity of muscles of the trunk during walking. J. Anat. (Lond.) 111 (1972) 191–199

Witschel, H., R. Mangelsdorf: Geschlechtsunterschiede am menschlichen Brustbein. Z. Rechtsmed. 69 (1971) 161–167

Taylor J. R.: Growth of human intervertebral discs and vertebral bodies. J. anat. (Lond.) 120 (1975), 49–68

Zaki, W.: Aspect morphologique et fonctionnel de l'annulus fibrosus du disque intervertebral de la colonne cervicale. Bull. Assoc. Anat. 57 (1973) 649–654

Upper Limb

Ashley, G. T.: The manner of insertion of the pectoralis major muscle in man. Anat. Rec. 113 (1952) 301–308

Basmajian, J. V., W. R. Griffin Jr.: Function of anconeus muscle. An electromyographic study. J. Bone Jt. Surg. 54-A (1972) 1712–1714

Basmajian, J. V., A. Travill: Electromyography of the pronator muscles in the forearm. Anat. Rec. 139 (1961) 45–49

Bearn, J. G.: An electromyographical study of the trapezius, deltoid, pectoralis major, biceps and triceps, during static loading of the upper limb. Anat. Rec. 140 (1961) 103–108

Bojsen-Møller, F., L. Schmidt: The palmar aponeurosis and the central spaces of the hand. J Anat. (Lond.) 117 (1974) 55–68

Christensen, J. B., J. P. Adams, K. O. Cho, L. Miller: A study of the interosseous distance between the radius and ulnar during rotation of the forearm. Anat. Rec. 160 (1968) 261–271

Čihák, R.: Ontogenesis of the Skeleton and the Intrinsic Muscles of the Hand and Foot. Springer-Verlag, Berlin 1972

Clarke, G. R., L. A. Willis, W. W. Fish, P. J. R. Nichols: Assessment of movement at the glenohumeral joint – Orthopaedics (Oxford) 7 (1974) 55–71

Dempster. W. T.: Mechanisms of shoulder movement. Arch. Phys. Med. 46 (1965) 49–70

Doody, S. G., L. Freedman, J. C. Waterland: Shoulder movements during abduction in the scapular plane. Arch. Phys. Med. 51 (1970) 595–604

Dylevsky, I.: Ontogenesis of the M. palmaris longus in man. Folia Morphol. (Prague) 17 (1969) 23–28

Franzi, A. T., E. Spinelli, G. Ficcarelli: Variazione del muscolo palmare lungo: Contributo alla casistica. Quad. Anat. prat. 25 (1969) 71–76

Garn, S. M., C. G. Rohman: Variability in the order of ossification of the bony centers of the hand and wrist. Am. J. Phys. Anthropol. NS. 18 (1960) 219–230

Glasgow, E. F.: Bilateral extensor digitorum brevis manus. Med. J. Aust. 54 (1967) 25

Hohmann, G.: Hand und Arm, ihre Erkrankungen und deren Behandlung. Bergmann, München 1949

Jonsson, B., B. M. Olofsson, L. C. Steffner: Function of the teres major, latissimus dorsi and pectoralis major muscles. A preliminary study. Acta Morphol. Neerl. Scand. 9 (1972) 275–280

Kaneff, A.: Über die wechselseitigen Beziehungen der progressiven Merkmale des

M. extensor pollicis brevis beim Menschen. Anat. Anz. 122 (1968) 31–36

Kapandji, A.: La rotation du pouce sur son axe longitudinal lors de l'opposition. Rev. Chir. Orthop. 58 (1972) 273–289

Kauer, J. M. G.: The articular disc of the hand. Acta Anat. (Basel) 93 (1975) 590–605

Kauer, J. M. G.: The interdependence of carpal articulation chains. Acta anat. (Basel) 88 (1974) 481–501

Kiyosumi, M.: New ligaments at articulationes manus. Kumamoto Med. J. 18 (1965) 214–227

Krmpotic-Nemanic, J.: Über einen bisher unbeachteten Mechanismus der Fingergrundgelenke. Gegenseitige Längsverschiebung der Finger bei der Flexion. Z. Anat. Entwicklungsgesch. 126 (1967) 127–131

Kuczynski, K.: Carpometacarpal joint of the human thumb. J. Anat. (Lond.) 118 (1974) 119–126

Landsmeer, J.: Atlas of the Hand. Churchill Livingstone, Edinburgh 1976

Landsmeer, J.: Fonctions des lombricaux. C. R. Assoc. Anat. 138 (1967) 735–739

Lewis, O. J., R. J. Hamshere, T. M. Bucknill: The anatomy of the wrist joint. J. Anat. (Lond.) 106 (1970) 539–552

Long, C.: Intrinsic-extrinsic muscle control of the fingers. Electromyographic studies. J. Bone Jt. Surg. 50-A (1968) 973–984

McClure, J. G., R. Beverly: Anomalis of the scapula. Clin. orthop. (Phila.) 110 (1975) 22–31

McFarland, G. B., U. L. Krusen, H. T. Weathersby: Kinesiology of selected muscles acting on the wrist. An electromyographical study. Arch. Phys. Med. 43 (1962) 165–171

Mehta, H. J., W. U. Gardner: A study of lumbrical muscles in the human hand. Am. J. Anat. 109 (1961) 227–238

Mrvaljevic, D.: Sur les insertions et la perforation du muscle coracobrachial. C. R. Assoc. Anat. 139 (1968) 923–933

Murata, K., K. Abe, G. Kawahara et al.: The M. serratus anterior of the Japanese. The area of its origin and its interdigitation with the M. obliquus externus abdominis. Acta Anat. Nippon. 43 (1968) 395–401

Pauly, J. E., J. L. Rushing, L. E. Scheving: An electromyographic study of some muscles crossing the elbow joint. Anat. Rec. 159 (1967) 47–54

Poisel, S.: Die Anatomie der Palmaraponeurose. Therapiewoche, 23 (1973) 3337

Renard, M., B. Brichet, A. Fonder, P. Poisson: Rôle respectif des muscles sous-épineux et petit rond dans la cinématique de l'humerus. C. R. Assoc. Anat. 139 (1968) 1266–1272

Renard, M., A. Fonder, C. Mentre, B. Brichet, J. Cayotte: Contribution à l'étude de la fonction du muscle susépineux. Communication accompagnée d'un film. C. R. Assoc. Anat. 136 (1967) 878–883

Roche, A. F.: The sites of elongation of the human metacarpals and metatarsals. Acta Anat. (Basel) 61 (1965) 193–202

Shrewsbury, M. M., R. K. Johnson: The fascia of the distal phalanx. J. Bone Jt. Surg. 57A (1975) 784–788

Shrewsbury, M. M., M. K. Kuczynski: Flexor digitorum superficialis tendon in the fingers of the human hand. Hand 6 (1974) 121–133

Shrewsbury, M. M., R. K. Johnson, D. K. Ousterhout. The palmaris brevis. A reconstruction of its anatomy and possible function. J. Bone Jt. Surg. 54-A (1972) 344–348

Soutoul, J. H., J. Castaing, J. Thureau, E. De Giovanni, P. Glories, M. Jan, J. Barbat: Les rapports tête humérale-glène scapulaire dans d'abduction du membre supérieur. C. R. Assoc. Anat. 136 (1967) 961–971

Stack, H. G.: The Palmar Fascia. Churchill Livingstone, London 1973

Strasser, H.: Lehrbuch der Muskel- und Gelenkmechanik, Vol. 4: Die obere Extremität. Springer, Berlin 1917

Weston, W. J.: The digital sheaths of the hand. Aust. Radiol. 13 (1969) 360–364

Lower Limb

Altieri, E.: Aplasia bilaterale congenita della rotula. Boll. Soc. Tosco-Umbra Chir. 28 (1967) 279–286

Asang, E.: Experimentelle und praktische Biomechanik des menschlichen Beins. Med. Sport (Berlin) 13 (1973) 245–255

Aumüller, G.: Über Bau und Funktion des Musculus adductor minimus. Anat. Anz. 126 (1970) 337–342

Barnett, C. H.: Phases of the human gait. Lancet 2 (1956) 617–621

Basmajian, J. V., T. P. Harden, E. M. Regenos: Integrated actions of the four heads of quadriceps femoris. An electromyographic study. Anat Rec. 172 (1972) 15–20

Bojsen Møller, F., V. E. Flagstad: Plantar aponeurosis and internal architecture of the ball of the foot. J. Anat. (Lond.) 121 (1976) 599–611

Bowden, R. E. M.: The functional anatomy of the foot. Physiotherapy 53 (1967) 120–126

Bubic, I.: Sexual signs of the human pelvis. Folia med. (Sarajevo), 8 (1973) 113–115

Candiollo, L., G. Gautero: Morphologie et fonction des ligaments méniscofémoraux de l'articulation du genou chez l'homme. Acta anat. (Basel) 38 (1959) 304–323

Ching Jen Wang, P. S. Walker: Rotatory laxity of the human knee joint. J. Bone Jt. Surg. 56-A (1974) 161–170

Čihák, R.: Ontogenesis of the Skeleton and Intrinsic Muscles of the Human Hand and Foot. Springer-Verlag: Berlin 1972

Crock, H. v.: The Blood Supply of the Lower Limb Bones in Man. Churcill Livingstone, Edinburgh and London 1967

Detenbeck, L. C.: Function of the cruciate ligaments in knee stability. J. Sports Med. 2 (1974), 217–221

Didiio, B. J. A., A. Zappalá, W. P. Carney: Anatomico-functional aspects of the musculus articularis genu in man. Acta anat. (Basel) 67 (1967) 1–23

Elftman, H.: Biomechanics of muscle with particular application to the studies of gait. J. Bone Jt. Surg. 48-A (1966), 363–377

Emery, K. H., G. Meachim: Surface morphology and topography of patello-femoral cartilage fibrillation in Liverpool necropsies. J. Anat. (Lond.) 116 (1973) 103–120

Emmett, J.: Measurements of the acetabulum. Clin. Orthop. 53 (1967) 171–174

Gluhbegovic, N., H. Hadziselimovic: Beitrag zu den vergleichenden anatomischen Untersuchungen der Bänder des lateralen Meniskus. Anat. Anz. 126 Suppl. (1970) 565–575

Goswami, N., P. R. Deb: Patella and patellar facets. Calcutta Med. J. 67 (1970) 123–128

Heller, L., J. Langman: The menisco-femoral ligaments of the human knee. J. Bone Jt. Surg. 46-B (1964) 307–313

Hoerr, N. L., S. J. Pyle, C. C. Franciss. Radiographic Atlas of Skeletal Development of Foot and Ankle. Thomas, Springfield Jll. 1962

Hohmann, G.: Fuß und Bein, ihre Erkrankungen und deren Behandlung, 3rd Edition. Bergmann, München 1939

Jacobsen, K: Area intercondylaris tibiae: osseous surface structure and its relation to soft tissue structures and applications to radiography. J. Anat. (Lond.) 117 (1974) 605–618

Janda, V., V. Stará: The role of thigh adductors in movement patterns of the hip and knee joints. Courrier, Centre Internat. de l'Enfance 15 (1965) 1–3

Jansen, J. C.: Einige nieuwe functioneel-anatomische aspecten von de voet. Ned. Tijdschr. Geneeskd. 112 (1968) 147–155

Johnson, C. E., J. V. Basmajian, W. Dasher: Electromyography of sartorius muscle. Anat. Rec. 173 (1972) 127–130

Joseph. J.: Movements at the hip joint. Annals R. Call. Surg. Engl. 56 (1975) 192–201

Kaplan, E. B.: The iliotibial tract, clinical and morphological significance. J. Bone Jt. Surg. 40-A (1958) 817–831

Kaufer, H.: Mechanical function of the patella. J. Bone Jt. Surg. 53-A (1971) 1551–1560

Kennedy, J. C., H. W. Weinberg, A. S. Wilson: The anatomy and function of the anterior cruciate ligament. As determined by clinical and morphological studies. J. Bone Jt. Surg. 56-A (1974) 223–235

Knief, J.: Materialverteilung und Beanspruchungsverteilung im coxalen Femurende. Densitometrische und spannungsoptische Untersuchungen. Z. Anat. Entwicklungsgesch. 126 (1967) 81–116

Kummer, B.: Die Beanspruchung der Gelenke, dargestellt am Beispiel des menschlichen Hüftgelenks, Verh. Dtsch. Ges. Orthop. Traumatol. 55 (1968) 302–311

Kummer, B.: Die Biomechanik der aufrechten Haltung. Mitt. Naturforsch. Ges. Bern 22 (1965) 239–259

Kummer, B.: Funktionelle Anatomie des Vorfußes. Verh. Dtsch. Orthop. Ges. 53 (1966) 483–493

Lesage, Y., R. Le Bars: Etude electromyographique simultanée des differents chefs du quadriceps. Ann. Méd. phys. 13 (1970) 292–297

Loetzke, H. H., K. Trzenschik: Beitrag zur Frage der Varianten des M. soleus beim Menschen. Anat. Anz. 124 (1969) 28–36

Marshall, J. L., E. G. Girgis, R. R. Zelko: The biceps femoris tendon and its functional significance, J. Bone Jt. Surg. 54-A (1972) 1444–1450

Martin, B. F.: The origins of the hamstring muscles. J. Anat. (Lond.) 102 (1968) 345–352

Menschik, A.: Mechanik des Kniegelenkes. I. Z. Orthop. Ihre Grenzgeb. 112 (1974) 481–495

Menschik, A.: Mechanik des Kniegelenkes. II. Z. Orthop. Ihre Grenzgeb. 113 (1975) 388–400

Mörike, K. D.: Werden die Menisken im Kniegelenk geschoben oder gezogen? Anat. Anz. 133 (1973) 265–275

Morrison, J. B.: The mechanics of the knee joint in relation to normal walking. J. Biomech. 3 (1970) 51–61

Novozamsky, V., J. Buchberger: Die Fußwölbung nach Belastung durch einen 100-km-Marsch. Z. Anat. Entwicklungsgesch. 131 (1970) 243–248

Oberländer, W.: Die Beanspruchung des menschlichen Hüftgelenks.Z. Anat. Entwicklungsgesch. 140 (1973) 367–384

Olbrich, E.: Patella emarginata – Patella partita. Forschungen und Forscher der Tiroler Ärzteschule 2 (1948–1950) 69–105

Pauwels, F.: Gesammelte Abhandlungen zur funktionellen Anatomie des Bewegungsapparates. Springer, Berlin 1965

Pheline, Y., S. Chitour, H. Issad, G. Djilali, J. Ferrand: La région soustrochantérienne. C. R. Assoc. Anat. 136 (1967) 782–806

Ravelli, A.: Zum anatomischen und röntgenologischen Bild der Hüftpfanne. Z. Orthop. 113 (1975) 306–315

Renard, M. B. Brichet, J. L. Cayotte: Analyse fonctionelle du triceps sural. C. R. Assoc. Anat. 143 (1969) 1387–1394

Rideau, Y., P. Lacert, C. Hamonet: Contribution à l'etude de l'action des muscles de la loge postérieure de la cuisse. C. R. Assoc. Anat. 143 (1969) 1406–1415

Rideau, Y., C. Hamonet, G. Outrequin, P. Kamina: Etude électromyographique de l'activité fonctionelle des muscles de la loge postérieure de la cuisse. C. R. Assoc. Anat. 146 (1971) 597–603

Sick, H., P. Ring, C. Ribot, J. G. Koritke: Structure fonctionnelle des menisques de articulation du genou. C. R. Assoc. Anat. 143 (1969) 1565–1571

Sirang, H.: Ein Canalis alae ossis illii und seine Bedeutung. Anat. Anz., 133 (1973) 225–238

Stern, Jr. J. T.: Anatomical and functional specializations of the human gluteus maximus. Am. J. Phys. Anthropol. 36 (1972) 315–339

Strasser, H.: Lehrbuch der Muskel- und Gelenkmechanik, Vol. 3: Die untere Extremität. Springer, Berlin 1917

Strauss, F.: Gedanken zur Fuß-Statik. Acta anat. (Basel) 78 (1971) 412–414

Suzuki, N.: An electromyographic study of the role of muscles in arch support of the normal and flat foot. Nagoya Med. J. 17 (1972) 57–79

Takebe, K., M. Vitti, J. V. Basmajian: Electromyography of pectineus muscle. Anat. Rec. 180 (1974) 281–284

von Volkmann, R.: Wer trägt den Taluskopf wirklich, und inwiefern ist der plantare Sehnenast des M. tibialis post. als Bandsystem aufzufassen? Anat. Anz. 131 (1972) 425–432

von Volkmann, R.: Zur Anatomie und Mechanik des Lig. calcaneonaviculare plantare sensu strictiori. Anat. Anz. 134 (1973) 460–470

Zivanovic, S.: Menisco-meniscal ligaments of the human knee joint. Anat. Anz. 135 (1974) 35–42

Head and Neck and Peripheral Neurovascular Pathways

Buntine, J. A.: The omohyoid muscle and fascia; morphology and anomalies. Aust. N. Z. J. Surg. 40 (1970) 86–88

Burch, J. G.: Activity of the accessory ligaments of the mandibular joint. J. Prosthet. Dent. 24 (1970) 621–628

Campbell, E. J. M.: The role of the scalene and sternomastoid muscles in breathing in normal subjects. An electromyographical study. J. Anat. (Lond.). 89 (1955) 378–386

Carella, A.: Apparato stilo ioideo e malformazioni della cerniera atlo occipitale. Acta Neurol. (Napoli) 26 (1971) 466–472

Coleman, S. S., B. J. Anson: Arterial patterns in the hand based upon a study of 650 specimens. Surg. Gynecol. Obstet. 113 (1961) 408–424

Fortunato, V., St. D. Bocciarelli, G. Auriti: Contributo allo studio della morfologia ossea dell'area cribrosa dell'etmoide. Clin. Otorinolaringoiatr. 22 (1970) 3–15

Hadziselimovic, H., M. Cus, V. Tomic: Appearance of the sigmoid groove and jugular foramen in relation to the configuration of the human skull. Acta anat. (Basel) 77 (1970) 501–507

Hilty, H.: Die makroskopische Gefäßvariabilität im Mündungsgebiet der V. saphena magna des Menschen. Schwabe, Basel 1955

Honee, G. L. J. M. The Musculus pterygoideus lateralis. Thesis, Amsterdam 1970 1–152

Ingervall, B., B. Thilander: The human spheno-occipital synchondrosis. 1. The time of closure appraised macroscopically. Acta Odontol. Scand. 30 (1972) 349–356

Isley, C. L., J. V. Basmajian: Electromyography of human cheeks and lips. Anat. Rec. 176 (1973) 143–148

Lippert, H.: Arterienvarietäten, Klinische Tabellen. Beilage in Med. Klin. München 1967–1969, 18–32

May, R., R. Nißl: Die Phlebographie der unteren Extremität. 2nd Edition. Thieme, Stuttgart 1973

Melsen, B.: Time and mode of closure of the spheno-occipital synchondrosis determined on human autopsy material. Acta anat. (Basel) 83 (1972) 112–118

Miller, M. R., H. J. Ralston, M. Kasahara: The pattern of innervation of the human hand. Am. J. Anat. 102 (1958) 183–218

Nikolic, V.: Variations du trou sphénopalatin. Acta anat. (Basel) 68 (1967) 189–198

Oberg, T., G. E. Carlsson, C. M. Fajers,: The temporomandibular joint. A morphologic study on human autopsy material. Acta Odontol. Scand. 29 (1971) 349–384

Poisel, S., D. Golth: Zur Variabilität der großen Arterien im Trigonum caroticum. Wien. Med. Wochenschr. 124 (1974) 229–232

Porter, M. R.: The attachment of the lateral pterygoid muscle to the meniscus. J. Prosthet. Dent. 24 (1970) 555–562

Proctor, A. D., J. P. de Vincenzo: Masseter muscle position relative to dentofacial form. Angle Orthodont. 40 (1970) 37–44

Renard, M., M. Jandeaux, J. Cayotte: Corrélations cranio-sellaires. C. R. Assoc. Anat. 139 (1968) 1045–1052

Sato, S.: Statistical studies on the exceptional muscles of the Kyushu Japanese. 1. The muscles of the head (the facial muscles). Kurume Med. J. 15 (1968) 69–92

Shapiro, R., F. Robinson: The foramina of the middle fossa. A phylogenetic, anatomic and pathologic study. Am. J. Roentgenol. 101 (1967) 779–794

Sirang, H.: Ursprung, Verlauf und Äste des N. saphenus, Anat. Anz. 130 (1972) 158–169

Vitti, M., M. Fujiwara, J. V. Basmajian, M. Lida: The integrated roles of longus colli and sternocleidomastoid muscles: an electromyographic study. Anat. Rec. 177 (1973) 471–484

Wallace, W. A., R. E. Coupland: Variations in the nerves of the thumb and index finger. J. Bone Jt. Surg. 57 B (1975) 491–494

Weisengreen, H. H.: Observation of the articular disc. Oral. Surg. 40 (1975) 113–121

Wright, D. M., B. C. Moffett Jr.: The postnatal development of the human temporomandibular joint. Amer. J. Anat. 141 (1974) 235–249